Elaine R. Monsen, PhD, RD, Editor

research
Successful Approaches
Second Edition

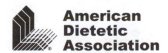

American Dietetic Association

Diana Faulhaber, Publisher
Elizabeth Nishiura, Production Editor

10 9 8 7 6 5 4 3 2

Library of Congress Cataloging-in-Publication Data

Research : successful approaches / Elaine R. Monsen, editor.— 2nd ed.
  p. ; cm.
Includes bibliographical references and index.
  ISBN 0-88091-199-9
  1. Nutrition—Research. 2. Dietetics—Research.
  [DNLM: 1. Nutrition. 2. Research Design. 3. Data Collection. 4.
Dietetics—methods. 5. Epidemiologic Methods. QU 145 R432 2003] I.
Monsen, Elaine R.
  TX367.R46 2003
  613.2′072—dc21

                                           2003005562

Contributors

Editor

Elaine R. Monsen, Ph.D., R.D.
Editor-in-Chief, *Journal of the American Dietetic Association*
Professor of Nutrition and Medicine
University of Washington
Seattle, Washington

Authors

Cheryl L. Achterberg, Ph.D.
Dean, Schreyer Honors College
Professor, Nutrition Department
The Pennsylvania State University
University Park, Pennsylvania

Sujata Archer, Ph.D., R.D.
Research Assistant Professor
Department of Preventive Medicine
Northwestern University Feinberg School of Medicine
Chicago, Illinois

Karil Bialostosky, M.S.
Nutrition Aide
U.S. Senate Committee on Agriculture, Nutrition, and Forestry
Washington, DC

Alma J. Blake, Ph.D., R.D.
Silver Spring, Maryland

Carol J. Boushey, Ph.D., M.P.H., R.D.
Assistant Professor and Director
Coordinated Program in Dietetics
Department of Foods and Nutrition
Purdue University
West Lafayette, Indiana

Ronette R. Briefel, Dr.P.H., R.D.
Senior Fellow and Nutrition Epidemiologist
Mathematica Policy Research, Inc.
Washington, DC

Lisa Brown, M.P.H., D.Sc.
Consultant

Jean C. Burge, Ph.D., R.D.
Manager, Metabolic Medical Outcomes
Medical Outcomes Research and Economics
Roche Laboratories, Inc.
Nutley, New Jersey

Carrie L. Cheney†, Ph.D., R.D.
Assistant Professor
Department of Epidemiology
Nutritional Sciences Program
University of Washington
Seattle, Washington
†Deceased.

Ronni Chernoff, Ph.D., R.D., F.A.D.A.
Associate Director, Geriatric Research Education and
    Clinical Center
Central Arkansas Veterans Healthcare System
Professor, Dietetics and Nutrition
University of Arkansas for Medical Sciences
Little Rock, Arkansas

Anne Dattilo, Ph.D., R.D., C.D.E.
Nutrition Research and Practice
Athens, Georgia

Barbara H. Dennis, Ph.D., R.D.
Research Associate Professor (retired)
University of North Carolina at Chapel Hill
Chapel Hill, North Carolina

Judith A. Ernst, D.M.Sc., R.D.
Associate Professor of Nutrition and Dietetics
Nutrition and Dietetics Program
Indiana University School of Medicine
Indianapolis, Indiana

Judith A. Gilbride, Ph.D., R.D., F.A.D.A.
Professor, Nutrition and Food Studies
New York University
New York, New York

Geoffery W. Greene, Ph.D., R.D., L.D.N.
Professor, Department of Nutrition and Food Sciences
University of Rhode Island
Kingston, Rhode Island

Mary B. Gregoire, Ph.D., R.D., F.A.D.A.
Department Executive Officer and Professor
Hotel, Restaurant, and Institution Management
Iowa State University
Ames, Iowa

Jean H. Hankin, Dr.P.H., R.D.
Researcher, Professor Emeritus
Cancer Research Center, University of Hawaii
Honolulu, Hawaii

Rachel K. Johnson, Ph.D., M.P.H., R.D.
Professor of Nutrition and Dean
College of Agriculture and Life Sciences
The University of Vermont
Burlington, Vermont

Mark Kestin, Ph.D., M.P.H.
Associate Professor
Nutrition Program
Bastyr University
Affiliate Associate Professor
Department of Epidemiology
University of Washington
Seattle, Washington

P.M. Kris-Etherton, Ph.D., R.D.
Distinguished Professor of Nutrition
The Pennsylvania State of University
University Park, Pennsylvania

Johanna W. Lampe, Ph.D., R.D.
Associate Member
Division of Public Health Sciences
Fred Hutchinson Cancer Research Center
Research Associate Professor
Department of Epidemiology
University of Washington
Seattle, Washington

Richard D. Mattes, M.P.H., Ph.D., R.D.
Professor, Foods and Nutrition
Department of Foods and Nutrition
Purdue University
West Lafayette , Indiana

Esther F. Myers, Ph.D., R.D., F.A.D.A.
Director, Scientific Affairs and Research
American Dietetic Association
Chicago, Illinois

Sara C. Parks, Ph.D., R.D.
Professor and Director
School of Hotel, Restaurant, and Recreation Management
The Pennsylvania State University
College of Health and Human Development
University Park, Pennsylvania

Ruth E. Patterson, Ph.D., R.D.
Associate Member
Fred Hutchinson Cancer Research Coordination
Research Associate Professor
University of Washington
Seattle, Washington

Jean A.T. Pennington, Ph.D., R.D.
Research Nutritionist

Division of Nutrition Research Coordination
National Institutes of Health
Bethesda, Maryland

Judy E. Perkin, Dr.P.H., R.D.
Associate Dean
College of Health
University of North Florida
Jacksonville, Florida

Cheryl L. Rock, Ph.D., R.D., F.A.D.A.
Associate Professor
Department of Family and Preventive Medicine
University of California, San Diego
La Jolla, California

M. Rosita Schiller, Ph.D., R.D., F.A.D.A.
Professor and Director
Medical Dietetics Division
The Ohio State University
Columbus, Ohio

Sandra K. Shepherd, Ph.D., R.D.
President
NutriLink
Stuart, Florida

Bettylou Sherry, Ph.D., R.D.
Epidemiologist
Division of Nutrition and Physical Activity
National Center for Chronic Disease Prevention and Health
    Promotion
Centers for Disease Control and Prevention
Atlanta, Georgia

Margaret D. Simko†, Ph.D., R.D., F.A.D.A.
Clinical Professor
Department of Family Medicine
Robert Wood Johnston Medical School
New Brunswick, NJ
†Deceased.

Jeannie Sneed, Ph.D., R.D.
Associate Professor
Iowa State University
Ames, Iowa

Patricia L. Splett, Ph.D., R.D., F.A.D.A.
Evaluation Consultant
Splett and Associates
St. Paul, Minnesota

Linda Van Horn, Ph.D., R.D.
Professor
Department of Preventive Medicine
Northwestern University Feinberg School of Medicine
Chicago, Illinois

Carol West Suitor, D.Sc., R.D.
Nutrition Consultant
Northfield, Vermont

Monica E. Yamamoto, Dr.P.H., R.D., F.A.D.A.
Nutrition Epidemiologist
Assistant Professor of Epidemiology
Graduate School of Public Health
Department of Epidemiology
University of Pittsburgh
Pittsburgh, Pennsylvania

Contents

Foreword

The Research Dietetic Practice Group of the American Dietetic Association (ADA) represents ADA members who promote the role of nutrition research in setting professional practice standards and health policy, and in determining the role of nutrition in health and disease prevention. Without strong dietetics-based research, dietitians and nutrition professionals would not have the tools needed to make responsible dietary and lifestyle recommendations to the consumer. As research dietitians, we recognize the importance of understanding and applying scientific principles to our profession. It is imperative that we appropriately collect, analyze, and interpret research data and make sound decisions based on these data.

Over the past 20 years, Dr. Elaine Monsen has been a strong advocate of the importance of research to our profession. As the editor-in-chief of the *Journal of the American Dietetic Association,* she has worked diligently to see that the journal publishes high-quality research articles. Her years as a highly successful scientist and as editor of the *Journal* have prepared her well to guide and refine this book, now in its second edition. Readers will benefit from her research knowledge and her ability to apply research techniques to the dietetics profession. In addition, the contributing authors, many of whom are dietitians, have strong research backgrounds and have published extensively in their respective research areas. They bring to the book their research experience and their knowledge of how research contributes to the growth of the dietetic profession.

The Research Dietetic Practice Group regards this book as an invaluable resource for all dietitians. *Research: Successful Approaches* will help research dietitians understand and interpret their own research data and clearly present their findings to other scientists and consumers. Furthermore, this book will help the practitioner understand and interpret the research they read. The dietetics profession is only as strong as the research upon which we base our recommendations.

Phyllis Bowen, Ph.D., R.D., 1998–1999 Chairman

Nancy Lewis, Ph.D., R.D., 1999–2000 Chairman

Melinda M. Manore, Ph.D., R.D., 2000–2001 Chairman

Linda A. Vaughan, Ph.D., R.D., 2001–2002 Chairman

Alana Cline, Ph.D., R.D., 2002–2003 Chairman

Introduction

The chapters presented here provide insights and guidance from experts in diverse areas of nutrition and dietetics research. The authors' excitement about and satisfaction from research is evident throughout their discussions of its challenges and rigor. The practical observations given by these experienced investigators will make research accessible to all readers.

This second edition of *Research: Successful Approaches* is organized in nine parts, plus a coda. It begins with an overview of research design: descriptive research designs, analytic research designs, statistical analysis, and presentation. Part 2, on the research environment, discusses ethical issues in conducting and presenting research and supplies useful information about preparing research proposals and funding applications. Parts 3 through 7 provide clear discussions of analytic, descriptive, integrative, and translational research, as well as important techniques used in research. Parts 8 and 9 discuss the use of numbers in research, specifically for sample size estimates and statistical analysis, and present processes for the effective presentation of research. A coda and the book's final chapter focus on the many beneficial interactions of practice and research. The book concludes with a detailed and thorough index, which will direct readers to discussions of key terms and allow examination of their use in context.

Each of the 31 chapters has benefited from the expertise and thorough review of individuals in each specialized area. The mammoth task of reviewing the entire collection of chapters was carried out by the various authors themselves and other capable reviewers. The final review was done by Judith Gilbride, Ph.D., R.D. The exceptional chapters of the 39 contributing authors have been transformed into this book through the diligence and steadying hands of Elizabeth Nishiura, production editor at ADA; Janet McGregor, assistant to the editor-in-chief, *Journal of the American Dietetic Association;* Gill Robertson, M.S., R.D.; and Judith Clayton, formerly ADA's managing editor.

Elaine R. Monsen, Ph.D., R.D.
Editor-in-Chief, Journal of the American
Dietetic Association

Part I

—⚬—

The Research Question

Chapters 1 through 3 present key research issues. The first step in any research project is to select the research topic and clearly state the question to be researched. Research is categorized by its purpose, that is, either to describe or to analyze.

Descriptive research (see Chapter 1) generates data, both qualitative and quantitative, that define the state of nature at a specified point (or points) in time. Among the methods used frequently to secure descriptive data are assessments of selected populations, well-constructed surveys, accumulated vital statistics, and observation and interviews of individuals or groups (see also Chapters 8 through 10). Often the objective is to obtain baseline data for use in decision-making or in monitoring changes over time. Descriptive research offers effective ways by which associations may be established and hypotheses generated; however, descriptive research can neither assess hypotheses nor ascertain cause and effect. Descriptive research often generates analytic research.

Analytic research techniques (see Chapter 2), through observational or experimental designs, allow the evaluation of hypotheses and the determination of causal relationships. (Case-control and cohort studies are two types of observational analytic studies.) Experimental research designs in which intervention is care-fully controlled by the researcher permit verification of causal relationships. Clinical trials are designed to evaluate clearly defined treatment groups in which the investigator manipulates the variables of interest and compares resulting data from the study groups with the data from a control group (see also Chapter 7).

Chapter 3 offers an overview of statistical analysis and the appropriate presentation of results. Standard deviation and standard error are clearly differentiated, and the chapter discusses how to handle outliers and missing values. Briefly described are various statistical methods, including cluster analysis, factor analysis, multiple regression and logistic regression analyses, survival analysis, path analysis, and meta-analysis.

Chapters 1 through 3 are pivotal ones and received the valued review and input of more than 40 experts in nutrition and dietetics research. Many of the individuals whose comments were solicited have actively participated as authors, reviewers, or members of the Board of Editors of the *Journal of the American Dietetic Association*. Their assistance is greatly appreciated.

ERM, Editor

1

—◆—

Descriptive Research Designs

Elaine R. Monsen, Ph.D., R.D., and Carrie L. Cheney, Ph.D., R.D.

Research is the backbone of nutrition and dietetics. It supports practice, innovation, and progress. Research allows objective measurement of complex environments and rigorous evaluation of the outcomes of procedures and treatments. Through research, associations can be observed, hypotheses tested, programs compared, and protocols evaluated. Research procedures can be used to document practice, to monitor activities, to ensure quality, and to assess cost-effectiveness. The strength of a discipline, whether in health sciences or management, is associated closely with its research base. Strong research supports a strong profession.

Dietitians are assuming an increasingly important role in research, both as leaders and as collaborators. In selecting specific areas for research, dietitians develop and extend their own areas of expertise. Research has an impact on all areas of dietetics. Dietetics and nutrition education are guided and updated by research findings. Practice-related research will continue to drive the future of dietetics professionals.

Research may be broadly classified according to its purpose as descriptive or analytic. Descriptive studies include qualitative research, case series (including case reports), and surveys. The designs of descriptive studies describe the state of nature at a specific point in time. They are useful for generating hypotheses regarding the determinants of a condition or disease or the characteristic of interest. Descriptive studies provide baseline data and can monitor change over time (for example, the nutritional status of a nation). These studies can establish associa-

tions among factors but do not allow causal relationships to be determined.

DESIGNING A DESCRIPTIVE RESEARCH STUDY

Descriptive research begins by identifying a relevant important topic and designing a well-considered research question. After the research design has been determined, the research protocol is prepared and a pilot study undertaken. Throughout each phase, researchers must consider the ethical implications of their actions.

Selecting the Research Topic

Research is a problem-solving, decision-making process involving a series of interrelated decisions. When the researcher focuses on one decision at a time, the research process becomes manageable. Each option can be considered, and the most appropriate option then can be selected. Research projects should be meaningful; they should expand current knowledge and enhance the practice of the profession.

As a researcher, initially choose issues important to your practice and thereby important to the field of dietetics. Research questions can evolve from many sources, including ideas to improve patient health, suggestions to increase the effectiveness of services and products, untested concepts in published literature, the application of business research methods (1,2), and uncharted boundaries in basic research in all areas of advanced study. Observe and thoughtfully consider the needs of your own practice. Then, in addressing the overall topic, break the problem down into its component parts, and single out a component that is feasible to study in your setting. Start with a simple question. Data generated in response to the initial question will lead to many other questions and aspects of the problem that subsequent studies can address.

Preparing for the Project

Review the published research literature related to your topic. In your review, emphasize both current scientific literature and seminal classic articles. A computerized literature search can speed and facilitate your review. A critical review of previous work in the field can be the base upon which to build solid new research projects. Shortcomings can be improved and suggested new areas developed. Contact people in the field. Discuss the problem with them by telephone or by electronic communication. Actively seek out information that may be useful to you from colleagues in related fields.

Assess available resources and personnel, such as patient population, laboratory and library facilities, foodservice equipment, nutrient databases, data-processing capabilities, computer facilities, personnel resources, statistical consultants, other consultants, and collaborative opportunities. Team efforts are invaluable, as they permit quality research that provides major benefits to the profession. Practicing dietitians can demonstrate leadership in research by directing team efforts.

The direct and indirect costs of performing the research need to be estimated. If a study is well designed and carefully developed, it may be implemented with existing personnel and facilities. If it is necessary to obtain funds, consider a variety of funding sources (3,4). Preparation for a research project involves both formulating the research question and evaluating its feasibility.

Clearly Stating the Research Question

A concise, simple, straightforward statement of the research question focuses the research design process. Clearly define the question, and strive to keep it uncomplicated. Use objective, measurable, operational terms, such as *identify, compare, differentiate, assess,* and *describe.*

Components of the research question include the following:

- *Who (which).* The subjects or units being assessed should be defined in broad terms (for example, *patients with diabetes, dietetics students, food items, tray lines,* or *foodservice costs*).
- *What.* The factor of interest should be stated specifically (for example, *body weight, knowledge, iron intake, tray error,* or *labor costs*).
- *How assessed.* The outcome to be assessed should be stated specifically (for example, *disease incidence, change in knowledge, alterations in food selection, tray errors per meal,* or *labor costs per patient day*).

Designing the Research Project

When the research question has been stated clearly, the research project can be designed more easily. Consider several research designs to see which design is best suited to the research question and the setting. Among items to consider are the dependent and independent variables, which are characteristics or attributes of the persons or objects that vary within the study population (examples could include serum cholesterol and fiber intake). The dependent variables are the outcome variables of interest (for example, serum cholesterol). The independent variables are the variables that are thought to influence the dependent variables and that are manipulated in experimental designs (for example, fiber intake).

Other study design characteristics relate to time and direction of data collection. These characteristics differentiate (1) the cross-sectional study (a study based on data collected from a group of subjects at a single point in time); (2) the longitudinal study (a study based on data collected at more than one point in time); (3) the prospective study (a study that begins with examination of presumed causes, such as fiber intake, and goes forward in time to observed presumed effects, such as cardiovascular disease); and (4) the retrospective study (a study that begins with manifestations of an outcome, such as cardiovascular disease, and goes back in time to uncover relationships with presumed causes, such as fiber intake).

Preparing the Research Protocol

Research protocols are essential to concentrate research efforts and to provide needed information to key parties.

Components to include in the research protocol are (1) a focused and concisely stated research question; (2) a literature review; (3) the importance and potential value of the research; and (4) the research design, which presents a clear outline of who, what, and how. The research design component should be composed of manageable subsections, including methods, data analysis, and appropriate statistical analysis.

When research funding is sought, research proposals must conform with the funding agency's guidelines. Many private and public agencies model their guidelines after those of the National Institutes of Health (NIH; see Chapters 5 and 7). The initial section of an NIH grant application includes a title page, an abstract of the research plan, a table of contents, biographical sketches of investigators and other key project personnel, other existing or pending sources of support, and an assessment of the availability of needed resources and the appropriateness of the environment in which the research will be conducted.

The second section of an NIH grant application comprises eight subsections. First, the specific aims and objectives of the research project are summarized succinctly. Second, the significance of the research is presented to support the practical and theoretical relevance of the project, and a critical, concise review of the literature is included. Third, published and unpublished preliminary studies (including pilot studies) done by the investigators are discussed.

Fourth, the research design and methods to be employed are given in detail. Within this subsection, it is customary to present the research question; methods of sample selection, including statements about selection bias; justification of sample size estimates; experimental intervention, if planned; instrumentation and the reliability and validity of planned measuring instruments; data collection procedures, including where and how data will be collected; plans for analysis of data; and a project schedule or work plan.

Fifth, human-subject approval procedures to ensure protection of subjects' rights and to disclose the potential risks undertaken are outlined. Prior approval obtained from the local institutional review board or boards can be included to support the research grant application. Sixth, if vertebrates are to be used in the research project, justification as to their need in the research and their welfare during the research must be provided.

Seventh, if consultants are to be used during the project, letters confirming their willingness to participate must be provided. Eighth, the literature cited within the application is listed.

Conducting a Pilot Study

A trial or pilot study is strongly advised. The pilot study provides the researcher with valuable experience prior to the full research project. It may suggest many refinements in methods and measuring instruments. Although it is tempting to design an instrument and immediately use it in collecting data, time is more effectively used if the instrument is tested before it is used in the major study. Making adjustments before instigating a major study can make data collection easier and more successful. In some cases, a researcher will wish to redraft the research question, as well as the research protocol. As a researcher, think through what data you need and what you will do with the data statistically. If you do not know what you will do with the data, ask yourself whether you need to collect them. Data and experience generated from the pilot study can be used to gain support and funding for the major project.

Ensuring Ethics in Research

Researchers must follow ethical procedures in all aspects of the design and conduct of their research (5,6). The choice of topics, the samples selected, the interventions designed, and the data collection procedures all involve ethical considerations. Ethics are also of great importance in the analysis and reporting of data (7).

All research involving human subjects requires prior approval by an institutional review board. These investigations must meet ethical guidelines to protect the rights, privacy, and welfare of the individuals. The Declaration of Helsinki, drafted in 1964 by the World Medical Association, serves as the basis for the ethical guidelines that are now detailed regulations issued by governmental agencies, such as the NIH. A local institutional review board has the task of reviewing all investigations using human subjects to ensure ethical conduct and evaluate potential risks and benefits.

A key principle for ethical conduct is the investigator's responsibility to explain to potential subjects the nature of the study, including the possible risks and discomforts they may experience. Following a full verbal and written description of the study, subjects are invited to participate. If they accept, they must sign a written consent. Confidentiality of all data is mandated by all review boards. Specific elements to be included in the informed consent procedure are designated by the local review board.

Check with administrative authorities about local review procedures of both the research site and the researcher's affiliated institution. The privacy of the information gathered must be protected during all phases of the study, including record keeping, data storage, data retrieval, follow-up, computing, reporting, and procedures. Procedures to ensure confidentiality prevent the identification of individual subjects. For example, code numbers are used as identifiers rather than names. Other steps to protect confidentiality should be planned in advance.

In studies that involve nonroutine tests or measures, informed written consent must be obtained from each subject. Even when routine tests are used, informed consent is frequently necessary to ensure that the data can be included in the study. (See Chapter 4 for a fuller discussion of this keystone of ethics in research.)

QUALITATIVE RESEARCH

A qualitative study often precedes other research designs. Its primary purpose is to explore the phenomenon of interest as a prelude to theory development (8). The design is necessarily flexible so the researcher can discover ideas, gain insight, and ultimately formulate a problem for further investigation. Kidder and associates (9) refer to qualitative studies as formulative or exploratory studies, characterized by a receptive, seeking attitude of the investigator and an intense study of the individuals or groups. One approach is grounded theory research, where data "grounded" in real-life observations are collected and analyzed with the purpose of developing theoretical propositions.

EXAMPLE. Grounded theory research can be used to explore and describe the major attributes of effective practitioners, such as foodservice administrators, dietetic technicians, or clinical dietitians. For example, the question "What specific dimensions are associated with an effective nutrition counselor?" was addressed initially by developing a set of criteria for selecting effective clinical dietitians. The criteria were based on existing research, role delineation studies, peer evaluation, student evaluation, recommendation by supervisors, peer recognition, and

award. Data were collected through systematic focused interviews and direct observations during daily activities in clinical settings. Individuals who interacted closely with the selected clinical dietitians—patients, students, peers, and supervisors—were interviewed. All data were treated as confidential. Commonalities and differences in patterns of behavior and cognitive and affective domains emerged. Using the results of the grounded theory research, prior theories were refined, and new hypotheses, to be tested quantitatively in future research, were generated.

Subjects are selected according to their experience with the phenomenon being explored. Thus, they have special characteristics and are not considered to be typical or representative of the population. Data are collected by such methods as observation, interviews, and questionnaires. The interview format may range from structured (restricting the range of responses) to less structured (permitting an unlimited range of responses). The less-structured or unstructured interview may focus on a particular topic or experience (a focused interview) or may have minimal direction (a nondirective interview) (9).

A focus group involves a group of respondents assembled to answer questions on a specific topic. Focus groups can be used to examine attitudes toward issues in consumer or other target populations (10–13). The Delphi technique utilizes a panel of experts who may answer separately; their judgments are collated and circulated to the panel members, who may then be questioned two or three more times until a consensus is reached. The process results in the reduction of the variability of judgments among panelists. The Delphi technique is useful in developing solutions to problems, planning, and forecasting. It is also effective in preparing the format and materials used in studies involving focus groups (10,11).

EXAMPLE. Priorities in nutrition and dietetics research can be examined using the Delphi technique with three cycles of question, analysis, feedback, and response. For example, panel members recognized for their interest and expertise in research were identified by dietetic practice groups. The first questionnaire requested each panel member to identify seven research areas of highest priority. Responses were analyzed, and the areas most frequently identified were sent back to the panel members, along with a questionnaire requesting that the areas be ranked as to importance and potential impact on the field. Responses were summarized and sent with the last questionnaire requesting further comment on areas in which the panelists disagreed. Final results were then sent to all panelists.

CASE SERIES

A case series is a report of observations on one subject (a case report) or more than one subject (a case series) that may be used in administrative, as well as educational and clinical, settings.

Uses of Case Series

The purpose of the case series is to describe quantitatively the experience of a group of cases with a disease or condition in common. Investigators using this research design attempt to identify the variables that are important to the etiology, care, or outcome of a particular condition.

A carefully prepared case series report helps generate hypotheses for future studies. The information gathered can provide evidence for an association between a disease or condition and a suspected etiologic or therapeutic factor. It also provides the data necessary to justify the need for future studies and can help determine the methods to be used in such studies. However, results from case series research cannot be generalized unless the cases are representative of the target populations. (See the discussion of survey subject selection later in this chapter.)

Case Series Features and Subject Selection

A case series comprises all cases of a specific disease or condition occurring or being presented to a particular clinic or locality during a specified time. For example, a series may consist of patients with gastric cancer who were referred to a nutrition support service for consultation during a 6-month period. It is important to recognize that this method of subject selection yields a convenience sample that cannot be considered representative of all gastric cancer patients; therefore, the results cannot be generalized to larger groups.

EXAMPLE. A case report was generated by evaluating opportunities for cost savings through private consultation in the operation of a long-term-care facility. Permission for quality assurance review was obtained from the administrator of the facility. Two areas were emphasized: (1) food production, with observation of sanitation procedures and the use of standardized recipes, and (2) an overview of the nutrition needs of the residents, as observed by a chart review of residents with decubitus, insulin-dependent diabetes mellitus, renal failure requiring dialysis, or severe or chronic weight loss. Medical records were reviewed for charting of height, weight, and energy intake. If residents were receiving parenteral or enteral feeding, records will be reviewed for charting of energy, protein, and fluid requirements and intake.

Data Collection in Case Series

Most commonly, existing records provide the data in case series; however, data generated concurrently may be collected. The advantage of concurrent data collection is the opportunity to obtain complete information in a standardized way, although that goal may also be obtained with the use of existing data.

EXAMPLE. A case series design was used to describe dietary intakes of a group of critically ill infants with viral infections of the lower respiratory tract. Infants were enrolled in the study at the time of admission for treatment of the infection. The typical pre-illness diet was assessed by the infant's diet history, obtained from the parent. Anthropometric measures were obtained and dietary intakes were measured throughout the period of hospitalization, allowing investigators to compare the nutrient intake during illness to usual intake and to current recommendations (14).

EXAMPLE. A concurrent case series determined the labor minutes per meal equivalent and the percentage of time spent in direct work, indirect work, delay time, and total time. A preliminary study identified 14 areas in which employees worked most frequently in the foodservice department, the average number of employees per work area, and an estimate of the required number of readings needed for the projected study on labor time. Data were collected from activity sampling studies of foodservice workers in the same community hospital for 7 days (Monday through Sunday) during the second week of February for 12 consecutive years. The longitudinal study provided an opportunity to assess trends in the distribution of labor time, examine patterns among work and delay activities, and identify factors in the foodservice environment that may have an impact on labor productivity (15).

Data concerning relevant factors are collected by chart or record review, questionnaires, interviews, or examination. A combination of collection methods may be used. The data usually cover a broad range of factors in depth, forming a detailed description of the cases. The variety and depth allow a number of factors to be considered but of necessity limit the number of subjects or objects under study.

EXAMPLE.   A case series was generated from all reports of food-borne illness received over the past 5 years by the regional public health department. Reports selected for review had to include a microbiological analysis of suspected foods. Descriptive analysis of the data allowed patterns related to food type and geographic distribution to emerge.

Statistical Analysis and Interpretation of Case Series

Simple descriptive statistics—such as means, medians, standard deviations, ranges, and frequencies—are appropriate in reporting the results of case series. Alternatively, the actual data for each subject may be presented for the most important variables, especially if the size of the series (for example, the number of subjects) is small. Regardless of sample size, statistical tests for inference are usually not appropriate, because hypotheses are not investigated in a case series.

When the researchers interpret the results of a case series report, they must acknowledge that the sample is not representative of a larger population of cases. The series of cases is selected by the investigators according to certain conditions and may consist of cases unique in certain characteristics. It remains to be shown in further study whether the results can be generalized beyond the individuals chosen for the study.

EXAMPLE.   In an effort to identify factors related to the use of albumin and to describe the outcome of its use, a series was generated from a chart review of all acute care patients who were given albumin infusions during hospitalization. The requisite for selection was the existence of records that included complete daily intake and output measurements and laboratory reports and that could be evaluated. Many important cases were omitted because records were incomplete. Some of the factors that resulted in an incomplete record were known, such as interruptions because of emergency procedures and incontinence in patients not catheterized. The number of patients omitted was listed, along with the known factors. However, the investigators suspected that other, unidentified reasons existed, because most of the omitted patients were on the gastrointestinal surgical service. These patients were likely to be different in other ways from the patients selected for study. Those differences may have related in some way to albumin use or outcome. The investigators were careful to describe the study patients thoroughly and refrained from generalizing the results.

SURVEYS

A survey is research designed to describe and quantify characteristics of a defined population. A survey lacks a specific hypothesis, although the investigator may suspect that certain relationships exist. The purpose of a survey is to obtain a statistical profile of the population (16). A survey, for example, may be designed to assess the nutrient content of the food supply.

EXAMPLE.   A survey was designed to describe clinical nutrition managers' perceptions of their access to sources of power (resources, support, information, and opportunity) and to explore the relationships of perceptions of power to variables such as time in the profession, years in management, education level, and work setting. Dietitians who were selected randomly from the American Dietetic Association (ADA) Clinical Nutrition Management dietetic practice group were sent a survey instrument designed to study empowerment in dietetic professionals (17).

EXAMPLE. To determine the variation in nutrient composition of fast-food fried chicken, a preliminary study was conducted to determine the design for a nationwide sampling for a descriptive study (a survey). From each selected city and vendor, 5 breast/wing and 5 thigh/leg units were purchased. Each sample was deboned, homogenized, coded, and frozen prior to analysis. Utilizing appropriate chemical and microbiological methods, replicate samples were analyzed for fat, protein, moisture, and vitamin content. Control samples were prepared by identical procedures and analyzed along with each laboratory run (18).

Uses of Surveys

A survey may be useful for establishing associations among variables or factors and often provides clues for further study. Surveys can also provide baseline data about the prevalence of a condition or factor of interest in the population. A major use of the survey method is for planning health and dietary services.

EXAMPLE. The clinical dietitian for a large prepaid health plan wants to know what proportion of the plan's enrollees are interested in weight reduction. The dietitian hopes to plan a weight-reduction clinic and needs the estimated participation rates for budget purposes. A random sample of enrollees will be selected to receive a pilot-tested questionnaire regarding their interests. The results will be used to tailor the clinic to the participants' needs; thus, questions will cover the kinds of help enrollees want for weight reduction.

EXAMPLE. A patient survey can be designed for quality assurance in a hospital's dietary services. For example, in one hospital randomly selected patients were questioned with regard to their satisfaction with tray presentation. Assessment of cold food, hot food, time of delivery, and tray appearance was included. The random survey was repeated periodically so that tray service could be monitored, trends could be observed, and actions could be taken to improve service.

Survey Subject Selection

It is usually not feasible to measure an entire population in a survey, so a sample is selected based on a probability design so that all individuals have an equal chance of being selected. The individuals who consent to participate in the sample are then questioned or examined for the disease or characteristic of interest and other relevant variables.

EXAMPLE. A survey was conducted to describe the food intake and food sources of macronutrients in the diets of older Hispanic adults in the northeastern United States, as well as to explore relationships between acculturation, years in the United States, and macronutrient intake. The 779 subjects in the Massachusetts Hispanic Elders Study sample were selected using a two-stage random cluster sampling technique that ensured a sample that was representative of the state of Massachusetts (19).

EXAMPLE. Foodservice managers in health care and educational institutions that applied computer technology to their operations were surveyed to examine the extent to which computers were applied to management and client service functions. The research questionnaire was designed to collect data on the characteristics of the institution, the types of computers in use, the applications for which computers were being used, and the reasons for not using computers. The questionnaire was pretested by a panel of experts using the Delphi technique. The expert panel was composed of specialists in foodservice management, computer systems, and survey research methods. The experts were asked a series of questions, the answers to which were used by the researcher to devise the final questionnaire, upon which the panel agreed. Questionnaires were mailed to 2,064 persons randomly selected from the membership listings of several professional organizations related to foodservice management (20).

Results of a survey can be generalized with confidence only if the sample is representative of the target population. Thus, the target population must be defined and enumerated; then a sample is drawn at random from it. A probability sample scheme is devised by which all the individuals in the target population have a known chance of being included in the sample; that is, the chances of being selected are specified in the sampling scheme. A probability sampling method allows the sampling errors to be calculated and increases the likelihood that the study is representative of the target population. A high rate of participation (response rate) increases the chances that the results are representative, as it is never certain that responders and nonresponders are similar.

Possible sampling schemes range from the simple random method to complex methods utilizing varying selection probabilities among subgroups (strata) of the population. Elwood (21) discusses the rationale for probability sampling in nutrition research, and Williams (22) provides details on methodology.

The appropriate sample size for a survey depends upon many factors, including how precisely the sample should estimate the population parameters. Methods for calculating sample size requirements are given by Cohen (23).

A survey based on an accidental or convenience sampling scheme is of limited value, because its results cannot be generalized. The reference population is undefined or is defined by the conscious or unconscious selection biases of the investigator. Further, the selection itself may be influenced by the condition or factor under study.

EXAMPLE. A survey was conducted to identify factors related to noncompliance to diet among patients treated for hypertension with medication plus diet. The study included a convenience sample of patients who returned for follow-up at a hypertension clinic. Unfortunately, this scheme selected those patients who were likely to be more compliant with the diet simply because they returned for follow-up. Investigators failed to meet the purpose of the research, because the study generated no information on the patients who did not comply with follow-up visits.

Survey Data Collection

Data in surveys are most frequently collected by questionnaires or interviews. They also may be generated by physical examination (for example, anthropometric measurement; laboratory evaluation of specimens, such as blood analysis for hemoglobin levels; or direct observation, such as employee productivity).

One of the most difficult aspects of survey methodology is designing a questionnaire (24). Depending on the research objectives, standard or tested instruments may be available. If questions must be developed, they must be unambiguous, yet concise and tactful. The length of the questionnaire, its format, and how it is to be administered are also important considerations. Polit and Hungler (25) present guidelines and suggestions for questionnaire development.

Consider how the questionnaire will be analyzed in the design phase. Once the instrument has been constructed, a pilot study helps detect problems. Subjects in the pilot test should be individuals similar to those eligible to participate in the formal study.

Questions can be administered by personal interviews, telephone interviews, or computer-assisted or self-administered questionnaires. Interviews allow questions to be clarified and more detailed information to be collected. The interviewers must be highly trained and objective and must adhere to a set questioning routine to minimize their influence on the subjects' responses.

Information about physical traits or symptoms can be collected by observation in some settings, particularly institutional or clinical settings. Criteria and definitions by which observations are made must be specific to improve accuracy. The observation technique should be standardized and each observer carefully trained to minimize intraobserver and interobserver variation. Laboratory methods must be reliable and standardized, and their accuracy should be quantified. Any laboratory analyses performed out of the researcher's laboratory should be done in select laboratories that are certified by a recognized agency, such as the College of Medical Pathologists. For any assessment that is dependent to some degree upon the judgment of the observer (for example, self-reports of appetite), assessment of a more objective, "hard" variable (for example, measured energy intake) is helpful. Such assessment is also an aid to establishing validity of a subject's self-report.

EXAMPLE. To assess whether women in a hospital obstetrics clinic meet recommendations for folate, vitamin B-12, and zinc intakes during pregnancy, investigators obtained 7-day food records from subjects at several time points during pregnancy and after delivery. On the day following each food record, blood samples were collected to measure red blood cell folate, serum vitamin B-12, and serum zinc levels (26).

EXAMPLE. To examine the entry-level role responsibilities in community dietetics programs, questionnaires were sent to randomly selected subjects consisting of 152 Plan IV representatives, 82 internship directors, and 740 dietetic interns. Postage-paid return envelopes were enclosed. A follow-up postcard was mailed 2 weeks later. Questionnaires were color-coded according to the seven geographic areas used by the ADA House of Delegates; all materials were otherwise anonymous. Data collected from dietetic interns were self-reports of perceived competence at two points in time: the current moment and the start of the dietetic internship experience. Data collected from internship directors used the same scale, but ratings were opinions as to the perceived degree of competence that students should possess at the completion of their academic work (27).

Validity, Accuracy, Reliability, and Precision

Four measurement qualities critical to all research are validity, accuracy, reliability, and precision; they relate to all research projects and data interpretation. Every research instrument must be pilot-tested, revised, and retested to ensure its validity and reliability.

The validity of a test or instrument refers to its ability to measure the phenomenon it intends to measure. The validity of an instrument can be readily assessed when the true state of the phenomenon can be measured. Unfortunately, if such a method exists, it is often costly and time-consuming.

A quantitative measure of the validity of an instrument is accuracy. The accuracy of an instrument is the measure of the systematic error in measurement (28). The difference between the measured and the true values expresses the accuracy of the instrument. Observer subjectivity also affects the accuracy of the instrument. For example, observers may be more likely to report even values when reporting the last digit of a caliper reading. An average of repeated readings may help to minimize the error in accuracy. Questionnaires requiring recall of diet or other events are particularly subject to inaccuracy. Supplementing responses with other types of information may help establish validity.

The reliability of a test instrument is determined by the consistency of its results when administered to the same specimen repeatedly by either the same individual or different persons. The reliability of clinical tests can be determined by repeated assays of aliquots taken from the same specimen. The reliability of observational reports or physical examinations can be assessed by comparing the data from the same subjects gathered by two or more observers. Follow-up questionnaires can be administered to a subset of the sample to determine whether the instrument elicits the same responses.

A quantitative measure of the reliability of an instrument is precision. The precision of an instrument is described by the amount of variation that occurs randomly, a measure of its random error (28). The dispersion (variation) of measurements around the true value expresses the precision. Less random variation results in greater precision in the measurement and greater reliability.

Sensitivity and Specificity

If a survey or other research protocol involves screening for a particular condition, both sensitivity and specificity must be addressed. For example, the intent of a survey may be to determine the prevalence of a certain condition or diagnosis, such as folate deficiency in pregnant women. Tests or observations are used to classify subjects as to the presence or absence of folate deficiency as defined by a cut-off value of 6 nmol/L (3 ng/mL) (29). How well the cut-off criteria categorize the population is quantified by two measures: sensitivity and specificity.

The sensitivity of a test or criterion is the proportion of affected individuals who test positive (for example, the proportion of individuals with folate deficiency whose serum folate level is less than 6 nmol/L [3 ng/mL]). The specificity of a test or criterion is the proportion of nonaffected individuals who are identified as nonaffected (that is, who test negative). Griner et al (30) review the principles of test interpretation, including calculating sensitivity and specificity. Begg (31) describes the sources of bias in diagnostic tests and critiques the measures of test efficacy, sensitivity, and specificity.

The choice of a single cut-off value to categorize individuals may not be clear when the test yields a continuous scale of values. A cut-off value chosen to maximize sensitivity will unavoidably cause the test to be less specific (24). The selection of an appropriate cut-off point is aided by use of a graph plotting true-positive against false-positive ratios, known as a "ROC curve" (receiver operating characteristic curve). The ROC curve graphically displays the reciprocal relationship between sensitivity and specificity for values of a test measured on a continuous scale, and it allows investigators to choose a cut-off point that maximizes the performance of the test for the needed levels of sensitivity, specificity, or both. Several authors discuss constructing and using a ROC curve (32–34).

Statistical Analysis and Interpretation of Survey Results

Results of surveys can be described using simple descriptive statistics, such as means, medians, standard deviations, and frequency distributions. Plot the frequency distributions of important variables to determine skewness, or departure from the normal bell-shaped curve. If skewness is present and the mean and median differ substantially, more information about the distribution must be presented, such as a histogram of the distribution. Relationships among variables are best presented as scatter plots and subsequently defined by mathematical models, such as correlation coefficients. Prevalence rates can also be calculated (18).

The National Health and Nutrition Examination Surveys (NHANES) provide examples of positive, or right-skewed, data. The mean intake of vitamin C for females, aged 6 months to 74 years, as assessed for 10,339 subjects in NHANES II, was 93 mg/day (35); the median intake was 63 mg/day. Because of such strong positive skewness, the presentation of the median intake with high and low percentiles (such as 10th and 90th, or 11 mg and 209 mg, respectively) provides a clearer picture of the intake of the study population than does the mean with either its standard deviation (163 mg) or its standard error (1.6 mg). (See Chapter 3.)

When survey results are interpreted, limitations inherent in the study methodology should be considered. An important limitation is a low response rate, because nonrespondents may differ in important ways from respondents. The response rate affects the confidence given the results and limits the degree to which the results can be generalized. Vigorous follow-up efforts should be made with nonrespondents to increase the response rate. A low response rate can seriously damage an otherwise well-designed study, as it increases the sampling error (error due to sampling only the responsive portion of the target population).

Another important limitation in the interpretation of survey results occurs because measurements are taken at one point in time (that is, cross-sectional design). Because all variables are measured simultaneously, no information is available about the temporal relationship between factors and the condition or disease of interest. For example, it is not clear that exposure to a suspected risk factor or causal agent preceded the onset of a disease. For the same reason, it is not possible to distinguish between a risk factor and a prognostic factor.

Researchers must use discretion in applying inferential statistical tests to data from survey research. Because survey studies are designed to be descriptive rather than analytic, formal tests of hypotheses are undertaken after the data are viewed, and the test result is likely to be biased toward a spurious statistically significant result. Such inferential tests should be regarded as exploratory and useful in generating questions for future analytic studies.

Ex Post Facto Analysis of Survey Results

Analysis of survey or other research results "after the fact," or ex post facto, should be made with caution. In ex post facto research, a research question is posed using data collected for another purpose. Because of this, the study design lacks scientific rigor; variations in the variable of interest have not been manipulated by the researcher but rather have occurred at various times prior to data collection in the natural course of events. Subjects have not been assigned randomly into treatment groups, and no control or comparison group has been studied.

Although ex post facto analysis does provide information regarding associations of variables, it cannot yield satisfactory answers regarding causal relationships, as previously discussed. The preferred approach in testing causal relationships is to devise an analytic study (for example, an experimental design), an observational analytic study (for example, a cohort, or follow-up, study, or a case-control study). (See Chapter 2.) If it is not possible to design an analytic research project, then ex post facto analysis may be considered. However, the results of this analysis should be viewed as exploratory and preliminary, and they must not be interpreted falsely as causal. Instead, ex post facto analysis can serve as the springboard for future analytic designs.

EXAMPLE.   Cross-sectional data on food consumption, supplement use, and bone density were obtained from one thousand postmenopausal women randomly selected from the Midwest. Ex post facto analysis of the data showed a statistically significant positive association between dietary calcium intake and bone density and between supplementary calcium intake and bone density. Thus, analytic studies could be designed to test the hypothesis that calcium intake affects the bone density of postmenopausal women.

An observational analytic study using a case-control design (see Chapter 2) could be developed from the existing survey data by identifying cases and controls and obtaining retrospective data from existing records, personal interviews, and questionnaires. A different analytic research study could be devised using an experimental design in which a subset of postmenopausal women with low bone density was randomly assigned to one of four treatment groups: placebo plus diet counseling to increase calcium intake, calcium supplementation plus diet counseling to increase calcium intake, placebo alone, and calcium supplementation alone. Changes in bone density of the subjects would be measured by dual photon absorptiometry at the initiation of the study, at 6 months, and at 1 year. The experimental design outlined is a double-blind, placebo-controlled, randomized controlled trial that conforms to a 2×2 factorial design (see Chapter 2).

REFERENCES

1. Cooper DR. *Emory CW Business Research Methods.* Toronto, Canada: Irwin Publishing; 1994. Irwin Series in Statistics.
2. Blank SC. *Practical Business Research Methods.* Westport, Conn: AVI Publishing Co; 1984.
3. Moragne L, ed. *Nutrition Funding Report.* Washington, DC: Nutrition Legislation Services; 1986.
4. *The Foundation Directory.* 22nd ed. New York, NY: Foundation Center; 2000.
5. Code of ethics for the profession of dietetics. *J Am Diet Assoc.* 1999;99:109–113.
6. *Honor in Science.* 2nd ed. New Haven, Conn: Sigma Xi, Scientific Research Society; 1986.
7. Angell M, Relman AS. Fraud in biomedical research: a time for congressional restraint. *N Engl J Med.* 1988;318:1462–1463.
8. Kerlinger FN, Lee HB. *Foundations of Behavioral Research.* 4th ed. New York, NY: Harcourt College Publishers; 2000.
9. Kidder L, Judd CM, Smith ER. *Research Methods in Social Relations.* 6th ed. New York, NY: Holt, Rinehart and Winston; 1991.
10. Geiger CJ. Communicating dietary guidelines for Americans: room for improvement. *J Am Diet Assoc.* 2001;101:793–797.
11. Satia JA, Patterson RE, Taylor VM, et al. Use of qualitative methods to study diet, acculturation, and health in Chinese-American women. *J Am Diet Assoc.* 2000;100:934–940.
12. Dahlke R, Wolf KN, Wilson SL, Brodnik M. Focus groups as predictors of dietitians' roles on interdisciplinary teams. *J Am Diet Assoc.* 2000;100:455–457.
13. Slawson DL, Clemens LH, Bol L. Research and the clinical dietitian: perceptions of the research process and preferred routes to obtaining research skills. *J Am Diet Assoc.* 2000;100:1144–1148.
14. Fitch CW, Neville J. Nutrient intake of infants hospitalized with lower respiratory tract infections. *J Am Diet Assoc.* 2001;101:690–692.
15. Matthews ME, Zardain MV, Mahaffey MJ. Labor time spent in foodservice activities in one hospital: a 12-year profile. *J Am Diet Assoc.* 1986;86:636–643.
16. Ferber R, Sheatsley P, Turner A, Wakesberg J. *What Is a Survey?* [American Statistical Association Web site]. Available at: http://amstat.org/sections/srms/brochures/survwhat.html. Accessed February 6, 2001.
17. Mislevy JM, Schiller MR, Wolf KN, Finn SC. Clinical nutrition managers have access to sources of empowerment. *J Am Diet Assoc.* 2000;100:1038–1043.
18. Bowers JA, Craig JA, Tucker TJ, Holden JM, Posati LP. Vitamin and proximate composition of fast-food fried chicken. *J Am Diet Assoc.* 1987;87:736–739.
19. Bermudez OI, Falcon LM, Tucker KL. Intake and food sources of macronutrients among older Hispanic adults: association with ethnicity, acculturation, and length of residence in the United States. *J Am Diet Assoc.* 2000;100:665–673.
20. McCool AC, Garand MM. Computer technology in institutional foodservice. *J Am Diet Assoc.* 1986;86:48–56.
21. Elwood PC. Epidemiology for nutritionists: 2. sampling. *Hum Nutr Appl Nutr.* 1983;37:265–269.
22. Williams WH. *A Sampler on Sampling.* New York, NY: John Wiley and Sons; 1978.
23. Cohen J. *Statistical Power Analysis for the Behavioral Sciences.* 2nd ed. Matwah, NJ: Lawrence Erlbaum; 1988.
24. Dillman DA. *Mail and Internet Surveys: The Tailored Design Method.* 2nd ed. New York, NY: John Wiley and Sons; 1999.
25. Polit DF, Hungler BP. *Essentials of Nursing Research: Methods, Appraisal, and Utilization.* 5th ed. Philadelphia, Pa: Lippincott Williams and Wilkins; 2000.
26. Berg MJ, Van Dyke DC, Chenard C, Niebyl JR, Hirankarn S, Bendich A, Stumbo P. Folate, zinc, and vitamin B12 intake during pregnancy and postpartum. *J Am Diet Assoc.* 2001;101:242–245.

27. Fruin MF, Lawler MR. Perceptions of competency attainment in community dietetics: academic plan IV vs. dietetic internship. *J Am Diet Assoc.* 1987;87:1025–1030.

28. Bland M. *An Introduction to Medical Statistics.* 3rd ed. New York, NY: Oxford University Press; 2000.

29. Huber AM, Wallins LL, DeRusso A. Folate nutriture in pregnancy. *J Am Diet Assoc.* 1988;88:791–795.

30. Griner PF, Mayewski RJ, Mushlin Al, Greenland P. Selection and interpretation of diagnostic tests and procedures. Principles and applications. *Ann Intern Med.* 1981;94:557–592.

31. Begg CB. Biases in the assessment of diagnostic tests. *Stat Med.* 1987;6:411–423.

32. McNeil BJ, Keeler E, Adelstein SJ. Primer on certain elements of medical decision making. *N Engl J Med.* 1975;293:211–215.

33. Hanley JA, McNeil BJ. The meaning and use of the area under a receiver operating characteristic (ROC) curve. *Radiology.* 1982;143:29–36.

34. Department of Clinical Epidemiology and Biostatistics, McMaster University. Interpretation of diagnostic data: 4. How to do it with a more complex table. *Can Med Assoc J.* 1983;129:832.

35. *Dietary Intake Source Data: United States, 1976-80.* Washington, DC: US Government Printing Office; 1983. DHHS publication PHS 83-1681.

2

Analytic Research Designs

Carrie L. Cheney, Ph.D., R.D., and Elaine R. Monsen, Ph.D., R.D.

The intent of analytic research is to test a hypothesis concerning causal relationships—perhaps a hypothesis generated from an earlier descriptive study. Experimental design is the gold standard of analytic research because in that design, all factors are held constant save those factors manipulated by the investigator. Some observational designs, such as cohort (follow-up) studies and case-control studies, are analytic but not experimental.

> **EXAMPLE.** The variation in nutrient composition of fast-food fried chicken described in a nationwide survey (see Chapter 1) could lead to further research to test the effects on fat content of two different frying techniques using an analytic study design.

EXPERIMENTAL DESIGN (CLINICAL TRIAL)

Experimental design is a powerful analytic research method, regardless of whether the subjects are human beings, experimental animals, or inanimate objects. In each case, criteria for subject selection need to be established, the appropriate sample size needs to be estimated, the treatment or treatments must be clearly defined, and end points must be established. After a preliminary study has been conducted and the experiment has been designed, data need to be collected and analyzed suitably (see Chapter 3) to permit appropriate interpretation and application.

Randomized Clinical Trials

Uses of the Randomized Clinical Trial

The experimental design in medical research, referred to as a clinical trial, is the most powerful design for evaluating practices and medical treatments. It is used to prove the feasibility and safety of a treatment. After safety has been established, a randomized clinical trial may be designed to determine the optimal treatment regimen to obtain the desired effect. Most commonly, a clinical trial is employed to compare the efficacy of two or more treatments or practices.

> **EXAMPLE.** The efficacy and safety of a new lactose-free infant formula based on bovine protein were evaluated in a randomized, double-blind, controlled multicenter trial. The new lactose-free cow's milk–based infant formula was compared with a standard cow's milk-based formula containing lactose in this trial with two parallel groups of healthy term infants. Weight, length, and occipitofrontal circumference assessments were the primary means of determining efficacy. Safety was evaluated by comparing the numbers and types of adverse events (1).

Features of the Randomized Clinical Trial

There are three general features of the randomized clinical trial. First, prospective subjects are informed about the study purposes and risks and are asked to participate. Second, people consenting to participate are assigned randomly to one of two or more treatment or intervention groups. The group randomized to receive the standard treatment or treatments constitutes the control group. The key feature is random assignment; that is, chance determines treatment assignment. Third, subjects are observed for the occurrence of particular outcomes or end points following or concurrent with intervention or treatment.

EXAMPLE. By randomly assigning dietetics students to a group that received a short curriculum in death education or to a group who did not, the effectiveness of the curriculum could be assessed. This analytic research was a logical extension of a prior quasi experiment (to be discussed later in the chapter) that used a pretest/posttest format for a single group of students who received the curriculum in death education. The prior study provided baseline data and testing of the evaluation instruments that measured the students' change in knowledge of the grief process, personality traits of empathy and dogmatism, fear of death, fear of interacting with the dying, and attitudes toward working with terminally ill clients. Clinical performance of empathic counseling was assessed by direct observations (2).

Selection of Subjects

In a randomized clinical trial, the degree to which a study group is representative of a reference population determines whether the results can be generalized. This fact must be reconciled with the equally important requirement of a high degree of probability that the treatment effect can be seen. In general, the researcher should select subjects who are relatively homogeneous in major characteristics (for example, diagnosis and nutrition status) so that extraneous sources of variation are eliminated. Other factors to consider when selecting subjects are subject compliance, ease of follow-up, and cost of enrolling and monitoring the subjects (3).

Compliance to the study protocol may be enhanced by offering appropriate incentives to all participants, such as special information or health care. Assessment of compliance prior to the start of the study may also be helpful; it can be done by including a pre-study requirement for all potential subjects. Repeated 24-hour urine collections or several days of dietary intake records are useful requirements for judging compliance. Subjects who are unable to complete the pre-study tasks are less likely to comply with study demands and should be excluded from the study before it begins. The resulting sample is necessarily biased, composed as it is of persons selected for their compliant behavior.

The ease of follow-up is related, in part, to the study setting. Follow-up is facilitated in highly restrictive settings or in settings in which the subject can be readily observed, such as in hospital settings. Unless the research question is relevant in such restricted settings, however, imposing severe restrictions on subjects can impair the study's ability to correspond to a natural setting and can decrease its usefulness.

The cost of enrolling and monitoring subjects influences the number of subjects in the study. In many cases, investigators can lower the cost per subject by employing facilities and resources that are already available and using information that is collected routinely.

Choice of Intervention or Treatment

As with subject selection, the intervention in a randomized clinical trial is chosen to maximize the likelihood that an effect can be measured and detected statistically. The more the treatment of the intervention group differs from the treatment of the comparison or control group, within the range of safe or acceptable levels, the more likely measurable differences will be seen. As much as possible, the comparison or control treatment should have a reasonable expectation of benefit at least equal to that of the experimental treatment (3). An untreated group as a control is valid only if there is no recognized treatment. Otherwise, the control group should receive the standard treatment or an accepted treatment for the disease or condition of interest.

If there is no recognized treatment and it is thought that a psychological effect or observer bias is likely, a placebo is recommended (4). The result is a blind study in which the subjects are unaware of the treatment assignment. The placebo, or sham treatment, must be inert and identical to the experimental treatment in appearance and mode of administration. The efficacy of blinding should be evaluated before and during the trial to insure that blinding is maintained (5). If both subjects and investigators are unaware of the treatment assignment, the trial is a double-blind clinical trial—a powerful design because it eliminates expectation bias on the part of the subject and the investigative staff. The effect of expectation cannot be underestimated, as illustrated in the following classic example.

EXAMPLE. The National Institutes of Health conducted a double-blind randomized controlled trial (a trial in which neither subject nor investigator was informed as to which treatment group the subject was assigned) of the effectiveness of ascorbic acid on reducing the frequency and severity of the common cold. A lactose-capsule placebo that could be easily distinguished from a vitamin C tablet by taste was used, although the investigators gave little thought to the possibility that their subjects might actually bite into the capsules. Early in the study, the investigators learned that many of their curious volunteers had bitten into the capsules; as a result, a significant number of subjects knew which medication they were receiving. Although the study was no longer a double-blind study, it did illustrate an association between severity and duration of symptoms and knowledge of the medication taken. Among those subjects who tasted their capsules, those receiving vitamin C had shorter, milder colds, whereas the converse was true for the placebo group. Among those subjects who remained blind to their treatment, no effect of vitamin C was seen (6).

Assignment to Treatment Groups

A random method of treatment assignment is essential in a randomized clinical trial. Researchers are advised to avoid any treatment assignment method that is not random, such as allocation procedures based on characteristics associated with patients (for example, birth dates or Social Security numbers) or odd-even or other systematic schemes (7). The random method eliminates the selection bias that can occur if the subject or the investigator selects the treatment. It also mitigates nonintentional bias, or the chance formation of groups that are not comparable because of differences in factors that affect the response to treatment, such as age or gender. The random method does not guarantee comparable groups, however, and a chance imbalance between groups is possible, especially if the sample size is less than two hundred (8). Restricted randomization is a method of randomization that ensures that groups are equal or similar in numbers of subjects with certain characteristics, such as age and gender.

A crossover design uses subjects as their own controls rather than using a separate control group. This design requires fewer subjects, because the within-subject variation is less than the between-subject variation. It is useful when the study involves conditions that are chronic and the treatment effects, if present, are not long lasting. In a crossover design, the subjects are randomly assigned to two groups differing in the sequence of treatments. This assignment method ensures that an effect due to order of treatment is eliminated from the observed treatment effect (9).

EXAMPLE. To investigate how the diet of people with diabetes is affected by the consumption of fat-modified foods, five low-fat or no-fat products or their regular-fat counterparts were provided to volunteers to take home and use for 3 days in a randomized crossover design. People with diabetes were case matched to people without diabetes. Subjects were provided low-fat or no-fat products. After a washout period of at least 9 days, subjects were provided with the same products in their regular-fat version. Treatment order was counterbalanced across type of product received, and subjects were randomly assigned to an order (10).

Although seemingly simple and appealing, the crossover design is difficult to justify in most circumstances because the validity of the comparison rests upon the assumption that the subject enters each time period—treatment and control—in an identical state. There can be no carryover effects of the treatment and no appreciable change in the subject's condition. The crossover design is not appropriate when the treatment acts systemically (11) or when the physical condition of the subjects is unstable over the period of the trial (12). The relevant issues are discussed by Hills and Armitage (9) and by Louis et al (13).

Instead of randomizing patients to a control group, it is often tempting to use a historical control group composed of subjects—usually patients—who were treated in some manner recognized as standard in the past. Unfortunately, it is difficult to establish the validity of historical controls. The biases present in such a series of patients are rarely completely identifiable and may irretrievably weight the outcome of the comparison in favor of the new treatment (14). It is not possible to ensure comparability between current and previous patients and the treatments used. A suggested alternative is to use both historical and concurrent randomized controls, but only when certain conditions are met, as outlined by Pocock (15).

Some clinical questions cannot be addressed by a randomized controlled trial because a comparison group of internal controls cannot be formed for ethical or logistic reasons. Other comparison groups—external controls—are necessary. If those controls are well chosen, the studies can make valuable contributions. General advice on the proper use and interpretation of studies using external controls is offered by Bailar et al (16).

Sample Size

The ability of a clinical trial to detect a difference between treatment and control groups depends, in part, on the sample size. Determining the sample size yields an estimate only and is based on several assumptions and judgments about circumstances of the study. The procedures for estimating the size of a study are detailed by Lachin and others (7,17). The procedure involves six steps:

1. Choose the main end point of interest and its method of measurement. The main end point selected should be the most important variable amenable to measurement of the variables studied.
2. Choose the statistical test to be applied to the data.
3. Specify the magnitude of the difference that is meaningful to detect. A smaller difference requires a larger sample size. The amount of difference specified should be meaningful, that is, significant in practice.
4. Estimate the expected variability using published research or results from pilot studies. Sometimes data are not available, and a best guess must be made.
5. Specify the acceptable chances of being wrong. Formally, these are the probability levels of type I and type II errors (17). A type I error (α error) is the probability that a difference will be detected when in truth there is no difference. A type II error (β error) is the probability that a true difference will not be detected. The power of a study, which is the probability that a difference in specified size will be detected successfully, is determined by $1 - \beta$.
6. Apply the appropriate calculations.

See Chapter 26 for details regarding the calculations and examples of approaches to sample size and power estimation.

If the resulting number is larger than is reasonable with available resources, the researcher should ask: Given the available resources and the sample size feasible to accrue, what is the chance that a meaningful difference can be detected (that is, what is the power of the study)? The answer can be calculated by the same methods, but solving for power instead of sample size. A study may not be worth doing if there is a low probability of detecting a relevant difference. If the final analysis shows that sufficient resources cannot be obtained, the project should be redesigned to require fewer assets.

End Points and Data Collection

The end point of a study is the variable by which the treatments are compared. The choice of a meaningful end point is often clear from the nature of the research question. However, the preferred end point for some research questions is not measurable; reasons may include the length of time required for the end point to occur or the sophisticated equipment necessary to measure the end point. In such cases, a surrogate for the end point is chosen, often an antecedent to the end point. The surrogate or antecedent condition must be highly predictive of the end point for it to serve as a valid answer to the study question (3). Collecting more than a single surrogate may be advisable to help corroborate findings.

EXAMPLE. In a study comparing two parenterally administered solutions differing in amino acid composition, the end point of interest was lean body mass (LBM), and the comparison was efficacy of sparing LBM. Because the study was done in an acute care setting, it was not possible to use the more accurate estimates of LBM given by neutron activation analysis or isotope dilution techniques. The investigators decided to measure urine creatinine excretion to estimate muscle catabolism and changes in muscle mass. This surrogate yielded an acceptable answer, to the extent that other factors bearing on creatinine excretion, such as renal function or creatinine intake, were measured and considered in the analysis of the data. Nitrogen balance was also measured. Neither urine creatinine excretion nor nitrogen balance is a direct measure of lean body mass, but the two measures did offer useful information in the absence of the true end point (18).

As Weiss cautions, the possibility exists that the treatment affects only the antecedent or surrogate and not the end point of interest (3). In choosing the surrogate, consider all available information to help prevent that problem from occurring.

The choice of end point may be between "hard" (objective) and "soft" (subjective) evidence or data. Serum cholesterol concentration and body weight are hard data; degree of headache pain and severity of flu symptoms are soft data. Hard variables are preferred because they are more objective, more reliable, and easier to measure. Relevant soft variables should not be dismissed, however, because they are frequently the most interesting and important outcomes and can be useful in interpreting hard data. A useful approach is to combine a few carefully chosen hard and soft variables.

EXAMPLE. A randomized intervention trial was designed to evaluate the effect of a farmer's market nutrition program, with or without coupons, on fruit and vegetable consumption behavior. Participants were randomized to education or education with farmer's market coupons. A self-administered questionnaire measured attitudes toward fruit and vegetable consumption and intake of fruits and vegetables before and after intervention. Records from the U.S. Department of Agriculture Women, Infants, and Children Program were used to document redemption of coupons (19).

The assessment and measurement procedures should be standardized and applied to all subjects equally and in the same manner. To minimize observer biases in evaluating the end point, the person who evaluates the end point should be unaware of the treatment assignment (blind evaluation). This precaution is especially important if the observation requires a subjective assessment.

Variation among observers is also a potential problem when the assessment method involves making a judgment. Suggestions to reduce variation among observers are given by Gore (20).

Variables other than the end point should be measured. Collect data on variables that help characterize the subjects or that are relevant to the study end point. Such variables have the potential to distort the treatment comparison (that is, confounding variables) if they differ in frequency or magnitude between groups. Randomization does not ensure that the groups are balanced in all factors, and some adjustment or stratification in the analysis may be necessary.

EXAMPLE. A study was conducted to compare the nitrogen-sparing effectiveness of two levels of parenterally administered solutions containing different concentrations of branched-chain amino acids in patients undergoing intensive and prolonged cancer treatment (18). Because it is known that physiological stress exacerbates nitrogen loss, the investigators collected information on the severity of stress the patients experienced during the study. Neither the investigators nor the patients were aware of the amino acid solution given, so there was little chance that one group would be scrutinized to a greater degree than the other or that symptoms would be more likely to be reported in one group. At the end of the study, one group had indeed experienced a greater frequency of severe stress than had the other group. The investigators were able to account for this difference in the analysis by adjusting for the severity of stress, thus controlling (to some degree) the influence of stress on the outcome measure. If that measure had not been taken, the estimate of the treatment effect would have been distorted by group differences in stress.

When measuring a numeric variable with the intent to categorize the levels, such as low and high serum cholesterol concentrations, retain the value intact in data collection (for example, 5.95 mmol/L [230 mg/dL] in measuring serum cholesterol). Doing so provides more information and greater flexibility than including only a single dimension or category.

Statistical Analysis and Interpretation

Several excellent references describe statistical procedures for testing hypotheses in experiments (7,21–23). A general review of selected tests can be found in Chapter 3. Among the major problems frequently encountered in analyzing and interpreting results of clinical trials are noncompliance and loss of subjects.

Even with the best efforts to maintain strict adherence to the treatment protocol, noncompliance often occurs. Adherence to treatment should be monitored to learn of practical aspects of the treatment. All subjects should be followed to the same extent, regardless of their compliance with treatment. At the time of analysis, retain subjects in their originally assigned treatment group whether or not they actually received the treatment (7). This comparison reflects how the treatments perform in practice (21). A selection bias is introduced if the subjects are excluded or analyzed in groups other than the group to which they were randomly assigned. A secondary analysis could evaluate the outcomes of the treatments actually received, but that analysis should not be given more weight or relevance than the primary "intent-to-treat" analysis.

Withdrawal of subjects presents another opportunity for selection bias to occur. Subjects who are withdrawn from the study should be followed in the same manner as study subjects, if possible (24). As in the problem of noncompliance, these subjects should be analyzed as part of the original treatment group. Report reasons for withdrawal, and compare them among groups. One treatment may favor withdrawal because it is less acceptable or has unexpected adverse effects.

Reporting adverse effects will aid in evaluating the practicality of the treatment and in planning future studies. If follow-up is not possible and the outcome is not known, compare the known characteristics of the withdrawn subjects with the characteristics of the subjects who complete the study. This comparison may help determine the nature of the bias introduced into the results by the subjects' withdrawal. As an additional step in estimating the effect of removing the subjects, a secondary analysis could be done assuming an unfavorable outcome for those subjects. Compare this "worst-outcome" result with the result obtained with known end points.

Factorial Design

The study designs previously described in this chapter consider only one study question and investigate only one factor. Their simplicity makes them preferred designs in most settings. If the facilities allow, however, it may be useful and efficient to study more than one factor in a single study using a factorial design. A factorial design includes study groups for all combinations of levels of each factor under study. For example, a two-factor factorial design with two levels per factor would have four treatment groups (see Figure 2.1).

The comparison of levels of factor A is achieved by comparing groups with factor A (cells 1 and 3) with groups without factor A (cells 2 and 4); the comparison of levels of factor B is achieved by comparing groups with factor B (cells 1 and 2) with groups without factor B (cells 3 and 4). These comparisons are made using two-way analysis of variance. This design also allows a synergistic effect (interaction) to be detected (21). Snedecor and Cochran (25) provide details for the design and analysis of factorial experiments.

EXAMPLE.   The impact of incentive programs on the effectiveness of employee training was assessed in a 2×2 factorial design in which a the awarding of a monetary bonus was compared with awarding bonus points. All employees were enrolled in a course on customer service, and each was given an audiocassette and a self-paced workbook. Employees were randomly divided into one of four groups receiving bonus points only, monetary bonus only, both bonus points and monetary bonus, or no bonus. Outcomes measured were knowledge and attitude scores before and after testing, reported customer satisfaction, and job performance evaluations before and 3 months after the course.

Partially Controlled or Quasi Experimental Designs

All research involves a balance of the ideal with the feasible. In certain situations randomized treatment assignment or assembly of an appropriate control group is impossible. Other study design options are available, although each has limitations, and none is as convincing as the randomized controlled trial. Experiments that compare groups that have not been randomized, or that lack a control group, are sometimes termed *quasi experiments*.

Although these studies do involve the manipulation of a treatment or intervention, they are weak in allowing causal inferences to be made. This drawback exists because these studies are far less satisfactory than the randomized controlled trial in controlling for the influence of confounding or distorting variables. Of particular concern is the problem of unmeasured confounding variables, such as lifestyle (26,27). Other research options to consider are the observational analytic study designs (that is, cohort and case-control studies).

COHORT (FOLLOW-UP) STUDIES

Cohort (follow-up) studies are observational analytic studies that are designed to mimic the randomized clinical trial. A cohort study does not involve investigator manipulation and thus is not categorized as experimental, but it does test a hypothesis of a causal relationship and thus is analytic in approach.

A cohort is a group of persons followed over time and having a common characteristic or factor of interest. A cohort or group is assembled on the basis of factors thought to relate to the development of the end point un-

FACTOR A

		YES	NO	
	YES	Cell 1 Yes–Yes	Cell 2 Yes–No	1 + 2
FACTOR B				
	NO	Cell 3 No–Yes	Cell 4 No–No	3 + 4
		1 + 3	2 + 4	A × B

FIGURE 2.1 An example of a 2p factorial design in which two factors are at two levels each. The effects of Factor A (cells 1 and 3 vs cells 2 and 4), Factor B (cells 1 and 2 vs cells 3 and 4) and the interaction of A × B may be calculated using two-way analysis of variance.

der study. This organization allows the investigation of a hypothesis concerning the etiology of the outcome of interest. The study involves following the group or cohort forward in time to observe its experience. The outcome studied most commonly is a disease; for convenience, the following discussion refers to the studied outcome as a disease. This design is by no means limited to the study of diseases, however. Many other conditions can be studied in the same manner. The possible causal factors under investigation, referred to as *exposures,* may cover a wide range of environmental and lifestyle characteristics.

Uses of Cohort Studies

A cohort design is useful to determine the frequency of a newly diagnosed disease or a health-related event and to assess the exposure-disease relationship. In the cohort design, exposure to a suspected risk factor is identified when individuals are free of detectable disease; that is, the cohort is identified on the basis of exposure to certain factors thought to affect risk but without the presence of disease. Exposure to the factor of interest clearly precedes the detection of disease. Because it helps establish the temporal sequence of risk factor and end point, the cohort design is appealing for the study of causes of disease. A drawback is that sufficient time must elapse between assessing the exposure and detecting the outcome, causing a typical cohort study to be long. Cohort studies are most useful when the time between exposure and detection of the end point is thought to be relatively short.

EXAMPLE. Investigators used a cohort design to assess the association between changes in nutrition status in hospitalized patients and the occurrence of infections, complications, length of stay in the hospital, and hospital charges. In patients admitted to the hospital inpatient service for a stay of longer than 7 days, nutrition status at the time of admission and discharge was measured, and change in nutrition status during hospitalization was assessed. Outcome measures included length of stay, complications, infections, and hospital charges (28).

Unless the disease studied is extremely common in the population to be studied, most individuals in a cohort will not develop it. Therefore, a large number of subjects is required to compare incidence between exposure groups. This design is more feasible for conditions that are relatively common in the population studied.

EXAMPLE. A cohort study design was used to examine demographic and psychosocial factors that predict healthful dietary change. Participants were recruited by random-digit dialing and were followed up with assessments 2 years later. At baseline, participants were interviewed to obtain demographic characteristics, attitudes and behavior related to cancer risk, and psychosocial factors related to diet. Dietary fat intake was measured at baseline and follow-up by the use of a validated 12-item questionnaire that asked about fat-related dietary habits over the previous 3 months. At the same time, fruit and vegetable intakes were assessed, using a validated 6-item questionnaire. Baseline characteristics were examined for their ability to predict changes in dietary fat-related behaviors and fruit and vegetable intakes (29).

Features of Cohort Studies

The subjects in a cohort are apparently free of the disease under study and are selected on the basis of the presence or absence of a factor of interest, or exposure. Subjects are then followed forward in time to determine the occurrence of the disease or of a specific end point serving as an indicator of the disease. The monitoring process can be concurrent or nonconcurrent. The direction of the study is always prospective, because the exposure is identified before the disease is detected. However, the follow-up period may be concurrent or nonconcurrent. Follow-up may proceed at the same time as the study is conducted (concurrent follow-up); current records generate data on disease occurrence. Alternatively, follow-up may have occurred earlier (nonconcurrent follow-up); existing records yield data on disease occurrence. Clearly, the latter scheme alleviates the need to wait for the cohort to go through time.

EXAMPLE.   A nonconcurrent cohort design was used to determine if stature is a useful prognostic factor in cystic fibrosis survival. The cohort was assembled from the national registry maintained by the Cystic Fibrosis Foundation in the United States. The registry maintains records on numerous variables related to patient morbidity and mortality. Individuals were included in the cohort if they were born between 1980 and 1989, had a minimum of four records each, were alive at age 7 years, and had a recorded height measurement at age 7 to 8 years. Vital status, along with the date of death if it had occurred, was obtained from the registry (30).

Selection of Subjects in Cohort Studies

The subjects making up the cohort must be at risk for developing the disease or outcome of interest but free of the disease at the start of the study. The subjects may be members of a single cohort and classified according to their exposure to the factor of interest, or the subjects may be members of different cohorts, selected from special exposure groups so that the exposed cohort can be compared with the nonexposed cohort. The validity of the comparison between cohorts depends upon the assumption that the cohorts are comparable in all relevant factors other than the exposure.

Sample Size in a Cohort

The size of the cohort required for study is related to the frequency that the end point of interest occurs. A low frequency requires a large sample size. Most cohort studies involve hundreds to thousands of individuals. Several authors address the issues and procedures of estimating sample size (31–35). The basic concepts for estimating sample size for cohort studies are similar to those covered in the discussion of sample size in randomized clinical trials.

Assessing Exposure Status

Exposure to the factor of interest is observed or measured for each subject at the start of a cohort study. The technique of assessment should be standardized to improve reliability (see the discussion of statistical analysis and interpretation of randomized clinical trials earlier in this chapter and in Chapter 3). Information relating to exposure and other important characteristics can be collected from direct measurement, existing records, personal interviews, and questionnaires.

Assessing dietary intake poses special problems. Dietary intake methodology is the subject of continuing investigation, as no single method has been shown to be reliable and valid for all types of research. When selecting the method for collecting dietary data, the researcher should review three issues thoroughly.

First, the researcher should study the limitations and use of available dietary intake collection methods—for example, an in-depth food history, a 3-day food record, or a 24-hour dietary recall (36–41). Second, review should cover the uses to which the data are to be addressed, such as comparisons of an individual subject's nutrient intake and laboratory values. Third, the researcher should review specific research goals, such as estimating intakes of individuals or of groups (42–50). Instead of relying solely on dietary intake assessments, investigators also measure biomarkers of intakes of nutrients or specific food groups, such as plasma carotenoids for fruit and vegetable intakes or erythrocyte fatty acids for diet quality indexes (51–53).

A difficulty of cohort studies is that a change in exposure status may occur during the follow-up period. A change in exposure status may dilute the study's ability to detect a difference in risk between exposed and unexposed groups. If possible, measure the factor again during the follow-up period (54).

EXAMPLE. A cohort study was designed to determine whether higher juice intakes are related to poorer growth in young children. Because of the potential for juice intakes to change over time, investigators measured juice intake during seven in-home interviews when the children were 24 to 72 months of age. Growth parameters, including height, weight, body mass index, and ponderal index, were measured at 72 months. The association between juice intake over time (longitudinal observations) and growth and overweight indexes was evaluated (55).

Assessing End Points (Diseases)

The end point in a cohort study should be defined in detail to be an unambiguous and reliable definition. The method and type of follow-up should be identical for all subjects, regardless of exposure status. Achievement of this goal is facilitated by making the evaluators unaware of the subjects' exposure status (that is, blind assessment). Blinding ensures that the efforts for follow-up and the assessment methods used will be applied equally and will not be biased by the investigators' expectations.

The end-point events are counted as they occur during the follow-up period. However, end points occurring immediately after assessment of the exposure status cannot be counted when it is not clear that the exposure preceded the end point. This decision depends upon what is known or believed to be true about the length of the induction or latent period for the disease or end point in question.

It is often useful to supplement the information about the end point. Record the date of detection of the end point, as well as its occurrence, depending upon the nature of the factor under study.

Complete follow-up on all members of the cohort is vitally important. Loss of subjects can seriously distort the results. Make vigorous efforts to assess the outcome of each subject at the end of the follow-up period.

The length of follow-up depends on the hypothesis and related knowledge of the latency period or the mechanisms of action of the risk factor. The longer the follow-up

period, the more difficult the follow-up becomes because of changes of residence, death from other causes, changes in exposure status, and the added staffing expenses for monitoring subjects and collecting data. Those considerations must be balanced with the need to allow sufficient time for the proposed effect to become manifest.

Statistical Analysis and Interpretation

Baseline characteristics of the cohort are described using descriptive statistics. The usual inferential comparative analysis of cohort studies involves determining the incidence of disease and estimating the incidence ratio for exposed versus unexposed subjects. The incidence ratio is known as the relative risk and measures the strength of the association between the exposure factor and the disease. Various authors discuss the rationale and provide methods for calculating the statistics (22). Often it is necessary to adjust for the effects of confounding variables by stratification (22); a more complex analysis is indicated if several variables must be adjusted simultaneously (56). Researchers unfamiliar with the techniques are advised to seek statistical consultation.

The weakness in this observational design is that a relationship is not clearly causal. All factors are not held constant, as they are in an experiment. Factors other than the exposure of interest may affect the outcome, and those factors may not be measured or known. The population may experience changes in environment or lifestyle that modify exposures and responses, yet such changes cannot be controlled by the investigators. Furthermore, the end point may be related to the factors that determine the exposure status rather than to the exposure itself. The results are interpreted in light of other known evidence. The criteria for examining factors associated with disease risk are outlined by Hill (57).

CASE-CONTROL STUDIES

Case-control studies are observational analytic designs that investigate hypotheses of causal relationships. These designs are retrospective, historically oriented studies, also known as *case-referent studies* or *case-comparison studies*. Because case-control designs do not involve intervention by the investigators, they are not experimental but do adhere to as many principles of experimental design as possible.

Uses of Case-Control Studies

A case-control design is used to explore etiology by comparing the prevalence of the exposure to factors of interest in persons who have a disease with that of a group without disease. The design is useful in studies of rare diseases or end points. In general, case-control studies are less expensive to conduct and require less time than cohort studies. An entire issue of the *Journal of Chronic Diseases* is devoted to the use and methods of the case-control design and is a classic reference (58).

Features of Case-Control Studies

The case-control study design assesses exposure status after disease status is known and thus is retrospective. The comparison groups are formed on the basis of disease or outcome status, either with disease diagnosis (cases) or without disease diagnosis (controls). Subjects are then investigated for the current presence of, or previous exposure to, a factor or factors of interest. The prevalence of the factor or factors is compared between cases and controls.

EXAMPLE.   Inadequate antioxidant defenses against free-radical toxicity have been implicated in the etiology of amyotrophic lateral sclerosis (ALS). A case-control study was designed to assess diet as a predisposing factor for the development of ALS. Over a 4-year study period, 180 new patients diagnosed with ALS met study criteria. Controls were identified by random-digit dialing of households in the same residential areas (counties) as the cases. An in-person structured interview and a self-administered food frequency questionnaire were used to obtain information on lifestyle and diet exposures (59).

Selection of Cases

In a case-control study, the goal in selection of cases is to obtain a sample that is representative of cases arising from a defined target population. This goal is difficult or impossible to attain in most circumstances. The ideal compromise is to select all incident (newly developed or detected) cases arising in a defined population over some specified period. Selecting incident cases rather than existing (prevalent) cases is preferred because factors related to survival, and thus to selection for the study, may differ from causal factors but cannot be distinguished from one another when prevalent cases are used. The definition of a case should be specific and objective to minimize the bias of personal judgment.

EXAMPLE.   To investigate the hypothesis that a low intake of dietary fiber contributes to the risk of developing cholelithiasis, a case-control study was planned in a prepaid health care setting. During a 2-year period, all newly diagnosed patients with cholelithiasis were asked to participate. The control group was randomly selected from the health care enrollee population and frequency matched for age group and gender. Patients who agreed to participate were interviewed in their homes to learn their usual intake of dietary fiber using a food frequency questionnaire administered by trained interviewers who did not know whether the subjects were cases or controls. The reported fiber consumption (both quantity and type) was compared between cases and controls.

Selection of Controls

Selection of an appropriate comparison group in a case-control study depends largely upon the hypothesis. The goal in selecting the control subjects is that controls should be representative of the population from which the cases arose. A random probability sample is ideal and is feasible if information is available on the sampling units (or community) (see also Chapter 1). A random probability sample is also feasible if the population is a closed one, such as a prepaid health plan or institution. Samples of convenience are often used, but the validity of the study rests upon the assumption that the subjects are similar to the reference or target population with regard to the factors of interest; this assumption may or may not be reasonable.

Considerations in choosing a control group are cost, response rate, and interview setting. Compromises may have to be made to reduce the cost of accessing a control subject while maximizing the response rate. Insofar as possible, the interview setting should be comparable to the setting for cases. Much of the information is elicited by recall and self-report, and factors bearing on those methods should be as identical as possible between the groups.

A selection bias in controls is undesirable but possible. Minimize bias by planning a structured selection system with established criteria for selecting control subjects. The criteria should be applied without the investigators' knowledge of the individuals' exposure status. Other sources of bias, such as age, gender, or socioeconomic status, may be eliminated by matching in the selection or by stratification in the analysis. How to select appropriate controls is not always clear; several authors review problems and give suggestions (60–63).

EXAMPLE. Recent studies have suggested that tea may be protective against cancers of the urinary tract. Using a case-control design, investigators examined the association between usual adult tea consumption and risk of bladder and kidney cancers in a population-based study. Newly diagnosed cases of bladder and kidney cancer were identified through the Iowa Cancer Registry. Controls younger than 65 years were selected from Iowa drivers' license records, whereas controls aged 65 years and older were selected from U.S. Health Care Financing Administration records. Cases were frequency matched to controls by gender and 5-year age group. Usual tea intake, as well as intakes of coffee and other beverages, was assessed by self-report using a mailed questionnaire. Subjects who were reluctant to complete the detailed questionnaire (5.8 percent) were offered a 15-minute abbreviated telephone interview. Tea use was categorized into four levels of intake, and distribution of tea use was compared between cases and controls using odds ratios, adjusted for potential confounding factors (64).

Assessing Exposure to the Factor of Interest

In case-control studies, the historical information, including the exposure to the factor of interest, is obtained from existing records, examinations, direct measurements, and personal interviews or questionnaires. Schlesselman (61) provides guidelines for developing the research instrument, noting that the starting point for developing any data-gathering tool is a list of all pertinent variables, including the extent of detail needed. The methods for assessing past diet in case-control studies have been studied in a variety of settings. Investigators should review the literature before choosing the intake method (7,37–42, 65–68).

EXAMPLE. A population-based case-control study was conducted to examine the association between selected nutrients, foods, and diet behaviors and bladder cancer. Bladder cancer cases diagnosed within a 4-year period were identified from the Surveillance, Epidemiology, and End Results Program cancer registry for Western Washington State. Controls were identified through random-digit dialing for the same residential area. A food frequency questionnaire was used to estimate usual food intake. Subjects were asked to estimate this intake for the year that was the midpoint of the 10-year reference period (that is, 7 years prior to diagnosis for cases and a similar reference period for controls) (69).

Regardless of the instrument used, the procedure for gathering information should be the same for cases and controls. The comparability of the procedure is increased if the interviewer or evaluator does not know whether the subject is a case or a control. This goal may not be possible in a personal interview but may be feasible for a person gathering other objective data.

The sample size considerations discussed in the section on randomized clinical trials pertain to case-control studies as well. In addition, a detailed discussion is provided by Schlesselman (61).

Statistical Analysis and Interpretation

In a case-control study, the frequencies of the exposure of interest are presented for cases and controls. The association between the exposure and the disease is expressed by estimating the odds ratio, a statistical comparison of the prevalence of exposure between cases and controls (22). A typical analysis proceeds from the simple to the complex, involving stratification and possibly multivariate methods. Detailed presentations are given by Schlesselman (61) and Breslow et al (60).

The observational methodology and retrospective nature of the case-control study present limitations that should be kept in mind in the interpretation of the results. Sackett (70) reviews the possible biases and their effect on the interpretation of case-control studies. There are always alternatives to a causal explanation for an association (61). Chief among the alternatives are the following:

1. In a case-control study, it may be unclear whether the factor preceded the disease or resulted from it.

2. Recall bias is likely to be present; the self-report is influenced by the presence of the disease, especially if the subject is aware of the hypothesis being tested. If present, the observed association will overestimate the actual association.

3. The comparability of cases and controls may be questionable. The choice of control group is crucial to a valid study

REFERENCES

1. Heubi J, Karasov R, Reisinger K, et al. Randomized multicenter trial documenting the efficacy and safety of a lactose-free and a lactose-containing formula for term infants. *J Am Diet Assoc.* 2000;100:212–217.

2. Oakland MJ. The effectiveness of a short curriculum unit in death education for dietetic students. *J Am Diet Assoc.* 1988;88:26–28.

3. Weiss NS. *Clinical Epidemiology: The Study of the Outcome of Illness.* 2nd ed. New York, NY: Oxford University Press; 1996.

4. Gore SM. Assessing clinical trials—trial discipline. *Br Med J.* 1981;283:211–213.

5. Farr BM, Gwaltney JM Jr. The problems of taste in placebo matching: an evaluation of zinc gluconate for the common cold. *J Chronic Dis.* 1987;40:875–879.

6. Karlowski TR, Chalmers TC, Frenkel LD, Kapidian AZ, Lewis TL, Lynch JM. Ascorbic acid for the common cold. A prophylactic and therapeutic trial. *JAMA.* 1975;231:1038–1042.

7. Meinert CL, Tonascia S. *Clinical Trials: Design, Conduct, and Analysis.* New York, NY: Oxford University Press; 1986.

8. Gore SM. Assessing clinical trials—why randomise? *Br Med J.* 1981;282:1958–1960.

9. Hills M, Armitage P. The two-period cross-over clinical trial. *Br J Clin Pharmacol.* 1979;8:7–20.

10. Rodrigues LM, Castellanos VH. Use of low-fat foods by people with diabetes decreases fat, saturated fat, and cholesterol intakes. *J Am Diet Assoc.* 2000;100:531–536.

11. Gore SM. Assessing clinical trials—design I. *Br Med J.* 1981;282:1780–1781.

12. Willan AR, Pater JL. Using baseline measurements in the two-period crossover clinical trial. *Control Clin Trials.* 1986;7:282–289.

13. Louis TA, Lavori PW, Bailar JC, Polansky M. Crossover and self-controlled designs in clinical research. *N Engl J Med.* 1984;310:24–31.

14. Sacks H, Chalmers TC, Smith H. Randomized versus historical controls for clinical trials. *Am J Med.* 1982;72:233–240.

15. Pocock SJ. The combination of randomized and historical controls in clinical trials. *J Chronic Dis.* 1976;29:175–188.

16. Bailar JC, Louis TA, Lavori PW, Polansky M. Studies without internal controls. *N Engl J Med.* 1984;311:156–162.

17. Lachin JM. Introduction to sample size determination and power analysis for clinical trials. *Control Clin Trials.* 1981;2:93–113.

18. Lenssen P, Cheney CL, Aker SN, et al. Intravenous branched chain amino acid trial in marrow transplant recipients. *JPEN J Parenter Enteral Nutr.* 1987;11:112–118.

19. Anderson JV, Bybee DI, Brown RM, et al. 5 a day fruit and vegetable intervention improves consumption in a low income population. *J Am Diet Assoc.* 2001;101:195–202.

20. Gore SM. Assessing clinical trials—between-observer variation. *Br Med J.* 1981;283:40–43.

21. Matthews DE, Farewell V. *Using and Understanding Medical Statistics.* 2nd ed. New York, NY: Karger; 1988.

22. Fleiss JL. *Statistical Methods for Rates and Proportions.* 3rd ed. New York, NY: John Wiley and Sons; 2001.

23. McTavish DG, Loether HJ. *Social Research: Achieved Design.* Boston, Mass: Allyn and Bacon; 1999.

24. Gore SM. Assessing clinical trials—rash adventures. *Br Med J.* 1981;283:426–428.

25. Snedecor GW, Cochran WG. *Statistical Methods.* 8th ed. Ames, Iowa: Iowa State University Press; 1989.

26. Hulley SB, Cummings SR. *Designing Clinical Research: An Epidemiological Approach.* Baltimore, Md: Williams and Wilkins; 1988.

27. Polit-O'Hara DF, Hungler BP. *Essentials of Nursing Research: Methods, Appraisal, and Utilization.* 5th ed. Philadelphia, Pa: Lippincott Williams and Wilkins; 2000.

28. Braunschweig C, Gomez S, Sheean PM. Impact of declines in nutritional status on outcomes in adult patients hospitalized for more than 7 days. *J Am Diet Assoc.* 2000;100:1316–1322.

29. Kristal AR, Hedderson MM, Patterson RE, Neuhouser ML. Predictors of self-initiated, healthful dietary change. *J Am Diet Assoc.* 2001;101:762–766.

30. Beker LT, Russek-Cohen E, Fink RJ. Stature as a prognostic factor in cystic fibrosis survival. *J Am Diet Assoc.* 2001;101:438–442.

31. Fleiss JL, Tytun A, Ury HK. A simple approximation for calculating sample sizes for comparing independent proportions. *Biometrics.* 1980;36:343.

32. Greenland S. Power, sample size, and smallest detectable effect determination for multivariate studies. *Stat Med.* 1985;4:117–127.

33. Munoz A, Rosner B. Power and sample size for a collection of 2×2 tables. *Biometrics.* 1984;40:995.

34. Palta M, McHugh R. Planning the size of a cohort study in

the presence of both losses to follow-up and non-compliance. *J Chronic Dis.* 1980;33:501–512.

35. Browner WS, Black D, Newman TB, Hulley SB. Estimating sample size and power. In: Hulley SB, Cummings SR. *Designing Clinical Research: An Epidemiological Approach.* Baltimore, Md: Williams and Wilkins; 1988:139–150.

36. Algert S, Stumbo P. *Validity and Reliability in Dietary Methodology: An Annotated Bibliography.* Chicago, Ill: Research Dietetic Practice Group; 1986.

37. Tran KM, Johnson RK, Soultanakis RP, Matthews DE. In-person vs telephone-administered multiple-pass 24-hour recalls in women: validation with doubly labeled water. *J Am Diet Assoc.* 2000;100:777–783.

38. Morgan KJ, Johnson SR, Rizek RL, Reese R, Stampley GL. Collection of food intake data: an evaluation of methods. *J Am Diet Assoc.* 1987;87:888–896.

39. Craig MR, Kristal AR, Cheney CL, Shattuck AL. The prevalence and impact of 'atypical' days in 4-day food records. *J Am Diet Assoc.* 2000;100:421–427.

40. Jonnalagadda SS, Mitchell DC, Smiciklas-Wright H, et al. Accuracy of energy intake data estimated by a multiple-pass, 24-hour dietary recall technique. *J Am Diet Assoc.* 2000;100:303–311.

41. Yaroch AL, Resnicow K, Khan LK. Validity and reliability of qualitative dietary fat index questionnaires: a review. *J Am Diet Assoc.* 2000;100:240–244.

42. Cullen KW, Baranowski T, Baranowski J, Hebert D, de Moor C. Behavioral or epidemiologic coding of fruit and vegetable consumption from 24-hour dietary recalls: research question guides choice. *J Am Diet Assoc.* 1999:99:849–851.

43. Haines PS, Siega-Riz AM, Popkin BM. The Diet Quality Index revised: a measurement instrument for populations. *J Am Diet Assoc.* 1999;99:697–704.

44. Block G. A review of validations of dietary assessment methods. *Am J Epidemiol.* 1982;115:492–505.

45. Byers T, Marshall J, Fiedler R, Zielezny M, Graham S. Assessing nutrient intake with an abbreviated dietary interview. *Am J Epidemiol.* 1985;122:41–50.

46. Willett WC, Sampson L, Stampfer MJ, et al. Reproducibility and validity of a semiquantitative food frequency questionnaire. *Am J Epidemiol.* 1985;122:51–65.

47. Jain M, Howe GR, Johnson KC, Miller AB. Evaluation of a diet history questionnaire for epidemiologic studies. *Am J Epidemiol.* 1980;111:212–219.

48. Rider AA, Calkins BM, Arther RS, Nair PP. Diet, nutrition intake, and metabolism in populations at high and low risk for colon cancer. Concordance of nutrient information obtained by different methods. *Am J Clin Nutr.* 1984;40 (suppl):906–913.

49. Freudenheim JL, Johnson NE, Wardrop RL. Misclassification of nutrient intake of individuals and groups using

50. Morgan KJ, Johnson SR, Rizek RL, Reese R, Stampley GL. Collection of food intake data: an evaluation of methods. *J Am Diet Assoc.* 1987;87:888–896.

51. Polsinelli ML, Rock CL, Henderson SA, Drewnowski A. Plasma carotenoids as biomarkers of fruit and vegetable servings in women. *J Am Diet Assoc.* 1998;98:194–196.

52. Rock CL, Moskowitz A, Huizar B, et al. High vegetable and fruit diet intervention in premenopausal women with cervical intraepithelial neoplasia. *J Am Diet Assoc.* 2001;101:1167–1174.

53. Gerber MJ, Scali JD, Michaud A, et al. Profiles of a healthful diet and its relationship to biomarkers in a population sample from Mediterranean southern France. *J Am Diet Assoc.* 2000;100:1164–1171.

54. Van Beresteyn EC, van't Hof MA, van der Heiden-Winkeldermaat HJ, ten Have-Witjes A, Neeter R. Evaluation of the usefulness of the cross-check dietary history method in longitudinal studies. *J Chronic Dis.* 1987;40:1051–1058.

55. Skinner JD, Carruth BR. A longitudinal study of children's juice intake and growth: the juice controversy revisited. *J Am Diet Assoc.* 2001;101:432–437.

56. Breslow NE. Elementary methods of cohort analysis. *Int J Epidemiol.* 1984;13:112–115.

57. Hill AB. *Principles of Medical Statistics.* 9th ed. London, England: Oxford University Press; 1971.

58. The case-control study: consensus and controversy. *J Chronic Dis.* 1979;32:1–144.

59. Nelson LM, Matkin C, Longstreth WT, McGuire V. Population-based case-control study of amyotrophic lateral sclerosis in western Washington State. II. Diet. *Am J Epidemiol.* 2000;151:164–173.

60. Breslow NE, Day NE, Davis W. *Statistical Methods in Cancer Research: The Analysis of Case-Control Studies.* New York, NY: Oxford University Press; 1993.

61. Schlesselman JJ. *Case-Control Studies: Design, Conduct, and Analysis.* New York, NY: Oxford University Press; 1982.

62. Hayden GF, Kramer MS, Horwitz RI. The case-control study: a practical review for the clinician. *JAMA.* 1982;247:326–331.

63. Horwitz RI, Feinstein AR. Methodologic standards and contradictory results in case-control research. *Am J Med.* 1979;66:556–564.

64. Bianchi GD, Cerhan JR, Parker AS, et al. Tea consumption and risk of bladder and kidney cancers in a population-based case-control study. *Am J Epidemiol.* 2000;151:377–383.

65. McKeown-Eyssen GE, Yeung KS, Bright-See E. Assessment of past diet in epidemiologic studies. *Am J Epidemiol.* 1986;124:94–103.

66. Hankin JH, Nomura AMY, Lee J, Hirohata T, Kolonel LN.

Reproducibility of a diet history questionnaire in a case-control study of breast cancer. *Am J Clin Nutr.* 1983;37:981–985.

67. Jensen OM, Wahrendorf J, Rosenqvist A, Geser A. The reliability of questionnaire-derived historical dietary information and temporal stability of food habits in individuals. *Am J Epidemiol.* 1984;120:281–290.

68. Willett WC, Sampson L, Browne ML, et al. The use of a self-administered questionnaire to assess diet four years in the past. *Am J Epidemiol.* 1988;127:188–199.

69. Bruemmer B, White E, Vaughan TL, Cheney CL. Nutrient intake in relation to bladder cancer among middle-aged men and women. *Am J Epidemiol.* 1996;144:485–495.

70. Sackett DL. Bias in analytic research. *J Chronic Dis.* 1979;32:51–63.

3

Statistical Analysis, Data Presentation, Conclusions, and Applications

Carrie L. Cheney, Ph.D., R.D., and Elaine R. Monsen, Ph.D., R.D.

Graduate students in nutrition sciences often say that the most fun they experience during research projects is in analyzing their data. All the hard work of planning and conducting a study begins to pay off when they see results, even if the results are the most basic of descriptive statistics. The rewards are in the numbers, tables, *P* values, charts, and graphs. Many seasoned investigators express this same level of satisfaction at the data analysis stage of the research process.

STATISTICAL ANALYSIS AND PRESENTATION OF RESULTS

Preanalysis Planning and Consultation

To help ensure that the data analysis stage of a research project is enjoyable, it is important to design the analysis approach during the planning stage of the research effort. Obtain professional statistical consultation during planning and thereafter as needed. When communicating with a statistician, it helps to be familiar with important fundamental statistical issues and terms. This chapter briefly introduces these concepts and suggests a useful approach to statistical analysis and presentation.

Statistical analysis is driven by the study hypothesis. Before beginning the analysis, review the hypothesis for the study. What is the question of interest, and how is the study designed to answer it? Resist the temptation to answer all possible questions with the data or to suggest unrealistic applications (see Chapters 1 and 2).

Steps in Analysis: Description and Inference

Simply stated, statistical analysis is used to (1) describe the study sample and (2) make inferences (estimates) about the underlying population. Usually, the likelihood (probability) that these inferences are true (or due to chance) is also determined.

Describe characteristics of the sample and values of important variables by plotting first, usually by the use of a frequency histogram. Such plots usually allow errors to be detected. Nominal and ordinal variables, such as gender and anthropometric percentiles, can be presented simply in this manner or tabulated as proportions within categories or ranks. Continuous variables, such as age and weight, are customarily presented by summary statistics describing the frequency distribution. The choice of statistics depends on the symmetry of the plotted frequency histogram. The mean and standard deviation may be used when the distribution is relatively symmetrical. The median and a percentile range, such as the 25th and 75th percentiles, are preferable when the distribution is asymmetrical (1,2).

After the data have been described, the hypotheses are evaluated by statistical inference, which involves estimating parameters and testing statistical significance.

Conceptually, this technique compares the expected distribution with the observed distribution. The expected distribution is defined by the null hypothesis that there is no association or no effect of the factors under study. The null hypothesis specifies values for parameters that describe the underlying distribution. For most of the common tests, this is the normal distribution, and the parameters are the mean and the variance. The sample is used to estimate these parameters for the population. The question then is, How likely is it to observe the mean and standard deviation given by the sample if the null hypothesis is true?

Many of the frequently used statistical tests are presented in Table 3.1. Refer to a basic statistics text before applying any test in order to review the assumptions and constraints for its use.

The validity of most standard tests depends upon the assumptions that (1) the data are from a normal distribution and (2) the variability within groups (if these are compared) is similar. Tests of this type are termed *parametric* and are to some degree sensitive to violations of those assumptions. Check whether the data meet conditions by plotting histograms of key variables; histograms will display evidence of skewness and other characteristics of nonnormal distributions. Other options should be considered if the conditions are not met. Data may be transformed (for example, logarithmically) to reduce skewness and minimize variation across groups (3). Alternatively, nonparametric or distribution-free tests, which do not depend on the normal distribution, can be used (4). Nonparametric tests are also useful for data collected in categorical or interval form (for example, severity of illness ranked on a 4-point scale or acceptability rated on a 5-point scale). Relative to their parametric counterparts, nonparametric tests have the advantage of ease but the disadvantage of less statistical power.

One-Sided and Two-Sided Significance Tests

A two-sided (two-tailed) significance test evaluates departures in either direction from the mean, whereas a one-sided (one-tailed) significance test is sensitive to differences in only one direction. For most situations, a two-sided test of significance is appropriate. The one-sided test is justified only in those rare situations in which the difference is expected to be in a specified direction and a difference in the opposite direction is of no interest. One-sided tests are less rigorous and thus should be avoided if conclusions would change when a two-sided test was applied. A rule of thumb is to use two-sided tests unless advised otherwise by a statistician.

Standard Deviation and Standard Error

The standard deviation (SD) is descriptive and is used to describe the characteristics of the sample. The standard error (SE) is inferential and is used to indicate confidence in the population estimates. The SD indicates the distance from the center or mean, and it describes the spread, or variation, around the sample mean. The SE describes the

TABLE 3.1   Statistical Tests Appropriate for Data Analysis

Relationship Among Samples	Type of Data	Normal Distribution	Statistical Test	
			Two Samples	> Two Samples
Independent	Binary/classification	—	x^2	x^2
	Ordinal/ranked	—	Wilcoxon rank sum	Kruskal-Wallis
	Continuous/measured	Yes	t-test	One-way analysis of variance
		No	Wilcoxon rank sum	Kruskal-Wallis
Related	Binary/classification	—	x^2	x^2
Paired, repeated measures, replicate measures	Ordinal/ranked	—	Sign test Signed rank test	Friedman's test
	Continuous/measured	Yes	Paired t-test	Two(N)-way analysis of variance
		No	Signed rank test	Repeated measures analysis of variance Friedman's test

variation relative to the sample size; that is, the SE is the SD of a sampling distribution. The SE is a measure of the precision of the sampling estimate of a population parameter (that is, how accurate the estimate is likely to be). Researchers should present the most appropriate statistic, not the smallest one (see Chapter 3).

EXAMPLE. In a controlled dietary intervention study, Jonnalagadda et al sought to determine the accuracy of reported energy intake using multiple-pass 24-hour recall techniques with energy intake required for weight maintenance, as assessed by measuring actual food intake of the study foods provided to maintain weight. Among participants, mean ± SD energy intake as recalled was 2,358 ± 802 kcal, whereas actual measured energy intake (mean ± SD) was 2,691 ± 528 kcal. The mean ± SE difference between recall and actual energy intakes was −333 ± 84 kcal. Note that investigators correctly used mean ± SD when describing distributions of intake for both recall and measured values, and they used mean ± SE when presenting the estimate of the difference between the two conditions. In the latter case, the important values are the estimate of the difference and the statistic (SE) showing how precise that estimate is, given the sample used. Alternatively, the investigators could show the mean difference, along with its 95 percent confidence interval (see the next section) (5).

Confidence Intervals

Key results of statistical analyses should be presented along with descriptive data. Important among the details to present are the test statistic (for example, $t = 2.45$ or $X^2 = 14.7$), the degrees of freedom, and the P value. The estimate of the parameter (such as the mean difference or relative risk) should be given as a point estimate and confidence interval of that estimate.

The two products of any statistical test are (1) an estimate of the quantity of interest (for example, mean difference) and (2) the probability that this estimate is a chance occurrence. The two are usually presented as a mean difference and a P value. That method provides only a single value to describe the difference, along with a single value describing its likelihood. An estimate of the population parameter is more meaningfully presented as a range of values within which the true value probably exists: a confidence interval. The confidence interval is the range from the smallest to the largest value that is plausible for the true population value, with a certain degree of confidence (usually 95 percent). It is calculated using the estimated value and its SE.

EXAMPLE. In a study of vitamin A status of Indonesian preschool children, Humphrey et al used confidence intervals to show the range of possible values within which the median intake of vitamin A was likely to be. Using the 24-hour history, researchers found the mean ± SD intake to be 234 ± 489 μg RE among children with normal ocular status, indicating a highly skewed distribution of intake. Humphrey et al estimated the median population vitamin A intake to be 122 μg RE with a 95% confidence interval = 86, 153 μg RE. This shows that the point estimate for the median is 122 μg RE, indicating that 50 percent of the population values are greater than this level, and 50 percent of the values are less than 122 μg RE. The confidence interval values indicate that with 95 percent probability, the true population median is not less than 86 μg RE and not greater than 153 μg RE. The Recommended Dietary Allowances recommendation for children aged 1–3 years is 300 μg RE (6).

Besides describing the possible magnitude of the value, the confidence interval provides information about the certainty in the estimate (precision). Gardner and Altman (7) present the rationale and methods for calculating the confidence interval for a number of statistical tests.

Repeated and Replicated Measurements

It is common to repeat measurements of a variable at several points in time. The simple approach for analysis is to calculate the mean and SD for each period and present them graphically by a line joining the means. Differences among the means are sometimes tested by several t tests. However, these methods are not the most satisfactory ones for analysis of serial measurements (2,8). The mean curve may not accurately summarize the data, especially if substantial individual variability is present. Furthermore, multiple significance tests are likely to yield false-positive results, as will be discussed later in the chapter. Likewise, usual regression and correlation analyses are not appropriate, because the observations are related rather than independent.

A more useful analysis would be to evaluate some

characteristic of individual curves, such as rate of change or time required to attain a specified level (2,8). Another approach to use is a repeated measures analysis of variance, using time as a main factor, to determine whether groups differ in their responses over time. If there are missing values during the period, some adjustment is necessary to account for different amounts of information per subject. Statistical advice is recommended.

Replicate measurements, or several measures taken without regard to time, are also related observations, and the analysis must account for the fact that they were obtained from a single subject. Analysis of variance can be used for replicate measurements of a continuous variable, provided the number of measurements is the same for each subject. If the number of observations varies among subjects, the analysis is more complex (2,8,9). Statistical advice should be obtained.

Multiple Significance Tests

A common problem in nutrition literature is multiple significance testing (10), as often occurs in studies of nutrient intakes when results from many subgroups are compared or many variables are analyzed. The chances of finding a spurious significant result increase as the number of tests increases. The significance tests relating to the hypothesis serving as the basis for the study carry the greatest weight; other tests should be considered only as exploratory (2). If other tests are done, the chances for false-positive results can be minimized by adjusting the criterion of statistical significance (that is, α, usually 0.05) downward, using a procedure such as the Bonferroni procedure (11).

It is often necessary to compare the means of several groups. If multiple t tests are used, the multiple comparison problem arises. Other methods to consider are analysis of variance and multiple-comparison methods specially designed to make several pairwise comparisons, such as the Tukey, least significant difference, Scheffe, and Walker-Duncan tests (12).

EXAMPLE. Investigators presented descriptive anthropometric reference data for older Americans derived from adults aged 60 years and older who were examined in the third National Health and Nutrition Examination Survey. Because the researchers examined differences among racial/ethnic groups for men and women by age groupings, many statistical tests were applied. Researchers recognized the problem of multiple comparisons and used the Bonferroni approach to calculate the critical significance value (13).

Outliers

Outliers are extreme observations that are not consistent with the other observations. They cannot be excluded from the analysis unless there are other reasons to question their credibility (14). Analyze the data with and without outliers to assess their effect on conclusions.

Missing Values

There is no single way to analyze data if there are missing values; consultation with a statistician is recommended. Missing values can have a pronounced impact on the results. They may be unavoidable, but they must not be ignored. The sample sizes of groups at each measurement period should be clearly presented, and the reasons for missing these observations should be given by group. The discussion should include an evaluation of how the missing values might affect the conclusions.

Regression and Correlation Analysis

The relationship between continuous variables is often expressed by a mathematical model describing a straight line, known as *simple linear regression analysis*. Regression analysis is commonly used to determine the association between two variables and to make predictions based on the linear relationship.

Results of regression analyses that may be presented include the fitted regression equation, variances of the slope and intercept coefficients, the variance of the residuals, and the proportion of the variation in the dependent variable explained by the regression equation (2,15). When a plot is used to describe the relationship, include the regression line and the confidence interval curves on both sides of the line.

Correlation analysis and regression analysis differ in purpose, although they are related in technique. In correlation analysis, linear regression is used to yield only a measure of the strength of the association between the independent and dependent variables, the correlation coefficient. The presentation need not include the regression equation and associated variances but can present the correlation coefficient alone, along with the probability that the coefficient occurred by chance, or the 95 percent confidence interval for the coefficient.

Complex Statistical Methods: Brief Descriptions

Cluster Analysis

The term *cluster analysis* refers to several multivariate statistical techniques used to classify into groups a set of previously unclassified objects or subjects, in order to identify patterns in complex data (16).

EXAMPLE. Wirfalt and Jeffery used cluster analysis to identify groups of persons with unique patterns of food energy consumption. Researchers collected data on usual dietary intake by food frequency questionnaire, physical activity measures, body mass index, and demographic characteristics in 526 men and women. From these measures, cluster analysis identified six patterns of food energy sources that differed among persons in regard to nutrient intake, body mass index, and gender (17).

Factor Analysis

Factor analysis constructs new independent factors to explain the relationships among several related variables. These new factors are then used in other analyses instead of the several related variables (9).

EXAMPLE. Kristal et al proposed that 4 dimensions of dietary behavior could be used to describe the process of selecting lower-fat foods and wanted to develop a behavioral measure that could quickly assess these behaviors. Researchers developed a questionnaire to assess the behavioral dimensions and collected dietary intake measures on a large sample of women. From the large amount of data collected by these instruments, they used factor analysis methods to produce a model that had 5 factors consisting of 18 items. They then tested the model for validity and reliability, and results yielded a brief scale that measured dietary patterns related to selecting low-fat diets (18).

Discriminant Analysis

Discriminant analysis provides a mathematical model that discriminates between two populations on the basis of several independent variables. The populations are classi-fied previously, such as those persons with and without cardiovascular disease. The method uses a linear model to describe the relationship between several independent variables and one nominal dependent variable (9).

Multiple Regression Analysis

Multiple regression is used to describe the relationship between several independent variables considered simultaneously and a single dependent variable (9). Multiple regression analysis is commonly used to identify factors related to, or predictive of, some outcome of interest, such as dietary factors and blood pressure. An important use of multiple regression analysis is to adjust for the influence of several factors while assessing the independent relationship of another factor.

EXAMPLE. Kalkwarf et al conducted a longitudinal study to assess the relationship between fiber intake and insulin requirement in pregnant women with insulin-dependent diabetes mellitus. Researchers used multiple regression analysis to adjust for energy and carbohydrate intakes, body weight, duration of disease, and other variables that would potentially alter their assessment of the independent relationship between fiber intake and insulin requirement (19).

Logistic Regression Analysis

Logistic regression adapts the multiple regression model for a binary response variable, such as mortality or the presence/absence of disease. This analysis yields estimates of relative risk while adjusting for covariates and is useful in cohort and case-control designs (20).

EXAMPLE. Hartman et al conducted a case-control study to examine the associations between serum levels of selected B vitamins and risk of lung cancer within the large Alpha-Tocopherol, Beta Carotene Cancer Prevention Study. Men who developed lung cancer were matched with controls from the same study group; serum levels of selected B vitamins were assessed at baseline, before cancer was diagnosed, for both cases and controls. Researchers used logistic regression to determine the risk of lung cancer associated with baseline serum vitamin concentrations. Logistic regression analysis allowed investigators to adjust for potentially confounding variables, such as body mass index and age, while evaluating the association between vitamin status and lung cancer (21).

Survival Analysis

Survival analysis techniques determine the distribution of survival times (that is, death or other dichotomous event) for a cohort. From the survival distribution, the probability of survival (or death) for each specific period can be derived. Survival analysis methods include the life table (actuarial) method for grouped data and the Kaplan-Meier method for ungrouped exact times of death (22).

Path Analysis

Path analysis extends multiple regression analysis to examine a limited number of causal hypotheses or to build theoretical explanations for the observations (23).

EXAMPLE. Schnoll and Zimmerman conducted a randomized study of the effectiveness of incorporating two self-regulatory strategies (goal setting and self-monitoring) into a nutrition education class to enhance dietary fiber consumption. Researchers used path analysis to determine whether the effects of goal setting and self-monitoring on postintervention dietary fiber intake were mediated through the intervening variables knowledge and self-efficacy, as well as to control for preintervention levels of these variables (24).

Meta-analysis

Meta-analysis combines and analyzes the results of previous reports. Such analysis is particularly useful when several small studies but no larger studies of the hypothesis of interest are available and none of the small studies is acceptably large or acceptable with regard to α and β errors. The product has both quantitative and qualitative aspects and allows conclusions to be drawn and new studies to be planned. To ensure quality meta-analysis, great care must be exercised in study design, choice of previous studies to combine, control of bias, statistical analysis, sensitivity analysis, and application of results (25,26).

RESEARCH DATA CONCLUSIONS AND APPLICATION

At that exciting moment when the research data have been collected and analyzed, the researcher is ready to present the data to, and interpret the data for, the scientific and professional community (27). This time is a thoughtful one of introspection, hope, concern, and truthfulness.

When drawing conclusions from research data, the investigator needs to recognize the limitations of the study design and its execution. Among factors to consider are violations of the research protocol, sources of bias, subject selection, sample size, response rate, compliance, subjects lost to follow-up, and missing values. These limitations determine how clearly the research data answer the research question and, of great importance, whether and to what extent the answer can be generalized to populations beyond the study population.

The data can have great practical use when applied to the study population or used to document the investigator's practice, even if extension to other populations is inappropriate. If the integrity of the study was maintained, if the study population was representative of the general population, if the sample size was sufficient, if response rate and compliance were high, if few subjects were lost to follow-up, if few values were missing, and if the differences observed were both statistically significant and of significance in practice, then the results can be applied with confidence to the larger population.

The distinction between statistically significant differences and differences of practical significance is very important. For example, a change in serum cholesterol concentration of 0.05 mmol/L (2 mg/dL) may be highly statistically significant, but for an individual or subgroup of the population, such a change may not be important. It is only from practical differences that meaningful recommendations may be made.

Studies that yield statistically nonsignificant results, or negative studies, may be important to report. A negative study is especially important if it is of sufficient statistical power that a relevant difference could have been detected, suggesting that the true difference may be of impractical magnitude. At the least, negative studies provide valuable suggestions and show errors to avoid in future research.

The only overall conclusions and recommendations drawn from the research data should be those that can be supported by the data. Further research may be needed before more global and more diverse recommendations can be supported, and thus offered.

With the successful completion of the research project, many ideas and questions appear. The researcher at this point will see new avenues of research ahead. It is a time to evaluate thoughtfully the completed research project and consider ways to better execute the next project.. As the completed research project was devised after viewing the original research topic as a composite of its many component parts (see Chapter 1), the opportunities for future research are obvious. The advantage now is that the researcher can use the recent research project as a guide for the next project.

REFERENCES

1. Altman DG, Gore SM, Gardner MJ, Pocock SJ. Statistical guidelines for contributors to medical journals. *Br Med J.* 1983;286:1489–1493.
2. Lang TA, Secic M. *How to Report Statistics in Medicine.* Philadelphia, Pa: American College of Physicians; 1997.
3. Gore SM. Assessing methods—transforming the data. *Br Med J.* 1981;283:548–550.
4. Marascuilo LA, McSweeney M. *Nonparametric and Distribution-free Methods for Social Sciences.* Monterey, Calif: Brooks/Cole; 1977.
5. Jonnalagadda SS, Mitchell DC, Smiciklas-Wright H, et al. Accuracy of energy intake data estimated by a multiple-pass, 24-hour dietary recall technique. *J Am Diet Assoc.* 2000;100:303–311.
6. Humphrey J, Friedman D, Natadisastra G, Muhilal. 24-Hour history is more closely associated with vitamin A status and provides a better estimate of dietary vitamin A intake of deficient Indonesian preschool children than a food frequency method. *J Am Diet Assoc.* 2000;100:1501–1510.
7. Gardner MJ, Altman DG. Confidence intervals rather than *P* values: estimation rather than hypothesis testing. *Br Med J.* 1986;292:746–750.
8. Matthews JN, Altman DG, Campbell MJ, Royston P. Analysis of serial measurements in medical research. *Br Med J.* 1990;300:230–235.
9. Klenbaum DG, Kupper LL. *Applied Regression Analysis and Other Multivariable Methods.* 3rd ed. Montery, Calif: Brooks/Cole; 1997.
10. Ried M, Hall JC. Multiple statistical comparisons in nutritional research. *Am J Clin Nutr.* 1984;40:183–184.
11. Rimm AA, Tukey JW. Some thoughts on clinical trials, especially problems of multiplicity. *Science.* 1977;198:679.
12. Godfrey K. Statistics in practice. Comparing the means of several groups. *N Engl J Med.* 1985;313:1450–1456.
13. Kuczmarski MF, Kuczmarski RJ, Najjar M. Descriptive anthropometric reference data for older Americans. *J Am Diet Assoc.* 2000;100:59–66.
14. Van Beresteyn ECH, van'T Hof MA, van der Heiden-Winkeldermaat HJ, ten Have-Witjes A, Neeter R. Evaluation of the usefulness of the cross-check dietary history method in longitudinal studies. *J Chronic Dis.* 1987;40:1051–1058.
15. Godfrey K. Simple linear regression in medical research. *N Engl J Med.* 1985;313:1629–1636.
16. Everitt B. *Cluster Analysis.* 2nd ed. New York, NY: Halsted Press; 1980.
17. Wirfalt AK, Jeffery RW. Using cluster analysis to examine dietary patterns: nutrient intakes, gender, and weight status differ across food pattern clusters. *J Am Diet Assoc.* 1997;97:272–279.
18. Kristal AR, Shattuck AL, Henry HJ. Patterns of dietary behavior associated with selecting diets low in fat: reliability and validity of a behavioral approach to dietary assessment. *J Am Diet Assoc.* 1990;90:214–220.
19. Kalkwarf HJ, Bell RC, Khoury JC, Gouge AL, Miodovnik M. Dietary fiber intakes and insulin requirements in pregnant women with type I diabetes. *J Am Diet Assoc.* 2001;101:305–310.
20. Kleinbaum DG, Kupper LL, Morgenstern H. *Epidemiologic Research: Principles and Quantitative Methods.* New York, NY: Van Nostrand Reinhold Co; 1982.
21. Hartman TJ, Woodson K, Stolzenberg-Solomon R, et al. Association of the B-vitamins pyridoxal 5'-phosphate (B6), B12, and folate with lung cancer risk in older men. *Am J Epidemiol.* 2001;153:688–694.
22. Matthews DE, Farewell V. *Using and Understanding Medical Statistics.* New York, NY: Karger; 1985.
23. McTavish DG, Loether HJ. *Social Research: Achieved Design.* Boston, Mass: Allyn and Bacon; 1999.
24. Schnoll R, Zimmerman BJ. Self-regulation training enhances dietary self-efficacy and dietary fiber consumption. *J Am Diet Assoc.* 2001;101:1006–1011.
25. Sacks HS, Berrier J, Reitman D, Ancona-Berk VA, Chalmers TC. Meta-analyses of randomized controlled trials. *N Engl J Med.* 1987;316:450–455.
26. Stroup DF, Berlin JA, Morton SC, et al. Meta-analysis of observational studies in epidemiology: a proposal for reporting. Meta-analysis of Observational Studies in Epidemiology (MOOSE) group. *JAMA.* 2000;283:2008–2012.
27. Monsen ER. Communicating ethically and professionally. In: Chernoff R, ed. *Communicating as Professionals.* 2nd ed. Chicago, Ill: The American Dietetic Association; 1994.

Part 2

—ɯ—

The Research Environment

Research opens many doors and windows. Preparing for research is an unusually exciting, creative time—a time of opportunity. During planning, one focuses on the research question and looks forward to the answers and applications. Chapters 4 and 5 are designed to help create a productive environment conducive to research.

Chapter 4, on ethics, considers two interrelated topics: human error and research errors. Human error may be the consequence of inadvertent actions, negligence, or fraud. Professionals circumvent human error through responsible, truthful behavior. Research errors may result from inappropriate sampling, nonresponse, measurement error, or improper representation of oneself, one's research design, or one's data. Through careful research design, conduct, statistical analysis, and presentation, research errors may be prevented. "Data dredging" and fragmentation of reports (for example, into least publishable units, or LPUs) are two easily avoidable problems.

Strategies to minimize research errors are extremely important and are discussed not only in Chapter 4, but throughout the book. For example, sampling strategies are also discussed in Chapters 6, 7, and 13.

The use of human subjects and the need for appropriate consent forms are considered in Chapter 7. Reduction of measurement error is detailed in the various chapters of Parts 3, 4, 6, and 7. Appropriate uses of statistical analyses are described in Chapter 27. Strategies to enhance the presentation of research findings are considered in Chapters 28 through 30. Issues of authorship are incorporated into Chapters 4 and 30.

Chapter 5 guides the reader in writing research proposals and securing funding for research projects. Devising research questions, reviewing the literature, identifying collaborators and advisers, and locating funding sources are discussed. The detailed sections on preparation of the proposal, the timeline, the budget, and the budget justification include pertinent checklists.

First-time investigators and experienced researchers alike may want to read Chapter 5 once for an overview of the topic and again to study the specific points. It is a road map, complete with encouragement and instructions, for commencing and continuing the adventure of research.

ERM, Editor

4

—ᄿᄿ—

Conducting and Presenting Research Ethically

Elaine R. Monsen, Ph.D., R.D.

"Ethics and Science need to shake hands."

—Richard Clarke Cabot, in
The Meaning of Right and Wrong

The concept of ethics encompasses the principles of conduct governing an individual or group, and as such, it pervades all aspects of personal and professional life. The American Dietetic Association has adopted a voluntary, enforceable code of ethics, as have other responsible professional groups. The current version of the code, which became effective in 1999, delineates 19 principles to guide dietetics professionals in their conduct, commitments, and obligations to "self, client, society, and the profession" (1). According to the code of conduct, practitioners act with objectivity and respect for the unique needs and values of individuals; avoid discrimination; maintain confidentiality; base practices on scientific principles and current information; conduct professional affairs with honesty, integrity, and fairness; and remain free of conflicts of interest.

Not all judgments are ethical judgments; many evaluations and decisions are based on considerations of practicality, aesthetics, or professional values. Furthermore, diversity exists within ethical deliberations (2,3). Ethical judgments reflect divergent opinions. Each case can be evaluated on an individual basis; indeed, case analysis is a major pillar of moral reasoning (4). Nonetheless, despite this disparity, people of all cultures and eras are found to agree on which actions are basically constructive—or destructive—to human interaction. Ethical conduct underscores behavior that supports positive relationships between persons and facilitates scientific progress.

At each step of research, ethical issues arise. Designing, conducting, reporting, and interpreting research, as well as planning future research, all involve decisions in which professional ethics are pivotal (5). Whenever human subjects are involved in research, the bioethics of the research must be recognized and carefully considered. The field of bioethics, a major component of professional ethics, includes the ethics of human experimentation (6,7). Issues related to authorship and to conflicts of interest are also critically important in research ethics. These various ethical issues will be addressed in this chapter; the key errors in research design and presentation—and practical strategies—will also be discussed.

RESEARCH ERROR, HUMAN ERROR, AND FRAUD

Scientific errors can seriously deflect scientific progress, whether the errors are consequences of flawed design, improper conduct of research, or unintentional or intentional human error. Repercussions of error are manifold. Time and finances can be lost in pursuing blind alleys, misapplication can be damaging to society, scientific careers can be severely thwarted, and education of future professionals in the field can be flawed. Tainted literature, like an ocean blackened by an oil spill, requires time to be cleansed (8). Poor and inadequate supervision is not acceptable in scientific enterprises. It is critical that researchers assume responsibility and enable investigation if misconduct is charged in any research projects in which they have participated.

Researchers need to, and generally can, circumvent research errors: those of design, execution, analysis, and presentation (9). Research errors may be categorized into six types: sampling errors; noncoverage errors; nonresponse errors; measurement errors; errors of data distortion and overgeneralization; and errors of misrepresentation to human subjects, in authorship, and in conflicts of interest. Quality research demands that research errors be minimized; moreover, allowing such errors may cause major ethical dilemmas in the future. This chapter discusses the six research errors and proposes strategies to avert them.

Human errors are generally more hidden and less readily detectable than research errors. Human errors are an unfortunate—and, it is hoped, infrequent—occurrence in research. Three sources of human error need to be differentiated: inadvertent behavior, negligence, and intentional actions.

Because scientists are fallible, inadvertent errors can occur. An honest mistake is tolerable to the scientific community and the public if it is promptly and properly handled when uncovered. However, preventable mistakes attributable to carelessness or negligence are not tolerable to either science or society; sloppy science is a form of intentional error. It is critical, therefore, for researchers to be vigilant and maintain a strong leadership role throughout the research process.

Fraud, or intentional deception, destroys science by eroding trust and integrity. The scientific method is built upon hypotheses and honest observation; deception is anathema to science. Fraud comes in varying degrees, including concealing data not supportive of a hypothesis and presenting only supportive data ("selective" reporting or "cooking" data), revising observed data to conform to a hypothesis ("trimming" data), and blatantly fabricating data. Each deception is intentional, though the extent of misconduct differs dramatically. Researchers rarely falsify or fabricate data, but when they do it has a calamitous impact that can annihilate laboratories and cripple participating institutions. Plagiarism is a further category of intentional fraud. The real authors and subjects feel its damaging effects keenly, and the perpetrators can face severe criticism from both the scientific community and the public.

ETHICS IN RESEARCH INVOLVING HUMANS

Nuremberg Code and Declaration of Helsinki

Current guidelines and regulations regarding human experimentation have evolved since the middle of the 20th century, in reaction to public and scientific outcry over a few individual cases of gross human injustice. One of the first areas to receive public scrutiny was the heinous behavior of physicians toward the inmates of Nazi concentration camps in Germany during World War II. Following the war, 20 doctors were tried in Nuremberg before an international tribunal for war crimes and crimes against humanity. The resulting Nuremberg Code of 1947 established 10 principles that must be followed in human experimentation to satisfy moral, ethical, and legal concepts (10). These principles, for the first time, established that the informed voluntary consent of human subjects was essential.

The second major international code of ethics was the Declaration of Helsinki adopted by the World Medical Association in 1964, with a proviso that the text be reviewed periodically. The basic principles in the Declaration of Helsinki were extended by the 29th World Medical Assembly in Tokyo in 1975 and further revised in 1983 (11). The 12 basic principles delineated the concept of submitting experimental protocols to an independent committee for consideration, comment, and guidance. This concept was the genesis of the institutional review board, which has become a major force in ensuring the rights of human subjects. The Helsinki Declaration also counseled researchers to exercise caution in conducting research that could affect the environment and to respect the welfare of animals used for research.

Belmont Report

A third important document supporting the rights of human subjects is the 1978 Belmont Report, issued by the National Commission for the Protection of Human Subjects of Biomedical and Behavioral Research (12). This president's commission was formed in 1974 in a rapid response to the disclosure of two scandalous research studies of the 1930s (13). The first study, which concerned the immune response, involved the injection of live, malignant cells into several elderly patients in a chronic disease hospital without the patients' prior consent. The second study concerned long-term observation of the "natural" course of syphilis in men who were recruited into the study without informed consent. The men were observed for several decades but did not receive penicillin, even though its effectiveness in the treatment of syphilis was established several years after the initiation of the study.

Respect for persons, beneficence, and justice are the three basic principles evoked by the Belmont Report. This critically important report addresses the ethical conduct of research involving human subjects and argues for balancing society's interests in protecting the rights of subjects with its interests in furthering knowledge that can benefit society as a whole. The Belmont Report argues that "respect for persons" incorporates at least two basic ethical convictions (or assurances): that individuals be treated as autonomous agents and that individuals in need of protection because of diminished autonomy are entitled to protection. Beneficence is understood to encompass acts of kindness and charity that go beyond strict obligation. Beneficent actions extend from doing no harm to maximizing possible benefits and minimizing possible harms. Justice, the third principle set forth in the Belmont Report, demands that each person be treated fairly. Justice requires that burdens and benefits be shared with equity, and that those who may reap the benefits of the research are also those who should shoulder the risk. Collectively, these ethical convictions serve as the foundation of effective team-based research that benefits human beings.

The reports issued by the National Commission for the Protection of Human Subjects of Biomedical and Behavioral Research established recommendations for the protection of special categories of human subjects, including human fetuses, children, prisoners, and people institutionalized as mentally infirm. To protect the rights of subjects, institutional review boards were empowered through federal regulations.

In all aspects of human experimentation, it is critical that researchers avoid misrepresentation to human subjects. The paramount strategy to avoid this research error relies on the three ethical principles of respect, beneficence, and justice. These principles affirm full and comprehensible disclosure to subjects; noncoercive consent; confidentiality (14); protection of privacy; equity in subject selection; autonomous right of free choice, in-

cluding the right of the subject to terminate participation without penalty; and the termination of the research project at any point if the data warrant such action. For example, if a study is scheduled to end at 7 years, but before then benefits from the treatment protocol become apparent, the research must be terminated so that control subjects or subjects in ineffective treatments may benefit from the effective treatment protocol.

ETHICS IN DESIGNING, CONDUCTING, AND ANALYZING RESEARCH

Confidentiality of medical and personal information is a pillar of scientific ethics. Participants agree, through the informed consent process, to have specific clinical, psychological, or physiological data collected. Researchers must manage the data in a manner that maintains subject anonymity. Once the data have been collected, the "contract" of informed consent is concluded, and further testing or analysis of samples is prohibited. After a specified period of time to allow for final data analysis, samples should be destroyed. Only when additional consent can be, and is, obtained may further analysis be done. Any records involving identity of subjects must be maintained securely, with restricted access.

Whereas using "banked samples" for new analysis may be of scientific interest, there can be no assumption of consent. Moreover, "blanket consent" is not ethical. A participant cannot agree to tests and analyses not in the original consent agreement. For example, some analyses may be developed after the research has been designed and approved; it is conceivable that subsequent analyses not governed by the consent agreement could bring to light medical conditions that could have a major impact on subjects' lives, as in influencing insurance, medical, and employment decisions.

The scientific method is the basis for research design (9). Initially, the existing body of scientific knowledge is carefully assessed. Questions important to science and society are formulated, and in response to the research questions a vigorous and rigorous research design is crafted. Ethical scientific conduct includes accurate recording of data in such a way that they are readily available and understandable to current and future colleagues. To ensure appropriate data accessibility, the data need to be recorded at the time they are generated both correctly and in the detail necessary for ready comprehension. Original data books need to be carefully secured and retained, and they must be made available if request-ed. Subject anonymity must be maintained as well.

Throughout the research process, careful attention needs to be paid to details of subject selection, method choice, and execution (15). If critical details are disre-garded and if sloppy science is allowed, ethical predica-ments may, and indeed usually do, develop.

Dillman (16), who is recognized for his research on survey methodology, outlined four potential research er-rors that invalidate research: sampling error, noncover-age error, nonresponse error, and measurement error. The impact of such errors extends beyond survey design to other descriptive research techniques and to analytic re-search as well. By minimizing and, it is hoped, eliminat-ing these sources of error, research will be substantially more useful.

Sampling Errors

Errors of sampling result from the differences between the study sample and the actual population (15,16). To have a true probability sample, each individual in the study population must have an equal chance of being se-lected as a subject. Sampling errors may be random; that is, they may occur by chance as samples from the same populations are drawn. Ensuring that each individual within the study population has the same likelihood of participating will minimize random sampling errors.

Another key element in minimizing sampling error is ensuring that the sample size is appropriate for the goals of the research (see Chapter 26). Random sampling errors generally decrease as the sample size increases. A rule of thumb is that random sampling error will be re-duced by one-half if the sample size is quadrupled (16).

Noncoverage Errors

Noncoverage errors result from a sampling format that excludes some individuals within the study population in the selection of subjects. Noncoverage errors, in general, are systematic and difficult to overcome (16). They are caused by bias in specifying or selecting the study sample (15). For example, the subjects may be selected from out-dated lists that exclude recent additions; from published telephone listings that exclude people with unlisted num-bers; or from a group of people who are able to attend lectures in the evening, excluding people who work at that time. Bias generally occurs when samples of conve-nience are selected—for example, members of a group,

volunteers responding to advertisements, or people from different health care institutions in whom a specific dis-ease is diagnosed. Such biases affect the degree to which the data generated may represent the population at large. Bias is of concern in both qualitative and quantitative re-search. When bias cannot be eliminated, it is particularly important to recognize it and declare it to the people who are considering the results of the study.

Other examples of sampling bias include the fol-lowing:

- Differences in access to diagnostic procedures be-cause of geographic, time, or economic factors.
- Differences in treatment modalities that are stan-dard for specific localities.
- Differences resulting from the fact that people with specific disorders or exposures gravitate toward certain health care facilities.
- Differences in diagnostic labels or treatment plans for the same condition at different points in space or time. (Secular changes in definitions, exposures, diagnoses, and treatments may make noncontem-poraneous controls noncomparable.)
- Differences in exposure or outcome between "early comers," volunteers, or respondents (who tend to be "healthier") and "late comers," nonvolunteers, or nonrespondents.
- Membership in certain groups (for example, em-ployed, college graduates, or bicyclists), which may imply a degree of health or health awareness that systematically differs from that of the general population.
- Previous history that if not reported and taken into account may bias outcome because of the affect of prior diagnostic or treatment tactics.

Noncoverage error, like any systematic sampling er-ror, distorts results. Because the bias of systematic errors is usually difficult to assess, the findings from the study become clouded. It cannot be assumed that the data col-lected from the flawed sample adequately represent the entire population. Thus, generalizations of the results to either the study population or other populations must be limited by the constraints of the actual subjects sampled.

Nonresponse Errors

The third category of error is that of nonresponse. In sur-veys, the response rate is the percentage of people who actually answer the survey queries (16). A low response rate raises serious questions as to whether the observed data accurately represent the study population—whether the nonresponders differ significantly from the responders. In many studies, researchers strive to improve response rate by devising various strategies to motivate, remind, and cajole subjects to respond.

Unfortunately, researchers may pay little attention to a modest response rate unless there is a marked disparity between projected and actual observations. One way to quiet some of the concern over a low response rate is to evaluate demographic and other available data of both nonresponders and responders to ascertain whether important differences exist between the two groups. A further dilemma results when responders provide incomplete data sets, for example, omitted or partial responses to some questions in a survey. Researchers can decrease inadequate responses to survey questions by evaluating and pilot testing the survey carefully, ensuring clarity of the questions and ease of reply.

A corollary of nonresponse in clinical trials is error resulting from loss of subjects to follow-up. To minimize such loss, researchers make valiant efforts to complete the data sets. For example, to secure 25 years of follow-up data, some researchers have commissioned private detectives to investigate the whereabouts and life or death status of individuals in cohorts. Other sources of nonresponse errors are missing data for either laboratory values or anthropometric measurements, or incomplete food intake records. In each case, the complete and incomplete data sets must be evaluated to ascertain whether the missing data skew the apparent results.

Unless the researcher can be confident that the inclusion of incomplete data does not misguide, the complete and incomplete data sets should be handled separately, rather than as a single, blended group of data.

Measurement Errors

Measurement error is the fourth type of research error. Whereas the first three types of error result from nonobservation, measurement error is an error of observation (16). As such, errors in conducting or executing the research are akin to measurement error. For example, if a question is worded in such a way that it cannot be answered accurately or if a questionnaire is structured so that unequal emphasis is placed on certain questions, measurement error will result. The impact of the placement of questions is influenced by whether the respon-

dent receives the questions verbally or visually. In all cases, it is critical to recognize that biased questions and biased organization produce biased answers. Characteristics of the subjects may also produce measurement error.

Other Sources of Bias Error

Other biases (15) in executing research projects need to be avoided. One frequent error results when the experimental group and control group are treated differently in ways beyond what is designated by the specified intervention, as in giving additional attention or care to the experimental group. When the control group does not receive care and attention equal to what the experimental group receives, differences in outcome may be inaccurately attributed to the intervention. A masked study design in which subjects and researchers are blinded to treatment and control group assignments can help avoid treatment biases. However, it is difficult to maintain the masked design if certain end points (for example, body weight or blood pressure) are monitored during the study as a component of usual patient care.

Another type of research bias occurs when issues of efficacy become confounded with those of compliance, as may occur when the experimental design requires patients to adhere to specified therapies. For example, some subjects may have a low rate of attendance at the education sessions of a program being evaluated. As suggested in the section on nonresponse error, the researcher should compare the complete data sets with the incomplete data sets to determine whether the data can be merged. Similarly, subjects who either withdraw or are withdrawn from an experiment may differ systematically from those subjects who remain, causing withdrawal bias. Furthermore, preconception bias is likely to occur unless the experimental design is masked, or blinded, striving to allow the investigation to proceed and data to be collected without influence or bias from either subject or investigator.

Well-Crafted Design

The well-crafted research design minimizes research errors. All people in the population the investigator wishes to observe have an equal probability of being subjects, avoiding noncoverage error. Individual subjects within that population are randomly selected, and the number selected is sufficiently large to provide the desired precision, minimizing sampling error. Subject sampling criteria are guided by official research policies; for example, *children* are defined by set standards. Every subject selected responds and is not lost to follow-up, avoiding response error. The techniques for estimating response are precise, accurate, reproducible, and equally valid for each subject; each subject complies fully to the assigned regimen, limiting measurement error; and all data are truthfully and fully recorded.

Thoughtful and adequate supervision is essential in all research projects to ensure that the data are properly collected. Each person in a research team must assume responsibility for all aspects of the research in his or her domain and maintain awareness of the project in its entirety. The team involves graduate students, research assistants, intradisciplinary and interdisciplinary professionals, and faculty. Although the chief supervisor must assume ultimate accountability, responsibility for ethical conduct falls on everyone's shoulders.

ETHICAL PRESENTATION AND INTERPRETATION OF RESEARCH

Honesty, truthfulness, and full disclosure are necessary in presenting research. It is the researcher's obligation to publish valid data, to analyze the data objectively and dispassionately, and to present a fair and unbiased interpretation to readers (17,18). Inference must be supportable by the data. Authors must recognize the power of inference and avoid misleading the reader.

As a parallel, readers are obligated to use data ethically, without distortion (19). The Council of Biology Editors contends that equal care must be exercised by researchers and authors as to the message they send and by readers as to the message they receive and use (18).

Presentation of the Whole Truth, and Nothing but the Truth

The ethical investigator truthfully reports and fully discloses research data and the methods whereby the data were generated. Limitations of the study design—for example, subject bias—should be clearly stated. The ethical investigator objectively evaluates the data and provides a fair interpretation. To do more or less is ethically insupportable. At all times, scientific proof must be rigorous and without bias (20).

Several practices in handling data are considered unethical and may be considered errors of data distortion:

data dredging, selective reporting of findings, fragmentation of reports, redundant publication, and inappropriate statistical tests (18). Data dredging is the process of combing through a large pool of data to pick up "significant findings" from research that was not designed to produce those results. Data dredging is particularly noxious when only "positive" results are reported and "negative" results are ignored, thus making the former appear to be important rather than merely significant by chance. Because the accepted level of statistical significance is a probability of .05 or less, the chance that a relationship would be considered significant is 1 in 20. Thus, if the number of comparisons were many, as could occur if data collected from 10 laboratory values and the dietary intake of 10 nutrients were compared, the potential comparisons would undoubtedly yield several "significant relationships" (perhaps 5 out of 100, in the example), most of which would be by chance and would lack relevance.

The relationships that are appropriate to evaluate are those decreed by the original research design, driven by the research question and hypothesis. Chance observations may encourage further research, and if the new research question results in data that replicate the earlier "positive" results, publication of the findings would be justified.

Selective reporting of research findings is a form of intentional fraud, often motivated by efforts to support a hypothesis when the data do not clearly provide adequate support. Such actions as concealing data, presenting solely favorable data, or in any other way shaping or trimming data to accommodate the hypothesis disregards scientific and ethical principles. Such conscious acts are ignoble, premeditated efforts to distort data and mislead colleagues and the public.

Research findings that are fragmented and published in multiple small units are a disservice to readers. The whole picture is not visible, and interrelationships are lost. Scientific editors discourage submission of "least publishable units," commonly called LPUs, and refer to such fragmentation as "salami science." A similar wasteful practice is duplicate or redundant publication—presentation of essentially the same study in more than one place with little, if any, modification.

Statistics in Data Interpretation

Statistics is the art and science of interpreting quantitative data. It includes framing questions that are answerable, designing the study, exercising quality control of the data to reduce both variance and bias, drawing inferences from data, and generalizing results to other situations (15,18,20).

Fienberg (21) suggests that the following eight points be addressed in a statistical review of a submitted manuscript. The points are of equal usefulness in designing, conducting, and reporting research.

1. What are the original data? How have they been transformed for use in the statistical analyses?
2. Is information given on uncertainty and measurement error?
3. How were the statistical analyses done, and are they accurately described in the paper?
4. Are the statistical methods used appropriate for the data?
5. Have the data or analyses been "selected," and does such selection distort the "facts"?
6. What population do the data represent? Does the design for data collection allow for the inferences and generalizations made?
7. Are there additional analyses that would be enlightening?
8. Are the conclusions sensitive to the methodological and substantive assumptions? If so, is this fact acknowledged? Do reported measures of uncertainty reflect this sensitivity?

The core of the scientific method, and hence of science, is inference: learning about unobserved phenomena by studying and interpreting relevant data on observed phenomena. (15,18,20). Inference must be protected, not abused by such distorting actions as selective reporting and data dredging. Data need to be honest and honestly presented.

ETHICS IN PUBLICATION

"All knowledge attains its ethical value and its human significance only by the human sense in which it is employed."

—Hermann Nothnagel

It is an author's responsibility to submit manuscripts that are appropriate for publication consideration and peer review; in other words, the data need to be accurate, responsibly analyzed, and responsibly interpreted. The research design and the materials and methods used need to be clearly and fully presented. All relevant sources need full and accurate citation. As has been discussed, it is unethical and deceptive to present data selectively, to withhold contradictory data, or to revise data for their impact.

Questions often arise as to how much data should be presented in a manuscript. The goal should be to proffer the optimal publishable unit, not to disperse the data in a variety of LPUs. As tenure evaluations are turning toward quality per unit published and away from number of units published, LPUs will be a negative factor in a researcher's list of publications. When a researcher is allowed to offer five original publications for tenure consideration, the advantage will go toward a well-crafted and reasoned article rather than a single fragment of a research project.

Peer review is the prime way that science monitors itself. The scientist accepts the dual professional responsibility of submitting research for peer review and serving as an objective, ethical peer reviewer for the work of others. Reviewers assume the responsibility of ensuring the scientific integrity of published literature, and their confidentiality is necessary to ethical behavior toward an author. Should legitimate conflicts of interest be apparent to peer reviewers, they should decline to review rather than jeopardize a sound review process. It is obviously unethical to take advantage of authors by invading the confidentiality of the peer review process or by using their work before its official publication.

When interpreting and applying data, it is tempting to overpresent them to the media and the public (22). The desire to make a point or to support a bias or preconception must not override accurate use of scientific data. As discussed, research errors resulting from sample bias and noncoverage, nonresponse, and measurement errors determine, in large part, whether the data may be generalized to other populations or even to the entire study population. For example, a research study showing lower serum cholesterol concentrations in men who consumed a diet low in saturated fat cannot be generalized to the population at large (all other men), let alone to infants, children, adolescents, women, or the elderly. The error of overgeneralization is an error of misrepresentation to colleagues and to the public. To overgeneralize erodes the credibility both of the researcher and of science (23). It is particularly disturbing when data are overgeneralized in an effort to perpetrate prejudices or patronage. Honest differences of opinion exist; they should be stated clearly, while recognizing opposing views. However, inappropriately representing one's own data or the data of others is scientifically reprehensible, as it misleads others.

ETHICAL ISSUES RELATED TO AUTHORSHIP

Authorship implies a substantial contribution to a published article and conveys responsibility for the content. Collaboration in research allows input from the vantage of each participant. As such, collaboration can benefit research design, conduct, presentation and dissemination. Also, effective collaboration sets the stage for further joint research endeavors (23).

The Uniform Requirements for Manuscripts Submitted to Biomedical Journals delineates three criteria to determine whether someone has contributed sufficiently to be designated as an author. The criteria, all of which are to be satisfied, are substantial contributions to (1) design or analysis and interpretation of the data, (2) drafting or revising the article critically for important intellectual content, and (3) final approval of the version to be published (24). The error of misrepresentation in authorship can be avoided if the three criteria are used to determine author status.

Authorship cannot be justified for a person whose participation is limited to the acquisition of funding, administration of the department or unit, or the collection of the data. General, as opposed to specific, supervision of the research group is also considered inadequate to warrant authorship. Each section critical to the main conclusions of the article must be the responsibility of one or more of the designated authors. For an article consisting of the contributions of researchers from diverse fields, only the key people responsible for the article should be specified as authors; other contributors should be recognized and thanked in an acknowledgment. Gratuitous or honorary authorship is neither appropriate nor ethically acceptable. Authorship is not a gift, but a right founded on substantial contribution to the resulting manuscript.

An author must make major contributions to the genesis and presentation of the research data. In addition, an author is not only responsible for the published data but also must be prepared to defend the data and the interpretation of the data. Discussion continues on how extensive an individual's contribution must be to qualify as an author, and how accountable to both peers and the public an author must be for the paper in its entirety. One of the obvious dilemmas is the extent of accountability an author assumes when collaborating with scientists and professionals in diverse fields. At minimum, individual authors are responsible for all aspects of work that are within and proximate to their fields of expertise.

The primary or lead author has a special position that is determined from having made the major intellectual input to the article. The primary author also should have made outstanding, positive, and creative contributions; provided the major intellectual input; participated actively in the work, data tabulation, and interpretation; and provided key scientific leadership throughout the research design, conduct, analysis, and presentation (18).

CONFLICTS OF INTEREST

Conflicts of interest occur in any situation in which financial or other personal considerations may compromise, or appear to compromise, an investigator's professional actions in designing, conducting, or reporting research. Conflicts of interest may also bias other aspects of an investigator's research activities, such as the choice of methods, length of time subjects are studied, purchase of materials, hiring of support staff, or choice of statistical analyses. Other scholarly activities are affected by conflicts of interest; for example, in the preparation of review articles, financial and personal interests may interfere with professional objectivity.

It is customary for investigators to disclose any and all possible conflicts. Professional journals expect acknowledgment of each author's funding sources and institutional and corporate affiliations on the title page of articles submitted for publication. In addition, consultancies, stock ownership, or other equity interests or patent licensing should be disclosed to the journal editor in a cover letter at the time articles are submitted (18,25). The error of misrepresentation of conflicts of interests is averted when such interests are disclosed to the readers of any related publication. It is important for full disclosure to be made, because the appearance of conflict may be as professionally damaging as known conflict (26). Many reputable scientists have one or several actual or perceived conflicts of interest. Their disclosure provides a platform for unbiased, open evaluation.

Fear of conflicts of interest should not deter an investigator from seeking ethical financial and corporate relations. Problems develop when financial interests are not disclosed. It is ethically irresponsible for a scientist, because of a personal conflict of interest and thus a potentially desirable or undesirable financial impact, to repress negative data, to expose only selected findings, or to distort the presentation of data in any way. Financial interest should neither impinge upon professional objectivity nor drive professional activities.

RESEARCH IN AN ETHICAL CLIMATE

Discovering the unknown, expanding horizons, updating perceptions and techniques, and devising and evaluating new applications all make research exciting. The investigator's profession and society are advanced concurrently. Ethical scientific conduct of research ensures the acceptance of new data and the positive assessment of the data's interpretation.

Throughout the many steps of research (5), highly ethical behavior is imperative. In selecting important questions and designing effective research protocols in which research errors are minimized, it is essential to keep in mind that the execution and presentation of the research must be accomplished in an ethical fashion. The three principles of respect for persons, beneficence, and justice are excellent guides, not only when considering human subjects but also when interacting with close colleagues, professional peers, clients, the public, and the media. Conflicts of interest require full disclosure to avoid misleading others. In such an ethical climate, research accomplishments will grow and survive. As Sir Peter Brian Medawar states in *The Art of the Soluble,* "The scientist values research by the size of its contribution to that huge, logically articulated structure of ideas which is already, though not yet half built, the most glorious accomplishment of mankind" (27).

REFERENCES

1. American Dietetic Association. Code of Ethics for the profession of dietetics. *J Am Diet Assoc.* 1999;99: 103–113.
2. Fieber LK. Practice points: ethical considerations in dietetics practice. *J Am Diet Assoc.* 2000;l00:454.
3. Dalton S. What are the sources and standards of ethical judgment in dietetics? *J Am Diet Assoc.* 1991;91:545–546.
4. Jonsen AR, Toulmin S. *The Abuse of Casuistry: A History of Moral Reasoning.* Berkeley, Calif: University of California Press; 1988.
5. Monsen ER, Vanderpool HY, Halsted CH, McNutt KW, Sandstead HH. Ethics: responsible scientific conduct. *Am J Clin Nutr.* 1991;54:l–6.
6. Emanuel EJ, Wendler D, Grady C. What makes clinical research ethical? *JAMA.* 2000;283:2701–2711.
7. Silverman WA. *Human Experimentation: A Guided Step Into the Unknown.* Oxford, England: Oxford Medical Publications; 1986.
8. Garfield E, Welljams-Dorf A. The impact of fraudulent research on the scientific literature. The Stephen E. Breuning case. *JAMA.* 1990;263:1424–1426.
9. Committee on the Conduct of Science, National Academy of Sciences. *On Being a Scientist.* Washington, DC: National Academy Press; 1995.
10. *Trials of War Criminals Before the Nuremberg Military Tribunal Under Control Council Law No. 10.* Vol 2. Washington, DC: US Government Printing Office; 1949.
11. 18th World Medical Assembly. The Helsinki Declaration of 1964. In: Reich WT, ed. *Encyclopedia of Bioethics.* Vol 4. New York, NY: Free Press; 1978:1770–1771.
12. National Commission for the Protection of Human Subjects of Biomedical and Behavioral Research. *The Belmont Report: Ethical Principles and Guidelines for the Protection of Human Subjects of Research.* Washington, DC: US Government Printing Office; 1978. DHEW Publication No. (OS) 78-0012; Appendix I, DHEW Publication No. (OS) 78-0013; Appendix II; DHEW Publication (OS) 78-0014.
13. Levine RI. *Ethics and Regulation of Clinical Research.* 2nd ed. New Haven, Conn: Yale University Press; 1988.
14. Botkin JR. Protecting the privacy of family members in survey and pedigree research. *JAMA.* 2001;258:207–211.
15. Riegelman RK. *Studying a Study and Testing a Test.* 4th ed. Philadelphia, Pa: Lippincott Williams & Wilkins; 2000.
16. Dillman DA. *Mail and Internet Surveys: The Tailored Design Method.* 2nd ed. New York, NY: John Wiley and Sons; 1999.
17. Block BH. Ethical and legal issues in medical writing. *J Am Podiatr Med Assoc.* 1998;88:45–46.
18. Council of Biology Editors. *Ethics and Policy in Scientific Publication.* Bethesda, Md: Council of Biology Editors, Inc; 1990.
19. Kagarise MJ, Sheldon GF. Translational ethics: a perspective for the new millennium. *Arch Surg.* 2000;135:39–45.
20. Huth EJ. *Writing and Publishing in Medicine.* 3rd ed. Baltimore, Md: Williams & Wilkins; 1999.
21. Fienberg SE. Statistical reporting in scientific journals. In: *Ethics and Policy in Scientific Publications.* Bethesda, Md: Council of Biology Editors, Inc; 1990.
22. Fahmy S. *Research Integrity and the Media. CBE Views.* Vol 22. Bethesda, Md: Council of Biology Editors, Inc; 1999:151.
23. Gardner JK, Rall, LC, Peterson, CA. Lack of multidisciplinary collaboration is a barrier to outcomes research. *J Am Diet Assoc.* 2002;122:65–71.

24. International Committee of Medical Journal Editors. Uniform requirements for manuscripts submitted to biomedical journals. *Ann Intern Med.* 1988;108:258–265.

25. Krinsky S, Rothenberg LS. Financial interest and its disclosure in scientific publications. *JAMA.* 1998;280: 225–226.

26. Inbody T. *Conflicts of Interest in Relation to Articles. CBE Views.* Vol 22. Bethesda, Md: Council of Biology Editors, Inc; 1999:188.

27. Medawar PB. *The Art of the Soluble.* London, England: Metheun; 1967.

5

How to Write Proposals and Obtain Funding

M. Rosita Schiller, Ph.D., R.D., F.A.D.A., and Jean C. Burge, Ph.D., R.D.

The proposal-writing skills of researchers at all levels of professional development can be enhanced. Early success at obtaining approval for research studies often triggers a lifelong pattern of grant activity characterized by increasingly larger or more prestigious awards, publications in highly reputed journals, and invitations to evaluate others' research.

This chapter offers guidelines for developing proposals that will ultimately receive both approval and funding. The information can be used in a variety of ways. Investigators new to the research arena can carefully follow each point to ensure optimal results. Researchers who have unfunded proposals can use the chapter as an evaluation checklist to identify weaknesses and pitfalls. Project leaders can offer the information as a guide to new researchers, who can use it to gain valuable experience. For researchers who need a refresher course, this chapter may offer new insights for better preparation of proposals. Proposal writers who seek renewed motivation may find new ideas on how to prepare a high-quality proposal that deserves full funding.

THE RESEARCH PROPOSAL

Proposal development is ordinarily divided into three distinct phases: preparation, writing, and review. It takes about 6 months to develop a good proposal from start to finish.

Proposal Preparation

The preparation of a proposal begins with the simple desire to conduct research—to contribute to the development of new knowledge. The preparation phase may require at least 3 weeks to 4 weeks, depending on time spent at the library and proposal-related meetings.

Identifying the Problem Area

The first challenge in preparing a research proposal is the generation of an idea that is clearly focused and merits investigation. Saunderlin (1) and Weekes (2) noted several stimuli that can fuel the thinking process and lead to viable research topics: personal interest and experience, clinical problems encountered, completed research of others, a sudden insight, and a practical need. Dietetics professionals might also generate research ideas by mulling over four key forces for research enumerated by Monsen (3):

1. Unexpected observations (something atypical that happens in the practice setting).
2. Potential for building on what is already known or expanding prior observations.
3. Shifts in thinking or application of present knowledge to emergent realities.
4. Response to public concerns, cultural and ethnic interests, or sociopolitical issues.

Key research areas have been identified by several authors. Suggested topics for exploration include clinical

49

practice (4), public policy (5), foodservice (6), women's health (7), food and nutrition science (8), outcomes measurement (9), aging (10), and nutrition care (11).

Successful researchers hone in on one area of study. All their work contributes in some way to further understanding the specified area. They follow the advice of Kahn (12), who encourages researchers to "focus, focus, focus." A defined focus has several advantages. It simplifies becoming familiar with current literature and staying abreast of new developments. It helps establish the researcher as an authority on the subject. A history of successful research projects along the same theme lends credibility to a new study and verifies the importance of the work. Once an area of study is defined, one investigation easily leads to another. Findings often suggest further unanswered questions and the need to pursue new paths of inquiry.

Surveying the Literature

After a problem area has been identified, an initial review of literature from the past 4 or 5 years is needed to explore recent work on the topic. Numerous databases are available from which nutrition professionals can retrieve information (13). Reading both review articles and original reports steeps the researcher in the subject, determines whether a germinating question has been tested previously, and identifies experts in the area. Such study also enables the researcher to conceptualize the theoretical framework, formulate research objectives, and delineate hypotheses (14).

The initial survey of literature may be cursory. In time it will become part of an extensive literature review required for the written proposal, a topic that will be addressed later in this chapter.

Identifying Potential Collaborators

It is possible, but difficult, to conduct research in total isolation. Dietitians can find others with similar research interests to share the process, stimulate new ideas, challenge poorly conceived research designs, or serve as research mentors. The best research teams are made up of people with differing backgrounds and expertise. Practitioners often benefit from collaborating with university faculty members, who generally have more extensive research experience and better access to various resources. Alternatively, faculty members gain the advantage of expanded research opportunities in practice settings. Interdisciplinary medical or health care research teams often

welcome the nutrition expertise of dietitians. Membership on a multidisciplinary team generally enhances research productivity, stimulates development of research protocols, and encourages ongoing involvement in focused research studies.

Collaboration offers many other benefits (15). Working together spreads the responsibilities and speeds implementation of the project. Representation from various backgrounds, such as biostatistics, epidemiology, pharmacology, nursing, or medicine, may be required to answer the research question satisfactorily. Some funding agencies give priority to interdisciplinary studies because of the complex nature of investigations involving human subjects and health care delivery systems. Collaboration with an established researcher enhances funding potential, because grant awards are usually given to researchers with a strong track record. Most funding agencies require affiliation with a university or institutional research institute, a characteristic frequently achieved when researchers join forces.

Collaboration also has drawbacks; however, by addressing these adverse effects up front, they can be minimized (16). For example, a system for frequent interaction with team members is imperative; loss of contact usually results in the termination or significant delay of the project. Commitment to the research is essential; collaborators who are lack it may disrupt momentum, impede progress, and cause missed deadlines. Divergent thinkers who lack commitment to the research question may introduce new ideas or force compromises that are not fully acceptable to other team members. Collaborators must decide early who will serve as principal investigator and whose name will appear first on any publications. In addition, they must determine how the work will be divided and make sure everyone accepts accountability for designated assignments.

Defining Limits

After the problem area has been identified, the literature surveyed, and the research collaborators identified, these collaborators are ready to formulate the research question, decide on the magnitude of the study, and determine its feasibility. A key here is to dream big but start small (17). Pursue just one line of investigation rather than attempting to tackle simultaneously all dimensions of a multifaceted problem. The question should be as precise as possible, focusing on a single issue or group of research subjects. The examples in Table 5.1 illustrate research questions that are too broad or too poorly defined

TABLE 5.1 Sample Research Questions

Too General or Poorly Designed	Specific
Does malnutrition increase the cost of medical care?	Is malnutrition associated with increased length of hospitalization for patients admitted for elective hip and knee joint replacement?
Is there a positive relationship between blood sugar levels and dietary fiber?	Can blood glucose levels of tube-fed, nonstressed elderly patients with insulin-dependent diabetes mellitus be maintained within the normal range by the use of a fiber-containing enteral formula?
Are Recognized Young Dietitians characterized by a unique personality profile?	Is there a unique personality profile, as assessed by the Myers-Briggs personality inventory, differentiating Recognized Young Dietitians and Dietetic Technicians from other young practitioners in the field?
Does conversion from a 3-week cycle menu to a 1-week cycle menu save money?	Can total meal costs be reduced by more than $1 per patient per day by converting from a 3-week selective cycle menu to a 1-week selective cycle menu, keeping raw food costs within the present range?

and corresponding questions that are appropriately specific or clearly defined.

Time limits for the study also need to be established. Shorter studies help keep new researchers motivated and energized (18). Most proposals are funded for 1 year to 3 years. Investigators who have successfully managed a small research grant often receive long-term funding for subsequent studies that may extend to 5 years or longer. Formulate the research question to fit a realistic time frame. Graduate students and novice researchers usually select questions that can be answered in 1 or 2 years. Established investigators often frame complex questions that require longer for completion. Availability of research subjects also influences the length of a proposed study. Sufficient numbers of subjects and accessibility to the required data need to fit within the planned time frame. It may be necessary to reformulate a research question or sharpen the focus to accommodate a feasible sample population.

Developing an Advocate/Advisory Committee

It is helpful to develop a group of people who can assist in obtaining research funding. For graduate students, this group will include a research adviser and a thesis or dissertation committee. Others may find it helpful to identify a research mentor. Advisers or mentors can provide needed skills in writing and reviewing the research proposal. They may have access to needed resources, such as laboratory space or equipment. They may be able to provide introductions to individuals in federal or state agencies and foundations. Finally, they may be able to provide expertise in grant writing, a valuable attribute in the search for funding. It is also important to gain administrative support early in the planning process to ensure the success of a research proposal (19).

Choosing a Potential Funding Agency

Often a grant proposal is written in response to a specific request for proposals (RFP) or request for applications (RFA). In other cases, seeking out a potential funding agency is part of the grant preparation phase. It is important to identify potential funding agencies before actually writing a proposal (14). Early selection facilitates the process in several ways. Appropriate application forms and proposal guidelines can be obtained and followed right from the start. Submission deadlines are preset, enabling the group to pace its work. Eligibility can be determined and compliance with requirements confirmed in the application. The proposal can be tailored to fit funding limitations and agency priorities. Sources and techniques for identifying feasible funding sources are considered later in this chapter.

Contacting Potential Funding Agencies

Rather than immediately developing a full-blown proposal for submission to a granting agency, it is a good idea to contact potential grantors first to determine their interest in the topic. This contact can be made in one of three ways:

1. Call program staff at agencies and foundations to discuss the research idea with them. Make sure the proposal would be welcome. Heed any advice given regarding points to include in the proposal (17).
2. Submit a one- or two-page concept paper. The concept paper should include a succinct summary of the research idea, including the problem statement, specific aims, research methods, and significance of the study. Include a budget estimate, and ask if the agency might look favorably on such a proposal.

3. Write a letter of inquiry to the target agency, briefly outlining the research idea, giving cost estimates, and asking the likelihood of grant support for the project.

Some proposals receive funding on their merits alone; others are funded because the applicant has made personal contacts. Networking both inside and outside the funding agency is one way to gain recognition, to improve the proposal, and to ensure a match between the proposed project and the sponsor's expectations and priorities (20). Key contact names and telephone numbers are available on-line for nutrition-related research projects (21).

Contacts can help both to garner and to document support for a proposal. Influential contacts can introduce researchers to key people who may know someone at the targeted funding agency. Mentioning the person's name at the funding agency can facilitate scheduling a meeting or getting attention by telephone. Letters included in the proposal appendix from key supporters both inside and outside the institution lend credibility to a proposal. These letters may reflect support from such individuals as the medical director of a clinical research center, a statistician or director of a research consulting center, a department whose cooperation will be needed to conduct the study, a major administrator whose unit may benefit from the project, or a publisher interested in publishing results of the study.

Before writing a proposal, a personal conversation with a designated project officer or staff member in charge of receiving proposals is in order. Their names may be obtained from the RFP/RFA, agency annual reports, or foundation offices. The telephone call (or meeting) can provide clues regarding staff attitudes and evaluative criteria that may be used. The discussion can cover such things as preliminary research ideas, application forms, submission dates, budget targets and guidelines, the number of proposals anticipated, how much money has been appropriated, types of projects targeted to receive funding, or subtle characteristics desired in winning proposals (20).

A researcher can establish, maintain, and expand relationships at granting agencies in a variety of ways. Such networking is a lifelong process and may include meetings at the grantor's office, appointments to review panels, internships with granting agencies, attendance at meetings where grantors will be speaking, arranging for grantors to speak at the researcher's institution, and invitations to conduct site visits of the researcher's major research projects (22).

Writing the Proposal

Proposal writing is an act of persuasive communication (14,23). Proposals must present a clear, accurate, and complete picture of the activity to be funded. Kennicott (24) notes that the proposal must convince reviewers that the proposed activity has the following characteristics:

- The proposed activity is appropriate for support by the funding agency.
- The proposed activity is both worthwhile and highly desirable in light of funding alternatives.
- The proposed activity is both methodologically sound and likely to succeed.
- The proposed activity is in the hands of a well-qualified principal investigator who will complete the project if it is funded.

To ensure achievement of these aims, the grant preparation tips outlined in Figure 5.1 should be carefully followed. Although each funding agency has its own unique guidelines, general suggestions for developing proposals and conducting research are offered in a number of resources listed in the Further Reading at the end of this chapter.

Proposal Writing Tips

In the first draft, use the following writing and formatting techniques often employed by experienced grant writers (20,25):

- Use short, simple sentences, and write in the active voice.
- Use bold type to grab attention in headlines and key words.
- Expect to edit the proposal several times—to rearrange, rewrite, and reformat until the manuscript is both logical and pleasing to look at. Be sure to spell check and proofread the document carefully.
- Use headlines and subsections to shepherd reviewers through the proposal. Make it easy for them to determine if the proposal meets funding criteria.
- Use lists, figures, and tables to convey ideas succinctly and to break up pages of print.
- Use left-margin justification, and leave right margins ragged. This format facilitates reading the manuscript.
- Use transitions in writing to make a clear connection between ideas and sentences. Transitions may take one of four forms, each with an appropriate

- Grant writing is not a solo activity; seek consultation and collaboration from others.
- Follow the directions in detail, including margins, page limits, and the use of references or appendexes.
- Have the proposal reviewed by peers before submitting it for funding.
- Plan ahead, and develop a time frame for completing the grant proposal. Avoid the last-minute rush that will compromise the quality of the proposal.
- State ideas clearly and succinctly. Give attention to spelling and grammar.
- Use appendexes to include study instruments, procedures, or other supporting materials.
- Use letter-quality printing and a good-quality photocopier. Make sure to include the requested number of copies.
- Include support letters from individuals who are important to the success of the study. These individuals include medical staff, nursing administrators, consultants, and coinvestigators.

FIGURE 5.1 Grant preparation tips. Adapted from Ferrell BR, Nail LM, Mooney K, and Cotanch P. Applying for Oncology Nursing Society and Oncology Nursing Foundation Grants. *Oncology Nursing Forum*. 1989;16:728–730. Adapted with permission from the Oncology Nursing Press.

transitional word: (1) additions *(furthermore, next, likewise, moreover)*, (2) examples *(for instance, indeed, in fact, to illustrate)*, (3) results *(therefore, accordingly, as a result)*, and (4) summary *(hence, in brief, to conclude)*.
- Use the type style and type size indicated in the proposal guidelines. If the type style is not indicated, it is best to use a serif typeface, such as New Times Roman or Courier, in the text of the proposal.
- Use white space liberally. It helps segment ideas and make long copy more pleasing to the eye.

Cover Letter

As a matter of courtesy, a proposal should include a cover letter addressed to the grants coordinator, foundation president, or other appropriate individual. This letter should be brief and friendly, noting the attachment of a proposal and a designated number of copies. It also should specify whether the proposal is in response to an RFP/RFA, a follow-up to an approved concept paper or letter of inquiry, an unsolicited initiative previously discussed with individuals at the granting agency, or a brand-new idea in pursuit of funding.

Title Page

The title page should feature a project title that is descriptive and within limits set by the funding agency. It should relate directly to the proposal topic. Key words in the title provide an introduction to the study, and they often determine where the proposal will be sent for review. Avoid cute, magazine-type titles, because they tend to convey flamboyancy rather than serious research.

Most grant applications provide the format for a title page, and it should be used as is, with the information inserted as requested. Many agencies provide application forms on-line, and these forms can be completed electronically. Also, a scanner may be used so that the completed form will be identical to the one provided by the funding agency. Deviating from standard formats requires greater concentration from reviewers, and the inconvenience might tarnish perceptions toward an otherwise laudable research study.

Abstract or Summary

The abstract or summary is written last. It offers a concise but complete overview of the entire project, including the problem statement, research objectives, research design, methodologies, timetable, and requested budget. The abstract is generally limited to one page or the space designated in the application.

Depending on the review process, a majority of review panel members may read only the title, abstract, and significance of a proposal; they will depend on designated in-depth reviewers for accurate assessments of the strengths and weaknesses of the study (26). This fact accentuates the importance of drafting a descriptive title and a concise—but complete—abstract.

Problem Statement

The problem statement establishes the framework for the research question. The main purpose is to justify the proposed activity and show the apparent need for conducting the study (20). Contents may include a brief review of pertinent current literature, gaps in present knowledge of the subject, results of pilot studies, or needs assessments describing the target population. The problem statement should show how the proposed study relates to what is known and how it will advance both knowledge and practice. The problem statement also should delineate how this research will support the mission or values of the proposed funding agency. Examples of a written problem statement and other sections of a research proposal can be obtained from completed theses, dissertations, and some textbooks.

Specific Aims

This section on specific aims addresses the question, What will be accomplished? Aims should be stated as clearly and succinctly as possible. Aims, goals, objectives, hypotheses, and study questions should be obviously coherent, a goal often achieved through the use of an outline format.

The writer should move from the general to the specific, clearly describing expected outcomes. Overall aims and specific objectives need to be both reasonable and attainable; they should logically point toward research hypotheses, experiments, or study questions (27). Hypotheses should be stated for experimental studies in which relationships between variables are to be determined. A list of proposed experiments may be given under specific aims to illustrate how the desired outcomes will be achieved. Study questions or objectives, rather than hypotheses, are best used for descriptive or exploratory studies (20).

Significance

In this section on significance, the researcher builds a foundation to support the specific aims previously stated. A thorough but concise review of pertinent literature is essential to show the researcher's familiarity with the field, the relationship of the present study to the research area, and the importance of the proposed work in extending the current knowledge base. Mackenzie (25) suggests beginning this section with the words, "The proposed research is important because. . . ." This wording helps the researcher highlight immediately salient points that may otherwise get buried in the narrative. References relating to previous research in the area by the investigator or other team members will reinforce the expertise of the researcher.

Review of the Literature

A maximum of eight pages may be devoted to the section on review of the literature in applications for funding from the National Institutes of Health (NIH). This specification connotes the importance given to previous research or pilot studies related to the problem area. Results

of completed work can be used to report progress of previously funded projects; convey the likelihood that a project will be carried to completion; substantiate that the investigator is familiar with the techniques to be used and that he or she has the skill and qualifications to complete the proposed work; illustrate that the current study is a logical extension of earlier work; and estimate variability, experimental effect, and sample size needed for statistically significant results in the proposed study.

Various techniques can facilitate reviewer comprehension of preliminary work. For example, tables, graphs, and exhibits can present results of previous studies (27). The section can start with an outline if several studies are to be summarized. References for published reports can be cited.

Experimental Design and Methodology

The section on experimental design and methodology is the most critical section of the proposal. Reviewers give more weight to it than to any other section when evaluating the proposal and calculating the total score for priority ratings. Niederhuber (27) cautions that at least two-thirds of the time and effort of writing a proposal should be devoted to the section on research design and methodology.

This section should parallel specific aims and contain information regarding the experimental design, subjects, measurement of variables, methodology, and statistical analysis. It should begin with a declarative statement regarding the basic research method, followed by a diagram showing the flow of planned investigations (28). Subheadings may be used to highlight major components of the research design.

Research Design.　In the first sentence of the section on research design, state the name of the proposed research design, such as a double-blind, crossover, experimental study. If appropriate, a diagram may be used to illustrate the research model. Diagrams are especially helpful for experimental studies or proposals that contain a series of steps. Figure 5.2 illustrates the experimental protocol for a 49-day crossover study of colonic adaptation to fructooligosaccharides. The figure shows what happens on specific days of the study, including feedings, washout periods, and specimen collections.

Subjects.　The discussion of experimental design and methodology includes the type and number of subjects to be used, as well as their availability and accessibility to the investigator. It should also describe the research set-

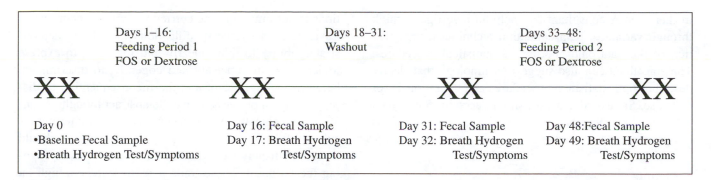

FIGURE 5.2   A research design: experimental protocol for a 49-day crossover study of colonic adaptation to fructooligosaccharides (FOS). Courtesy of Steven Hertzler, Ph.D., R.D., Assistant Professor, Medical Dietetics Division, The Ohio State University, Columbus, Ohio. Used by permission.

ting, subject selection criteria, how subjects will be assigned to a random or control group, an estimate of available subjects, and the sample size calculations (see Chapter 26). The number of subjects must be sufficient to achieve desired confidence levels and statistical power, as well as anticipated variance in the data. The number of subjects must be large enough to allow potential attrition; if possible, an estimate of attrition should be stated.

When a study requires the use of human subjects, prior approval of an institutional review board (IRB) or human research advisory committee is required. This review process may require 1 or 2 months. Many funding agencies stipulate that the approval number or a copy of the IRB review form be included in the proposal. The purpose of an IRB is to ensure compliance with the ethical principles for conducting research. All potential risks must be identified, even if the risk may seem remote. All materials that will be used for recruitment and any information that will be provided to the subjects must accompany the application for approval. The IRB considers the following (29):

- Methods of subject selection.
- Identification and minimization of risks (physical, emotional, and financial).
- Balance of risks and benefits.
- Informed consent procedures.
- Qualifications of investigators.
- Plans to terminate the study if it becomes apparent that subjects are being deprived of beneficial treatments or are being exposed to harm.
- Protection of subjects' privacy.
- Exclusion or steps to safeguard vulnerable groups, such as children, pregnant women, prisoners, and people with limited mental capacity.

Measurement of Variables.   The proposal should describe each variable and how it will be measured, as well as illustrate how each variable is linked to specific aims of the study. It is important to justify the use of measurement tools or techniques, outlining their previous use, standardization, and selection criteria over other available instruments or techniques. This section also should cover any measures used to ensure validity and reliability of the data. Copies of data collection instruments should be included in the appendixes.

Methodology or Procedures.   Having described what instruments or methods will be used and who will participate, the writer's next step is to explain all procedures in a step-by-step fashion, telling how data will be collected. Again, exhibits may be used to illustrate work flow, complex interventions, or the sequential use of various techniques.

The following questions illustrate the wide range of information needed for this section of the proposal:

- Will research assistants be employed to collect data?
- Who will train research assistants?
- What steps will be taken to enroll subjects, and when will consent be obtained?
- When and where will data be obtained?
- How will the data be recorded?
- How will confidentiality be maintained?
- In what sequence will activities occur?
- What statistical tests will be used, and why?

Statistical Analysis.   The use of a statistical consultant lends credibility to most research studies. A consultant is essential unless the researcher has documented expertise in this area. A consultant can help an investigator think through variables, data collection techniques, organization of the data, and appropriate statistical procedures. The consultant can also suggest terminology that clearly describes both statistical procedures and the rationale for their use. Statistical analyses should account for all data collected, and they should answer the research questions or hypotheses (see Chapter 27).

Timetable

Most proposal outlines require a timetable for completion of the work. If a timetable is not required as a separate section, it should be included in a description of procedures. Reviewers want to know how long various parts of the study will take. The timetable should specify such things as preparations needed, recruitment of subjects, training of research personnel, data collection, data analysis, preparation and presentation of reports and potential publications resulting from these studies. The timetable should include provisions for items included in specific aims and anticipated outcomes of the research. If not all the work can be completed within the funded time frame, the timetable should explain what provisions have been made for completing unfinished work.

Budget

Researchers who have not established a track record should keep their request for money in a conservative range. Frequently, internal funding can be obtained for a pilot study, which can serve the purpose of preparing a draft proposal, developing and testing procedures, providing preliminary data, and enhancing the qualifications of the researcher.

Consultants from a research office can provide invaluable assistance in preparing the budget. An extensive discussion on estimating costs and preparing a budget is provided in this chapter's discussion of budgets and budget justification.

Biographical Sketches

For NIH proposals, biographical sketches are standardized, and forms need only be filled in. For other agencies, biographical sketches are often limited to two pages. The reviewers will judge from the data provided whether they think the personnel can perform the proposed research. Therefore, a proposal should provide convincing information to help sway the judges. Evidence of qualifica-

tions is not limited to the curriculum vitae. According to Eaves (30), desirable qualifications include a "demonstrated ability to think clearly and logically, to express logical thought concisely and cogently, to discriminate between the significant and the inconsequential, to display technical prowess, to handle abstract thought, to analyze data objectively and accurately, and to interpret results confidently and conservatively." Researchers should be sure to display these desirable characteristics throughout the proposal. These traits place researchers high on the list for potential funding.

Other Support

Funding agencies want to know if and how much support is available from other sources and if a proposal for similar research has been submitted to another agency. They want to know what will happen if both proposals are funded. Also, if the percentage of time designated for multiple studies exceeds 100 percent of the investigator's time, an explicit plan must be provided showing how requirements for each study will be met.

Resources and Environment

Reviewers will not ordinarily be familiar with any specific work environment. Therefore, most proposals are strengthened by a description of the hospital, laboratory, community setting, or other factors that contribute to a supportive research environment. A proposal should give pertinent details, such as the availability of specific equipment needed to carry out the proposed study, access to important information, and institutional philosophy regarding research in relation to service requirements.

Appendixes

The appendixes may include data that support the proposal but that are too lengthy, detailed, or technical to be placed in the body of the proposal, for example, an letters of support and endorsements, related papers published by the researcher, curricula vitae, data collection forms, IRB approval, descriptive materials such as brochures and flyers, and pictures of unusual equipment or devices to be used in the study.

Appended material might not be copied for all reviewers (26). Therefore, any material crucial to understanding the proposed research should be placed in the main body of the proposal.

Internal Proposal Review

It is a mistake to hurry through writing a proposal and to send it to a funding agency immediately. Instead, two or three seasoned colleagues should be asked to read and evaluate it. Brakey (31) suggests including internal reviewers from other disciplines, because many panels are multidisciplinary. Internal reviewers can point out gaps or weaknesses in a plan, and they can give suggestions regarding organization and clarity of materials presented. Time should be provided during the development phase for peer assessment and completion of suggested revisions.

Before the application is submitted, be sure that a clear and documented relationship exists between the proposed research and stated priorities of the funding agency. Also, the proposal should state what will be done with the findings; for example, data may be used to generate new hypotheses for further study, develop a new treatment program, advance practice in the field, or extend development of an important database.

Make sure other guidelines have been followed. For example, if the proposal is written to support a graduate student thesis or dissertation, some institutions require that the faculty adviser be listed as the principal investigator, with the student serving as a coinvestigator.

As noted earlier, research involving humans or animals requires approval of an institutional ethics review committee. Sufficient lead time must be allotted for this review. The application should include an assurance of compliance with the ethical guidelines of both the funding agency and the institution.

Most funding agencies require the approval (in the form of signatures) of one or more institutional representatives, usually major administrators and a grants officer. These authorizations ensure tacit approval for the project, release time to conduct the work, employment of designated personnel if funding is received, and fiduciary responsibility for the use of any grant support. Again, the researcher must plan ahead for unforeseen circumstances, such as vacations and business trips, to be sure the needed signatures can be obtained prior to submission deadlines.

BUDGETS AND BUDGET JUSTIFICATION

The main purpose of writing a proposal is to obtain funding. Therefore, the budget is a critical segment of the proposal and should be given appropriate attention. Each agency has its own rules for what will be covered, various line-item categories, and dates for the fiscal year. These specific guidelines must be followed, and if the application materials include a form, it must be used. If no forms are provided, the funding agency should be contacted for guidelines (20). Involvement of grants officers early in the budgeting process can save valuable time and facilitate the budgeting process.

The budget should provide a detailed, precise estimate of anticipated expenses. A "padded" bottom line gives the impression of dishonesty; an inadequate budget conveys naiveté or incompetence (26). Poor budgeting can adversely affect a research study and may negatively bias future prospects for new grants. If a realistic budget exceeds the limits of a funding agency, one consideration is cost sharing, such as using donated time, equipment, or service. Multiyear projects should reflect annual increases to account for inflation.

Justification should be provided for each budget item. Sometimes justification can be included on the budget form; otherwise, explanations are given on a separate sheet following the budget page. Budgets ordinarily have two main sections: personnel and nonpersonnel.

Figure 5.3 contains the budget for year 2 of a 5-year project to study the effect of a planned intervention on bone health of teenaged girls, presented on the standard U.S. Department of Agriculture budget form. (This budget form is available on-line for easy completion.)

Personnel

Personnel costs include wages for all individuals needed to carry out the proposed work, including project directors, investigators, interviewers, research assistants, student employees, and secretaries. Fringe benefits are calculated as a percentage of the salary and are usually standard for the institution. Each participant's expertise, precise role, and estimated time required in relation to specific aims of the project must be specified. Personnel costs often account for a substantial portion of the budget.

"Release time" is often requested to free personnel from their regular duties, giving them time to conduct the proposed study. These monies may be used to employ temporary personnel. Funding may also be sought to pay fourth-quarter salaries to faculty members who conduct the research during the "off term" of a 9-month contract.

UNITED STATES DEPARTMENT OF AGRICULTURE
COOPERATIVE STATE RESEARCH, EDUCATION, AND EXTENSION SERVICE
BUDGET

OMB Approved 0524-0022
Expires 7/31/2001
Year 2

ORGANIZATION AND ADDRESS				USDA AWARD NO.	
1063 Hovde Hall West Lafayette, IN 47907-1140				Duration Proposed Months: **12**	Duration Awarded Months:
PRINCIPAL INVESTIGATOR(S)/PROJECT DIRECTORS(S)				FUNDS REQUESTED BY PROPOSER	FUNDS APPROVED BY CSREES (If Different)

		CSREES FUNDED WORK MONTHS				
A.	Salaries and Wages				$	$
	1. No. of Senior Personnel	Calendar	Academic	Summer		
	a. _1_ (Co)-PI(s)/PD(s)	12	0.00	0.00	$13,522	
	b. _0_ Senior Associates		0.00	0.00	$0	
	2. No. of Other Personnel (Non-Faculty)					
	a. _0_ Research Associates-Postdoctorates	0.00			$0	
	b. _0_ Other Professionals	1.00			$0	
	c. _1_ Graduate Students	**9 month stipend**			$9,270	
	d. _0_ Prebaccalaureate Students	. . . .			$0	
	e. _0_ Secretarial-Clerical	. . . .			$0	
	f. _0_ Technical, Shop and Other				$0	
	Total Salaries and Wages	. . . .			$22,792	
B.	Fringe Benefits (If charged as Direct Costs)				$4,443	
C.	Total Salaries, Wages and Fringe Benefits (A plus B)				$27,235	
D.	Nonexpendable Equipment (Attach supporting data. List items and dollar amounts for each item.)				$0	
E.	Materials and Supplies				$1,079	
F.	Travel					
	1. Domestic (Including Canada)	. . . .			$5,190	
	2. Foreign (List Destination and amount for each trip.)				$0	
G.	Publication Costs/Page Charges				$0	
H.	Computer (ADPE) Costs				$0	
I.	**All Other Direct Costs (Human Subject Payments)**				$9,750	
	Cost of DVD-ROMs				$1,500	
	DEXA Testing for 150 subjects				$18,750	
	1 GRAD FEE REMISSIONS	**3 quarters tuition**			$5,757	
J.	Total Direct Costs (C through I)		☐		$69,261	
K.	Indirect Costs If Applicable (specify rate(s) and Bases(s) for on/off campus activity. Where both are involved, identify itemized costs included in on/off campus bases.) 19% Total Federal Funds				$16,247	
L.	Total Direct and Indirect Costs (J plus K)		☐		$85,508	
M.	Other		☐		$0	
N.	Total Amount of This Request		☐		$85508	$
O.	Cost Sharing (If Required Provide Details)	$		$0		

NOTE: Signatures required only for Revised Budget		This is Revision No. 1	
NAME AND TITLE (Type or print)	SIGNATURE		DATE
Principal Investigator/Project Director **Steve Hertzler, PhD, RD**			
Authorized Organizational Representative **Daniel Sedmak, M.D.**			

Form CSREES-55 (6/95)

FIGURE 5.3 Sample budget showing the second year of a 5-year project funded by the U.S. Department of Agriculture. Courtesy of Steven Hertzler, Ph.D., R.D., Assistant Professor, Medical Dietetics Division, The Ohio State University, Columbus, Ohio. Used by permission.

Researchers are generally not paid supplemental wages to carry out a research project.

If graduate students are employed as research assistants, tuition and fees for designated terms may be included as expenses. Policies of the sponsoring institution should be followed.

Consultants

When weaknesses in the backgrounds or skills of the researchers are apparent, consultants can enhance the success of the project. The specific roles of consultants (for example, offering statistical assistance, training research assistants, conducting interviews, managing pharmaceutical administrations, or monitoring biochemical reactions) should be delineated, with approximate hours or days devoted to the project. An application is strengthened by the inclusion of a letter from each proposed consultant indicating willingness to contribute the time and expertise designated.

Equipment

Durable items costing more than $500 are considered equipment. Only equipment specifically needed to conduct the proposed research should be requested. Research equipment should be budgeted in the first year of a multi-year project; this budgeting reflects the needs for an item and allows greatest use of it. Equipment rental and service contracts may be itemized and often receive approval. Computers and other office equipment should not be requested unless they are integral to a project. The sponsoring institution is expected to support these items from general funds.

Costs of space rental and construction or remodeling to accommodate a specific project may be allowed by some funding agencies. It is best to clear such items prior to including them in a budget.

Materials and Supplies

Accurately calculating the cost of office, laboratory, and clinical supplies is often one of the greatest challenges in budgeting. If a study involves food items, meals, or formulas, these items will be a key segment of the budget, requiring careful cost projections. Funding agencies are not likely to give supplemental funding once a study has been approved; any shortfalls are the responsibility of the researcher.

Anticipated supply use must be analyzed thoroughly. It should include such things as stamps, printing, database (for example, MEDLINE) searches, videotapes, telephone and fax charges, long-distance calls, interview forms, computer time, laboratory tests, flasks and test tubes, kits for laboratory analyses, file folders, computer disks, printer paper, printer cartridges, letterhead, and envelopes. Researchers may wish to subcontract with a secretarial service to prepare, mail, and receive questionnaires. Specific items for the study—for example, postage and questionnaires for a survey—should be itemized. Other items can be grouped under the category "office supplies." Grants officers can offer advice on the best way to present and justify supply costs.

Subjects or Participants

Dietetics research often involves the use of human beings or animals. Subjects or study participants are frequently paid a stipend to ensure compliance with the study protocol, but stipends should not be so great as to influence voluntary participation (14). Stipends ordinarily cover the costs of travel and parking; time involved; baby-sitting; and other incidentals, such as newspapers or refreshments during waiting periods. On occasion, a study may require hospitalizations or overnight stays in a metabolic unit. If group sessions are planned, the funding request should cover room rental and refreshments. Other items are the costs of appropriate laboratory tests, clinical procedures, physician visits, physical examinations, and medications. Expenses for parking, mileage, bus fare, or taxi service should be included if subjects are not paid a stipend to cover these items.

Travel

Collaborative research may require travel for team meetings. For example, Bergstrom et al (32) describe a collaborative team comprising representatives from 5 states who met together annually over a 5-year study period. All related costs, including airfare and hotel accommodations, were covered in the research grant.

Travel expenses may be extensive. If home visits are planned, travel costs for them should be included in the budget. Travel expenses may also include going to a conference to present research results, attending a scientific meeting with others conducting similar studies, or visiting other sites to consult with experts in the field. These expenses should be described in detail, including the names of meetings or visitation sites, airfare, and per diem costs. Reviewers will carefully examine any unjustified expenses in this category (26).

Other Expenses

Other expenses may include costs of computer time, telephones, reprints of journal articles, publications, graphic design work, computer software, film, slides, photographic processing, manuals, poster exhibits, and photocopying. Sometimes these items can be moved between the "supply" and "other" sections of the budget to give balance to the overall budget.

Indirect Expenses

Some funding agencies have a policy of not paying any indirect expenses. Others designate a small percentage of the total budget as overhead, administrative, or indirect expense (20). Many institutions have a negotiated indirect expense rate, which may range anywhere from 25 percent to 67 percent or more of direct expenses for research studies and be around 8 percent for training grants. Some institutions exclude the cost of equipment or supplies from these overhead estimations. An institutional grants officer can assist in calculating appropriate indirect expenses.

Cost Sharing

Occasionally, a granting agency requires the institution to share the cost of conducting research. Institutions frequently bear the costs of release time, employee benefits, office supplies, travel, equipment maintenance and repair, remodeling space, and computer time. Cost sharing may be in the form of actual monetary support, for it can be represented as in-kind contributions of personnel in support of grant activities (20).

AGENCY REVIEW PROCESS

Although procedures differ from one agency to another, the review process generally undergoes similar steps. A grants coordinator first reviews the application for eligibility and completeness. Proposals that meet eligibility criteria are sent to a panel of 3 to 15 peer reviewers, who critique the proposal for its scientific merit following a preestablished list of evaluative criteria.

Usually the review panel meets to discuss all pro-

posals. One or two panel members are selected to conduct an in-depth review, prepare a list of strengths and weaknesses, and present an overview of the proposed study. The panel discusses each proposal and votes for its approval or disapproval based on soundness of research design and methodology, qualifications of the investigators, overall merit of the proposal, and how this research fits within the priorities of the agency's research mission. Approved proposals may be given a priority score, and one panel member is given the task of writing a summary statement of the review group's comments (33, pp 11–23).

After the initial review for scientific merit, applications are forwarded to a decision-making body such as a national advisory council, board of directors, or board of trustees. This second review body looks at proposals for their balance, and they endorse new initiatives (34). Projects approved for funding may be awarded the full amount requested, or the budget may be modified for a better fit with priorities and resources of the funding agency.

A staff member communicates final decisions to the principal investigators and sends them summary comments of the review panel. Researchers who receive funding are sent a formal notice indicating the amount of the award, starting date, and any reporting requirements. Researchers who are not approved also get a letter, which usually includes the priority score and a copy of the comments from reviewers.

MATCHING PROJECTS WITH FUNDING AGENCIES

A successfully funded proposal can start a lifelong career in nutrition research. Locating appropriate funding sources for a project enhances the potential for successful funding. Even a proposal that is superbly written and well thought out will not be funded if it arrives at the wrong agency. Funding priorities are a fact of life for every agency. It is part of the researcher's job to ascertain that each proposal meets the goals of the selected funding agency. Therefore, it is important to know as much as possible about the funding history of a particular agency. This information, as well as agency goals and priorities, is widely available, but it must be sought out. This section provides steps to follow when searching for an appropriate agency to fund a research proposal.

There are many different types of funding agencies, as shown in Table 5.2. A particular project idea usually

TABLE 5.2 Funding Agencies

Type of Agency	Examples
Federal	National Institutes of Health, Department of Health and Human Services, Agency for International Development
State and local	Department of Education, Department of Human Services, arts councils, local school districts
Foundation	Ford Foundation, Spenser Foundation, Rockefeller Foundation
Nonprofit organization	American Diabetes Association, American Dietetic Association
Industry	IBM, Eli Lilly, Ross Laboratories, Mead Johnson
Institutional	Local universities and hospitals

can be modified to match the funding priorities of more than one type of granting agency. A search for funding begins with development of the research idea.

Defining the Project

A research proposal should clearly identify the gap between what knowledge or technology already exists and what the proposed study will contribute. A project should be defined carefully, looked at in as many ways as possible, and related to other subject areas. This activity will help identify agencies that may benefit from funding the project and will simplify the next step.

A project that proposes to study the effect of early nutrition intervention on the birth weight of infants born to adolescent mothers, for example, might seem to be very clear-cut. However, looking at it in a different light might generate the following questions.

- Does the project involve nutrition education to the client or training physicians or other health professionals who might be asked to intervene? If it does, the proposal might be submitted to an agency that funds professional education in nutrition.
- Does the project involve the use of special supplements or the provision of additional nutrients to the mother? If so, a dairy association or pharmaceutical company might be a funding possibility.
- Will the project involve the school system in any way? If so, a department of education may support the study.
- Will the project involve public assistance pro-

grams? If it will, a department of health might be a source of possible funding.
- Is this a model project? If it is, a local foundation may be receptive to funding the project.

Identifying Constituency Groups

During the investigation of a project, it is important to identify who will benefit from its results. Funding agencies also have constituencies and will usually set funding priorities accordingly. The project on nutrition intervention described earlier would have several possible constituencies. The most obvious is infants born to adolescent mothers. The adolescent will also benefit. Agencies that serve these clients may be a less obvious constituency group. Health care institutions may be a constituency group, because efforts to improve birth outcomes will likely decrease the costs of neonatal care and related hospital costs. Early nutrition intervention may mean spending fewer federal dollars on postnatal care of these infants. Physicians and nurses may benefit by observing or participating in the project and therefore may become another constituency group. The task here is to identify numerous groups that may benefit from the proposed study. This delineation then can be used to determine potential funding agencies.

Searching for Key Words

Once the idea has been defined and the subject areas explored, it is important to begin searching for key words within funding databases. A project titled "The Effect of Early Nutrition Intervention on the Birth Weight of Infants Born to Adolescent Mothers" might generate the following key words: *nutrition, pregnancy, adolescent pregnancy, infants, birth weight,* and *prenatal nutrition.*

The process of identifying key words allows a researcher to begin searching for an appropriate funding source. Two major databases, IRIS (Illinois Research Information Services, Campus Wide Research Services Offices, University of Illinois at Urbana-Champaign, 901 S. Mathews Ave., Urbana, IL 61801) and SPIN (Sponsored Program Information Network, The Research Foundation of SUNY, PO Box 9, Albany, NY 12201), list both federal and private agencies that fund projects. Access to these agencies is based on a search for key words listed in agency descriptions of funding priorities and limitations. IRIS has a key word list of approximately 2,500 words.

Limitations of the database systems include the fact

that although both attempt to update their databases frequently, their information may not be current. Also, both databases are term sensitive and may list numerous funding agencies that in fact do not match given research criteria. Nevertheless, from the generated list, several agencies can be identified for potential research funding.

Access to these databases usually requires a university affiliation. Subscriptions are expensive, and few private institutions have the resources and need to justify purchasing access. Usually, as a service to the local community, universities are willing to make database information available.

When searching sources other than those listed in SPIN and IRIS for funding, two approaches can be used: referring to books that list funding sources or accessing computerized databases. As a service to researchers, several authors and organizations compile and publish information about foundations and agencies that fund research and other projects. See the Further Reading at the end of the chapter for a listing of such books and other resources. Researchers often use the World Wide Web to conduct electronic searches for information about funding sources. The Foundation Center's *Guide to Grantseeking on the Web* (35) contains information about hundreds of grant-maker Web sites, corporate grant making, and government funding sources. The Foundation Center's Web site (http://www.foundationcenter.org) provides access to numerous resources, including Foundation Finder, *Philanthropy News Digest,* and an on-line proposal writing course. Researchers can also find a virtual catalog of World Wide Web resources in the biomedical sciences at BioSites, a Web page sponsored by the National Network of Libraries of Medicine (http://www.library. ucsf.edu/biosites). Michigan State University maintains a Web site that includes information on grants for individuals in food science and nutrition (http://www.lib.msu.edu/ harris23/grants/3food.htm).

Another on-line service is the Community of Science (COS), found at http://www.cos.com. COS is a global network for scientists and research and development professionals. This Web site provides researchers with personalized electronic alerts for funding opportunities and MEDLINE publications, based on their professional interests. COS also offers a research database that enables researchers to track research activities and projects sponsored at the NIH, National Science Foundation, U.S. Department of Agriculture, and other agencies. Your institutional grants officer will be able to tell you if your university, company, or agency is a participating member of COS.

Targeting Appropriate Funding Agencies

Funding agencies can be separated into six distinct types, as shown in Table 5.2 and described in the following discussion. Mailing addresses for various agencies and some World Wide Web sites are provided in Further Reading at the end of the chapter.

Federal Agencies

Federal agencies provide the greatest proportion of research funding. Most nutrition research money comes from the NIH through its various individual institutes. Additional sources of federal funding include the Department of Agriculture, the Department of Health and Human Services, the Department of Education, the Agency for Healthcare Research and Quality, and the National Foundation for the Centers of Disease Control and Prevention.

Federal funding may be in the form of an investigator-initiated research grant submitted to an agency for consideration of funding or a response to an RFP/RFA developed by a research agency for the completion of specific research projects. For federal agencies, RFP guidelines are published in the *Federal Register*. These guidelines may be very specific, including a brief review of the literature and prescribed methodology. Other RFPs may be less specific in methodology, allowing the investigator more latitude in the implementation of the project. Researchers who follow carefully the *Federal Register* can obtain advance notice of pending RFPs. Preliminary guidelines frequently are published several months ahead so that public comment can be generated prior to finalizing the RFP guidelines. Attention to the preliminary guidelines and the discussions generated at public hearings can give valuable lead time to a research team wishing to respond. The submission date for an RFP is usually less than 2 months after the final guidelines are printed. However, researchers who learn of a proposed RFP at its first publication may have 6 months or more to respond.

State and Local Agencies

State and local agencies are another source of potential funding for research projects. The researcher who includes clear documentation on how a research project will uniquely benefit a particular local population will have a greatly improved likelihood of funding. Many state agencies also generate RFPs for projects important to a given local area. Personal contact should be established with personnel at state and local agencies that may

TABLE 5.3 Types of Foundations and Their Funding Priorities

Types	Approximate Number	Examples	Funding Priorities
Community	300	San Francisco Foundation	Generally, projects in local area only
National (multipurpose)	100	Ford Foundation	Large model projects that have national impact
Special purpose	100	National Kidney Foundation	Projects specific to discipline
Family	>10,000	Small Family Foundation	Diverse projects; each foundation operates independently, with its own set of criteria, which may change frequently
Corporate	>10,000	Burroughs Wellcome Foundation	Projects that have potential benefit to Marriott Foundation corporation profits and/or community image

potentially fund research. Such contacts often give researchers access to information regarding pending agency interests. They also provide the agency with potential researchers who may be contacted for projects under consideration.

Foundations

Foundations are an important source of research support, and their funding complements funding from various government and private sources. Identifying the appropriate foundation for a proposal takes homework. Table 5.3 identifies the different types of foundations and characterizes their usual funding priorities.

Several reference sources provide information about private foundations. *The Foundation Directory* is available on-line at http://www.fconline.fdncenter.org. At this site you can access Links to Nonprofit Resources. From there, click on "Grantmaker Information" for annotated links to more than 1,500 Web sites of granting organizations. Foundations are required to submit annual reports that include their net worth and the amount of funding provided in the past year. A foundation's mission statement, also found in these documents, offers a clue to funding priorities. If a report does not list grantees and titles of funded projects, such information usually can be requested from the foundation.

Foundations usually require less detailed proposals than those demanded by federal agencies. At the same time, foundations generally expect submission of a concept paper or letter of inquiry before the completed proposal. Contacts with, and personal visits to, a foundation may enhance funding. A researcher should begin with a telephone call to the foundation to obtain information about funding priorities and limitations. When planning a visit to a foundation, the researcher should organize an agenda beforehand to obtain information regarding funding priorities, size of grants funded, and evaluation criteria. Offering to provide service to the agency in the form of grants review will both give valuable insight into criteria for successful funding and demonstrate a researcher's willingness to support foundation goals.

Nonprofit Organizations

Nonprofit organizations, such as the American Dietetic Association (ADA) Foundation, ADA-affiliated practice groups, the American Society for Parenteral and Enteral Nutrition, and the American Diabetes Association, may also fund research. The dollar amount of funding varies, and the research must specifically benefit the association's constituency. Information regarding grant possibilities can be obtained by contacting the individual associations.

Industry

Industry also funds research by independent investigators. These funds may be either for investigator-initiated proposals or industry-funded RFPs. Reasons for industry support of research are many, from support of important clients and accounts to the need for credible verification of the efficacy or effectiveness of a product. Working with industry may involve a research proposal, but more often than not it involves a contract, a binding agreement to provide research in a specific area for a specific amount of money. Although it may be similar to a research proposal, it may have strings attached (36). Contracts may provide for delay of publication of research results to give the corporation time to patent the findings. Difficulties and delays in publication may develop in situations where the findings do not support the corporation's products. It is frequently easier to obtain funding in situations where the likelihood of negative findings poses little risk to the proposed industry. It is important to define clearly the research to be done and the publication rights and procedures prior to accepting the contract. University grants officers can be very helpful when researchers need to prepare a contract.

Funding companies have unique interests that must be considered when developing an industry-funded proposal. Credibility of the researcher and of the institution doing the research are important aspects from the funding company's perspective. Ethical companies may ask for first review of the manuscript, but they will seldom prevent publication. Companies desire an initial review of the manuscript so that they can check the accuracy of the statistical analysis and prepare in advance a response to possible media questions. When doing an initial proposal review, a company will use the opportunity to assess possible elements of the design that would produce negative findings.

Most industry grants are for smaller dollar amounts and cover a shorter period than do federal and foundation grants. However, industry can provide products and services that may make up an important dimension of research in nutrition and dietetics.

Institutional

Many universities and hospitals have a research fund for their staff members. Sometimes only pilot studies will be funded. Institutions that have a strong commitment to research often fund initial studies to begin developing potential for a sustained research program. Often internal awards are based on the likelihood that the proposed project will lead to further funding from external sources.

COPING WITH REJECTION

Every successful investigator has had to deal with a rejected proposal, and usually several. In fact, a researcher who has never had a proposal rejected probably has never submitted one. The ability to deal with rejection may be the difference between a successful investigator and one who is not successful. A researcher who receives a rejection letter should take several positive steps before deciding to abandon the proposal.

Avoiding Discouragement

Rejection of a proposal to which numerous hours and untold personal energy have been committed can be devastating. After all, how could an agency not recognize the effort and the uniqueness of the research proposal? There are numerous reasons for rejections, and few, if any, pertain to a researcher personally. It is important for the successful investigator to realize that rejection of a proposal by an agency does not mean that the research is without merit. The first step after rejection of a proposal is to take action that may lead to future funding (20).

Asking for a Pink Sheet

Federal agencies provide a critique of each proposal they review for funding. This critique is printed on pink paper, so it is called a "pink sheet." This document is a valuable resource; it summarizes the strengths and—more important—the weaknesses of the proposal. If the funding agency has not provided a pink sheet, a researcher should ask for it. Careful review can provide suggestions to improve the proposal for a second submission. Subsequent submissions of improved proposals have a much greater chance of funding (37).

Figure 5.4 shows the most frequent problems with unfunded proposals (38), and Figure 5.5 offers character-

1. Lack of original ideas.
2. Diffuse, unfocused, or superficial research plan.
3. Lack of knowledge of published relevant work.
4. Lack of experience in essential methodology.
5. Uncertainty concerning future directions.
6. Questionable reasoning in experimental approach.
7. Absence of acceptable scientific rationale.
8. Unrealistically large amount of work.
9. Lack of sufficient experimental detail.
10. Uncritical approach.

FIGURE 5.4   The ten most common reasons for proposal failure. Adapted from Ogden TE, Goldberg IA. *Research Proposals: A Guide to Success.* 2nd ed. New York: Raven Press; 1995:20. Permission granted by Lippincott Williams & Wilkins.

- The proposal responds to the request for proposals.
- The proposal meets specific needs that are recognized by the funding source.
- The proposal utilizes knowledgeable individuals who have a history of success.
- The proposal directs the plan toward a population, not an organization. *Funding sources invest in programs to help people. They seldom give money to help organizations.*
- The proposal contains an innovative and well-organized plan of action with reasonable dates for objectives to be achieved.
- The proposal presents a workable management plan. The management plan is a good place to insert limited graphics (e.g., a chart showing the percentage of services vs. administrative costs).
- The proposal provides an evaluation plan that will measure and communicate (in plain English) outcomes or impacts.
- The proposal demonstrates support from the community with cooperative agreements for organizations to work together.
- The proposal outlines a realistic budget that is neither too high nor too low. A budget that is too low is a common mistake; nobody is funded on the basis of providing cheap labor. When working with a small organization that has not been audited, arrange for a complete financial audit.
- The proposal reflects well on the funding sources. Organizations invest in programs that are likely to bring a good return.
- The proposal is for research that is not dependent on a single source or type of funding and will not die when the current funding runs out.
- The proposal is carefully written, including the abstract (when an abstract is required). The reviewer's response to the abstract may set the tone for the entire proposal.

FIGURE 5.5 Characteristics of successful proposals. Adapted from Kemp C. A practical approach to writing successful grant proposals. *Nurse Practitioner.* 1991;16(11):51,55–56. Used by permission of Lippincott Williams & Wilkins.

istics of successful proposals (39). By reviewing rejected proposals and qualities of both unfunded and successful proposals, a researcher can often pinpoint the problem area when funding has been denied. These clues can be specifically addressed when preparing subsequent proposals.

Obtaining a List of Funded Research

A list of successful grants funded by the agency in the current funding cycle is always available; however, a researcher may need to request it. Agency priorities can usually be identified from this list. The list can help determine if the research question needs to be refocused or funding needs to be sought from a different source.

Successful grantees are usually willing to share their proposals. They may provide insight into problem areas and possible revisions that could increase funding potential.

Asking for a List of Reviewers

Granting agencies will also provide a list of proposal reviewers. By identifying the individuals who may read their proposals, researchers may be able to determine if the proposals were written in the appropriate language. A proposal may be too technical for the reviewers to understand. Reviewers with very little nutrition background, for example, may not appreciate the significance of the research. Knowing the reviewers greatly improves the possibility of effective and persuasive communication. See Miner and Miner (20) for a list of questions that might be posed to past reviewers.

Both new and experienced researchers in dietetics can improve their grant-writing skills and their ability to receive research funding. Diligent adherence to techniques for preparation, writing, and internal review can improve chances for positive external reviews for proposed investigations. An accurate, precise, complete, and reasonable budget adds to the merit of a persuasive proposal.

The likelihood of being funded can be improved by the effective use of strategies for establishing and maintaining strong ties with funding agencies, matching projects with funding priorities, and targeting sources most likely to fund specific projects. If at first a proposal is not funded, it is appropriate to find out why, take steps to address problem areas, and resubmit the proposal. Good research requires tenacity; sustained funding for research demands both persistence and ingenuity.

REFERENCES

1. Saunderlin G. Writing a research proposal: the critical first step for successful clinical research. *Gastroenterol Nurs.* 1994;17(2):48–56.
2. Weekes DP. Developing a research question: where to start? *J Pediatr Oncol Nurs.* 1992;9:187–191.
3. Monsen ER. Forces for research. *J Am Diet Assoc.* 1993;93:981–985.
4. Coulston A, Rock C. A summary of the current state of knowledge in clinical nutrition and dietetic practice: suggestions for future research. In: *The Research Agenda for Dietetics Conference Proceedings.* Chicago, Ill: American Dietetic Association; 1993:1–24.
5. Sims L. Research aspects of public policy in nutrition: generating research questions to determine the impact of nutritional, agricultural, and health care policy and regulations on the health and nutrition status of the public. In: *The Research Agenda for Dietetics Conference Proceedings.* Chicago, Ill: American Dietetic Association; 1993:25–38.
6. Lafferty L, Dowling R. Effectiveness of foodservice systems. In: *The Research Agenda for Dietetics Conference Proceedings.* Chicago, Ill: American Dietetic Association; 1993:60–66.
7. Kim SK. Dietetics professionals and women's health research at the National Institutes of Health. *J Am Diet Assoc.* 1998;98:133–136.
8. Thomas PR, Earl R. Creating the future of the nutrition and food sciences. *J Am Diet Assoc.* 1994;94:257–259.
9. Dwyer JT. Scientific underpinnings for the profession: dietitians in research. *J Am Diet Assoc.* 1997;97:593–597.
10. Position of the American Dietetic Association: nutrition, aging, and the continuum of care. *J Am Diet Assoc.* 2000;100:580–595.
11. Splett P, Myers EF. A proposed model for effective nutrition care. *J Am Diet Assoc.* 2001;101:357–363.
12. Kahn CR. Picking a research problem. *N Engl J Med.* 1994;330:1530–1533.
13. MEDLINE Plus Health Information: Databases: NLM/NIH Resources. Available at: http://www.nlm.nih.gov/medlineplus/databases.html. Accessed March 15, 2001.
14. Hodgson C. Tips on writing successful proposals. *Nurse Pract.* 1989;14(2):44–54.
15. Engebretson J, Wardell DW. The essence of partnership in research. *J Prof Nurs.* 1997;13:38–47.
16. Ingersoll GL, Brooks AM, Fischer MS, et al. Professional practice model research collaboration. Issues in longitudinal, multisite designs. *J Nurs Adm.* 1995;25:39–46.
17. Grey M. Top 10 tips for successful grantsmanship. *Res Nurs Health.* 2000;23:91–92.
18. Schiller MR, Moore C. Practical approaches to outcomes evaluation. *Top Clin Nutr.* 1999;14(2):1–12.
19. Selby ML, Riportella-Muller R, Farel A. Building administrative support for your research: a neglected key for turning a research plan into a funded project. *Nurs Outlook.* 1992;40(2):73–77.
20. Miner JT, Miner LE. A guide to proposal planning and writing. In: Miner JT, Miner LE. *Directory of Biomedical and Health Care Grants 2001.* Phoenix, Ariz: Oryx Press; 2001:xxv–xxxvi.
21. Research: Centers, Grant Opportunities, News, Projects. Available at: http://www.nutrition.gov/home/index.php3. Accessed February 25, 2002.
22. Sladek FE, Stein EL. Funding agency contacts: letting them help. *Grants Magazine.* 1983;6:19–31.
23. Gitlin LN, Lyons KJ. *Successful Grant Writing: Strategies for Health and Human Service Professionals.* New York, NY: Springer Publishing Company; 1996.
24. Kennicott PC. Developing a grant proposal: some basic principles. *Grants Magazine.* 1983;6:36–41.
25. Mackenzie RS. Grant writing and review for dental faculty. *J Dent Educ.* 1986;50:180–186.
26. Bliss DZ, Guenter PA, Heitkemper MM. From proposal to publication: are you writing research right? *Nutr Clin Pract.* 2000;299–305.
27. Niederhuber JE. Writing a successful grant application. *J Surg Res.* 1985;39:277–284.
28. Ohtake PJ. Grant writing: toward preparing a successful application. *Cardiopulmonary Phys Ther.* 2000;11(2):69–73.
29. Norwood SL. *Research strategies.* Upper Saddle River, NJ: Prentice Hall Health; 2000.
30. Eaves GN. Preparation of the research-grant application: opportunities and pitfalls. *Grants Magazine.* 1984;7:151–157.
31. Brakey MR. Tips for the novice grantseeker: implications for staff development specialists. *J Nurs Staff Dev.* 1997;13(3):160–163.
32. Bergstrom N, Hanson BC, Grant M, et al. Collaborative nursing research: anatomy of a successful consortium. *Nurs Res.* 1984;33:20–25.

33. Reif-Lehrer L. *Grant Application Writer's Handbook.* Boston, Mass: Jones and Bartlett Publishers; 1995.

34. Mervis J. Anatomy of the NIH grant system, or how to play the game. *J NIH Res.* 1990;2:59–68.

35. The Foundation Center. *Guide to Grantseeking on the Web.* 3rd ed. New York, NY: The Foundation Center; 1998.

36. Loos FD, Shortridge HA, Adaskin EJ, Rock BL. When industry courts your clinical research skills, should you collaborate? *Clin Nurse Spec.* 1994;8(2): 85–89.

37. Cuca JM, McLaughlin WJ. Why clinical research grant applications fare poorly in review and how to recover. *Cancer Invest.* 1987;5:55–58.

38. Ogden TE, Goldberg IA. *Research Proposals: A Guide to Success.* 2nd ed. New York, NY: Raven Press; 1995.

39. Kemp C. A practical approach to writing successful grant proposals. *Nurse Pract.* 1991;16(11):51, 55–56.

Further Reading and Resources

General References for Proposals and Research

Bauer DG. *The "How To" Grants Manual: Successful Grant Seeking Techniques for Obtaining Public and Private Grants.* 3rd ed. Phoenix, Ariz: Oryx; 1999.

Geever JC. *Guide to Proposal Writing.* 3rd ed. New York, NY: The Foundation Center; 2001.

Gitlin LN, Lyons KJ. *Successful Grant Writing: Strategies for Health and Human Service Professionals.* New York, NY: Springer Publishing Company; 1996.

Ireton-Jones CS, Gottschlich MM, Bell SJ. *Practice-Oriented Nutrition Research: An Outcomes Management Approach.* Gaithersburg, Md: Aspen Publishers; 1998.

Lefferts R. *Getting a Grant in the 1990s: How to Write Successful Grant Proposals.* New York, NY: Prentice Hall Press; 1990.

Miner LE, Griffith J. *Proposal Planning and Writing.* Phoenix, Ariz: Oryx Press; 1998.

Miner JT, Miner LE. *Directory of Biomedical and Health Care Grants 2001.* Phoenix, Ariz: Oryx Press; 2001.

National Institute of Allergy and Infectious Diseases. The original how to write a research grant application. Available at: http://www.niaid.nih.gov/ncn/toolmain.htm. Accessed February 25, 2002.

Ogden TE, Goldberg IA. *Research Proposals: A Guide to Success.* 2nd ed. New York, NY: Raven Press; 1995.

Reif-Lehrer L. *Grant Application Writer's Handbook.* Boston, Mass: Jones and Bartlett Publishers; 1995.

Schlein AM. *Find it on line: the complete guide to online research.* Tempe, Ariz: Facts on Demand Press; 1999.

Sources of Information on Funding Agencies

Foundations

IRIS, Campus Wide Research Services Offices, University of Illinois at Urbana-Champaign, 901 S. Mathews Ave, Urbana, Ill 61801

Miner JT, Miner LE. *Directory of Biomedical and Health Care Grants 2001.* Phoenix, Ariz: Oryx Press; 2001.

Sponsored Programs Information Network (SPIN), The Research Foundation of SUNY, PO Box 9, Albany, NY 12201

The Foundation Center, 79 Fifth Ave, New York, NY 10003 (800/424-9836)

The Foundation Directory

The Foundation Grants Index

The National Directory for Corporate Giving

The National Guide to Funding in Aging

Government

Catalogue of Federal Domestic Assistance, Superintendent of Documents, Government Printing Office, Washington, DC 20402

Federal Register, Superintendent of Documents, Government Printing Office, Washington, DC 20402

Commerce Business Daily, Superintendent of Documents, Government Printing Office, Washington, DC 20402

NIH Guide for Grants and Contracts, Grants Information, Division of Extramural Outreach and Information Resources, Office of Extramural Research, Room 499, Westwood Building, NIH Bethesda, MD 20894. Phone: 301/435-0714; Fax: 301/480-0525; e-mail: grantsinfo@nih.gov.

National Institute for Occupational Safety and Health, Center for Disease Control, 255 E. Paces Ferry Rd NE, Room 321, Atlanta, GA 30305 (404/262-6575)

Other

The Grants Register 1999. The Complete Guide to Postgraduate Funding Worldwide. 17th ed. New York, NY: St. Martin's Press; 1998.

GrantsNet, your one-stop resource to find funds for training in the biomedical sciences and undergraduate science education. Available at: http://www.grantsnet.org. Accessed February 25, 2002.

Selected World Wide Web Sites for Nutrition Researchers

Agencies

Agency for Healthcare Research and Quality
Web site: http://www.ahrq.gov

American Federation for Aging Research
  Web site: http://www.afar.org
Centers for Disease Control and Prevention
  Web site: http://www.cdc.gov
Department of Agriculture
  Web site: http://www.usda.gov
Department of Health and Human Services
  Web site: http://www.hhs.gov/grantsnet/
  Web site includes access to CRISP and to grant-writing
    tools on-line.
Federation of American Societies for Experimental Biology
    (FASEB)
  Web site: http://www.faseb.org
  Web site includes information from FASEB with links to its
    member societies and other biology Web sites.
Health Resources and Service Administration
  Web site: http://www.bhpr.hrsa.gov
HRSA Maternal and Child Health Bureau
  Web site: http://www.mchb.hrsa.gov
National Academy of Sciences (home page for the National
    Research Council and the Institute of Medicine)
  Web site: http://www.nas.edu
  Web site includes links to NRC report summaries and mem-
    ber directories.
National Center for Research Resources
  Web site: http://www.ncrr.nih.gov
National Dairy Council
  Web site: http://www.nationaldairycouncil.org
National Science Foundation
  Web site: http://www.nsf.gov

Web site includes program announcements and funding in-
    formation.
NIH Information
  Web site: http://www.nih.gov
  Web site includes funding announcements and a searchable
    telephone directory.
Office of Research on Women's Health
  Web site: http://www.nih.gov/orwh

Foundations

California Wellness Foundation
  Web site: http://www.tcwf.org
Canadian Foundation for Dietetic Research
  Web site: http://www.dietitians.ca/cfdr/index/htm
Robert Wood Johnson Foundation
  Web site: http://www.rwjf.org
Henry J. Kaiser Family Foundation
  Web site: http://www.kff.org
  Click on "Links" and then on "Foundations" to obtain a
    descriptive list of foundations and their funding
    priorities.
Life Sciences Research Foundation
  Web site: http://www.lsrf.org/lsrfgeninfo.html
Metropolitan Life Foundation
  Web site: http://www.metlife.org
Pew Charitable Trusts
  Web site: http://www.pewtrusts.com
Alfred P. Sloan Foundation
  Web site: http://www.sloan.org

Part 3

—ᴡ—

Analytic Research

Hypotheses can be evaluated and cause and effect studied through analytic research (see Chapter 6). Observational analytic research encompasses case-control and cohort (follow-up) studies. Experimental analytic research, including clinical trials, allows cause and effect to be examined.

Observational research designs generate measures of association (relative risk and odds ratios) and measures of effect (attributable risk). Relative risk is calculated from cohort studies and odds ratios, from case-control studies. Attributable risk indicates a public health impact or an effect on the population.

Experimental analytic research designs involve investigator-controlled interventions. Well-designed and carefully conducted clinical trials provide strong scientific evidence of causal relationships. The advantages and limitations of randomized clinical trials are discussed in Chapter 6. Chapter 7 discusses issues important in designing clinical trials to ensure that the statistical power is sufficient to detect differences among the study groups (see also Chapter 26) and that the data generated are generalizable (see also Chapter 4).

Chapter 7 provides practical guidelines for designing and conducting clinical trials and suggests techniques for the effective and ethical recruitment, screening, and retention of human subjects. The researcher is obligated to secure approval from the institutional review board, as well as voluntary consent from all subjects, before initiating the clinical trial (see also Chapter 4). In addition, Chapter 7 provides recommendations for carefully assessing food composition by both accurate calculation and chemical analyses (see also Chapter 16) and the development of data collection forms. Pilot tests are strongly endorsed. Future research is needed to construct efficient strategies for subject recruitment and retention, to devise objective methods for assessing compliance, and to expand food formulations suitable for controlled diets.

Through future research we will be able to clarify the associations between diet and chronic disease. In so doing, we need to identify clearly the foods and dietary factors that alter risk of chronic disease; determine mechanisms of action; improve methods for collecting and evaluating data on dietary exposures to foods; identify both biomarkers of dietary exposure and early indicators of risk; assess and quantify beneficial and adverse effects of diet; determine the optimal range of intake for macronutrients, micronutrients, and other dietary constituents; access the potential for reduction of chronic disease risk through clinical trials; and develop and evaluate public health programs that incorporate knowledge of diet and chronic disease. This valuable research will require effective analytic, descriptive, and integrative research designs (Chapters 6 through 9).

ERM, Editor

6

Analytic Nutrition Epidemiology

Monica E. Yamamoto, Dr.P.H., R.D., F.A.D.A.

Analytic epidemiologic methods have a long history in nutrition research. Early investigations of nutrition deficiency diseases, such as scurvy and pellagra, used epidemiologic methods (1). Epidemiology, the investigative basic science for health questions, studies "the distribution and determinants of health-related states or events in specified populations and the application of this study to control of health problems" (2). Nutrition epidemiology, a subdiscipline of epidemiology, addresses the fundamental question, Does diet or nutrition make a difference to health and disease? Analytic nutrition epidemiology investigates whether nutrition status or dietary intake is significantly associated with, or has a causal linkage with, the risk, progression, or prognosis of disease.

Findings from descriptive epidemiology provide the basis for analytic epidemiologic investigations. Descriptive epidemiology focuses on a triad of key common disease pattern features: the time of occurrence, the geography of the occurrence, and the characteristics of the persons affected. Descriptive epidemiology findings, although important, are not definitive for disease associations or causal relationships. An analytic framework allows these descriptive findings to be more rigorously examined and tested. Potential etiologic hypotheses can be generated from this descriptive information and its correlational studies. These etiologic hypotheses are the focus of analytic epidemiologic work.

This chapter provides an introduction to analytic nutrition epidemiology. First, an overview of analytic epidemiology is presented, with a focus on analytic goals and measures. Next, key issues in designing and implementing analytic nutrition epidemiologic studies are discussed. Finally, analytic epidemiology study designs are covered, including their uses, advantages, limitations, implementation issues, analytic considerations, findings, and diet and nutrition examples.

WHAT IS ANALYTIC NUTRITION EPIDEMIOLOGY?

Analytic nutrition epidemiology attempts to explain the described occurrence of disease or disease-related phenomena (3). It studies diet and nutrition as potential determinants of population disease patterns identified through descriptive epidemiology (4). It asks, What factors independently contribute to, or are likely to cause, the pattern of disease identified in the population?

Analytic epidemiologic studies can generally be classified as either observational or experimental. Observational designs study potential health-related relationships as they occur in nature (3), and most examine evidence to explain why diseases are distributed the way they are (3). Observational analytic epidemiology studies include cross-sectional studies, surveillance studies, cohort studies, and case-control studies. In experimental (etiologic) studies, the investigator intervenes and examines the effect of the intervention on one or more specific health or disease outcomes. Experimental analytic epidemiology studies include randomized controlled trials (RCTs), group-randomized trials, and multicentered RCTs.

Nutrition observational investigations test the hypotheses that health risks are significantly associated with diet and nutrition exposures (4). Nutrition experimental investigations test the hypotheses that diet or nutrition exposures are causally linked with health or disease outcomes. Finally, all analytic epidemiology studies include four groups: subjects who have the disease, subjects who do not have the disease, subjects with a particular exposure, and subjects without a particular exposure (5).

GOALS OF ANALYTIC EPIDEMIOLOGY

Analytic epidemiology includes two specific goals (Figure 6.1). One goal is to establish whether a significant association exists between a specific factor and a disease outcome. The other goal is to generate evidence for a causal effect of a specific factor on a disease outcome.

Establishing Association

What Is an Association?

The first step in identifying a factor's importance to health or disease is to test whether an association exists between this specific factor and the disease in question (2). The analysis examines whether the risk associated with a particular disease is significantly different based on the presence or level of the factor. It tests the hypothe-

sis that the specific risk factor is associated with a higher-than-normal or lower-than-normal risk of having a particular disease, disease prognosis, or disease progression.

What Are Measures of Association?

Epidemiology expresses disease association as risk of disease (Figure 6.2). *Relative risk* is a proportion of subjects with the disease in exposed versus nonexposed groups. The *etiologic fraction* is the proportion of subjects exposed (exposed-unexposed/exposed) who have the disease. The *odds ratio,* or *relative odds,* is an estimate of relative risk that is calculated when the disease is rare. *Attributable risk* is the amount of risk that can be assigned to a particular factor. *Population attributable risk* is the proportion of the disease incidence in a total population (both exposed and nonexposed) that can be attributed to a specific exposure (2).

What Study Designs Are Used to Study Associations?

Observational study designs are used to study associations. These designs include cross-sectional studies, surveillance studies, cohort studies, and case-control studies. Cross-sectional studies, as the name implies, are studies completed at one point in time. Surveillance studies are cross-sectional studies completed at designated intervals for monitoring purposes. Cohort studies examine the same group of individuals repeatedly over time, with a focus on exposed and nonexposed individuals. Case-control studies examine individuals with a particular disease (cases) and those without the disease (controls) to identify disease associations with particular exposures or risk factors. Observational studies compare exposed and nonexposed groups for case status (cohort studies) or cases and noncases (case-control studies) for potential risk factors, or they study populations for both case status and potential risk factors (cross-sectional studies and surveillance studies) (2). Measures of association are derived from these analyses.

Establishing Causation

What Is Causation?

Etiologic epidemiologic studies (that is, studies of disease causation) build on evidence for a significant association between a specific factor and a disease outcome where a possible causal relationship has been suggested. An experimental study is designed to test whether a

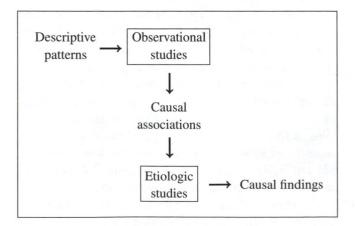

FIGURE 6.1 Epidemiologic research approach.

$$\text{Relative Risk (RR)} = \frac{\text{Cumulative Incidence in the Exposed}}{\text{Cumulative Incidence in the Nonexposed}}$$

$$\text{Attributable Risk (AR)} = \left[\begin{array}{c}\text{Cumulative Incidence}\\\text{in the Exposed}\end{array}\right] - \left[\begin{array}{c}\text{Cumulative Incidence}\\\text{in the Nonexposed}\end{array}\right]$$

$$\text{Population Attributable Risk (PAR)} = \left[\begin{array}{c}\text{Cumulative Incidence}\\\text{in the Population}\end{array}\right] - \left[\begin{array}{c}\text{Cumulative Incidence}\\\text{in the Nonexposed}\end{array}\right]$$

$$\text{Odds Ratio (OR)} = \frac{\text{Exposed Cases} \times \text{Nonexposed Controls}}{\text{Unexposed Cases} \times \text{Exposed Controls}}$$

FIGURE 6.2   Measures of association.

causal relationship actually exists between the factor and the disease.

Criteria for Causation

Specific causal criteria have been suggested for epidemiologic studies. Hill's eight criteria are commonly cited for this purpose (Figure 6.3) (4). Hill's first criterion is consistency of the association. Similar associations are found in a variety of studies (with different populations, study designs, and statistical methods). His second criterion is strength of the association. The magnitude of the association between the factor and the disease is significant. As illustrated in Figure 6.4, a relative risk of 1 indicates that the risk of a disease outcome is the same as expected. A relative risk with factor exposure substantially greater or less than 1 indicates that the disease outcome is

likely to be associated with the factor. Hill's third criterion is specificity of association. A single cause results in a single outcome. As for the fourth criterion, the temporal relationship, the exposure or factor precedes the disease outcome. The fifth criterion is a biologic gradient. A dose relationship is seen with a specific threshold, or an increased effect is seen with an increased dose. The sixth criterion is biological plausibility. There should be biological evidence from relevant experiments (for example, in vitro cell systems, animal models, or human metabolic and clinical studies). Hill's seventh criterion is coherence. This causal relationship is congruent with existing knowledge about the disease or condition (7). The final criterion is evidence from experimentation; specific evidence is provided through controlled experiments, including , laboratory studies, animal models, and randomized clinical trials (4).

1. Association's consistency.[a]
2. Association's strength.[a]
3. Association's specificity.[a]
4. Association's temporality.
5. Biological gradient (dose/response).[a]
6. Biological plausibility.[a]
7. Coherence.
8. Experimental evidence.

[a]Reduced criteria for diet and nutrition studies agreed upon by both Potischman and Weed (6) and the Committee on Diet and Health, Food and Nutrition Board, National Research Council (7).

FIGURE 6.3   Hill's criteria for causation. Adapted from reference 4.

EXAMPLE.   A highly significant association between salt intake and rise in blood pressure has been widely reported (strength of association). This finding

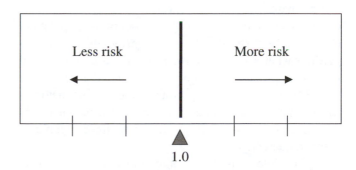

FIGURE 6.4   Relative risk.

is consistent regardless of the population studied (consistency of association). This association has been found regardless of other potential confounding influences, such as obesity or hypertensive versus normal blood pressure. (specificity of association). Higher salt intakes have been shown to lead to higher blood pressures and a reduction in salt intakes, to a lowering of blood pressures (temporal relationship). A dose-response relationship has been shown with salt intakes, with higher intakes resulting in higher blood pressures and lower intakes with lower blood pressures (biological gradient). Several well-known mechanisms for this relationship have been documented (biological plausibility). This association and its underlying mechanisms fit well with existing knowledge about blood pressure response (coherence). Finally, there is a large body of experimental evidence from animal studies and human clinical trials that has documented this relationship (evidence from experimentation). An important caveat to this summary is that several key questions remain unresolved regarding the relationship between salt intake and blood pressure (9), and ongoing research on this relationship continues to be pursued (6,10).

Diet and nutrition studies pose unique challenges in applying causal criteria (6,7). Evaluation of associations for causal effects in diet and nutrition studies (1) is complex, because frequent exceptions to the Hill criteria are encountered. Diet and nutrition factors have built-in measurement difficulties (for example, measurement error, lack of intake variation in population, and intake distributions unrelated to disease processes). Measurement problems can lead to serious underestimates of causal effects or evidence for causal effects that do not exist. Because everyone eats (that is, dietary exposures are common), somewhat small relative risks of 0.7 to 1.5 could be important (1). In contrast, exposures due to environmental contaminants or occupation would be "uncommon," because they would involve only a subset of the population. (It should be noted that there is considerable debate regarding what size of relative risk should be considered important. Some epidemiologists argue that risks less than 3.0 are likely to be spurious. Others argue that relative risks as low as 0.2 may be important if the factor has widespread exposure and is likely to have significant measurement error.)

Absolute consistency of findings is not a realistic expectation (1), and perfect specificity of associations is likely to be rare (7). This imperfect consistency and specificity could be due to the complexity of the disease process, the imprecision of diet measures, or the specific effects of diet components on organ systems or the disease processes (7). Dose-response relationships are likely to be "nonlinear or almost any shape depending on the starting point on a hypothetical spectrum of exposure" (1). Thus, typical analytic approaches may not detect underlying relationships. Also, a clear dose-response relationship might easily be the result of bias or confounding (1).

Biological plausibility, "post hoc, should be viewed cautiously because they can usually be developed for most observations, including those that are later refuted" (1). There is a lack of well-defined mechanisms for most cancers and many other chronic diseases (1). This fact hampers the ability to meet criteria for biological plausibility and coherence. Finally, experimental studies, particularly in human beings, would provide key evidence for causal relationships. Several practical considerations (time and money commitments) and ethical considerations limit the ability to carry out such investigations.

In light of these many concerns, it has been strongly suggested (6,7) that the Hill criteria are too stringent to apply to diet and nutrition studies. Instead, it has been recommended that a minimum set of causal criteria be used for these studies: consistency of findings, strength of association, dose response, biological plausibility, and temporality. This reduced set of criteria was used by the Committee on Diet and Health (Food and Nutrition Board of the National Academy of Sciences) for its landmark publication *Diet and Health: Implications for Reducing Chronic Disease Risk* (see Figure 6.3) (7).

EXAMPLE.   The Food and Drug Administration reviewed evidence for the relationship between periconceptional folic acid intake and neural tube defects (NTDs) in the early 1990s and subsequently implemented a policy for folic acid fortification of flours and cereals in the United States. Evidence from case-control studies and a prospective cohort study supported a consistent and strong association between occurrence of NTD and lower folic acid intakes, status, or both. A dose-response relationship was supported for prevention of NTD in both women who have never had a child with NTD and women who previously delivered a child with NTD. The temporality criterion was met, because folic acid supplementation appeared effective only when given during the specific critical neural tube fetal developmental period. Some experimental data were available from human studies (a British study and a Chinese study). Both provided credible evidence that folic acid supplementation in the periconceptional period significantly reduced the occurrence of NTD in women with previous NTD deliveries (the British study) and those without such a history (the Chinese study).

A recent critique of these studies has pointed to shortcomings, however. The British study provided a multivitamin supplement with or without folic acid; the Chinese study was nonrandomized, and supplements had to be purchased by the participant. Biomarkers of folic acid in the British study showed implausibly elevated serum levels, suggesting that multiple doses were taken just prior to blood drawing. Nonetheless, randomized double-blind supplement studies of folic acid alone are unlikely to be done because of ethical considerations (11).

Study Designs to Study Causation

As is typical of any scientific discipline, epidemiology uses experimental designs to study causation. In this type of study, the investigator randomizes individuals to treatment or no treatment (control group). General study designs (and relevant issues) for examining causation are discussed in detail in Chapter 2 and elsewhere in this monograph. In addition to the general design, epidemiologic investigations include designs that involve multiple study centers and extended follow-up, as well as designs that randomize groups rather than individuals to treatment or control groups. In the case of the multicentered studies with long-term follow-up, disease outcomes are compared for each randomization group usually controlled for center-specific effects. In the case of studies that randomize groups, disease outcomes are compared for each group.

ISSUES IN ANALYTIC NUTRITION EPIDEMIOLOGIC STUDIES

General issues relevant to any analytic nutrition epidemiology study design include the analytic nutrition epidemiology question, diet and/or nutrient exposures, problems resulting from poor exposure measurements, potential for other biases, and potential for confounding and multivariate relationships of diet and disease.

The Analytic Nutrition Epidemiology Question

From an epidemiologic perspective, nutrition can be viewed as a key factor affecting health and as a specific health/disease outcome. Nutrition studies often examine diet/nutrition as an outcome and analyze data for determinants of those outcomes. In epidemiologic studies, diet and nutrition are commonly studied as independent contributing factors (association) or independent causal factors (causation) of health/disease outcomes.

Diet and/or Nutrient Exposure

The term *exposure* refers to a factor's dose (that is, amount and concentration). A method of measurement is needed that will sufficiently capture differences that truly exist (1). The method needs to capture measurements of potential active agents and their doses. Dietary exposure measurements are challenging and have been an active area of research for more than four decades. Investigations of food safety problems can use food information from one point in time. Investigations of chronic diseases, which are major causes of debilitation and death, require diet and/or nutrient exposures that capture an extended period of intake behavior. The term *usual intake* is often used to connote this type of diet exposure. "Usual" intake is difficult to capture in the heterogeneous U.S. population, given its rapidly changing food marketplace and Americans' enthusiasm for food choice change. Given existing measurement problems, many investigators include more than one dietary assessment method and/or use other related measures of exposure, such as biological (for example, blood or urine) or molecular (for example, genetic) markers (12). Newer approaches are being developed and studied. Measurement methods for diet and/or nutrient exposures are discussed in Chapters 15 and 17.

The goals of the exposure measurement are to provide a reliable, accurate, and valid measurement of diet and/or nutrient exposure. Reliability is the characteristic in which repeated measurements done in a steady-state period yield similar results. Accuracy indicates that systematic error is minimized in the measurement (13). Validity is the degree to which a test is capable of measuring what it is intended to measure (13). None of these qualities can be corrected by increased sample size. To increase confidence in the reliability of the test, each subject can be tested at least twice (4). Random error may be mitigated through careful measurement and large sample size. However, random error cannot be completely eliminated and may be due to individual biological variation or residual sampling or measurement error (13).

Other diet and/or nutrient exposure considerations are important to the study design. Prior to mounting the study, evidence for sufficient variation in the diet or nutrient intake is needed. If everyone ate the same way, no differences in outcome with diet would be detected (1). Information about the latency period between diet exposure and disease is needed. A negative result from a 5-year cohort study might be due to a latency period of 10 years or longer between diet exposure and disease outcome. There may be a critical exposure period for a particular diet-disease relationship. For example, the critical period may be in childhood, with the disease manifesting itself in adulthood (1). Finally, the effects of diet and/or nutrient exposure may be acute and transient rather than long term.

Problems Resulting From Poor Exposure Measurements

In analytic epidemiology studies, poor measures in both comparison groups will make it impossible to detect existing associations. Poor measures in one of the groups can lead to findings of an association where none exists or association in the opposite direction (12). Diet and disease studies have inherent problems. Because of limited range of variation in the diet within most populations, in combination with the inevitable error in measuring intake, very modest relative risks (0.5 to 2.0) are usually found for diet effects. Because dietary intakes are an obligatory human behavior (in other words, everyone eats), even small risks associated with diet should be important (1). If risks were large, rougher exposure measures would capture those differences. However, smaller risks would require more refined exposure measures. Willett notes that typical dietary intake differences between cases and controls is only about 5 percent, and even a systematic error of 3 percent to 4 percent would seriously distort such a relationship (1). Furthermore, measurement errors would dilute or conceal any effect of diet on health/disease outcomes in experimental studies.

Potential for Other Biases

Systematic errors are also possible in epidemiologic studies through selection bias, other measurement bias, and analytic bias. Methodological sources of bias can obscure an existing relationship (1). Selection bias occurs when there is a systematic difference between the characteristics of people selected for the study and people who are not selected. For example, having some diseases may reduce a person's chance of being selected for a study (13). Several other subject selection biases are possible. The healthy-workers bias can be encountered in occupational epidemiology studies, where workers are likely to be healthier than people not working. There may be an increased likelihood of healthier and/or health-conscious and motivated individuals agreeing to participate in studies (volunteers bias). An incidence-prevalence bias (Neyman's bias) can also occur. This bias occurs where there is a loss of cases (by death or recovery) due to significant periods of time between exposure and development of the disorder. Finally, spurious differences between exposure and the disease can be due to differential hospitalization of cases and noncases with the exposure (Berkson's bias).

Measurement bias occurs when individual measurements or classifications of disease or exposure are inaccurate. Measurement bias that occurs equally in the groups being compared (nondifferential bias) almost always results in an underestimate of the true strength of the relationship (13). Recall bias can occur when the subject is aware of the study hypothesis. An information bias can occur where different quality and/or extent of information is obtained from exposed versus nonexposed subjects (2). A related problem is the Hawthorne effect, where the subject's performance changes because he or she is being studied. Measurement implementation problems can also occur (for example, quality control bias and nonstandardized measurement bias) (4). Blinding (where subjects are unaware of whether they are assigned to the treatment or the control group) is used in experimental studies to obviate subject measurement bias. Because knowledge about exposure status may bias assessment, outcome assessors may also be blinded to subject assignments or exposure status (2).

Bias may also be encountered in the analysis phase. Unintentional bias may occur in the data analyses and in interpretations of study findings if the investigators have strong study preconceptions (2).

Potential for Confounding

As illustrated in Figure 6.5, confounding relationships are relationships where the factor of interest is related to another factor that is also influencing the outcome of interest. Here the association can be explained by another factor associated with both the exposure and the disease

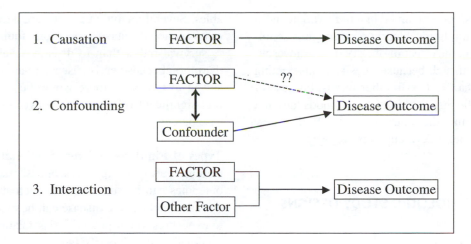

FIGURE 6.5 Comparison of predictive values.

(12). Confounding is not strictly a type of bias, because it does not result from systematic error in research design (13). Confounding occurs when there is a nonrandom distribution of risk factors in the source population that also occurs in the study population. For example, smoking can confound a relationship between coffee drinking and a disease outcome, because people who drink coffee are also more likely to smoke (2). Confounders can obscure or exaggerate existing associations (4). Another possibility is that an unmeasured third variable was related to the exposure and disease in an opposite direction, resulting in negative confounding (1).

The inability to control for confounding is a major limitation of descriptive epidemiologic findings. Analytic studies are designed to consider potential confounding factors when testing associations or causal relationships between key factors and disease outcomes. Analytic studies accomplish this goal through design features (for example, randomization, restriction, and matching) and analysis strategies (for example, stratification and statistical modeling). Randomization used in experimental studies can be designed to randomly distribute confounders to treatment and control groups. Restriction limits the study to people who have particular characteristics. Matching used in case-control studies selects controls to match cases by potential confounding factors to ensure that confounders are evenly distributed in the two groups being compared (13).

Potential for an Effect Modifier

An effect modifier (that is, an interaction) is a third variable that alters the association between an exposure and a disease outcome (see Figure 6.5) (14). With effect modi-

fication, the exposure may not have the same effect in all settings or subgroups of the population (12). For example, diet studies often separate gender and age groups, because diet may have a different effect on a particular outcome for these subgroups. Gender and age, in these cases, are considered effect modifiers. Another effect modifier may be genetic factors. A design strategy would be to randomize subjects to ensure that groups are balanced or to match controls on effect modifier variables (4). In large studies, it is usually preferable to control for confounding in the analytic phase. Stratified analyses are performed where measures of the strength of association are examined in well-defined and homogeneous categories (strata) of the confounding variable (13).

Multivariate Relationship of Diet and Disease

Willett (1) reminds us that diet and disease relationships are likely to be "extremely complex for both biologic and behavioral reasons." Food and nutrients are biologically complex. Nutrients are largely provided by food, so specific nutrients tend to be intercorrelated. There are nutrient-to-nutrient interactions where the effect of one nutrient depends on the level of another. What we eat and the quantity eaten are related to other health-related but nondiet factors such as age, gender, occupation, and behaviors (for example, smoking and exercise). All of these can distort, modify, or confound relationships of diet and disease.

Multivariate methods are needed to tease out and clarify the effect of diet and nutrition on outcomes. However, even these effects are complicated. Willett points to the example of the effect of obesity on cardiovascular disease. When obesity is examined in a multivariate model that includes serum lipids, blood pressure, glucose tolerance, and body fat, the effect of obesity on cardiovascular disease is diminished, because obesity is also acting through the other factors (1). In other words, because of inherent data problems, multivariate methods are not foolproof in discerning diet/nutrient effects. Rather, new study designs and future developments are needed.

ANALYTIC EPIDEMIOLOGIC STUDY DESIGNS

Study Designs for Examining Associations—Observational Studies

Cross-Sectional Studies

Cross-sectional epidemiologic studies, also called *prevalence studies* or *surveys* (15), are studies in which subjects are measured at approximately the same point in time. Both the exposure to a particular risk factor and disease outcome (case status) are determined at the same time (2,4). Although generally used for descriptive studies, they can also provide suggestive analytic information. Cross-sectional study data are commonly used to provide evidence for possible risk factors for disease outcomes (2).

Advantages and Disadvantages of Cross-Sectional Studies.   The key advantage of cross-sectional studies is that they are relatively simple and inexpensive, because neither follow-up measures nor treatment is required (4).

However, because of several inherent problems, cross-sectional studies are of limited utility in studying causal inference (16). Because measurements are made only at one point, the temporal relationship between exposure and disease outcomes cannot be tested (2). The problem of reverse causality bias can occur (16) where the disease outcome appears to precede the exposure in time (16). Furthermore, cross-sectional studies are likely to include survivors and new cases, (2) with early disease-related deaths missed.

Cross-Sectional Study Implementation Issues.   Key challenges in implementing cross-sectional studies include (1) the ability to ensure and verify reasonable sample representativeness, (2) the ability to capture "cases" (those with the disease outcome of interest), and (3) the ability to capture adequate variation in key exposure variables. Several analytic cautions are needed in examining cross-sectional data. Associations found may be related to survival rather than to disease development (2). Furthermore, because early disease-related deaths would result in lost "cases," there would be a reduced ability to find significant relationships between exposure and disease outcome.

Types of Findings in Cross-Sectional Studies.   Associations between exposures or risk factors and disease outcomes can be suggested. In such studies, individuals with and without the disease can be examined in relation to exposures, other potential risk factors, or both. Cross-sectional studies identify factors that may affect the level of a risk factor (5).

EXAMPLE.   The International Study of Salt and Blood Pressure (INTERSALT), conducted in 52 population samples worldwide, tested whether salt intake (as assessed by urinary sodium levels) was associated with higher blood pressures (17). INTERSALT found a linear positive relationship between sodium and blood pressure regardless of whether the individual was normotensive or hypertensive. Also, it found a rise in blood pressure with age only in those samples with higher salt intakes.

Suggestive evidence for the influence of other nutrients (for example, protein) on blood pressure led to the subsequent International Population Study on Macronutrients and Blood Pressure (INTERMAP). INTERMAP is a population-based epidemiologic investigation in 20 diverse samples from 4 countries (Japan, China, the United Kingdom, and the United States) from men and women aged 40 years to 59 years. It is currently in the data analyses phase.

Cohort Studies

Cohort studies track health information of individuals over a period of time (18). They provide a focus on disease development (19) and allow the study of the natural history of disease (16). An important feature of the cohort design is its time perspective on exposures. Concurrent cohort designs assess exposures as they occur during the study but are the most expensive (2). Retrospective studies examine exposures backward in time, and prospective studies look forward in time for exposures. A combined approach determines past exposure and provides follow-up of future exposures (2). Cohort studies are feasible for the study of common diseases where the exposure to risk factor(s) results in a measurable disease outcome within a reasonable time following the exposure. For practical reasons, cohort studies are not suitable for diseases with long latency periods (for example, 20 years) or for rare diseases requiring extraordinarily large sample sizes (18).

Advantages of Cohort Studies. Cohort studies offer several advantages. They can examine whether there is a temporal relationship between exposure and the disease. Furthermore, they can provide direct information on the temporal sequence of events (18) and can establish timing and directionality of events (4). Prospective cohort studies enable the measurement of diet before disease onset (1). They are easier and less costly than experimental studies (4). Finally, many diseases and exposures can be studied simultaneously (18).

Disadvantages of Cohort Studies. Cohort study designs have several disadvantages. Although they are less complex and costly than experimental studies, cohort studies are nonetheless expensive, resource intensive, and difficult, because they require the monitoring of large numbers of subjects over an extended period (18). They are ill suited for studies with long latency (16).

Cohort selection and recruitment is challenging, and sample randomness can be a problem (4). For example, people who refuse to volunteer may have particular characteristics, and their nonparticipation may bias the results (5). It may be difficult to find "nonexposed" individuals if exposure is popular (4). Groups may differ at the beginning of the study (the problem of confounding) (16).

Over the course of the study, subjects may change their behavior because of their being studied, and their exposure to the factor of interest may change (18). With long studies, subject nonresponse and loss to follow-up are likely problems (2). If the loss to follow-up is correlated with disease, risks associated with exposure will be diminished. If this loss is correlated with exposure, risk estimates will be biased (5).

Cohort Study Implementation Issues. Cohort studies are warranted (2) when there is good evidence for exposure leading to disease (clinical observations, case-control studies, and so on) and a relatively short interval between exposure and development of disease. However, there may be disagreement on what constitutes strong evidence, and diseases of interest may have low rates of occurrence (2). To obviate problems with participant recall

of exposures (18), retrospective studies are possible if there are appropriate and adequate past records (2). There are practical limits, however, because even common diseases such as heart disease require a cohort size in the thousands (1).

It is becoming increasingly common for large intervention studies to mount postintervention follow-up studies of participants after the main studies have been completed. Examples of these types of cohort studies include participants in the Multiple Risk Factor Intervention Trial, the Modification of Diet in Renal Disease Study, and the Trials of Hypertension Prevention Study. For example, 7 years after the completion of the Trials of Hypertension Prevention Phase 1 Study, Baltimore investigators (19) recontacted Baltimore participants and ascertained their hypertension status; measured their blood pressures, heights, and weights; and collected 24-hour urine samples for sodium and creatinine measurement. About 40 percent had developed hypertension. However, the investigators found that previous weight loss and sodium reduction participants had lower odds of developing hypertension compared with controls (OR = 0.23 and 0.65). Approximately 19 percent of weight-loss participants and 22.4 percent of sodium-reduction participants had developed hypertension (20).

Among the analytic considerations in cohort studies, assessment of the disease outcome and the selection of the nonexposed comparison group are key. Because there may be changes over time in relevant criteria and methods of assessment, ensuring comparability of repeated measures will be crucial (2). Key information on subjects lost to follow-up (for example, disease occurrence or death) is important to capture. Specific analyses are required to account for such losses.

Types of Findings in Cohort Studies. In cohort studies, exposed and nonexposed groups measured at baseline and followed over time are compared for disease incidence or deaths. Data are collected at two or more distinct time points (at baseline and in follow-up) (21). Subjects presumably are comparable from one period to the next (21). Data are compared between and among these periods (21), specifically for the incidence of disease (or new occurrence of the disease outcome) in those individuals exposed and not exposed to the risk factors of interest. Measurements generated express the proportion of the exposed who get the disease (or die) compared with those not exposed (2). These measurements can be in terms of relative risks, odds ratios, and attributable risk ratios (2).

EXAMPLE. The Iowa Women's Study, which began in 1986, was a prospective cohort study of randomly selected (from Iowa driver's license lists) women aged 55 years to 69 years. Of the approximately 98,000 selected women, 41,837 completed a mailed health questionnaire (on smoking, family cancer history, breast cancer risk factors, reported height and weight, and measured waist and hip circumference) and a Willett food frequency questionnaire (22). After 10 years of follow-up, 438 subjects had died of coronary heart disease and 131 of strokes. Flavonoids, phenolic compounds with antioxidant properties found in fruits and vegetables (23), were found to reduce the relative risk of coronary heart disease (but not strokes) by 40 percent in the subjects in the highest, as compared with the lowest, quintile of intakes, after controlling for age and energy intake.

Case-Control Studies

The case-control design is very popular among epidemiologists examining diet and nutrition questions. Case-control studies examine cases (individuals with disease) and controls (those without disease) for risk factor or prior exposure differences (2,4,18). Controls are matched with cases on characteristics correlated with possible disease causes. These characteristics are not independent causes but are involved in the pathway through which the possible causes of interest lead to disease. As compared with the cohort study, which starts with exposure, the case-control study starts with identification of diseased individuals. In other words, case-control studies compare diseased and nondiseased individuals, whereas cohort studies examine exposed and not-exposed individuals. Case-control studies are well suited for studies of rare disorders and studies where the lag time between exposure and outcome is long (16).

Advantages of Case-Control Studies. Case-control studies offer several advantages. They are relatively quick and inexpensive, and they require smaller sample sizes than cross-sectional or cohort studies. Because investigators can set the criteria for selecting controls, they can untangle potential confounding factors and interactions more precisely (2,18,19). Matching increases reliability and decreases the costs of study (19).

Disadvantages of Case-Control Studies. Case-control studies have a number of disadvantages. By design, case-control studies can investigate only one disease outcome

(18). Information about relevant exposures may be problematic. There may be significant differences in quality of information with cases researched more thoroughly (18). Cases and controls are likely to have different recall of specific exposures and events relevant to the studied disease outcome (16). For example, illness can affect recall of diet (1). Reliance on records to determine exposure may be equally inadequate for exposure determination (18). Furthermore, because case-control studies do not involve a time sequence, it would not be possible to demonstrate temporal causality between specific exposures and disease outcomes (18).

Other disadvantages of case-control studies arise from their intrinsic complexity. The selection of cases and controls, although seemingly straightforward, is challenging. Case-control studies can suffer from bias error, given the problem of sampling of controls (18). The selection of controls is an ongoing area of methodological concern (16). Finding suitable control matches is especially difficult where multiple matching factors are required. Additionally, there is the temptation to overmatch (2), or use unnecessary matching. Here the matching variable is related to the risk factor or disease under study but is not a true confounder or is so highly correlated with other matching variables as to be superfluous. Overmatching results in loss of efficiency and may also result in bias (18).

Another disadvantage is that specific complex analyses are required for case-control data. Data analysis for matched analyses is more complex to compute and understand. Furthermore, any variable used as a matching variable cannot be estimated (2,18). For example, if controls were matched on age and race, it would not be possible to examine the effect of age or race on the disease studied.

Case-Control Study Implementation Issues. The selection of cases and controls for case-control studies is a critical but complex issue. Given the problem of case misclassification, investigators need to specify how cases are identified or ascertained (2,19). Case selection should be based on a formulated, precise disease definition (18) with inclusion and exclusion criteria specified to increase the likelihood of exposure to the risk factor of interest (2,18). New (incident) cases are preferred, because the risk factor being studied may be avoided by those who already have the condition—that is, existing cases. For example, diet changes may occur following diagnosis. Additionally, cases may be lost prior to or soon after being diagnosed, and cases found may reflect survival rather than sickness (2,18).

A reliable source (18) for cases needs to be identified. Potential sources include hospitals, primary care practices, clinics, and health maintenance organizations. Disease-specific patient registries are an additional case source. However, case selection from a single source can be problematic. The patient population is likely to reflect referral patterns or other local factors and limit the ability to generalize study findings to other patients with that disease. For example, cases from a hospital that is a tertiary care facility may be severely ill (2), whereas other cases may be less ill or have less complicated illnesses.

Controls are defined as individuals who had an equal chance of exposure to a risk factor, had some potential for getting the disease, but do not have the disease (18). Ideally, controls are similar to cases in all respects other than having the disease in question. Conceptually, controls are representative of people without the disease from the same population as the cases. Controls are selected to "match" specific characteristics of cases, such as age, race, gender, or socioeconomic status (2). The purpose of matching is to adjust for potential confounding. There may be many differences between cases and controls beside exposure. Matched characteristics are those that potentially influence the disease outcome and are also related to the exposure being studied. For example, age and gender are commonly used matching factors, because they often influence disease status. Controls are selected to match case characteristics that are of concern. Matching, by direct control of confounders, may reduce the required sample size or use a shorter exposure period for a risk factor.

Ideally, the selection of controls would be a probability sample of the population. Such recruitment can be resource intensive, because only 60 percent to 70 percent of control eligibles are likely to complete study interviews (1). In practice, controls are recruited from various sources. Hospital controls and controls drawn from patient care lists are convenient, are inexpensive, and presumably can provide comparable medical data. However, this source is not foolproof, given the likelihood of differential rates of hospitalization (Berkson's bias) and potentially similar exposure to risk factors with different diseases (18)—for example, the use of antioxidant supplements for cardiovascular disease and cancer.

Community controls are presumably from the same population as cases. Community sources include school rosters, selective service lists, and insurance company lists. Random-digit dialing is frequently used to draw a random community sample, because the first three digits of telephone numbers generally match neighborhood boundaries. Nonetheless, the random-sampling frame is difficult to obtain and is expensive and time-consuming

(18). Whatever recruitment frame is used, volunteers tend to be health conscious (1) and are not actually representative of the population. A "best friend" control is usually similar in age and other demographic and social characteristics. Alternatively, spouses or siblings (genetic controls) are sometimes used.

Multiple controls are used per case in some studies. They can be the same type of controls or controls of a different type (2). In general, the greater number of controls per case, the greater precision in estimates and tests (2). Power (one measure of precision) increases as the number of controls increases for a fixed number of cases (18). Nonetheless, precision improvements are small beyond a case-to-control ratio above 1:4. Controls of a different type might be used for specific analyses (2). For example, the investigator might be interested in using hospital controls to control for the effect of hospitalization but would also want neighborhood controls to control for social and/or environmental influences.

Alternate Case-Control Study Designs. Other approaches to the case-control design have been used. One is the nested case-control study; the other is the frequency matching approach. In the nested case-control study design, cases are identified from an ongoing cohort study, with controls drawn from that same study (18). Baseline and follow-up data on exposures, risk factors, and disease status are collected from the cohort study. Cases are identified during the course of follow-up, and controls are selected from the cohort (2). This design combines the efficiencies and strengths of both the cohort and case-control designs. The Harvard studies (the Physicians' Health Study, the Nurses' Health Study, and the Health Professionals' Health Study) and other cohort studies (the Western Electric Study and the Cardiovascular Health Study) have used the nested case-control design with their cohorts.

Technically, frequency matching is not a case-control design. As such, it does not require the stringent analyses procedures of that type of design. This approach ensures that the control sample and the case sample have a similar makeup (18). Control matching is done so that the proportion with a certain characteristic is similar among cases and controls (group or frequency matching)—for example, both cases and controls are 50 percent women (2). With this type of matching, controls are selected after all of the cases are identified (2).

Analytic Considerations in Case-Control Studies. The drawback to matching is that the matching factor's effect on the outcome cannot be estimated. For example, if marital status is a matching factor, distribution of marital status between cases and controls would be the same. Specific techniques for the analysis of case-control data are detailed in several epidemiology methods texts. The reader is referred to these for in-depth instructions in performing more advanced analyses beyond general odds ratios. (See the Further Reading at the end of the chapter.)

Types of Findings in Case-Control Studies.   The case-control analysis generates an estimate of relative risk known as the *odds ratio*. It gives the odds of having the disease with a specific exposure level or risk factor. Additionally, it can provide an estimate of the attributable risk associated with the specific exposure level or risk factor (16).

EXAMPLE.   Ascherio et al conducted a case-control study of 239 patients with myocardial infarctions who were admitted to 6 local hospitals, and 282 population controls. Using a food frequency assessment, they found that after controlling for age and energy intake, the highest quintile (compared with the lowest quintile) of *trans* fatty acid intakes was associated with a significantly higher (odds ratio = 2.4; confidence interval = 1.4 to 4.2) risk of coronary heart disease (CHD). This relationship was still significant after controlling for other CHD risk factors and other dietary variables, including other fats, dietary cholesterol, vitamins C and E, carotene, and fiber. Because the intakes of cases were assessed after the patients had been hospitalized, the authors assessed the possibility that the hospitalization and diagnosis of myocardial infarction may have influenced recall of the "usual" diet. The investigators excluded cases who reported that they had had "high cholesterols" prior to their myocardial infarction who had changed their intake of butter to margarine in the previous 10 years, or who were on a "special diet" (24).

EXAMPLE.   Many prospective cohort study investigators have taken the opportunity to conduct nested case-control studies. Cases that develop within the cohort are matched with controls from the same cohort. Measures of key variables prior to the disease occurrence are available for controls and cases. Controls are usually selected based on specific characteristics that are likely to be confounders.

An example of such a study was one conducted

with data from the Physicians' Health Study. Chasan-Taber et al investigated whether folate and vitamin B-6 levels, cofactors in homocysteine metabolism, influenced the risk of myocardial infarction in this cohort. Cases occurring within 7.5 years' follow-up (n = 333) were matched by age and smoking status with controls (no prior myocardial infarction at the time of the case's diagnosis). Baseline plasma samples were assayed for folate and pyridoxal phosphate (a form of vitamin B-6) levels. After controlling for other known risk factors for myocardial infarction, low folate and vitamin B-6 levels were found to contribute to the risk of myocardial infarction, but not significantly. The authors suggest that weak folate and vitamin B-6 measurements (that is, a single measure insufficient to characterize long-term status) and the small proportion of physicians who might have low intakes severely limited their ability to detect significant relationships (25).

Study Designs for Examining Causation—Etiologic Studies

Randomized Controlled Trials

The clinical trial or randomized controlled trial (RCT) is the most efficient design for investigating a causal relationship between a treatment and its effect and is considered the gold standard for testing the effectiveness of clinical and public health therapeutic and preventive measures (2). Its essential features are the planned allocation of subjects to treatment (that is, randomization) (18) and the experimenter-controlled level of exposure (4). Randomization is used to overcome selection bias and to ensure that confounders are equally distributed among groups. In other words, randomization's goal is to ensure that the observed difference at the study's end can be directly attributable to the study factor (16), that is, the experimental treatment. Other specific features of the RCT are discussed in Chapter 7 and elsewhere in this monograph.

Group-Randomized Trials

Group-randomized trials are clinical trials where identifiable groups rather than individuals are allocated to treatment or control conditions (18,26). More trials of this type are likely to be fielded as effective prevention strategies are identified through usual RCT methodology. In the 1980s, three well-designed community trials for heart disease prevention were conducted in the United States: the Minnesota Heart Health Trial, the Stanford Five-City Project, and the Pawtucket Heart Health Program. Each of these trials included a comprehensive intervention focusing on established risk factors and using state-of-the-art behavioral strategies (27). The risk factors included cigarette smoking, hypertension, and elevated serum cholesterol levels. In the early 1990s, physician practice–based randomized clinical trials for heart disease prevention were conducted. (28,29) Neither the community trials (30) nor the physician practice–based trials (28,29) showed significant treatment effects. Building on that experience, substantial methodological research on group-randomized trials has accelerated (26) and continues to be pursued.

Advantages of the Group-Randomized Trial. The group-randomized trial design allows the investigator to examine the effects of interventions that operate at the group level, where the physical or social environment is manipulated or cannot be delivered to individuals (26). For example, the physician practice trials previously mentioned tested the efficacy of heart disease prevention interventions delivered by randomly selected physician practice groups as compared with control practice groups. The group-randomized trial provides the opportunity to directly test the experimental treatment in its "natural" environment. Thus, group-randomized trials are more likely to provide key information on the generalizability of the intervention (that is, its external validity). They offer an experimental framework to test public health strategies.

Disadvantages of the Group-Randomized Trial. Although group-randomized trials seem simple and straightforward, recent methodological work has uncovered serious pitfalls in carrying them out. Important among these pitfalls are design and analysis issues. Given its inherent statistical properties, the group-randomized trial requires a larger sample size, careful attention to potential subgroups and outcomes, and a sophisticated analysis plan. Because of these previously underappreciated complexities, studies with null findings are common. Additionally, there is a need for stronger interventions that can produce detectable significant effects. Pooled analysis of the three community-based trials previously mentioned found that results were still below expectations even when adequate power was available (30). Results below expectations were also found in subsequent

group-randomized studies with strong design and analytic plans (for example, the Child and Adolescent Trial for Cardiovascular Health) (26,31).

Statistical Issues in Group-Randomized Trials. The specific statistical considerations for group-randomized trials are crucial. However, they are beyond the scope of this chapter. Instead, the reader is referred to Murray's seminal textbook (26) and the current literature in this area. Finally, although most research design and implementation would benefit from statistical advice, this type of input is a requirement for group-randomized trials because of the complexity and evolving nature of this methodology.

More research is needed to understand the best approaches to collecting outcome data that are likely to capture significant differences. Some investigators have suggested the use of end point data at the community level (indicators) rather than measurements at the expensive individual level. Another approach is the use of more frequent, small surveys of randomly selected samples of the population or subgroups rather than infrequent, large surveys to capture end point trends (26).

Rooney and Murray (32) found that stronger intervention effects were detectable in studies with greater methodological rigor. These studies were characterized by the use of appropriate group-randomized trial methods; that is, they were planned from the start to use the assignment unit for the analysis unit, they used a sufficient number of randomized assignment units for each condition, they adjusted for baseline differences in important confounding variables, they had extended follow-up, and they limited dropout and loss to follow-up. Also, smaller identifiable groups for assignment units (for example, worksites, physician practices, schools, and churches) may be better for detecting intervention effects. This makes sense, because it is likely to be more difficult to change the "health behavior and risk profile of an entire heterogeneous community rather than in smaller identifiable groups" (26).

EXAMPLE. The Child and Adolescent Trial for Cardiovascular Health (CATCH) was a multicenter group-randomized trial conducted in four field sites (San Diego, Houston, New Orleans, and Minneapolis) over a 3-year period. Each of the four field sites recruited 24 eligible schools that had agreed to randomization to intervention or control groups and to completing study measurements and intervention activities. Fifty-six of the 96 schools were randomized to intervention, with half receiving a school-based intervention alone and the other half receiving a family intervention as well. The primary end points were individual serum cholesterol levels and, at the school level, amounts of fat and sodium in school lunches and time spent in vigorous physical activity. A baseline survey was completed of 60.4 percent of eligible third graders ($n \approx 5,000$ students) in the CATCH schools. Follow-up individual measures were done when these children completed the third, fourth, and fifth grades with about 80 percent completing final measurements. School measurements for school lunches and physical activity were completed at the same intervals. CATCH found a significant improvement in school measurements and a nonsignificant improvement in serum cholesterol measurements. The investigators suggested that the limited time and resources for the intervention resulted in a weaker-than-desirable effect (26,31).

Multicentered Randomized Controlled Trials

The essential and obvious difference between the standard single-center RCT and the multicentered RCT is the number of involved centers. The multicentered RCT offers the capability of examining questions that would be impractical for single-center RCT due to sample size or resource limitations and for which there is an adequate pool of interested and qualified investigators (33). The questions addressed by multicentered RCTs arise from observational, basic science and evidence from small clinical trials, especially if these data are inconclusive or conflicting and indicate the need for a larger and/or more diverse subject pool (33).

Advantages of the Randomized Controlled Trial. Randomized controlled trials efficiently examine questions that require a larger number of subjects and/or study groups or subgroups (for example, minority inclusions, geographic spread, and rural/urban residence). They offer greater possibility for a more heterogeneous study population, thereby providing a broader basis for generalization of findings. Multiple centers are able to expedite the recruitment and follow-up of eligible subjects to meet trial requirements. Also, economies of scale are offered. RCTs can afford central laboratory and reading centers, as well as dedicated resource centers for quality control, performance monitoring, and data analysis (for example,

a data-coordinating center). Overall, these RCTs result in less cost per patient.

Disadvantages of the Randomized Controlled Trial. In the more heterogeneous sample that characterizes the RCT, it is more difficult to detect treatment differences. A larger sample size is required. The RCT is characteristically administratively complex; it often includes multiple principal investigators, a steering committee, a data-coordinating center, an external safety monitoring board, and specific central laboratory and other measurement reading and coding centers. The RCT requires a complex organizational structure to link centers. These administrative complexities are cumbersome, but essential. Although there is less cost per subject, the overall cost of these studies is large.

Randomized Controlled Trial Implementation Issues. The RCT is collaborative and requires cooperative work, which is not easily accomplished. Study personnel are located at various centers. It is necessary to maintain communications and decision-making structures because the study requires uniformity in study procedures. Performance of study methods and procedures requires supervision and documentation. Quality control requires standard application of measurements and intervention in multiple sites with multiple staff over several years.

Randomized Controlled Trial Findings and Analyses Issues. In RCTs, issues of findings and analyses are similar to the single-centered RCT. The one exception is the likely need to adjust for center-specific effects in the analyses.

EXAMPLE. An example of a multicentered RCT was the Trial of Hypertension Prevention (TOHP) Phase I Study. Ten geographically dispersed centers recruited 2,182 participants aged 35 years to 54 years with high-normal blood pressures (diastolic blood pressure of 80 mm Hg to 89 mm Hg). Phase I tested lifestyle interventions (weight loss, sodium reduction, and stress reduction) over an 18-month period and nutrient supplements (potassium, calcium, magnesium, and fish oil) over a 6-month period for their blood pressure effect compared with controls. An average weight loss of 3.2 kg resulted in a significant blood pressure reduction (diastolic/systolic) of 2.9/2.4 mm Hg, and a sodium reduction of 44 mmol resulted in a significant 2.1/1.2 mmHg reduction. Neither the stress reduction nor the supplements demonstrated a significant short-term blood pressure reduction. TOHP Phase II tested sodium reduction and weight loss alone in combination as compared with controls for their long-term blood pressure effects (34,35).

REFERENCES

1. Willett W. Overview of nutritional epidemiology. In: *Nutritional Epidemiology*. 2nd ed. New York, NY: Oxford University Press; 1998:3–17.
2. Gordis L. *Epidemiology*. Philadelphia, Pa: WB Saunders; 1996.
3. Kelsey JL, Petitti DB, King AC. Key methodologic concepts and issues. In: Brownson RC, Petitti DB, eds. *Applied Epidemiology*. New York, NY: Oxford University Press; 1998:35–70.
4. Streiner DL, Norman GR. *PDQ Epidemiology*. 2nd ed. St. Louis, Mo: Mosby-Year Book, Inc; 1996.
5. Freudenheim JL. A review of study designs and methods of dietary assessment in nutritional epidemiology of chronic disease. *J Nutr*. 1993;123:401–405.
6. Potischman N, Weed DL. Causal criteria in nutritional epidemiology. *Am J Clin Nutr*. 1999;69(suppl): 1309–1314.
7. Committee on Diet and Health. Methodologic considerations in evaluating the evidence. In: Food and Nutrition Board, Commission on Life Sciences, National Research Council, eds. *Diet and Health: Implications for Reducing Chronic Disease Risk*. Washington, DC: National Academy Press; 1989:23–40.
8. Chrysant GS, Bakir S, Oparil S. Dietary salt reduction in hypertension—what is the evidence and why is it still controversial? *Prog Cardiovasc Dis*. 1999;42:23–38.
9. Chobanian AV, Hill M. *Summary Report: The NHLBI Workshop on Sodium and Blood Pressure: A Critical Review of Current Scientific Evidence*. Bethesda, Md: National Institutes of Health, NHLBI; 1999.
10. Elmer PJ, Grimm RH Jr, Flack J, Laing B. Dietary sodium reduction for hypertension prevention and treatment. *Hypertension*. 1991;17(suppl):I182–189.
11. Rayburn WF, Stanley JR, Garrett E. Periconceptional folate intake and neural tube defects. *J Am Coll Nutr*. 1996;15:121–125.
12. Brownson RC. Epidemiology: the foundation of public health. In: Brownson RC, Petitti DB, eds. *Applied Epidemiology*. New York, NY: Oxford University Press; 1998:3–34.
13. Beaglehole R, Bonita R, Kjellstrom T. *Basic Epidemiology*. Geneva, Switzerland: World Health Organization; 1993.
14. Freudenheim JL. Study design and hypothesis testing: issues in the evaluation of evidence from research in nutritional epidemiology. *Am J Clin Nutr*. 1999;69(suppl): 1315–1321.
15. Gerstman BB. Measures of association and potential impact. In: *Epidemiology Kept Simple: An Introduction to Classic and Modern Epidemiology*. New York, NY: Wiley-Liss, Inc; 1998:120–138.
16. Gerstman BB. Analytic study designs. In: *Epidemiology Kept Simple: An Introduction to Classic and Modern Epidemiology*. New York, NY: Wiley-Liss, Inc; 1998:139–160.
17. Stamler J. The INTERSALT Study: background, methods, findings, and implications. *Am J Clin Nutr*. 1997;65(suppl):626–642.
18. Woodward M. Fundamental issues. In: *Epidemiology: Study Design and Data Analysis*. Boca Raton, Fla: Chapman & Hall/CRC; 1999:1–30.
19. Friedman GD. *Primer of Epidemiology*. 4th ed. New York, NY: McGraw-Hill; 1994.
20. He J, Whelton PK, Appel LJ, Charleston J, Klag MJ. Long-term effects of weight loss and dietary sodium reduction on incidence of hypertension. *Hypertension*. 2000;35:544–549.
21. Sempos CT, Liu K, Ernst ND. Food and nutrient exposures: what to consider when evaluating epidemiologic evidence. *Am J Clin Nutr*. 1999;69(suppl):1330–1339.
22. Zhang S, Folsom AR, Sellers TA, Kushi LH, Potter JD. Better breast cancer survival for postmenopausal women who are less overweight and eat less fat. *Cancer*. 1995;76:275–283.
23. Yochum L, Kushi LH, Meyer K, Folsom AR. Dietary flavonoid intake and risk of cardiovascular disease in postmenopausal women. *Am J Epidemiol*. 1999;149:943–949.
24. Ascherio A, Hennekens CH, Buring JE, Master C, Stampfer MJ, Willett WC. Trans fatty acids intake and risk of myocardial infarction. *Circulation*. 1994;89:94–101.
25. Chasan-Taber L, Selhub J, Rosenberg IH, et al. A prospective study of folate and vitamin B_6 and risk of myocardial infarction in US physicians. *J Am Coll Nutr*. 1996;15:136–143.
26. Murray DM. *Design and Analysis of Group-Randomized Trials Design and Analysis of Group-Randomized Trials*. New York, NY: Oxford University Press; 1998.
27. Shea S, Basch CE. A review of five major community-based cardiovascular disease prevention programs. Part I. Rationale, design, and theoretical framework. *Am J Health Promot*. 1990;4:203–213.
28. Caggiula AW, Watson JE, Kuller LH, et al. Cholesterol-lowering intervention program. Effect of the step I diet in

community office practices. *Arch Intern Med.* 1996;156:1205–1213.

29. Keyserling TC, Ammerman AS, Davis CE, Mok MC, Garrett J, Simpson R Jr. A randomized controlled trial of a physician-directed treatment program for low-income patients with high blood cholesterol: the Southeast Cholesterol Project. *Arch Fam Med.* 1997;6:135–145.

30. Winkleby MA, Feldman HA, Murray DM. Joint analysis of three U.S. community intervention trials for reduction of cardiovascular disease risk. *J Clin Epidemiol.* 1997;50:645–658.

31. Luepker RV, Perry CL, McKinlay SM, et al. Outcomes of a field trial to improve children's dietary patterns and physical activity: The Child and Adolescent Trial for Cardiovascular Health (CATCH). *JAMA.* 1996;275:768–776.

32. Rooney BL, Murray DM. A meta-analysis of smoking prevention programs after adjustment for errors in the unit of analysis. *Health Educ Q.* 1996;23:48–64.

33. Meinert CL, Tonascia S. *Clinical Trials: Design, Conduct, and Analysis.* New York, NY: Oxford University Press; 1986.

34. Whelton PK, Kumanyika SK, Cook NR, et al. Efficacy of nonpharmacologic interventions in adults with high-normal blood pressure: results from phase 1 of the Trials of Hypertension Prevention. *Am J Clin Nutr.* 1997;65(suppl): 652–660.

35. The Trials of Hypertension Prevention Collaborative Research Group. Effects of weight loss and sodium reduction intervention on blood pressure and hypertension incidence in overweight people with high-normal blood pressure. The Trials of Hypertension Prevention, phase II. *Arch Intern Med.* 1997;157:657–667.

Further Reading

Brownson RC, Petitti DB, eds. *Applied Epidemiology.* New York, NY: Oxford University Press; 1998.

Kushi LH. Vitamin E and heart disease: a case study. *Am J Clin Nutr.* 1999.69(suppl):1322–1329.

Lilienfeld DE, Stolley PD. *Foundations of Epidemiology.* New York, NY: Oxford University Press; 1994.

MacMahon B, Trichopoulos D. *Epidemiology: Principles and Methods.* Boston, Mass: Little, Brown & Co; 1996.

Rothman KJ, Greenland S. *Modern Epidemiology.* Philadelphia, Pa: Lippincott-Raven Publishers; 1998.

Schlesselman JJ. *Case-Control Studies: Design, Conduct, Analysis.* New York, NY: Oxford University Press; 1982.

Szklo M, Nieto FJ. *Epidemiology: Beyond the Basics.* Gaithersburg, Md: Aspen Publishers; 1999.

Willett W. *Nutritional Epidemiology.* 2nd ed. New York, NY: Oxford University Press; 1999.

7

Designing, Managing, and Conducting a Clinical Nutrition Study

Barbara H. Dennis, Ph.D., R.D., and P.M. Kris-Etherton, Ph.D., R.D.

A clinical nutrition study is a specialized scientific approach used to examine many questions related to effects of dietary components on metabolic parameters and health outcomes. The results of these studies are important for making dietary recommendations for healthy populations, for individuals at high risk for certain diseases, and for persons with medical conditions that require medical nutrition therapy. In this chapter, a controlled clinical nutrition study is an intervention in which dietary modification is the independent or predictive variable. The number of subjects studied can vary and is dependent on the end points selected and power calculations that are used to establish the appropriate number of subjects required to test the hypothesis rigorously. Some small clinical studies are adequately powered with as few as 4 to 6 subjects, whereas other studies may require 20 to 30 subjects or more. The intervention may take the form of a well-controlled feeding study where all food is carefully measured and monitored, nutrient supplements are added to the subjects' usual diet, prepackaged diets are delivered to the subjects, or food is selected by subjects according to specified guidelines. Clinical studies are designed to have one or more treatment groups, as well as a control group (1).

Whatever the site of the clinical nutrition study—in an inpatient facility, academic setting, or other research setting—dietitians play a key role in designing, implementing, analyzing, and interpreting the results. This chapter explores issues involved in designing a controlled clinical nutrition study using techniques and methods covered in detail elsewhere in this book. Specifically, it discusses the essential components necessary to design and conduct a well-controlled, small clinical nutrition study, most frequently conducted in a single center. The interested reader is referred to an excellent reference that presents an in-depth overview of all aspects of conducting well-controlled diet studies in humans (2). In addition, unique situations that may be encountered in clinical nutrition studies are discussed in-depth by Most et al (3).

Designing a clinical nutrition study involves a series of steps that specify exactly why, how, and with whom the study will be carried out, as well as how the results will be interpreted. This process culminates in the study protocol (Figure 7.1). The protocol contains all the necessary information for carrying out the study. It is the written agreement between the investigator, the participant, and the scientific community (4), and it forms the basis for informed consent and institutional review board decisions on human subject safety. In the following sections, each aspect of the protocol is discussed in detail.

JUSTIFICATION FOR THE STUDY

The first step in planning a controlled clinical nutrition study is to identify and document the need for the study. What currently unavailable information will such a study yield, and why will the information be important? Various sources provide information on important and timely nutrition research needs. Agencies of the Public Health Service, the U.S. Department of Agriculture, and the

Introduction
- Inclusion and exclusion criteria
- Recruitment
- Screening procedures

Diet
- Precisely defined diet, menus, and feeding protocol

Study procedures
- Sample size
- Randomization
- Monitoring, compliance, retention, and termination
- Measurements and methods

Statistical statement
- Data variables
- Data collection
- Analyses

FIGURE 7.1 Protocol for a controlled clinical nutrition study.

Bureau of the Census frequently publish statistical reports for national and specialized populations. In addition, similar information is often available at the state level in health departments (see Further Reading). Workshop proceedings and task force reports, such as the *Third Report on Nutrition Monitoring in the United States* (5), the National Academy of Science publication *Diet and Health* (6), and *Healthy People 2010* (7), identify research needs. The National Institutes of Health *Guide for Grants and Contracts*, published weekly and available on-line (http://www.nih.gov/grants/guide), identifies specific research topics of interest to particular institutes. Once the need for a clinical trial has been identified, a thorough literature review will establish the extent of knowledge and activity in the area and provide information about promising ideas for further research.

STUDY OBJECTIVES AND HYPOTHESES

The objectives of the study should be clearly defined at the outset. Objectives are statements of the research question the study is designed to answer. They determine the design and duration of the study, selection of subjects, and statistical analysis of the results.

A hypothesis is an assertion that an association between two or more variables or a difference between two or more groups exists in the larger population of interest (8). The statistical test is performed on the null statement—that is, no association exists. Examples of hypotheses and null statements are shown in Table 7.1.

STUDY DESIGN

The clinical study should be designed to test at least one major hypothesis. This hypothesis plays a seminal role in guiding the design of the study, as well as the number of subjects studied. The resultant data are an important feature of the ensuing publications. Multiple hypotheses increase the number of statistical tests that are required. They can reduce the power of the study (the probability of rejecting the null hypothesis if it is false) by increasing the number of statistically significant findings that can occur by chance alone (4). Typically, this problem is addressed by identifying primary and secondary hypotheses. Primary hypotheses test the most important question or questions, and the inclusion of secondary hypotheses provides an opportunity to address additional questions with the ongoing study in a way that does not compromise the primary hypotheses. An example of a primary hypothesis is the effect of specific micronutrients on blood pressure; a secondary hypothesis that could be addressed is how the experimental diet affects other risk factors for cardiovascular disease.

Objectives and hypotheses of the study determine the degree of dietary control. In general, studies designed to evaluate the effects of individual nutrients on regulation of metabolic pathways require tighter control and more extensive resources than studies where behavioral components, such as compliance, are part of the study

TABLE 7.1 Examples of Hypotheses and Null Statements

Hypothesis	Null Statement
Myristic acid impairs insulin sensitivity compared with linoleic acid.	Myristic acid does not impair insulin sensitivity compared with linoleic acid.
A high-protein, hypocaloric, calorie-controlled diet results in greater weight loss than a low-fat, high-carbohydrate, hypocaloric, calorie-controlled diet.	A high-protein, hypocaloric, calorie-controlled diet does not result in greater weight loss than a low-fat, high-carbohydrate, hypocaloric, calorie-controlled diet.

aims. An example of a highly controlled feeding study is one that examines how the type and amount of dietary fat affects plasma lipids, lipoproteins, and hemostatic factors; in such a study it is important to weigh all sources of dietary fat (9). In contrast, in a study designed to evaluate the effects of macronutrient composition on satiety, foods could be measured using household measures and not weighed to the nearest milligram.

Statistical expertise is critical in the design phase of the study, as well as in the analysis of results. Thus, it is essential to seek the advice of an experienced statistician in the early planning stages of the study. It is also essential to have a statistician actively involved while the study is ongoing. This latter point is particularly important because decisions made as the study is conducted will affect the eventual data analysis.

STUDY PROCEDURES

Study procedures are the detailed specifications for carrying out the protocol. The procedures selected for use are determined by the study hypotheses, specific objectives, and the study design selected. The procedures will vary from being very intensive to less intensive. The procedures that are chosen will have a large impact on the resources that are required for the study, as well as the budget that is needed to conduct the study. Thus, it is critical that study procedures be defined in detail prior to the start of the study. Investigators can then assess the feasibility of conducting the study.

RESOURCES

The next step is to assess the resources needed to carry out the study. This assessment usually involves obtaining approval of the institutional review board and determining the level of administrative support needed for the study. Intervention studies based on self-selected diets need facilities for instruction, cooking demonstrations, and diet assessment; office space; and computer support. At the other end of the spectrum, well-controlled feeding studies require facilities for food storage, preparation, serving, and cleanup. In studies that do not involve feeding subjects on site, it will be necessary to have a facility for the storage of meals, foods, or supplements that are picked up by, or delivered to, the subjects. Location, accessibility, and ambiance of the feeding site, as well as of the facility where subjects pick up the meals, foods, or supplements, are important factors in the recruitment and retention of study participants. Interventions employing supplements must have facilities for preparation and packaging, either in-house or through contractual arrangement with the manufacturers.

Most studies involve some clinical or biochemical measurements, which may be as simple as measuring body weight and skinfold thickness or be more complex procedures involving biochemical analyses of body fluids, tissue samples, or whole-body procedures such as dual-energy X-ray absorptiometry. Resources must be available for carrying out these measurements either directly or through contractual arrangements with other laboratories with established quality assurance procedures.

BUDGET

The development of a realistic budget that covers all costs of the study is essential. Although the actual cost depends on the design, scope, and duration of the study, some general guidelines can be given. The major budget categories are personnel, supplies (including food costs), laboratory assays and procedures (which may be contracted out), and equipment. In most cases, a specified percentage of the direct cost of the project must be added to cover overhead. The research and grants office of the sponsoring institution supplies this information.

The following are functional considerations in the budget for personnel. Some persons may assume several responsibilities, which should be identified and incorporated into their job descriptions.

Senior professional staff members have responsibility for scientific decisions and control of the budget. They also have an important role in compliance and building morale over the course of the project. Consistent day-to-day management by a study coordinator is necessary to supervise kitchen operations (where applicable), the laboratory, and data collection. In studies involving diet instruction, dietitians are needed to provide the intervention. In feeding studies, personnel are needed for preparation of food and food aliquots for assay.

Well-controlled feeding studies require more extensive resources, especially if food is prepared and served on site. These resources may include leasing kitchen and dining facilities and the rental of food storage and freezer space. High-precision scales for weighing food, high-powered blenders for preparing aliquots, and other specialized equipment may be required. Food in general is the most costly item in controlled feeding studies. Dennis et al includes a detailed discussion of resources required for this type of study (2).

Most studies also require equipment and supplies for clinical, anthropometric, and laboratory measurements. Shipping costs and containers for shipment of laboratory samples also need to be considered. In all studies, statistical assistance is essential during the design and analysis phases. Both statistical and computer capabilities are required to manage and analyze the data. Specialized software may be needed for certain aspects of the study, such as nutrient calculations. Clerical activities include preparation of recruitment materials and forms, communication, scheduling potential recruits, and preparation of reports. General-purpose office equipment may need to be leased or purchased to meet the clerical demands of the study.

Laboratory supplies may be incorporated in the fees charged by the laboratory if laboratory measurements are contracted out. Forms, duplicating costs, and participant incentives make up other supply costs. Miscellaneous costs include transportation, parking for participants, social activities, closeout costs (celebration), and computer costs.

The duration of a clinical study is determined by the time required either to see a treatment effect or to ensure that there is not a treatment effect. Moreover, it is imperative that the duration of the treatment be sufficient to establish a stable end point response. It may be necessary to conduct a pilot study to determine the length of the treatment period needed to ensure that the response has stabilized. Another determinant of the duration of a clinical study is the number of diets studied. Thus, the time required to see a treatment effect, the number of diets studied, and the length of the washout periods or breaks between treatments are factors that affect the duration of the study.

STUDY SUBJECTS

Results from human studies are frequently difficult to interpret because of the heterogeneity in human populations and variability in free-living conditions. Therefore, a concerted effort must be made to control for these factors in the design of a small clinical study, beginning with the subject selection criteria. Controlling as many potential confounding factors as possible in the selection process may limit the generalizability of the results, but it

makes interpretation of the results easier. Random assignment into treatment and control groups also eliminates many sources of bias.

Subjects should be well defined in terms of the parameters relative to the study, such as age, sex, body weight, and health status. For example, if the objective of the study is to determine the effect of diet composition on weight loss, subjects should meet similar body mass criteria. It would also be important to control for physical activity and conditioning: marathon runners should not be grouped with sedentary people. Other potential confounding variables in a study of this type might include smoking status, fat distribution pattern, and duration of excess weight.

Careful thought about the study subject's eligibility and effects of the nutrition intervention are critical. For example, consider subjects who begin a weight-loss study with the same body mass index and achieve the same rate of weight loss and total weight loss, but who have initial body weights that vary considerably such that the weight loss represents a markedly different percentage of starting body weight. In this scenario it would be important to control for starting body weight, as well as body mass index. Outcome variables delineated in the study objectives and their possible confounding factors form the basis for making decisions with respect to defining the study sample.

Recruitment of Subjects

Recruiting subjects for a clinical study is a task that can range from being relatively easy to being very difficult. Many factors affect the recruitment process, such as the number of subjects required, exclusion criteria for participation in the study, study requirements, length of participation, subject remuneration, and perceived benefits to subjects. Recruiting a sufficient number of subjects is essential for the power of the study. Expeditious recruiting controls the cost of the study and keeps interest high in potential subjects. Problems that investigators typically encounter include overly optimistic recruitment goals and the lack of well-defined and realistic recruitment strategies. With effective planning, however, recruiting problems can be avoided.

Recruitment begins with a well-defined and organized plan containing realistic short-term and long-term goals. Accordingly, the number of subjects needed and the time frame for recruitment has to be clearly defined. (See Chapter 26 for a discussion of sample size calculation.) It is important that recruitment goals take into account a realistic estimate of dropouts. A dropout rate of 10 percent to 20 percent is to be expected in a relatively short-term clinical nutrition study (a study shorter than 6 months). A higher dropout rate can be expected for longer studies and for studies that demand subjects' time or unpleasant measurements, such as daily urine collections. For controlled feeding studies, it is often helpful to have a short (few days') run-in feeding period to help determine if any potential subjects find the requirements of the study (for example, eating only the food provided to them) too demanding. This run-in period gives potential subjects a taste of the intervention and a chance to back out before the start of the study, which should help lower the dropout rate.

Initial recruitment goals may be unrealistic and often are not met, so a contingency plan should be ready for immediate implementation. Staff responsibilities for recruitment should be clearly defined and effectively coordinated. Whatever the size of the recruitment staff, its members should be characterized by perseverance, flexibility, endurance, and commitment. Staff members must be scheduled to contact potential subjects at convenient times (that is, evenings and weekends). A small pilot study is very useful and highly recommended to identify and resolve weaknesses in the recruitment effort. Detailed information about recruiting study subjects is described by Kris-Etherton et al (10).

Subject recruitment depends on effective advertising. Numerous strategies are useful. For example, newspaper advertisements that appear in different sections, including the classified advertisements, usually reach a large audience, as do other mass media strategies, such as radio and television. Some radio and television stations advertise a study as a public service message. Occasionally, newspaper writers feature a story about a planned study and include important recruitment information. To initiate this approach, the investigator can contact science or health editors at newspapers. Announcements posted on bulletin boards in the community and physicians' offices are another effective recruitment strategy, as are announcements to community groups and classes. Mailing lists, which may be obtained from various individuals or groups, allow potential subjects to be contacted personally. Word-of-mouth recruitment also can be effective, especially if done by people who have served as experimental subjects. Hospital patients also may be a source of potential subjects. For established investigators, the pool of previous participants can be an important source of potential subjects.

Incentives for Subjects

Incentives are important for recruitment and participation in screening activities that are required before enrolling subjects in a study. Monetary incentives can be effective, though other types of incentives also encourage participation in the screening procedures. Examples of low-cost nutrition-related incentives include dietary assessment, a nutrition counseling session, a chronic disease risk profile, a calorie counter, and recipes. Other low-cost incentives include prizes, T-shirts, cosmetics, movie and raffle tickets, coupons, and gift certificates.

The primary purpose of incentives is to facilitate participant recruitment. Thus, incentives should be age and gender specific, and they should be appropriate for the time and effort required to participate in the screening process. Incentives should not be so grand that they encourage people with no intention of serving as study subjects to participate in the screening process, and they should not imply or be perceived as coercion. Negative implications of incentives include selection bias and a lack of subject commitment to the study.

A distinction should be made between incentives for recruitment and incentives for retention. Incentives may be given periodically throughout the study, but the bulk of the incentives should be reserved for those who successfully complete the study.

Screening Subjects

Screening ensures that participants meet eligibility criteria and are able to comply with the requirements of the study. This process does not bias the results of the study, because subjects are randomly allocated to treatment and control groups. In fact, a rigorous screening process is critical to the success of the study. In addition to ensuring that potential subjects meet eligibility criteria, screening provides an opportunity to evaluate subjective data—such as attitude, behavior, interest, commitment, maturity, and so forth—which are important attributes in retaining participants and maintaining compliance.

The complexity of the screening process depends on the specificity of subject exclusion criteria. Some studies require only a simple questionnaire, whereas others may require anthropometric, dietary, and laboratory data, as well as information on lifestyle practices, such as smoking and exercise behavior, and a medical examination to rule out underlying disease. It is particularly important that the screening process not prompt subjects to make any behavior changes prior to the initiation of the study. The interval between screening and the commencement of the study should be minimized.

Various strategies can be used to screen prospective subjects. Screening methods include questionnaires that can be mailed or completed by the recruitment team, telephone interviews, personal interviews, group meetings, and sessions in which data (for example, laboratory, psychosocial, or dietary data) are collected. Frequently, it may be necessary to have subjects participate in more than one screening session. Multiple screening sessions typically involve an initial telephone interview or a screening questionnaire followed up (if the subject is eligible, based on the initial interview) by one or more subsequent screening visits, which often include a clinic visit. Additional information about screening can be found in Kris-Etherton et al (10).

Informed Consent

Federal law mandates that all people who elect to participate in a scientific study give their written consent. They also have the right to withdraw from the study at any time. In addition, their anonymity must be guaranteed. Before consenting to participate, subjects must be informed of the objectives, the potential treatments, and all inherent risks of the study. The consent form should be simple and easy to understand, and it should describe procedures so that the general public can understand them (Figure 7.2). For example, the amount of blood taken should be stated in household measurements (tablespoons rather than milliliters). This information can be presented without biasing the study. When the Informed Consent Form effectively and comprehensively communicates the study purpose and protocol as well as potential risks to the subjects, their confidence in the study increases and they are more apt to become full partners in the research project. An emerging issue that needs to be addressed relates to whether DNA analysis is going to be conducted on the samples. It is mandatory to inform subjects that DNA analyses will be conducted and what the fate of the stored samples will be. Some Institutional Review Boards require that a defined term of sample storage be established prior to the start of the study.

STUDY PLAN

The study plan includes the timetable, randomization procedures, management plan, and methods for measuring all the variables collected in the study. This document is often referred to as the *manual of operations* or *procedure manual*. If the study is carried out in an existing clinical research unit, it is staffed with trained personnel. Many of the general procedures governing controlled dietary studies already should be in place, and only the procedures that are specific to the study need to be documented.

Randomization Procedures

Random assignment of subjects to either the treatment or the control group is a key feature of clinical studies. Through the random assignment procedure, one subject has an equal probability of being assigned to either the treatment or the control group. It is important that potential subjects be completely willing to accept assignment to either the treatment or control group and be willing to accept the blinded study design. In some studies, subjects will be assigned to all treatment groups, including the control group. The assignment should be blinded to the investigators as well. Double-blind assignment, in which neither subject nor investigator knows the assignment, is preferable; however, it is often difficult to blind a dietary modification to the experimental subjects.

Random assignment ensures that unmeasured, potentially confounding variables do not bias the study results. Techniques for randomly assigning subjects are available. There may be instances where investigators need to employ stratified randomization procedures to ensure that the baseline characteristics of the study groups are similar and to avoid introducing a confounding variable into the study. This procedure is done by the study statistician.

Forms

The design of forms and their use are essential for implementation of the study. Forms serve various purposes, and several functions may be combined in a single form. Data forms include questionnaires and dietary assessment, laboratory, and clinical forms. They make up the record of the data that are collected, and thus control the scope of the data analysis. Unlike medical records and other narrative-type documents, standard forms impose structure and help ensure completeness, consistency, and comparability of all data collected throughout the study. Therefore, considerable thought must be given to their development and testing during the planning phase. It is often useful to construct dummy tables of data that will

This is to certify that I, (subject's name), agree to participate as a volunteer in a scientific investigation as part of the nutrition research program of (name of institution) under the supervision of _____.

The investigation and my part in the investigation have been defined and fully explained to me by _____, and I understand his/her explanation. A copy of the procedures of this investigation and a description of any risks and discomforts have been provided to me and have been discussed in detail with me.

I have been given an opportunity to ask whatever questions I have had, and all such questions have been answered satisfactorily.

I understand that I am free to deny any answers to specific items or questions in interviews or questionnaires.

I understand that any data or answers to questions will remain confidential with regard to my identity.

I understand that in the event of physical injury resulting from this investigation, neither financial compensation nor free medical treatment is provided for such a physical injury, and that further information on this policy is available from

_____.

I certify that, to the best of my knowledge and belief, I have no physical or mental illness or weakness that would increase the risk to me of participation in this investigation.

I further understand that I am free to withdraw my consent and terminate my participation at any time.

_____ Date	_____ Subject's Signature
_____ Date	_____ Investigator's Signature
_____ Date	_____ Investigator's Signature
_____ Date	_____ Witness's Signature

FIGURE 7.2 Sample consent form.

be needed for analysis and interpretation of the results and then relate them back to the data collection forms.

Administrative forms are also used in the management of the study. These forms include food inventories, menu calculations, food preparation instructions, and work schedules. A study flow sheet is valuable for ensuring complete data collection on all subjects.

Quality assurance forms include forms used to certify that the appropriate food was received and consumed by the participant (compliance checks) and records of dietary adjustments, adverse reactions, and protocol deviations, such as failure to consume the prescribed diet.

Inherent to the development of different forms for the study is the fact that they are used to collect meaningful data. Figure 7.3 presents general guidelines for designing forms, designated as SLIPPS (space, logic, instruction, parsimony, pretest, and security). Information on designing forms is available in a variety of publications (11–13).

THE DIETARY INTERVENTION

Two critical factors in the design of the dietary intervention are control of the composition of the diet and

Space

- Allow appropriate format and space to facilitate data collection.

Logic

- Present questions in logical sequence.
- Use consistent response codes.

Instruction

- Print instructions on the forms when possible.
- Print units and decimals on the forms.

Parsimony

- Collect only as much data as necessary.
- Ensure that each item has a specific purpose.

Pretest

- Field test and revise the form before the trial.

Security

- Make duplicate copies and electronically back up data forms.
- Include a confidentiality assurance system.

FIGURE 7.3   Principles of form design (SLIPPS).

compliance with the diet. These factors, in turn, are directly related to the objectives and hypotheses of the study.

Consider the following situations. Investigator A wishes to test the effect of prescribing oat-bran supplements on serum cholesterol levels. A protocol is formulated in which the members of a control group of participants follow their regular diet, and the members of the intervention group follow their regular diet, but in addition are given oat-bran supplements with instructions and recipes for using them. Both groups keep records of their food intake at intervals specified by the investigator. Serum cholesterol level and body weight are measured at baseline and at regular intervals during the study. At the conclusion of the study, the investigator finds that the mean cholesterol level of the intervention group is 0.13 mmol/L lower than the control group, a statistically significant difference. The intervention group also reports eating less total fat and more carbohydrate than the control group. Both groups maintained their weight.

What does the investigator conclude? The investigator does not conclude that oat bran per se lowers serum cholesterol levels, because other dietary variables changed as well. The investigator also cannot conclude that prescribing oat bran causes people to eat less fat and hence lower their cholesterol, because there is no way of knowing the accuracy of the reported intake during the course of the trial. Thus, the investigator can conclude that the intervention followed by the subjects led to a reduction in serum cholesterol levels but cannot establish with certainty that the addition of oat bran to the diet caused the effect.

Investigator B, however, wishes to determine the effect of oat-bran supplements on serum cholesterol levels. A protocol is designed in which a specified amount of oat bran is incorporated into a diet of fixed composition. The foods for both control and intervention groups are prepared and served to the subjects. The only difference in the two treatment diets is the amount of oat bran fed to the subjects. The energy content of the diets is adjusted to maintain body weight. Subjects eat all their meals in a specified location. At the end of the trial, the investigator observes that the mean serum cholesterol level in the intervention group is statistically different from that of the control group. The investigator concludes that oat bran lowers serum cholesterol in people with characteristics similar to those of the study subjects.

Both investigators have made valid conclusions with respect to oat bran, but the research questions were quite different. In investigator A's study, the strategy of intervention (that is, the prescription of oat bran) was being tested, whereas in investigator B's study, the metabolic effect of oat bran was being tested. Investigator B's study required a much greater degree of dietary control and compliance than investigator A's study.

Estimating Energy Requirements

In controlled feeding studies, an important consideration in planning the diet is the anticipated energy requirements of the participants. This characteristic will affect the quantity of food needed and hence the budget. Energy requirements can be estimated using various methods (14). One commonly used method is to determine basal energy expenditure (BEE) with the Harris-Benedict equation and multiply the BEE by an activity factor to determine total energy expenditure (Figure 7.4). It is important to note that these estimates are not completely accurate for individuals, and often the energy level of subjects' diets must be adjusted. However, the estimates are sufficient to be used as a guide for planning for groups.

1. Calculate the BEE:
   Use the Harris-Benedict equation

Men:	**66.5 + 13.8W + 5.0H − 6.8A**
Women:	**655.1 + 9.6W + 1.8H − 4.7A**

2. Calculate the TEE:
   Multiply the BEE by one of the following activity factors:
   1.2 for patients confined to bed
   1.3 for ambulatory patients
   1.3–1.5 for most normally active people[a]
   1.75 for extremely active people
   2.0 for competitive athletes

   [a]Typically, 1.5 is used initially to calculate energy needs and then adjusted if necessary.

FIGURE 7.4   Determining energy requirements. BEE indicates basal energy expenditure; W, weight in kilograms (kg); H, height in centimeters (cm); A, age in years; and TEE, total energy expenditure.

The Experimental Diet

There are numerous approaches for delivering test diets. For example, subjects can be fed all foods in a metabolic ward setting or in a free-living environment setting. In the latter, subjects can be fed some or all of their meals on site or take some or all of them home for consumption. A frequent approach involves adding the nutrient of interest to a food source that is given to subjects for consumption either as part of a controlled diet or with instructions for inclusion in their habitual diet. The approach taken is often determined by the research question being addressed. For example, some studies are designed to evaluate treatment effects in free-living populations whereas others (those in a controlled setting) are designed to assess the maximal effect that can be achieved with diet.

Moreover, some studies are designed to evaluate the effects of single nutrients, whereas others are designed to assess the effects of dietary patterns on end points of interest. In the latter experimental approach, the emphasis is not on controlling specific nutrients but rather on identifying the effects of a different food group distribution.

The DASH Study is an example of the latter; the experimental diet was high in fruits, vegetables (9 to 10 servings per day), and low-fat dairy products (2 to 3 servings per day) (15). An example of a less dramatic change in the overall quality of the diet is substituting one fat or oil for another. In both examples, more than one nutrient would change in the experimental diet. This experimental paradigm represents a public health approach for evaluating the effects of diet. This approach does not allow investigators to identify the nutrients dietary factors that account for the effect observed but does assess how changes in an overall diet would affect health. In contrast, studying changes in only one nutrient reflects an experimental approach, and investigators can identify specific effects of single nutrients.

The design of the intervention must take into account a number of trade-offs. As shown in Figure 7.5, the greater the dietary control, the more costly the study and the less attractive to potential subjects. The use of formula diets or synthetic mixtures provides the greatest degree of consistency and facilitates the precise delivery of nutrients of interest (16). However, the results obtained with formula diets may differ compared to results obtained with a whole food diet, although there is some evidence that results are comparable between whole food and liquid diets (16). Thus, investigators should identify the most appropriate vehicle for the delivery of experimental diets. Again, the objectives of the study must be clearly formulated and, if necessary, revised to meet the limitations imposed by feasibility and reality. Then the investigator can decide whether the attainable objectives justify doing the study. At the other end of the scale, studies that are more feasible in terms of cost and recruitment are more difficult to interpret, because the results are confounded by issues of compliance and variability in dietary composition.

A more detailed classification system for various degrees of dietary control in clinical research has been described by St. Jeor and Bryan (17). Table 7.2 defines clinical research diets and describes conditions for their use.

Determining the Composition of the Diet

Once the dietary prescription has been determined, the next step is to calculate the composition of the diet. Factors that need to be considered in addition to the composition are the distribution of nutrients over the day, variability in the nutrient composition of foods that will be

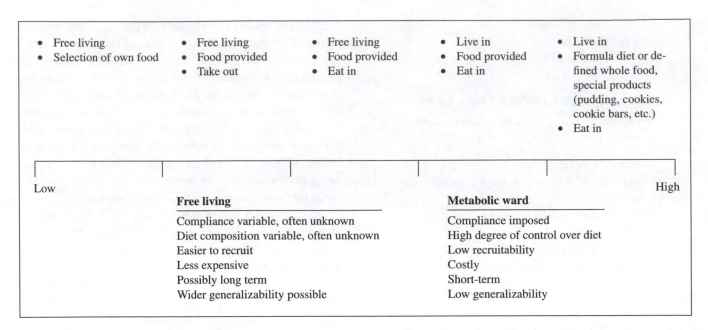

FIGURE 7.5 Degrees of dietary control.

used in the diet, palatability, and stability. Again, there are trade-offs. Palatability is related to variety, and variety increases nutrient variability. For example, the composition of an egg is related to the size and the relative proportions of white and yolk, as well as feed and season. Purchasing all the eggs needed for a study, homogenizing them, weighing out individual portions, and freezing them for future use would provide the best control of variability, but it would be monotonous for the participant. Likewise, canned or frozen foods from a single packing lot would be more uniform than fresh foods purchased daily. In addition, there is less nutrient variability in a 3-day versus a 7-day cycle menu.

The level of precision determines the ability to define specific effects of a dietary factor on an outcome variable. The level of precision needed again depends on the objectives of the study. For example, a study of the effects of fat and cholesterol intake on lipoprotein metabolism would require greater control of those nutrients and less control of variation in vitamins and minerals. By contrast, studies involving heat-labile vitamins would require greater attention to controlling food sources and preparation techniques. Clevidence et al (18) and Phillips and Stewart (19) offer detailed discussions of diet design and nutrient variability.

Many commercial software packages are available for estimating the nutrient composition of foods, and guidelines are available for evaluating them. Chapter 16 discusses this issue in detail. Nutrient databases, howev-

er, are derived from average composition values, which may not reflect what is actually being consumed. For studies in free-living subjects who may select food freely, average nutrient database values may be sufficient, but as a study moves toward greater control of the diet, the need for analytic values increases.

A good plan is to analyze aliquots of the calculated diets and to make adjustments, if necessary, before the study is started. If differences are identified between calculated and assayed values, then the food sources that account for the error must be identified and modified. This process can be challenging and time-consuming. It also can be a hit-or-miss procedure, because it is based on best-guessed estimates of food sources that are contributing to the error. Aliquots then should be collected and analyzed periodically throughout the study to assure that diet composition remains unchanged.

Preparation of Food Samples for Chemical Analysis

Chemical verification of the nutrient composition of diets or dietary supplements may be done in-house or by other laboratories. No matter where it is done, preparation of food samples for chemical analysis requires careful attention to many details. It must be done by trained personnel according to written procedures if assay values are to reflect the true composition of the food consumed by study subjects. Details of these procedures are beyond the scope of this chapter. Considerations that must be taken into account in developing the written protocol for sampling are summarized later in this chapter. Phillips and Stewart (19) provide details on sampling and the preparation of composites.

Selection of Food

The food selected for chemical analysis should be identical to that served to subjects. The most convenient method is to prepare an extra serving of each food item and then randomly select the complete day's meals and snacks. Water and noncaloric beverages generally are not included but may be analyzed separately if indicated by the study objectives. The foods should be sampled concurrently with the meal service to avoid deterioration of the sample in storage.

Food samples should be collected using fat-free, powder-free disposable gloves. Samples should be transferred quantitatively from serving dishes and stored frozen in airtight food collection containers until they are homogenized and subsequently aliquoted for analysis. The food samples should be clearly labeled using cryogenic markers.

Preparing Composites

Homogenizing the food samples is the most critical step in preparing the samples for analysis. Factors that must be considered include completeness of the sample (no lost food), storage of the sample, and uniformity of the homogenate. Nutrients susceptible to degradation or modification during processing require special procedures. Phillips and Stewart describe nutrient-specific precautions that should be taken in the preparation of composites (19).

Preparation of Subsamples and Analytic Aliquots

Factors to consider in preparing subsamples from the total homogenate include temperature and adequate mixing before sampling. Testing the homogeneity of the composites is a critical and often overlooked step. Phillips and Stewart explain this process in detail (19).

Storage and Shipment

Adequate facilities should be available to store food samples and subsamples of the homogenates at –20 degrees Celsius or lower. Samples and subsamples shipped to another laboratory should remain frozen according to the instructions of the laboratory.

Selection of a Food Analysis Laboratory

The most important criterion in selecting an analytic laboratory is the assurance of quality analyses. Inaccurate results at any price are not a bargain. Quality assurance ensures accurate analytic results related to sampling, sample handling, storage, preservation methods, validation, quality control procedures (to obtain valid and reliable results), skills of personnel, calibration of equipment, documentation of performance, reporting of results, and adequacy of the laboratory facilities.

Quality control includes such laboratory activities as calibrating laboratory instruments, maintaining quality control standards charts, and running recovery studies. Also important is a commitment to performing replication analyses, participation in proficiency testing, and use of certified standards.

Professional organizations such as the American Oil Chemists' Society (AOCS) (20) and the Association of Official Analytical Chemists (AOAC) (21) are a valuable resource for information about nutrient analysis of foods. For example, the AOCS examination board provides a list of AOCS-certified laboratories. For approval as a certified laboratory, there are two essential requirements. First, the laboratory must have on its full-time staff an AOCS-approved chemist, who is approved based on a recurring test of proficiency using samples submitted by the AOCS. Second, the laboratory must perform at an acceptable level on 12 additional lipid analyses each year using blind samples submitted as "referee" materials by the AOCS.

Not all laboratories are proficient in analyzing food matrixes. Before selecting a laboratory, it should be established that it performs well on food matrixes for the nutrients of interest in the study. Analysis of the diet is the common feature of most dietary intervention clinical trials, and hence it has been discussed in detail in this chapter. Methods for measuring outcome and intervening variables, however, are specific to the objectives of a study and are beyond the scope of this chapter.

POTENTIAL PROBLEMS WITH SUBJECTS

Subject Retention and Compliance

Retaining subjects and maintaining compliance throughout a study is important in ensuring the success of any clinical investigation. Many potential problems can be

TABLE 7.2 Clinical Research Diets—Definitions of Terms

Classification	Intake Calculated	Measurement of Diet	Food Source	Water Source	Food Preparation Procedures	Food Refusals	Laboratory Analysis of Diet	Advantages	Disadvantages	Application
Estimated	Daily (after intake charted), using equivalency lists or tables of averages	Estimated in household measures	Varied	Varied	Varied	Estimated	No	Closest to "free diet"; ease and speed of estimation; most accurate observational data	Least reliable nutritive data; biased by change of setting, different foods, etc	Estimate of patient's preferred intake; data to supplement dietary history
Weighed	Daily (charted sometimes before and always after intake), using standard tables	Weighed (gram scale) portions (usual or calculated)	Varied	Varied	Varied or controlled	Weighed	No	Minimal inconvenience to patient; more reliable nutrition data	Increased work with some increase in accuracy of data	More accurate idea of patient's preferred intake; more reliable observational data; general test diets
Controlled nutrient	Daily (before and after serving to patient), using standard tables, special references, or laboratory analyses	Weighed (torsion balance), controlled portions	Varied	Controlled or varied	Controlled or varied	Weighed, calculated, and perhaps replaced	Rarely	Flexible, food variety; offers some variety and flexibility to patient	Expensive dietitian's time unless computer available; constant monitoring for replacements	Diets with focus on desired maximum or minimum quantity or quality of nutrients; investigative diets

| Constant | Before study, using analyzed laboratory data, reliable manufacturers' data and nutrient databases, *USDA Handbook No. 8*, or other tables and references | Weighed (torsion balance), controlled portions | Constant | Controlled or constant | Constant | Discouraged, replaced if possible; otherwise weighed, calculated, and perhaps analyzed | Occasionally | Highly accurate; dietitian's time used more efficiently; minimal calculations | Lack of variety and flexibility; requires a research kitchen, properly trained personnel, and standardized food preparation procedures; requires trial period for acceptability | Diagnostic diets, research diets |
| Metabolic (balance) | Before study, using analyzed laboratory data, reliable manufacturers' data and nutrient data bases, *USDA Handbook No. 8*, or other tables and references | Weighed (torsion balance), controlled portions | Constant | Constant | Constant | Discouraged, replaced if possible; otherwise weighed, calculated, and analyzed | 2–3 times per menu | Most reliable data; supported by actual laboratory analyses; dietitian's time used most efficiently; minimal calculations | Requires analyses of all intake and sometimes excreta; only as accurate as collections and laboratory analyses; lack of variety and flexibility; requires research kitchen, properly trained personnel, and standardized food preparation procedures; requires trial period for acceptability | Metabolic (balance) studies only |

Adapted from St Jeor ST, Bryan GT. Clinical research diets: definition of terms. *J Am Diet Asooc.* 1973;62:47–51. Used with permission.

minimized or prevented by careful planning. A formal protocol and adequate resources for retention and compliance activities should be incorporated into the planning phase. Many problems with subject retention, compliance, and dismissal can be avoided by meticulous screening of potential subjects to identify people who will be cooperative and committed. In addition, it is important to provide continuous support and encouragement throughout the investigation. Criteria for subject dismissal must be established prior to the investigation and shared with study subjects at that time.

Accurate measurement of compliance with the experimental protocol is important for meaningful interpretation of the treatment effects (22). In some studies, compliance may be an important outcome variable, because the treatment effect may be biased by noncompliance. In either case, noncompliance must be accounted for in the final data analysis. For example, if a clinical study is designed to evaluate the effects of iron supplementation on measures of iron status, and one-half of the treatment group takes only 50 percent of the prescribed supplement, this must be quantified and considered in the data analyses. A common approach to the analysis of clinical trials is called *intent to treat*. In this analysis, all data that are available for an individual are evaluated, even if the individual drops out early or is noncompliant. This analysis tests the effect of the mode of intervention, but not the factors that could explain the effect. It is important in generalizing the results to other groups.

The actual assessment of compliance must consider several variables that vary as a function of the type and design of the investigation. In some studies, measurement of compliance may entail a very simple, straightforward approach, whereas other studies may depend on measuring some biological variable that requires a more complex assay (for example, platelet phospholipid fatty acids). Likewise, the sensitivity of the methods selected for assessing compliance may range from very sensitive (for example, measuring a urinary metabolite) to relatively insensitive (for example, subjects' self-assessment of compliance). Another consideration is whether compliance is assessed objectively or subjectively. Subjective assessment can be as simple as merely asking subjects if they are adhering to the protocol. This approach is successful when the investigator and subjects have established a friendly and trusting relationship. Often, investigators can ascertain compliance surprisingly well merely on the basis of subject attitude and behavior (level of participation, punctuality, and so forth). If there is any suspicion that subjects are not complying with the experimen-

tal protocol, they should be confronted. If noncompliance becomes a problem, the subject must be dismissed from the study.

Ideal compliance is the goal of all studies, but it is essential in metabolic studies. Not only must the subjects consume all the allotted food (and not lose any through emesis); they also must refrain from consuming any other food or substances that might bias the results of the study. However, it is seldom feasible to maintain study subjects in an enclosed, supervised environment 24 hours a day over an extended period. Therefore, proxy measures are often employed, with varying degrees of sensitivity.

Once energy equilibrium has been established, body weight changes may signal compliance problems. These changes, however, can be seen only as a gross indicator. This method would not differentiate changes in energy expenditure, nor would it detect small deviations in food intake that nevertheless could have a large effect if certain foods were systematically omitted or consumed outside the protocol.

When a complete collection of excreta is obtained, metabolites and other substances may be measured. For example, a constant sodium intake should be reflected in a constant sodium excretion (23). The validity of using excretion as an index of intake depends, of course, on the completeness of the collections. Complete 24-hour collections with a diet of constant composition are useful in determining urinary creatinine excretion (24); *p*-aminobenzoic acid administered in tablet form has been used to assess the completeness of urine collections (25) and, added to food, to monitor dietary compliance (26).

A detailed description of various methods for assessing compliance is beyond the scope of this chapter. For more information, the reader is referred to Bingham (27). Finally, it is important to note that human frailties and social needs being what they are, compliance is not likely ever to be perfect. It can be enhanced if overall morale is high and attempts are made to build into the protocol some free choices—for example, diet beverages that may be consumed at social gatherings.

Subject Morale

Subject morale can wane quickly in response to various factors, including increasing length of the study and other constraints. It is essential to maintain a high level of morale throughout the study, and reaching this goal requires commitment by the investigative team. The importance of time and resources devoted to this goal should not be underestimated. Continuous social support of the subjects by the investigators will be efforts well spent in the long run. Subjects need to feel valued and highly regarded by the investigators. Every effort should be made to ensure that the subjects are comfortable, are happy, and feel a sense of ownership of the study. Effective techniques include sending birthday and other greeting cards, recognition of significant events, providing entertainment during the study, and conducting raffles. In controlled feeding studies where food is provided, paying attention to details such as serving high-quality food, providing good service, and making newspapers and magazines available in comfortable surroundings is important. In some studies, contests are appropriate motivational stimuli.

Dismissal of Subjects

The criteria for subject dismissal must be clearly identified before the study begins, and they must be communicated to potential subjects. During the study, any behavior that compromises the results of the study is basis for dismissal. For example, the primary reason for dismissing a subject from a clinical nutrition trial is usually noncompliance with the test diet or other study procedures or disruptive behavior. Change in body weight, missed meals, and food records suspected of being falsified are indicators of noncompliance. It is imperative that this policy be consistent, enforced, and generally not modified.

At the onset of a study, the investigators have made considerable plans and are typically enthusiastic. They now must remember that sustained attention to the daily management and quality assurance of the study are essential. Providing this attention becomes more challenging, especially during larger and longer-term studies in which the treatment period is long, several different treatments are implemented, or subjects enter the study slowly (perhaps one at a time). A strong management plan and capable investigative team are the keys to avoiding problems that may be detrimental to the study.

MANAGEMENT PLAN

Components of a good management plan include organization, communication, clear delineation and coverage of duties and responsibilities, contingency plans, and proce-

dures for dealing with problems. It is also important that the management plan deal with monitoring the study in regard to the study goals. Questions such as the following should be asked regularly throughout the study to ensure that the goals of the study are met:

- Has a comprehensive management plan been developed from a detailed study protocol and made available to the investigative team and staff?
- Have subject recruitment and retention goals been met?
- Is subject retention still acceptable?
- Have data been collected from all subjects at designated times?
- Has the study been conducted as planned?

The staff can vary in size for a clinical study or trial, depending upon the scope of the study. Regardless of the magnitude of the study, there is always a principal investigator (or co-principal investigators) who is responsible for the conduct of the study. A project director may manage the day-to-day activities of the investigation. In any clinical study, it is important for the chain of command to be established and for each staff member to report to someone. Likewise, it is important that staff members be supervised, although some staff members may require only minimal supervision. A written work plan that includes specific goals, action plans, and a time line is useful in completing various tasks associated with the study.

Staff communication is essential for all studies. Frequent meetings at regular intervals are useful for keeping the staff informed about the progress of the study. Other effective types of communication include message books and logbooks, newsletters, blackboards, bulletin boards, and the use of computer networks. Committed, experienced, and enthusiastic leaders or supervisors avoid communication breakdowns by maintaining close contact with the project staff. They continually solicit information about the progress of various aspects of the study from staff members. Written reports submitted periodically and/or oral reports given at staff meetings summarizing each staff member's accomplishments facilitate communication among the project staff in achieving the goals of the study.

An often neglected but necessary consideration is planning for the unwanted, but inevitable, problems that are bound to happen during the course of the study. Problems may include the illness or emergency absence of staff and subjects, severe weather, mishaps in the kitchen and laboratory, lost or mislabeled samples, and noncompliance. Procedures for dealing with these situations should be thought out in advance and contingency plans developed. The timing of the study may have an adverse effect not only on recruitment but also on retention and compliance if it encompasses major holidays or school breaks.

QUALITY ASSURANCE

No study is better than the quality of its data (4). The quality assurance program is a continuous process of assessment and evaluation according to predetermined criteria, feedback, and correction. A well-designed quality assurance system incorporates quality control procedures at every point in the study where information is transferred. The quality control component is part of an overall management strategy that includes written and oral progress reports, budget monitoring, and morale building of staff and participants.

Quality assurance begins with the selection of methods with the highest degree of accuracy and precision attainable. Whenever possible, standards should be used, and routine monitoring should be included to ensure the continued accuracy of the methods. (An internal quality control system allows for reanalysis of samples at different times.)

Quality assurance includes training of personnel, regular maintenance and calibration of equipment, monitoring the performance of personnel and equipment, application of data-editing criteria, and documentation of the quality of corrective feedback throughout the collection and processing of data. A well-trained staff is important for ensuring that data are collected and managed without bias and variability.

Training, however, is only the first step; regular monitoring is also necessary. Subtle changes in the procedure over time can cause considerable drift, which could bias the results. The same is true for equipment. The tools for quality assurance are developed in the planning phase, and they include the protocol, procedure manuals, forms for data collection, and data management. Data management incorporates documentation of data quality, including protocol violations and missing and spurious values. Visual inspection of completed forms, ranges for acceptable values, logic, and consistency checks are applied as the data are collected so that problems can be detected and corrected early (Table 7.3). Ideally, the quality assurance program prevents problems before they occur.

TABLE 7.3 Quality Assurance Considerations in a Clinical Study

Aspects of the Study	Recommended Quality Control Procedures
Methods	Validate for accuracy Establish performance standards Provide staff feedback
Training staff and monitoring	Establish protocols
Performance	Establish written procedures Determine performance standards Provide staff feedback
Forms	Design forms Pilot test forms for validity and reliability
Data	Verify accuracy of data and data entry Adjudicate questionable data

DATA MANAGEMENT

It is important to realize that even in a small clinical study a considerable amount of data will be collected, typically from many sources at different times. Management of this aspect of the study includes the coordination of the collection of the data, data entry, controlling access to the data, ensuring the safety of the data, and monitoring quality control procedures. Although several members of the project staff should know these procedures, management should be the sole responsibility of one person. The data manager should possess specific training in statistics and computer science. Assuming that the data are collected according to the specified protocol, it is important that the data be secured against unauthorized access to protect the privacy of the subjects and to avoid damage and loss. Data should be entered into a secure computer file, and duplicate copies of data files (both paper and computer copies) stored in a safe, secure place in another location. There are different formats for storing data. The format selected should be consistent with the data analysis protocol established prior to the initiation of the major study.

PILOT STUDIES

Major clinical studies benefit greatly from a pilot study, which is a scaled-down version of the larger investigation. The pilot study allows the staff to practice implementing the experimental procedures of the major investigation, anticipate and fix problems, identify pitfalls, and simply determine whether the clinical trial, as planned, is feasible. Staffing issues such as size, scheduling, and necessary skills can also be assessed. A pilot study is useful for evaluating subjects' potential acceptance of the experimental protocol and diet. Problem areas can be identified and resolved so that the major study proceeds smoothly. Frequently, simple changes in the experimental protocol of diet (for example, substituting baked potatoes for baked sweet potatoes) will facilitate subject compliance and satisfaction with the study, the diet, or both.

A pilot study also provides perspective about the outcome of the major study. The variation in the subjects' responses to the treatment can be determined so that sample size adjustments for the major study can be made. In addition, the pilot study can be used to determine the length of time required for the major study (that is, the time needed for the parameters measured to stabilize in response to the treatment).

The overall benefits of a pilot study are worth the effort and costs. Because the pilot study implements every aspect of the clinical trial, most problems can be identified and resolved. A pilot study provides an excellent opportunity to ascertain whether the goals (recruitment, retention, compliance, response measurements, data collection, and analysis) of the major study are realistic and attainable. This information may be critical to the success of an application for funding of the larger study.

DATA ANALYSIS AND PUBLICATION

Results of the study are obtained by subjecting the data to statistical testing of the primary and secondary hypotheses defined in the initial study design. It is important that the data analysis be done carefully, rigorously, and by individuals who are experienced and knowledgeable in statistical methodology and analysis. Issues such as deciding which subjects to include in the analysis (that is, how to deal with exclusions and withdrawals and noncompliance), deciding what to do about poor quality and missing data, subgroup analyses, and comparison of multiple variables are of critical importance in interpreting the results (4).

Because of the problems that have been identified with the reporting of randomized controlled trials, especially those concerning the ability of readers to identify the number of participants assessed for eligibility, the number found to be eligible, the number randomized per group, the number who received the specific intervention/treatment, the number who are lost to follow-up, and the number included in the statistical analyses, a Consolidated Standards for Reporting of Trials (CONSORT) Statement has been published (28). The goal of CONSORT is to encourage the use of a flow diagram to enable readers to follow the progress of participants through various stages and treatments of the study (29) and thereby assess a study's conduct and assess validity of the results reported (30). The flow diagram specifies information that should be included on the passage of subjects through the four stages of the trial/study: enrollment, intervention allocation, follow-up, and analysis (30). Moher et al evaluated 211 randomized clinical trials published in 1994 and 1998 in the same journals and reported that the use of CONSORT improved the quality of reports (31). Consequently, it is essential to comply with CONSORT standards if one seeks to publish findings in a top-tier journal.

Analysis is part of the statistical design of the study that must be addressed during the planning phase of the study and specified in the protocol.

Dissemination of the study findings and conclusions should be the result of any scientific inquiry. In-house publications are useful in disseminating information about the study to colleagues, staff, and other interested persons in the institution where the investigation was conducted. Presentations at scientific meetings and submission of the study report to peer-reviewed journals provides valuable critical appraisal. Often, this appraisal leads to new insights in the interpretation of the study and new research directions. Chapter 30 provides guidance on preparing a manuscript for publication. When a work is presented at a scientific meeting, the popular press may wish to develop a story about the findings. In this case, make sure that the findings are not overinterpreted or generalized to make a good story. A single study, no matter how good, does not make policy, especially as it pertains to the highly selected samples enrolled in controlled nutrition trials. Reporting and interpreting the results to the subjects in a study should be done as early as feasible, and certainly before they hear about it in the popular media.

REFERENCES

1. Lilienfeld DE, Stolley PH. *Foundations of Epidemiology.* New York, NY: Oxford University Press; 1994.
2. Dennis BH, Ershow AG, Obarzanek E, Clevidence BA. *Well-Controlled Diet Studies in Humans. A Practical Guide to Design and Management.* Chicago, Ill: American Dietetic Association; 1999.

3. Most MM, Fishell VA, Binkoski A, et al. Clinical Nutrition Studies: Unique Applications. In: Berdanier CD, ed. *Handbook of Nutrition and Food.* Boca Raton, FL: CRC Press; 2002:435–452.

4. Friedman LM, Furberg CD, DeMets DL. *Fundamentals of Clinical Trials.* 3rd ed. New York, NY: Springer Verlag; 1998.

5. Life Sciences Research Office, Federation of American Societies of Experimental Biology. *Third Report on Nutrition Monitoring in the United States.* Washington, DC: US Government Printing Office; 1995.

6. National Research Council. *Diet and Health: Implications for Reducing Chronic Disease Risk.* Washington, DC: National Academy Press; 1989.

7. US Department of Health and Human Services. *Healthy People 2010.* Washington, DC: US Government Printing Office; 2000.

8. Riegelman RK. *Studying a Study and Testing a Test.* Boston, Mass: Little, Brown & Co; 1981.

9. Dennis BH, Stewart P, Wang CH, et al. Diet design for a multi-center controlled feeding trial: the DELTA program. *J Am Diet Assoc.* 1998;98:766–776.

10. Kris-Etherton PM, Mustad VA, Lichtenstein AH. Recruitment and Screening of Study Participants. In: Dennis BH, Ershow AG, Obarzanek E, Clevidence BA, eds. *Well-Controlled Diet Studies in Humans. A Practical Guide to Design and Management.* Chicago, Ill: American Dietetic Association; 1999:76–95.

11. Wright P, Haybittle J. Design of forms for clinical trials (1). *Br Med J.* 1979;2:529–530.

12. Wright P, Haybittle J. Design of forms for clinical trials (2). *Br Med J.* 1979;2:590–592.

13. Wright P, Haybittle J. Design of forms for clinical trials (3). *Br Med J.* 1979;2:650–651.

14. St. Jeor ST, Stumbo PJ. Energy needs and weight maintenance in controlled feeding studies. In: Dennis BH, Ershow AG, Obarzanek E, Clevidence BA, eds. *Well-Controlled Diet Studies in Humans. A Practical Guide to Design and Management.* Chicago, Ill: American Dietetic Association; 1999:255–262.

15. Sacks FM, Obarzanek E, Windhauser MM, et al. Rationale and design of the Dietary Approaches to Stop Hypertension Trial (DASH): a multicenter controlled-feeding study of the dietary patterns to lower blood pressure. *Am J Epidemiol.* 1995;5:108–118.

16. Mustad VA, Jonnalagadda SS, Smutko SA et al. Comparative lipid and lipoprotein responses to solid-food diets and defined liquid-formula diets. *Am J Clin Nutr.* 1999;70:839–846.

17. St. Jeor ST, Bryan GT. Clinical research diets: definition of terms. *J Am Diet Assoc.* 1973;62:47–51.

18. Clevidence BA, Fong AKH, Todd K, et al. Designing Research Diets. In: Dennis BH, Ershow AG, Obarzanek E, Clevidence BA, eds. *Well-Controlled Diet Studies in Humans. A Practical Guide to Design and Management.*

Chicago, Ill: American Dietetic Association; 1999:155–178.

19. Phillips KM, Stewart KK. Validating Diet Composition by Chemical Analysis. In: Dennis BH, Ershow AG, Obarzanek E, Clevidence BA, eds. *Well-Controlled Diet Studies in Humans. A Practical Guide to Design and Management.* Chicago, Ill: American Dietetic Association; 1999:336–367.

20. American Oil Chemists' Society. *Official Methods and Recommended Practices of the American Oil Chemists' Society.* 5th ed. Champaign, Ill: American Oil Chemists' Society; 1997.

21. Association of Official Analytical Chemists. *Official Methods of Analysis of the Association of Official Analytical Chemists International.* 17th ed. Washington, DC: Association of Official Analytical Chemists, Inc; 2000.

22. Windhauser MM, Evans MA, McCullough ML, et al. Dietary adherence in the Dietary Approaches to Stop Hypertension trial. DASH Collaborative Research Group. *J Am Diet Assoc.* 1999;99(suppl 8): 76–83.

23. Schachter J, Harper PH, Radin ME, Caggiula AW, McDonald RE. Comparison of sodium and potassium intake with excretion. *Hypertension.* 1980;2:695–699.

24. Jackson S. Creatinine in urine as an index of urinary excretion rate. *Health Phys.* 1966;12:843–850.

25. Bingham S, Cummings JH. The use of 4-amino benzoic acid as a marker to validate the completeness of 24 h urine collections in man. *Clin Sci.* 1983;64:629–635.

26. Roberts SB, Morrow FD, Evans WJ, et al. Use of P-amino benzoic acid to monitor compliance with prescribed dietary regimens during metabolic balance studies in man. *Am J Clin Nutr.* 1990;51:485–488.

27. Bingham S. The dietary assessment of individuals: methods, accuracy, new techniques and recommendations. *CAB International.* 1987;57:705–74.

28. Egger M, Juni P, Bartlett C for the CONSORT Group. Value of flow diagrams in reports of randomized controlled trials. *JAMA.* 2001;285:1996–1999.

29. Rennie D. CONSORT revised—improving the reporting of randomized trials. *JAMA.* 2001;285:2006–2007.

30. Moher D, Schulz KF, Altman DG for the CONSORT Group. The CONSORT Statement: revised recommendations for improving the quality of reports of parallel-group randomized trials. *Ann Intern Med.* 2001;134:657–662.

31. Moher D, Jones A, Lepage L for the CONSORT Group. Use of the CONSORT Statement and quality of reports of randomized trials. A comparative before-and-after evaluation. *JAMA.* 2001;285:1992–1995.

Further Reading

Books

Dennis BH, Ershow AG, Obarzanek E, Clevidence BA. *Well-Controlled Diet Studies in Humans. A Practical Guide to Design and Management.* Chicago, Ill: American Dietetic Association; 1999.

Pocock SJ. *Clinical Trials: A Practical Approach.* New York, NY: John Wiley & Sons; 1984.

Sources of Data

Centers for Disease Control (CDC). *Morbidity and Mortality Weekly Report.*

CDC, Public Health Service (PHS), Department of Health and Human Services (DHHS). *Pediatric Nutrition Surveillance System.*

Food and Drug Administration (FDA), PHS, DHHS. *Health and Diet Survey.*

Gable CB. A compendium of public health data sources. *Am J Epidemiol.* 1990;131:38 1–394.

Human Nutrition Information Service, US Department of Agriculture (USDA). *Continuing Survey of Food Intakes by Individuals (CSFII)*

Life Sciences Research Office, Federation of American Societies of Experimental Biology. *Assessment of the Nutritional Status of the U.S. Population Based on Data Collected in the Second National Health and Nutrition Examination Survey, 1976–1980.* Bethesda, MD: Federation of American Societies for Experimental Biology; 1984.

National Center for Health Statistics (NCHS), CDC, PHS, DHHS. *Hispanic Health and Nutrition Examination Survey.*

NCHS. *Health Statistics on Older Persons:* United States, 1986. DHHS publication PHS 87–1409, series 3, no. 25.

NCHS, CDC, PHS, DHHS. *National Health and Nutrition Examination Survey (NHANES) III.*

NCHS, CDC, PHS, DHHS. *National Health Interview Survey (NHIS).*

NCHS, CDC, PHS, DHHS. *National Vital Statistics.*

Part 4

——ɯɯ——

Descriptive Research

Descriptive research is an effective way to obtain information used in devising hypotheses and proposing associations. As stated in Chapter 1, descriptive research cannot test or verify; analytic research is required to evaluate hypotheses or ascertain cause and effect. Important examples of descriptive investigations are descriptive epidemiologic research and qualitative research studies.

Epidemiologic research is descriptive when data detailing person, place, and time are collected (Chapter 8). Descriptive epidemiologic research encompasses correlational studies, case reports, case series, surveys, surveillance systems, demographics, and vital statistics.

Researchers often consider two distinctly different parameters: *incidence* and *prevalence*. Incidence, also referred to as *incidence density* or *cumulative incidence*, is the number of new cases over a given period or the rate at which a certain event occurs. Prevalence is the total number of cases at a specified time point or period. These data are useful in describing populations and monitoring programs.

Two other sets of terms need differentiation: *reliability* versus *validity* and *sensitivity* versus *specificity*. *Reliability* indicates whether the results are repeatable or reproducible, and *validity* indicates whether the test measures what it is designed to measure and whether the measured value agrees with the "true" value. *Sensitivity* indicates the proportion of subjects with a given condition who test positive for that condition; greater sensitivity means that there is less likelihood that a negative result will misclassify an individual. *Specificity* indicates the proportion of subjects without the condition who test negative; there is less likelihood of misclassifying an individual with a positive test if the test has greater specificity.

Qualitative research generates narrative data—that is, data described in words instead of numbers (Chapter 9). A variety of techniques are suitable for securing qualitative data. Observation, in-depth individual interviews, focus-group interviews, nominal group process, the Delphi technique, free elicitation, concept maps, cognitive response tasks, and content analysis are among approaches specified in Chapter 10. Such data may produce graphic and dramatic responses to research questions. Impressive applications of descriptive research may be seen in program planning, identification of population needs, and development of educational materials. Methods—some of them computer-based—for analyzing, unitizing, coding, and comparing qualitative data are currently used to interpret qualitative data. Future research will explore strategies for appraising the "confirmability" of qualitative data (akin to evaluating the reliability of quantitative data) and further enhancing the usefulness of qualitative research in nutrition and dietetics.

ERM, Editor

8

Descriptive Epidemiologic Research

Bettylou Sherry, Ph.D., R.D., Sujata Archer, Ph.D., R.D., and
Linda Van Horn, Ph.D., R.D.

Epidemiology is defined as "the study of the distribution and determinants of disease frequency" (1). The epidemiologic methods for study design, data collection, and analysis provide the conceptual framework for describing the distribution of disease and for testing etiologic hypotheses for a disease or health consequence. This chapter focuses on descriptive epidemiologic research measurements and study designs applicable to nutrition and dietetics. The advantages and limitations of measurements and designs are presented.

Descriptive epidemiologic studies focus on the enumeration and description of person, place, and time. These studies can be used to quantify the extent and location of nutrition problems within a population and suggest associations between diet and disease that can be evaluated in analytic research.

Person-associated characteristics can provide valuable insights into disease etiology. By examining who gets a disease, one can determine whether a particular age, gender, racial, or cultural group is more likely to be at risk. Other person-associated attributes, such as socioeconomic status, family size, marital status, birth order, and personality traits, may be important to consider as well. For example, family income and education both show a strong inverse association with the prevalence of iron-deficiency anemia in women of childbearing age (2).

Place-associated characteristics may also provide valuable insights about potential risk factors for nutrition-associated problems. For example, there exist major geographic differences in international cardiovascular disease mortality rates. Japan and France have very low rates in comparison with northern European countries, New Zealand, and the United States. Among 27 industrialized countries, the United States ranks 15th for coronary heart disease (CHD) mortality in males and 11th in females. Such data lead researchers to investigate reasons for these differences to help identify possible risk factors. The importance of place can also be illustrated in that urban or rural living may affect the availability and price of food items. Even with today's food distribution system, the availability and price of highly nutritious, perishable foods such as fruits, vegetables, and fish vary dramatically by geographic region and by urban and suburban or rural setting. This variability may have a significant impact on the poor. For example, in poverty-stricken, inner-city areas, small neighborhood grocery stores charge higher-than-average prices for these perishable foods, making it difficult for the poor to include adequate amounts in their diets.

Time factors can also affect disease. Seasonal and interannual fluctuations in cumulative incidence, as well as secular trends, may indicate patterns that help elucidate causation. For example, exposure to sunlight has been reported to be one of the major determinants of circulating 25-hydroxy-D_3, the major form of circulating vitamin D, in elderly people with decreased concentrations in winter (3,4). Timing and length of exposure to a risk factor or the duration of latency period also may be important considerations.

DISEASE FREQUENCY

Disease frequency measures the amount of disease or morbidity in a population and is expressed as incidence or prevalence. In practice, the amount of disease translates into risk of disease and becomes the foundation for all descriptive and comparative work. For example, knowledge of the amount of a given disease in different populations can be used to compare the relative importance of this disease in these populations, or it may be used as a basis for comparing populations with different exposures to possible etiologic factors.

Measurement of Incidence

Cumulative Incidence

Cumulative incidence, or *incidence rate,* is the term used to describe disease frequency in a population. Cumulative incidence is the number of new cases of a disease occurring in a population at risk within a specified time interval. Frequently, the observed period is 1 year. It is defined as follows:

$$\begin{bmatrix} \text{Cumulative} \\ \text{incidence} \end{bmatrix} = \frac{\text{Number of new cases}}{\text{Population at risk}} \times \text{Time period}$$

Cumulative incidence is normally expressed as the number of cases per 100,000 per year; it can also be expressed as the risk of disease (Figure 8.1). The population at the midpoint in the study period is used as the population at risk.

When cumulative incidence is calculated, the denominator is based on population defined by geographic area, and it can have an even more specific focus, such as a particular gender, age, or ethnic group. For example, the population at risk could be the state of Washington or the number of African-American girls in Boston between the ages of 14 and 17 years.

Cumulative incidence is useful for documenting the relative importance of a disease in a population and for tracking changes in the occurrence of a disease over time. For example, changes in rates of premenopausal breast cancer are tracked by monitoring cumulative incidence over time. Cumulative incidence can also provide etiologic clues. A comparison of the cumulative incidence for populations that have different sex distributions, age groupings, ethnicity, or geographic locations can identify population groups with low or high rates of disease. This identification of high-risk groups can be used to target intervention programs where they are most needed.

A specific application of cumulative incidence for nutritionists and dietitians is quantifying the attack rate of an outbreak of food poisoning. *Attack rate* is the term substituted for *cumulative incidence* when the period of observation is short. In this situation, the population would be at risk for a short time, and the study period would encompass the entire epidemic. A good example would be an outbreak of *Salmonella* infection in a public school. An outbreak investigation would seek to identify the food contaminated with salmonellae by documenting what food was more likely to have been eaten by those who became ill in contrast to those who remained well.

Incidence density

Sometimes the study population in a research project is dynamic. Subjects may be lost due to death or migration, or they may have acquired the disease and therefore are no longer at risk. To account for this loss of subjects, the researcher can calculate incidence density, which is similar to cumulative incidence but calculated slightly differently. As in the calculation of cumulative incidence, the numerator in incidence density includes the number of new cases of a disease. The denominator, however, is different; it includes the total amount of time each person in the study is at risk for disease (Figure 8.2). Incidence density is calculated as follows:

$$\begin{bmatrix} \text{Incidence} \\ \text{density} \end{bmatrix} = \frac{\text{Number of new cases}}{\text{Person-time at risk}} \times \text{Time period}$$

where person-time at risk is the total amount of time all participants have been considered to be at risk for developing the disease, yet before they develop the disease, while they have been a part of the study. Good resources for more in-depth discussions on the calculation of incidence density include Rothman and Greenland (5) and Miettenen (6).

Incidence density calculations would be useful, for example, in studies of osteoporosis in postmenopausal women in which the subjects might die or move from the study area. The advantage of using incidence density is that it permits inclusion of all of the time that each person participates in the study. If cumulative incidence were

$$CI = \frac{\text{No. of persons in whom the disease develops}}{\text{Population at risk}} \times \text{Time period}$$

$$= \frac{\text{No. of new cases of colon cancer in county A}}{\text{Midyear population of county A}} \times 1 \text{ yr}$$

$$= \frac{20 \text{ new colon cancer cases in county A in 1991}}{995,000 \text{ population } 7/1/91} \times 1 \text{ yr}$$

$$= \frac{20}{995,000}$$

$$= \frac{2.01}{100,000}$$

or the risk of colon cancer in 1991 in county A is 0.002%.

FIGURE 8.1 Calculation of cumulative incidence (CI). An example of colon cancer CI being expressed as risk of disease is provided.

used, only the subjects enrolled in the study for the entire project period would be included in the calculation of the rate. Thus, incidence density calculations tend to use participant time in a study more efficiently.

Measurement of Prevalence

Prevalence is the proportion of the population that is affected by a certain disease or condition at a given time, and it includes both new and existing cases. Prevalence can be expressed either as point or period prevalence. Point prevalence depicts one point in time, as in a cross-sectional survey, and, unless otherwise specified, it is how the term *prevalence* generally is defined. Point prevalence is calculated as follows:

$$\begin{bmatrix} \text{Point} \\ \text{prevalence} \end{bmatrix} = \frac{\text{Number of new, existing,} \text{ and recurring cases}}{\text{Total population at risk}} \times \text{Time}$$

where time = one point in time.

In contrast, period prevalence is calculated as follows:

$$\begin{bmatrix} \text{Period} \\ \text{prevalence} \end{bmatrix} = \frac{\text{Number of new, existing,} \text{ and recurring cases}}{\text{Total population at risk}} \times \text{Time}$$

where time = a period of time.

Sometimes incidence data are not available for a disease, so prevalence data are calculated. This alternative is acceptable as long as the person interpreting the numbers clearly understands that incidence is the number of new cases within a specified period and that prevalence is the number of old and new cases within a period. A lack of understanding of the difference between incidence and prevalence is a common mistake in scientific writing (7).

Prevalence data are advantageous for assessing the frequency of diseases or conditions that do not have an acute onset. Anemia and obesity are good examples of illnesses or conditions that can be described best in this manner. Prevalence is applicable in monitoring control programs for chronic illnesses such as anemia. A series of cross-sectional studies that document point prevalence can be used to track changes in the burden of a disease to a population.

Prevalence is useful for identifying people at greatest risk and for planning health services, because

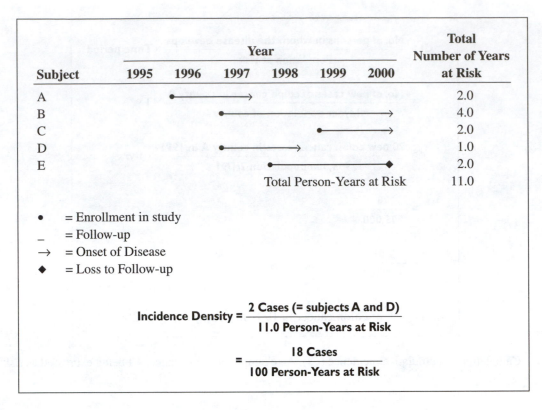

FIGURE 8.2   Calculation of person-time and incidence density.

prevalence describes the burden of a disease or condition to a population. For example, findings from the National Health and Nutrition Examination Surveys (NHANES) II (1976–1980) and II (1988–1994) indicate that the prevalence of overweight among children and adolescents is increasing. During this time period for children aged 6 years to 11 years, the prevalence among boys increased from 6.5 percent to 11.4 percent, and the prevalence among girls increased from 5.5 percent to 9.9 percent (8). For adolescents 12 years to 17 years of age, the prevalence among boys increased from 4.7 percent to 11.4 percent, and the prevalence among girls increased from 4.9 percent to 9.9 percent (8).

The difference between incidence and prevalence can introduce important sources of bias when evaluating the effect of a screening program where both the issues of identification of cases and the effectiveness of intervention need to be examined. For example, the prevalence of anemia prior to the implementation of a screening program may be compared with the prevalence found in a follow-up survey that includes both prevalent plus new incident cases. In addition, by the nature of the definition of *prevalence,* it is obvious that chronic conditions would

be more likely to be picked up in a survey than short-term acute conditions.

SCREENING TESTS

Screening tests are designed to identify people who either have a disease that can be effectively treated in the early stages or who are at high risk for a disease and therefore can benefit from intervention to reduce their risk. For example, dietitians and nutritionists use screening tests at the community level to target children with anemia for iron supplementation. In a clinical setting, the screening of newborns for phenylketonuria is a routine practice to prevent mental retardation. Also, a screening program that may include both dietary intake and biochemical indexes may be established in a clinical setting to identify patients at high risk for a poor nutrition outcome to target them for special care to either prevent or reduce their risk of nutrient depletion.

As will be discussed, the prevalence of a positive screening test and its reliability and validity, as well as the availability of a treatment for the disease or condition of interest, are key factors in determining whether the use of a screening test can be justified.

Reliability and Validity

Tests that are used for screening must be both reliable and valid. A reliable test gives the same results when the test is repeated on the same person several times. In other words, a reliable test gives reproducible results. A valid test measures what it is designed to measure.

Validity is used in epidemiologic studies to assess various methods of interest to dietitians, such as dietary assessment and anthropometric measures. For example, an epidemiologic study using the quantitative food frequency questionnaire could test the validity of its dietary instrument by comparing data with data obtained by other methods, such as multiple 24-hour dietary recalls. Yaroch et al compared results from administering a modified picture-sort food frequency questionnaire at two different time intervals with means of three 24-hour recalls among low-income, overweight, African-American adolescent girls (9). The investigators reported correlation coefficients between the second food frequency questionnaire and three recalls to exceed .50 for most nutrients. However, testing the reliability of their dietary instrument by test-retest within a 2-week period indicated poor relia-

bility. Therefore, the validity of a dietary assessment method does not always translate to a reliable instrument. It is recommended that studies examine the validity and reliability of each dietary assessment method by age, gender, and ethnicity to understand the best application of the tool (10).

Some biochemical markers are currently being used as surrogates for dietary assessment because validity studies have shown they provide an accurate assessment. For example, 24-hour urinary nitrogen excretion represents an approximate constant proportion of 80 percent of the total daily nitrogen ingested as protein (11). The INTERSALT study reported that urea was a valid marker of total dietary protein in population studies, because urea nitrogen was found to be highly correlated with total nitrogen concentration ($r = 0.984$) (12).

Sensitivity and Specificity

Two parameters used to assess the validity of a test are sensitivity and specificity. Sensitivity is the proportion of persons with the disease or condition who have positive test results. In contrast, specificity is the proportion of people without the disease or condition who have negative test results. The higher the specificity, the less likely it is that a positive test result will misclassify a person. These screening tests are schematically described in Figure 8.3.

		Test Result	
		Positive	**Negative**
Disease or Condition	**Yes**	a	b
	No	c	d

Sensitivity = Proportion of those with a disease who have a positive test

$$= \frac{a}{a + b}$$

Specificity = Proportion of those without a disease who have a negative test

$$= \frac{d}{c + d}$$

FIGURE 8.3   Schematic description of the screening test indices sensitivity and specificity and their calculation.

Sensitivity and specificity are used to establish cutoffs or reference interval limits for a test. The goal is to maximize both sensitivity and specificity in order to minimize false-positive and false-negative test results, but in reality there usually must be a compromise. Natural biological variability results in a spectrum of test values in any population. A few people with abnormal findings for a screening test will not have the disease. The converse will also occur: some people with normal test findings will have the disease. Where the normal reference range cutoff points are set will affect the sensitivity and the specificity. Detsky et al discuss how reference intervals are established to maximize sensitivity and specificity in their comparison of nutrition assessment techniques (13).

Predictive Value

The predictive value of a test is its ability to accurately distinguish people with or without the disease or condition. Thus, the positive predictive value is the probability of disease, given a positive test result, whereas the negative predictive value is the probability of no disease, given a negative test result (Figure 8.4).

Predictive values are strongly affected by the number of people with and without disease. For example, if sensitivity and specificity are constant, the differences in positive predictive values for a test for anemia in populations of different sizes with prevalences of 25, 3.3, and 0.3 percent are notable (Figure 6.5). This example using a highly sensitive and highly specific test shows that in a population where anemia is rare, this screening test has a very low positive predictive value. In this situation, a screening test may not be of value for public health purposes.

Effective Screening

For screening to be effective, it must have a major role in improving the outcome of illness. Thus, it is not enough for a screening test to have a high positive predictive value; there must be an effective treatment program for people identified as being at risk for, or having, the disease or condition. Diseases or conditions appropriate for screening are those that have serious consequences, a detectable preclinical phase, an effective treatment, and usually a high prevalence of preclinical disease in the population. It is also worthwhile to consider the practical qualities of a screening test. A suitable screening test is inexpensive; is easy to administer; provides minimal discomfort to the patient; and has reliable, valid results.

Phenylketonuria meets all the criteria for screening except that it has a relatively low incidence. The incidence varies by geographic area and ethnicity; for example, in the state of Georgia since 1979, the incidence has

		Positive	Negative
		a	b
		c	d

Test Result

Disease or Condition — Yes / No

Positive predictive value = Proportion of those with a positive test who have a disease

$$= \frac{a}{a + c}$$

Negative predictive value = Proportion of those with a negative test who do not have a disease

$$= \frac{d}{b + d}$$

FIGURE 8.4   Schematic description of the predictive values of a screening test.

		Population = 400 Prevalence = 25%		Population = 3100 Prevalence = 3.3%		Population = 30,100 Prevalence = 0.3%	
		Test Result		**Test Result**		**Test Result**	
		+	−	+	−	+	−
Anemia	+	97	3	97	3	97	3
	−	10	290	100	2900	1000	29000

Sensitivity $= \dfrac{97}{100} = 97\%$ $\dfrac{97}{100} = 97\%$ $\dfrac{97}{100} = 97\%$

Specificity $= \dfrac{290}{300} = 97\%$ $\dfrac{2900}{3000} = 97\%$ $\dfrac{29000}{30000} = 97\%$

Positive predictive value $= \dfrac{97}{107} = 90.6\%$ $\dfrac{97}{197} = 49.2\%$ $\dfrac{97}{1097} = 8.8\%$

FIGURE 8.5 Comparison of positive predictive values in populations of different sizes and different levels of prevalence of anemia.

been 1 in 17,209 live births (14). However, in affected infants, the elimination of all but the essential requirement of phenylalanine in the diet of an infant will prevent mental retardation. The social and economic costs of caring for a mentally retarded child are high; in contrast, the cost of screening all newborns is low, and the test is highly sensitive. In this example, a highly effective available treatment makes the cost of screening for a rare disease in a population justifiable.

Limitations of Screening Tests

If screening test results are to be used in analyses for public health planning and targeting programs, two potential biases must be considered. The first bias is that of volunteers or self-selection. On average, volunteers have a better health status than that of the general population. The second bias is that of lead time. *Lead time* refers to the amount of time the diagnosis is advanced by a screening program. Early diagnosis might make a treatment more effective and shorten the amount of time an affected person would have the disease. The benefits of early diagnosis are important to consider in the evaluation of the change in morbidity and mortality as a result of screening.

DESCRIPTIVE RESEARCH DESIGN

Descriptive studies are the simplest of all research designs. The most common types of descriptive studies include correlational studies, case reports or case series, surveys, and surveillance systems. They simply report the characteristics of person, place, and time of a disease or a condition of interest, and they are used to identify patterns of a disease or condition. They may report on countrywide populations, small geographic areas, small groups of people, or individual subjects.

Descriptive studies are also valuable for identifying potential associations between risk factors and a disease. Frequently descriptive studies are less expensive and take less time than analytic studies because they use precollected data, such as the National Food Consumption Survey; NHANES I, II, and III; vital statistics; or clinical records. Results from descriptive studies can form the basis of hypotheses for analytic research.

Correlational Studies

Correlational studies are beneficial for examining patterns relating a possible risk or causative factor in a disease. Often data from several countries are examined to identify these relationships. A good example of the application of this type of study to nutrition and dietetics is the international documentation of the relationship between diet and mortality from CHD by Keys et al (15). Using data from seven countries, the investigators found a significant positive correlation between the proportion of energy intake from saturated fat and death from CHD. Other examples of correlational studies are the large prospective studies that have reported a 40 percent lower rate of CHD correlated with consumption of vitamin E supplements of at least 100 IU/day for more than 2 years (16,17).

It is important to note that correlation studies show only associations between a factor and a disease or condition. They do not show causation or the effect of potential confounding factors, and they do not document the biological processes involved in a disease or condition.

Case Reports and Case Series

Unique experiences of one patient or a small group of patients with a similar diagnosis are reported in the literature as case reports or case series. These accounts can provide a basis for a more vigorous investigation and analytic approach to examining the factors of interest. This brief documentation also alerts health care professionals to possible, but not proved, beneficial or life-threatening aspects of a disease or its treatment. Case reports or case series may also be used to document the beginning of an epidemic. There are other uses for case reports, such as tracking toxicity reports of new foods. For example, there were two case reports of patients who had ingested the same botanical dietary supplement and experienced toxic concentrations of digoxin in the serum because the dietary supplement contained cardiac glycosides, natural components of *Digitalis lanata* (18).

A case series is of greater value than a single case report, because it gives more documentation of evidence for the suggested hypothesis. Case reports or case series are never conclusive in establishing cause and effect, but they are useful for the initial descriptions of a new disease or for documenting the biological processes of a disease or condition.

Surveys

Surveys can provide a wide variety of descriptive information about a disease or condition, but their important contribution is in providing a view of the people studied at one point or period of time. Many national surveys have been done and are repeated periodically. Examples include the Continuing Survey of Food Intakes by Individuals and NHANES I, II, and III. Currently the Continuing Survey of Food Intakes by Individuals and the NHANES have been combined and are being conducted annually (see http://www.cdc.gov/nchs/about/major/nhanes/current.htm). These surveys have sophisticated sampling frames to provide representative information from all segments of the population or special high-risk population groups.

The advantage of cross-sectional surveys is that they can offer a representative overview of the health of the population. Their limitation is that the data cannot provide answers to questions about disease etiology. When a population is surveyed at one point in time, it may be difficult to determine whether exposure to a risk factor came before a disease unless questions about timing are included. For further discussion of surveys and using these large databases, see Chapter 13.

Surveillance

Surveillance can be described as a systematic, ongoing survey designed to monitor specific health outcomes in a population (19). Surveillance systems are used to identify and monitor public health problems. In turn, this information can be used for public health planning, program evaluation, and policy development, as well as for research. Important components of a surveillance system include the cooperation and coordination of many individuals and groups, the collection of high-quality data, management of the data, and timely analysis and dissemination of the data for use.

Pertinent examples for dietitians include the Pediatric Nutrition Surveillance System (PedNSS) and the Pregnancy Nutrition Surveillance System (PNSS) managed by the Centers for Disease Control and Prevention (20,21). The PedNSS monitors growth indicators, anemia status, and breast-feeding status of children and includes minimal demographic data. The PNSS monitors prepregnancy weight, pregnancy weight gain, anemia status, behavioral risk factors, birth outcome, and infant feeding status, and it includes demographic data. These systems include data on low-income women, infants, and children who participate in publicly funded health and nutrition programs in states that participate in these surveillance systems.

Measurement of Vital Statistics and Demographics

Vital statistics are based on data from records such as birth certificates, death certificates, and census data. Vital statistics are really a type of surveillance data, as they routinely monitor vital events. By law, birth and death certificates must be filed by the birth attendant or attending physician at the local town or city clerk's office; these data are also forwarded to county and state offices for compilation and reporting. At the beginning of each decade, the federal government collects population census data. The calculation of commonly used indexes of vital statistics is summarized in Figure 8.6.

Birth and death certificate data are readily available from the vital records offices of counties or states. State vital statistics reports are published annually and can be obtained from the state office. These reports are available in the public documents area of public, college, or university libraries. National vital statistics reports are also available on the Internet from agencies such as the Cen-

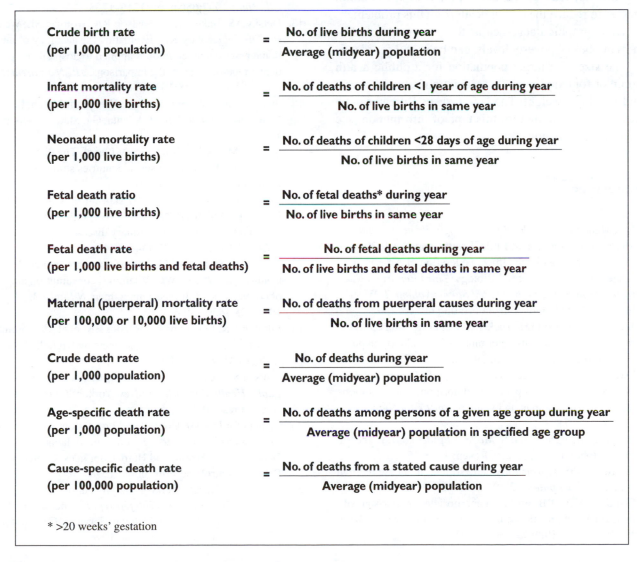

Crude birth rate (per 1,000 population)	=	No. of live births during year / Average (midyear) population
Infant mortality rate (per 1,000 live births)	=	No. of deaths of children <1 year of age during year / No. of live births in same year
Neonatal mortality rate (per 1,000 live births)	=	No. of deaths of children <28 days of age during year / No. of live births in same year
Fetal death ratio (per 1,000 live births)	=	No. of fetal deaths* during year / No. of live births in same year
Fetal death rate (per 1,000 live births and fetal deaths)	=	No. of fetal deaths during year / No. of live births and fetal deaths in same year
Maternal (puerperal) mortality rate (per 100,000 or 10,000 live births)	=	No. of deaths from puerperal causes during year / No. of live births in same year
Crude death rate (per 1,000 population)	=	No. of deaths during year / Average (midyear) population
Age-specific death rate (per 1,000 population)	=	No. of deaths among persons of a given age group during year / Average (midyear) population in specified age group
Cause-specific death rate (per 100,000 population)	=	No. of deaths from a stated cause during year / Average (midyear) population

* >20 weeks' gestation

FIGURE 8.6 Commonly Used Indices of Vital Statistics

ters for Disease Control and Prevention, National Center for Health Statistics, and the National Vital Statistics System. Examples of some data available are age-adjusted death rates for selected causes, such as diabetes mellitus or cardiovascular disease, by race and gender; data for births in the United States. according to maternal and demographic characteristics; and infant health status (see http://www.cdc.gov/nchs/nvss.htm).

Vital statistics data are especially useful for documenting person, place, and time characteristics of a disease or condition, as well as for documenting the relative importance of a disease or health problem in a population. For example, cause-specific maternal mortality rates can be used to identify the primary causes of maternal deaths. This information can be used to target major problem areas, such as maternal hypertension, and in turn, as part of the follow-up, lead to the development of intervention strategies to reduce the risk of death from this problem.

Demographic data, such as the percentage of children living below poverty levels, can be useful for identifying the size of a target population for a public health program or for examining the association between poverty and low birth weight. The U.S. Census Bureau can be accessed on the Internet for this type of information (see http://www.census.gov).

REFERENCES

1. MacMahon B, Pugh TF. *Epidemiology: Principles and Methods*. Boston, Mass: Little, Brown, and Co; 1970.
2. Life Sciences Research Office, Federation of American Societies for Experimental Biology. *Third Report on Nutrition Monitoring in the United States: Volume 1*. Washington, DC: U.S. Government Printing Office; 1995.
3. Jacques PF, Felson DT, Tucker KL, et al. Plasma 25-hydroxyvitamin D and its determinants in an elderly population sample. *Am J Clin Nutr.* 1997;66:929–936.
4. Dawson-Hughes B, Harris SS, Dallel GE. Plasma calcidiol, season, and serum parathyroid hormone concentrations in healthy elderly men and women. *Am J Clin Nutr.* 1997;65:67–71.
5. Rothman KJ, Greenland S. *Modern Epidemiology*. 2nd ed. Philadelphia, Pa: Lippincott-Raven; 1998:35.
6. Miettenen OS. Estimability and estimation in case referent studies. *Am J Epidemiol.* 1976;103:226–235.
7. Flanders WD, O'Brien TR. Inappropriate comparisons of incidence and prevalence in epidemiologic research. *Am J Public Health.* 1989;79:1301–1303.
8. Trioano RP, Flegal KM. Overweight children and adolescents: Description, epidemiology, and demographics. *Pediatrics.* 1998;101:497–504.
9. Yaroch AL, Resnicow K, Davis M, Davis A, Smith M, Khan LK. Development of a modified picture-sort food frequency questionnaire administered to low-income, overweight, African-American adolescent girls. *J Am Diet Assoc.* 2000;100:1050–1056.
10. McPherson RS, Hoelscher DM, Alexander M, Scanlon KS, Serdula MK. Dietary assessment methods among school-aged children: validity and reliability. *Prev Med.* 2000;31(suppl):11–33.
11. Kaaks RJ. Biochemical markers as additional measurements in studies of the accuracy of dietary questionnaire measurements: conceptual issues. *Am J Clin Nutr.* 1997;65(suppl):1232–1239.
12. Dyer A, Elliott P, Chee D, Stamler J. Urinary biochemical markers of dietary intake in the INTERSALT Study. *Am J Clin Nutr.* 1997;65(suppl):1246–1253.
13. Detsky AS, Baker JP, Mendelson RA, Wolman SL, Wesson DE, Jeejeebhoy KN. Evaluating the accuracy of nutritional assessment techniques applied to hospitalized patients: methodology and comparisons. *JPEN J Parenter Enteral Nutr.* 1984;8:153–159.
14. State of Georgia Comprehensive Newborn Metabolic Screening. *Annual Report*. Atlanta, Ga: State of Georgia; 1997.
15. Keys A, Menotti A, Karvonen MJ, et al. The diet and 15-year death rate in the seven countries study. *Am J Epidemiol.* 1986;124:903–915.
16. Stampfer MJ, Hennekens CH, Manson JE, Colditz GA, Rosner B, Willett WC. A prospective study of vitamin E consumption and risk of coronary disease in women. *N Engl J Med.* 1993;328:1444–1449.
17. Rimm EB, Stampfer MJ, Ascherio A, Giovannucci E, Colditz, GA, Willett WC. Vitamin E consumption and risk of coronary heart disease among men. *N Engl J Med.* 1993;328:1450–1456.
18. Silfman NR, Obermeyer WR, Aloi BK, et al. Contamination of botanical dietary supplements by Digitalis lanata. *N Engl J Med.* 1998;339:806–811.
19. Teutsch SM, Churchill RE. *Principles and Practice of Public Health Surveillance*. New York, NY: Oxford University Press; 1994.
20. Centers for Disease Control and Prevention. *Pediatric Nutrition Surveillance: 1997 Full Report*. Atlanta, Ga: US Department of Health and Human Services, Centers for Disease Control and Prevention; 1998.
21. Centers for Disease Control and Prevention. *Pregnancy Nutrition Surveillance: 1996 full report*. Atlanta, Ga: US Department of Health and Human Services, Centers for Disease Control and Prevention; 1998.

Further Reading

Abramson JH. *Making Sense of Data.* New York, NY: Oxford University Press; 1988.

Rothman KJ, Greenland S. *Modern Epidemiology.* 2nd ed. Philadelphia, Pa: Lippincott-Raven; 1998:35.

Weiss NS. *Clinical Epidemiology: The Study of the Outcome of Illness.* New York, NY: Oxford University Press; 1986:11.

9

—※—

The Philosophy and Role of Qualitative Inquiry in Research

Cheryl L. Achterberg, Ph.D., and Sandra K. Shepherd, Ph.D., R.D.

Qualitative research has always been an integral part of cross-cultural comparisons and descriptions of food habits in the nutrition and anthropology literature (1,2), but it has also become routine in food product development and sensory evaluation (3), food and nutrition marketing (4), materials development (5,6), program evaluation (7), dietary intake assessment (8), and nutrition education (9). It also offers a great deal of insight into nutrition and dietetics. The unique assumptions underlying qualitative research, the various approaches that may be used, and the types of information that it can produce are useful to dietitians in both research and practice. The purpose of this chapter is to define qualitative research, to describe when and why it should be conducted, and to correct some common misconceptions associated with it. Chapter 10 reviews qualitative methodologies.

WHAT IS QUALITATIVE RESEARCH?

Precise definitions for *qualitative research* are rarely found in the literature. Most of the definitions offered are discursive, complex, and based on philosophical perspectives. In addition, most define what each term is by contrast to what it is not (10,11). The distinction, however, is artificial (12), and a purely dichotomous approach (that is, quantitative research versus qualitative research) tends to obscure the similarities that exist between the two ap-

proaches, as well as the differences among methods within a given approach (11,13). The traditional or purist perspective is that an investigator can use only one approach or the other; the fundamental differences between qualitative and quantitative philosophies make it impossible to combine methods from the two traditions without violating the principles unique to each one. This chapter departs from that view, because nutrition or dietetics is an applied, and therefore pragmatic, science that almost always has as its goal intervention (as opposed to description for the sake of knowledge alone). In other words, researchers in nutrition and dietetics are more interested in identifying what works than in defending a particular methodology on philosophical grounds alone. Of course, the methodology also must be sufficiently rigorous to earn credibility for the results it produces.

Qualitative research may be defined as any data-gathering technique that generates narrative data or words rather than numerical data or numbers (14,15). For example, a qualitative approach to research on consumers' understanding of the word *cholesterol* would generate a large number of definitions in the consumers' own words, which might vary greatly from a quantitative approach that uses a set of definitions generated by dietitians in a multiple-choice survey questionnaire. The primary caveat in qualitative research is that the words must reflect the point of view of the study participant, not the researcher (16,17). In other words, qualitative research is based on the assumption that findings about human interaction, thinking, and behavior are better understood and more scientifically valid when seen from the inside out than when seen from the outside in.

THE RANGE OF QUALITATIVE RESEARCH

Qualitative research is not a homogeneous or one-size-fits-all enterprise. A multitude of qualitative approaches exist (11). Lincoln and Guba (10) allude to this fact in their discussion of a continuum between qualitative and quantitative research approaches, with pure analytic induction at one extreme and the standardized measures and statistical protocols of deduction at the other extreme. However, according to our pragmatic definition of qualitative research, standardized measures of words or word production and statistical protocols (as applied to the analysis of words or narratives) need to be used in certain qualitative inquiries. As Firestone and Dawson (18) noted, the question of when a study may properly be considered qualitative is becoming increasingly difficult to answer, especially when combined techniques are used. We prefer to depict qualitative and quantitative research approaches on separate, but parallel, continuums (Figure 9.1), where the two approaches vary greatly at the ends of their continuums but share many commonalities in between. From this perspective, the two approaches have obvious similarities, as well as differences.

The most important similarity between qualitative and quantitative research approaches is a shared e view that the world can be known through systematic, empirical observation. Both study approaches can provide information that will add to either the conceptual or methodological base of the field, contribute meaningful information to policy makers, or provide useful information to practitioners. However, the appropriateness, fit, and scope of the data produced by qualitative or quantitative studies vary according to the particular issue of interest. For example, qualitative approaches are seldom appropriate in engineering science, but they are often appropriate in the study of social behavior, such as food choices and eating.

As indicated in Figure 9.2, both qualitative and quantitative approaches—at least at certain points along the continuums—may be descriptive, evaluative, theory building, and context sensitive, and both approaches may be used to test hypotheses. Only at the extreme ends of the continuums are the differences between the research approaches greater than the similarities. It is also impor-

tant to point out that although qualitative researchers start out with words, they often end up using numbers to describe their results. By the same token, quantitative researchers may start out with numbers, but they end up using words to describe their results. Thus, researchers from both traditions use both words and numbers, and both use interpretive analyses in one form or another. One of the advantages of qualitative research, however, is that qualitative data can be analyzed as such. These data can also be converted subsequently to quantitative data for future analysis—for example, by simply ranking or counting the number of statements within each category. Quantitative data rarely, if ever, exhibit the converse versatility.

Strauss and Corbin (19) maintain the extreme position that qualitative research generates theory, whereas quantitative research does not. However, concept and observation are interdependent in both approaches (12). No qualitative researcher is able to observe from a blank slate, and no quantitative researcher should be blind to unanticipated data produced by a given experiment or study. The theory-generation value of both qualitative and quantitative studies depends on the particular data in hand, previous work done in the field, and the researcher's insight and creativity.

By the same token, research can be performed "atheoretically" in both qualitative and quantitative inquiries. In the atheoretical approach, the underlying theory is not made explicit before or after the study and thus is not open to verification, analysis, discussion, or development (20). Each study is designed and interpreted independently, with no common ground on which to base generalization. In contrast, theoretical research relies on theory to guide study design, interpretation of results, or both. The theory provides a conceptual framework for approaching the research problem, choosing the hypotheses, understanding the results, and relating them to the real world. Atheoretical research lacks that conceptual framework. For example, when no comprehensive theory exists as to why diet, smoking, stress, gender, age, and even beard growth are related to serum cholesterol levels and heart disease, it is not surprising that the results vary from study to study (21).

From a practical point of view, both qualitative and quantitative data can be used to build theory. Furthermore, it may be easiest to combine qualitative and quantitative approaches within a study in the area where the two continuums overlap (see Figure 9.3) and more difficult in the areas of no overlap.

WHY DO QUALITATIVE RESEARCH?

The most common reason investigators do qualitative research is that it "enables researchers to ask new questions, answer different kinds of questions and readdress old questions" (22). One of the main reasons the interest in qualitative research has grown in community settings is that the more traditional, quantitative methods are often impractical; hospitals and clinics have neither the staff, resources, nor expertise to mount a study with a sample size of thousands or controls sufficient to detect statistical significance. Even with large amounts of resources, however, problems arise. For example, people cannot be randomly assigned to different clinics in different communities to assess the impact of a new educational or counseling intervention. Qualitative methods often present a more pragmatic approach to conducting research in a natural setting. These methods also offer dietitians greater opportunities

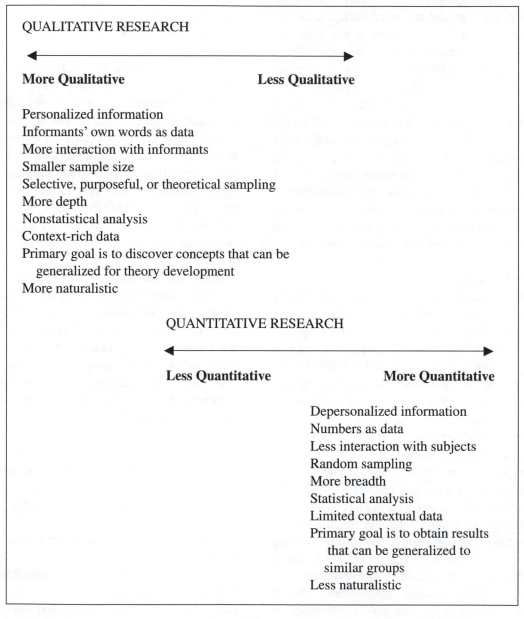

QUALITATIVE RESEARCH

More Qualitative   **Less Qualitative**

Personalized information
Informants' own words as data
More interaction with informants
Smaller sample size
Selective, purposeful, or theoretical sampling
More depth
Nonstatistical analysis
Context-rich data
Primary goal is to discover concepts that can be
    generalized for theory development
More naturalistic

QUANTITATIVE RESEARCH

Less Quantitative   **More Quantitative**

Depersonalized information
Numbers as data
Less interaction with subjects
Random sampling
More breadth
Statistical analysis
Limited contextual data
Primary goal is to obtain results
    that can be generalized to
    similar groups
Less naturalistic

FIGURE 9.1 Qualitative and quantitative research approaches depicted on separate, but overlapping and parallel, continuums, where both approaches seek to understand the world through observational methods.

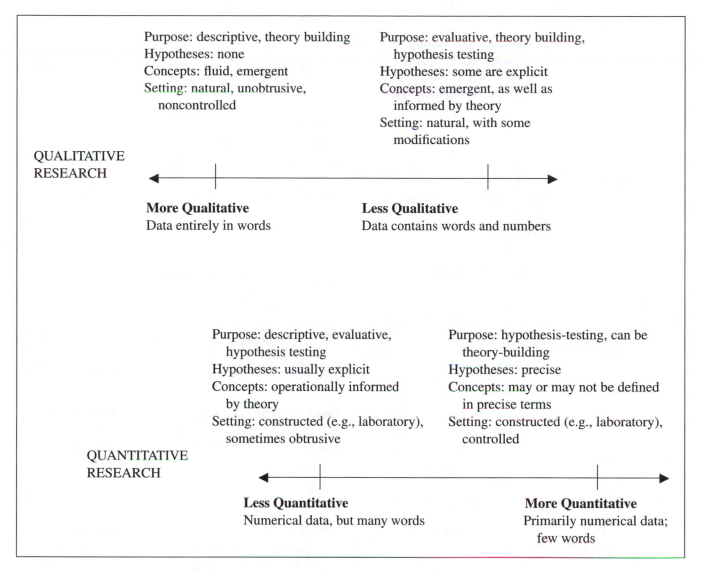

FIGURE 9.2 A comparison of qualitative and quantitative research approaches as defined by their purposes and settings.

to obtain information about clients' behavior, attitudes, beliefs, and social influences through the use of open-ended questions.

Qualitative and quantitative research designs have an important major difference. In qualitative research, the investigator retains the right to modify or alter the study design in the field according to the need to reassess issues that become apparent only in the field (16). The quantitative research design, in contrast, is seldom if ever altered, regardless of circumstances.

The most common situations in which investigators choose a qualitative research approach follow:

- The research problem is so new that it is "pretheoretical"—that is, not enough is known about the sit-

uation to formulate testable hypotheses or select a suitable theory to address it (23). An example might be the public reaction to genetically modified corn or rice in staple, core foods versus in occasional or "extra" foods, such as dessert items.

- The researchers are as interested in process variables as they are in outcome variables. In other words, evaluators wish to know how and why a given outcome happens. For example, dietitians may want to know why some clients adhere to a recommended diet plan and others do not.

- The evaluation needs to be extremely audience specific or very detailed in nature (for example, needs assessment for a group of women with both diabetes mellitus and bulimia).

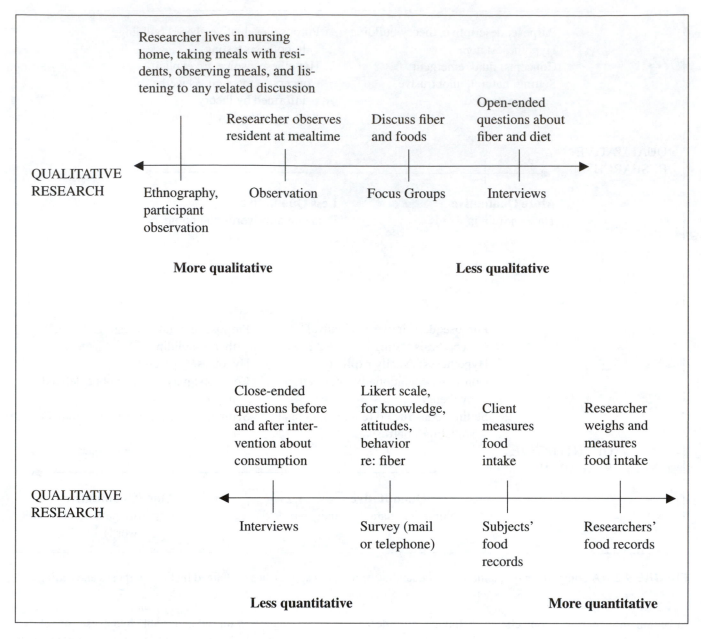

FIGURE 9.3 Qualitative and quantitative research approaches represented as parallel continuums and illustrated by hypothetical studies about increasing fiber intake in a nursing home.

- The researcher needs data on social context, structure, and interactions within which a particular behavior pattern can be understood. These data may be particularly important in understanding aberrant dietary behavior expressed by either individuals or groups, such as pica, anorexia, nonorganic failure to thrive, or binge eating.

Researchers may also turn to qualitative methods if they feel they are constantly trying to "force round data into square holes"(12), analyzing variables that are mea-

surable but irrelevant (24), ignoring categories of data that are important to the respondent but unanticipated by the researcher (for example, foods high in saturated fat are "spongy" and soak up fat), producing results that are not useful because they were generated under artificial or invalid conditions, or using theories that do not explain the measurable outcomes of interest (16). In some instances, researchers may suspect that they have fallen victim to type III error, the most common validity error made in research, by asking the wrong research questions (17). Tukey is quoted by Lincoln and Guba (10) as saying, it is better to have "an appropriate answer to the *right* question, which is often vague, than an *exact* answer to the wrong question, which can always be made more precise." In these situations, qualitative methods can be used to "discover" pertinent questions, variables, concepts, and problems, as well as to generate hypotheses or even theories that are more pertinent to the practitioner-researcher (19,25).

In some cases, quantitative survey data may be difficult to collect from certain groups of people, such as young children (26) and those who are functionally illiterate (27) or unfamiliar with the testing procedures (28). Other people may refuse to answer survey questionnaires because they distrust questionnaires, the source of the questionnaire (for example, private industry or government), or researchers in general. Yet all of these groups may readily participate in the more intimate and interactive data collection procedures offered by qualitative methodologies.

A small, in-depth qualitative study may also provide more useful information than a large-scale quantitative study during formative evaluations (that is, during the design and development testing of new products or programs), when the details provide insight as to how a future intervention program or product might be improved before further investments of time, personnel, and money are made. This kind of study can result in an economy of effort in the long run, whether the product is a new gastric tube, hospital menu, pamphlet, or weight-loss program.

Ideally, investigators should not use qualitative research methods unless they have training and experience with the methods or they have a consultant who can train and supervise staff appropriately. An in-depth study of the literature and some pilot work may also provide suitable background.

MYTHS AND MISCONCEPTIONS ABOUT QUALITATIVE RESEARCH

There are many widespread myths and misconceptions about qualitative research. This section discusses some that researchers might encounter.

Qualitative Research Is Not Objective

Objectivity is defined simply as the study of an object or fact independent of the thoughts, bias, prejudice, or mind of the observer (29). Some say that objectivity is the central goal of science.

Qualitative research is in some ways more objective than quantitative approaches and in some ways less objective, at least in terms of studying human behavior. In general, qualitative methods are more objective from the participants' perspective and less so from other researchers' perspective. For example, dietitians must constantly choose between weighed food records (which reflect accurate amounts but invalid intakes) and 24-hour recalls (which often reflect more accurate intakes but invalid amounts). Thus, the important issue is not whether qualitative research is objective but how its subjectivity is managed. If subjectivity is hidden or unrecognized, it can interfere with good science. For example, clients may change their diets or portion sizes when weighing their food to ease respondent burden, but then the results do not reflect their usual intakes. If, however, subjectivity is made explicit and systematically identified, its impact on the research should not be burdensome (30). An example might be having a client pour a serving of cereal out when he or she reports two servings of cereal per day to ascertain the accuracy of that person's self-reporting. The data then can be corrected accordingly.

Some people consider qualitative research "soft," or less reliable and therefore less desirable, than quantitative research, which is "hard." Numerical information is considered highly reliable because it is replicable, and therefore deemed more trustworthy. The fact that such data may not be valid is often overlooked. Qualitative data, in contrast, are rarely replicable (12,17). The authors take a pragmatic stand. Because this bias exists, it is useful to provide some numerical information with each study so that readers do not automatically dismiss the results produced in narrative form. For example, we have calculated interrater reliabilities based on the number of positive, negative, and neutral statements made in our interviews (31), focus groups (27), and cognitive response tasks (32). We have found that once these results are produced, most of the ensuing discussion turns on the substance of the qualitative results rather than on the appropriateness of our research methods. Kirk and Miller (17) may summarize it best, stating that qualitative work will "reasonably go ignored" if attention is not given to the issue of reliability.

Several authors, even within the qualitative research literature, have emphasized the need to standardize or objectify qualitative research data. Miles (33) sums it up nicely, saying that "the nuisances [of qualitative research] can be reduced by thoughtful methodological inquiry—most centrally into the problem of analysis and how it can be carried out in ways that deserve the name of science. Without more such inquiry, qualitative research . . . cannot be expected to transcend story-telling and we will be stuck with the limitations of numbers." Of course, qualitative research can improve its rigor at the design stage, too, selecting homogeneous samples using standardized guides, along with strict enrollment criteria.

Measures that can be used to minimize subjective bias include using a research partner who plays devil's advocate to question the researcher's analyses critically, searching constantly for negative cases, checking and rechecking the data for possible testing of rival hypotheses or alternative explanations of the data, devising tests to cross-check analyses, and making the data accessible so that other researchers can challenge and reanalyze the data (16).

Qualitative Research Is Easy and Takes Less Effort

Qualitative research may look deceptively simple at the outset. As is the case with most things in life, high-quality qualitative research requires commitment, understanding, highly developed skills, perseverance, and effort. Qualitative research conducted with integrity by a highly skilled researcher is at least as rigorous and demanding an intellectual effort as any other research approach. The sheer volume of data that qualitative studies typically produces often overwhelms the novice, and qualitative studies are perhaps abandoned more often before completion for that reason (19).

Qualitative studies are often challenging because they require parallel mental processing (as opposed to step-by-step or serial processing). For example, when conducting a focus group, the facilitator must simultaneously think about what question to ask next, what the respondents are saying, what needs further probing, how to manage the group so all feel "safe" to respond (and do so), how the facilitator's own demeanor is affecting the group (and the answers), and how to adjust to decrease bias (or increase objectivity) as much as possible. The development of such skills requires training, practice, monitoring, and hard work, but some people never develop the skills sufficient to conduct such research. Data analysis requires different cognitive skills, but no less discipline (see Chapter10). It presents special challenges to many researchers because the protocols are not given but must be developed in the process. Furthermore, the data from qualitative research must be processed and reprocessed multiple times, so, patience is needed (19).

Qualitative Research Can Be Performed Only in a Natural Setting

Natural context is central to the philosophy of qualitative research, because the qualitative approach tries to maximize validity by collecting data as close to real life as possible. However, *context* can be defined on a microlevel or macrolevel, and it should vary according to the phenomena of interest (34–36). If, for example, a researcher is interested in how a person reacts mentally to an educational brochure, the important data are the thoughts and feelings (in words) that the person has upon exposure, whether observed in a shopping mall, simulated physician's office, or the person's own physician's office. In this case, the natural setting is inside the respondent's mind. If, however, the researcher is interested in family interaction around the dinner table, the natural context and setting is probably the home or a fast-food restaurant, as opposed to an unfamiliar laboratory setting. Thus, natural settings are important in qualitative research, but depending on the research question, they can include laboratory studies, as well as field studies.

Qualitative and Quantitative Methods Are Incompatible

Sampling methods and sample sizes represent one critical area of difference between qualitative and quantitative methodologies. Quantitative studies tend to use larger sample sizes, which are predetermined by calculations of statistical power to estimate the number of subjects needed to ascertain statistical significance when certain discrete measures of change are used. Qualitative studies, however, rarely attempt to predetermine a sample size. How many study participants is enough is determined by data saturation rather than statistical significance. *Data saturation* refers to the phenomenon of hearing the same stories and seeing the same patterns of data over and over (19). In other words, qualitative research has an adequate sample size when no new data are produced (in as few as four focus groups in a homogenous sample and content). In contrast, quantitative research requires sufficient data points to detect statistical differences. Depending upon the magnitude of difference being detected and the variability of the factor of interest, large numbers of subjects may be required, ranging from 25 to 30 subjects per design cell to several thousand subjects per design cell.

Ideally, we suggest a three-stage research process to resolve most of the applied questions or interventions found in dietetics and nutrition: (1) qualitative research to define terms and issues from the respondents' perspectives; (2) quantitative research to verify the scope and incidence of the problem in various contexts, along with hypothesis testing regarding etiology; and (3) a follow-up qualitative study to verify the interpretation of the results produced in the second stage. For example, one author is conducting focus groups with underrepresented minorities to better understand the social climate in the workplace. The results will generate questions for a survey of all community members. Additional focus groups then will be held to probe the general responses from the survey in greater depth.

It Is Almost Impossible to Fund Qualitative Research

Quantitative research is more easily funded at this time. However, national funding agencies are becoming increasingly receptive to qualitative inquiry (24), and some have begun to require qualitative approaches in some instances. Many foundations and smaller agencies are more receptive to qualitative, grassroots evaluations and inquiries than they are to quantitative approaches. Our recommendation is to choose agencies and requests for proposals carefully. We also urge investigators to combine qualitative and quantitative methods (5,36,37). When agencies become acquainted with the usefulness of qualitative data, they often become more receptive to its methods on future inquiries. They may never learn to value qualitative data, however, unless researchers take a pragmatic approach and provide quantitative data along with the qualitative data.

Limitations of Qualitative Research

Qualitative research has its own limitations. Perhaps the most obvious is that generalizations cannot be made from any one data set to larger populations, and it is often difficult to compare qualitative studies because they are context bound. In addition, qualitative data do not at present lend themselves to meta-analysis, although researchers are pursuing ways to solve this problem. Data collection is very dependent on personnel (as opposed to equipment and statistical software), and data quality subsequently depends entirely on the quality and training of personnel. Data analysis tends to be time-consuming and tedious. In fact, when qualitative and quantitative methods are used together, it is sometimes difficult to complete the

qualitative analysis in time to be useful to the quantitative process.

In sum, qualitative research is for neither the lazy nor the faint of heart. It is demanding, is time-consuming, and takes great effort. The payoff in increased understanding, however, makes the effort a sound investment. Dietitians, therefore, should explore the variety of methodologies offered by the qualitative approach to research, especially to develop and evaluate interventions or programs in clinical or community environments.

REFERENCES

1. Pelto PJ, Pelto GH. *Anthropological Research: The Structure of Inquiry.* 2nd ed. Cambridge, England: Cambridge University Press; 1999.
2. Wilson CS. Food custom and nurture. *J Nutr Educ.* 1979;11(suppl):211.
3. Marlow P. Qualitative research as a tool for product development. *Food Technol.* 1987:74,76.
4. Kraak V, Pelletier D. How marketers reach young consumers: implications for nutrition education and health promotion campaigns. *Fam Econ Nutr Rev.* 1999;11(4):31–41.
5. Borra A, Kelly L, Tuttle M, Nevelle K. Developing actionable dietary guidance messages: dietary fat as a case study. *J Am Diet Assoc.* 2001;101:678–684.
6. Crockett S, Lytle L, Elmer P, Finnegan J, Luepker R, Laing B. Formative evaluation for planning a nutrition intervention: results from focus groups. *J Nutr Educ.* 1995;27:127–132.
7. Marino D, White C. Interviewing participants key to dietetic students' understanding of emergency food needs. *J Nutr Educ.* 1999;31:119A.
8. Shankar AV, Gittelsohn J, Stallings R, West KP, Gnywali T, Dhungel C, Dahal B. Comparison of visual estimates of children's portion sizes under shared-plate and individual plate conditions. *J Am Diet Assoc.* 2001;101:47–52.
9. Matheson D, Achterberg C. Description of a process evaluation model for nutrition education computer-assisted instruction programs. *J Nutr Educ.* 1999;31:105–113
10. Lincoln YS, Guba EG. *Naturalistic Inquiry.* Beverly Hills, Calif: Sage Publications; 1985:338.
11. Jacob E. Qualitative research traditions: a review. *Rev Educ Res.* 1987;57:1.
12. Bulmer M. Concepts in the analysis of qualitative data. *Soc Rev.* 1979;27:65.
13. Sandelowski M. The problem of rigor in qualitative research. *ANS Adv Nurs Sci.* 1986;27–37.
14. Knafl KA, Howard MJ. Interpreting and reporting qualitative research. *Res Nurs.* 1984;7:17.

15. Miles MB, Huberman AM. Drawing valid meaning from qualitative data: toward a shared craft. In: Fetterman DM, ed. *Qualitative Approaches to Evaluation Education: The Silent Scientific Revolution*. New York, NY: Praeger; 1988:222.

16. Rose K, Webb C. Analyzing data: maintaining rigor in a qualitative study. *Qualitative Health Rep*. 1998;8:556–562.

17. Kirk J, Miller ML. *Reliability and Validity in Qualitative Research*. Beverly Hills, Calif: Sage Publications; 1986:1.

18. Firestone WA, Dawson JA. Approaches to qualitative data analysis: intuitive and intersubjective. In: Fetterman DM, ed. *Qualitative Approaches to Evaluation in Education: The Silent Scientific Revolution*. New York, NY: Praeger; 1988:209.

19. Strauss A, Corbin J. *Basics of Qualitative Research*. Newbury Park, Calif: Sage Publications; 1998.

20. Achterberg CL, Novak JD, Gillespie AH. Theory-driven research as a means to improve nutrition education. *J Nutr Educ*. 1985;17:179.

21. Dean K. Nutrition education research in health promotion. *J Can Diet Assoc*. 1990;51:481–484.

22. Fetterman DM. Qualitative approaches to evaluating education. *Educ Res*. 1988:17–23.

23. Walker R. Evaluating applied qualitative research. In: Walker R, ed. *Applied Qualitative Research*. Brookfield, Vt: Gower Publishing Co; 1985:177–198b.

24. Patton MQ. *Qualitative Evaluation Methods*. 3rd ed. Newbury Park, Calif: Sage Publications; 2001.

25. Reeder LG. Social epidemiology: an appraisal. In: Jaco EG, ed. *Patients, Physicians, and Illness*. 3rd ed. New York, NY: Free Press; 1979:97–101.

26. Goodwin RA, Brulé D, Junkins EA, Dubois S, Beer-Borst S. Development of a food and activity record and a portion-size model booklet for use by 6- to 17-year-olds: a review of focus group testing. *J Am Diet Assoc*. 2001;101:926–928.

27. Achterberg CL, Van Horn B, Maretzki A. Evaluation of dietary guideline bulletins revised for a low literature audience. *J Ext*. 1994(4).

28. Shatenstein B, Claveau D, Ferland G. Visual observation is a valued means of assessing dietary consumption among older adults with cognitive deficits in long-term care settings. *J Am Diet Assoc*. 2002;102:250–252.

29. *The American Heritage Dictionary: Second College Edition*. New York, NY: Dell Publishing Co; 1987.

30. Peshkin A. In search of subjectivity—one's own. *Educ Res*. 1988;17.

31. Miller C, Achterberg C. Knowledge and misconceptions about the food label among women with NIDDM. *Diabetes Educ*. 1997;23:425–432.

32. Shepherd S, Sims LS. Employing cognitive response analysis to examine message acceptance in nutrition education. *J Nutr Educ*. 1990;22:215–228.

33. Miles MB. Qualitative data as an attractive nuisance: the problem of analysis. *Admin Sci Q*. 1979;24:590.

34. Bronfenbrenner U. *The Ecology of Human Development*. Cambridge, Mass: Harvard University Press; 1979.

35. Sallis JF, Owen N. Ecological models. In: Glanz K, Lewis FM, Rumer BK, eds. *Health Behavior and Health Education: Theory, Research, and Practice*. 2nd ed. San Francisco, Calif: Jossey-Bass; 1997.

36. Hamilton JA. Epistemology and meaning: a case for multimethodologies for social research in home economics. *Home Econ Forum*. 1989;4:12.

37. Morgan DL. Practical strategies for combining qualitative and quantitative methods: applications to health research. *Qualitative Health Res*. 1998;8:362–376.

10

—∿—

Qualitative Research Methods: Sampling, Data Collection, Analysis, Interpretation, and Verification

Sandra K. Shepherd, Ph.D., R.D., and Cheryl L. Achterberg, Ph.D.

The goal of qualitative research is to understand behavior from the study participants' frame of reference (1). During the last decade, much work has been done to clarify the theoretical underpinnings of qualitative research, illustrate its potential, and refine its methods (2). Dietitians use qualitative research for a variety of reasons. It is often used to explore learner needs and preferences in relation to nutrition education campaigns, programs, and materials (3–5). It is also used to understand how people conceptualize their diets (6), to develop and refine theories of food behavior (7), and to develop or validate quantitative measurement instruments (8,9). Qualitative research has been used less frequently in clinical settings than in community settings, even though qualitative methods can benefit clinical research in several ways (10). Qualitative methods can help increase understanding of important, but qualitative, between- and within-patient differences in clinical outcomes over time; detect unanticipated outcomes not detectable by measures developed from the researcher's perspective; and discover the burdens imposed by a treatment on patients and caregivers and how to alleviate them to improve compliance.

The goal of this chapter is to describe tools and strategies dietitians can use to conduct and evaluate qualitative research. It describes a variety of qualitative research methods and discusses how to develop observation forms and interview scripts; select, train, and monitor observers and interviewers; select a study sample; record and analyze data; and interpret and verify results. The

chapter concludes with a discussion of criteria that can be used to evaluate and improve qualitative research.

SELECTED METHODS OF DATA COLLECTION FOR QUALITATIVE RESEARCH

Two primary methods of qualitative data collection are observations and interviews (11). In their classic form, these methods are applied in naturalistic settings, where study participants live, work, and play in everyday life. Naturalistic settings are important because qualitative research hinges on the fundamental notion that events and observations can be understood only within the context in which they occur (12). Examples of naturalistic settings relevant in dietetics include hospitals, nursing homes, outpatient nutrition clinics, soup kitchens, supermarkets, restaurants and fast-food outlets, school cafeterias, home kitchens, and family dinner tables.

In their less classic form, observations and interviews are conducted in the researcher's setting. The loss of context that occurs when qualitative research is moved into the laboratory limits its potential, but data collected in nonnaturalistic settings can be useful nonetheless. The data can be especially useful if context is addressed methodologically by recreating it in the laboratory (for example, a simulated grocery store aisle, if the focus is on understanding food shopping) or by asking interview participants to envision and describe different situational contexts during the exchange.

Observations

Systematic observation of people and events in their natural settings is used to discover and describe behaviors and interactions in context (13). Observation can help researchers explore and understand the apparent gap between what people know or say and what they actually do (14). An important dimension of observation is the extent to which an observer interacts with the people observed. The continuum of interaction ranges from covert observation, where the people observed are not aware of the observer's presence, to participant observation, where the observer interacts freely with the people observed while collecting data (14). Examples of studies employing observation as the primary form of data collection include a study by Weber and Dalton (15) using participant observation to study the food habits of terminally ill men and a study conducted by Matheson and Achterberg (16) to explore children's use of a computer nutrition education program.

Interviews

Interviews are planned interactions in which one person systematically obtains information from one or more other people via questioning and discussion (17). As suggested by the definition, interviews may be conducted one to one with individual study participants or in a group setting with multiple participants interviewed together. Studies may vary widely with respect to the amount of time spent per interview and the number of interviews conducted with each individual or group (18).

Individual Interviews

The most common individual interviews are one-to-one verbal exchanges guided by the interviewer (19). Individual interviews have been used in dietetics to uncover perceptions of foodservice personnel in relation to school lunch programs (5); explore self-image among overweight adolescent girls (20); develop insights about food- and nutrition-related issues specific to Hispanic audiences (21); and describe beliefs about diet and health, weight perceptions, and weigh-loss practices among Lakota Indians (22). Individual interviews may vary in

depth, depending on the number of times each study participant is interviewed and the duration of each interview. In-depth interviews usually require multiple, extended sessions to explore issues in detail. The use of in-depth interviews in dietetics is illustrated by a study in which researchers explored women's perceptions and experiences of continuity and change in dietary behavior. For this study, each of 23 women were interviewed 3 times over a 13-month period (23).

Most individual interviews consist of guided conversations, but they may also involve specially designed activities. Examples include concept mapping and cognitive response tasks.

A concept map is a display of the network of concepts that constitute a person's top-of-mind understanding of a subject (24). A concept map is derived by offering participants a stimulus cue and asking that they respond with the first word or thought that comes to mind; this is called *free elicitation*. Stimulus cues used in free elicitation tasks are carefully selected and organized to reveal systematically the breadth and depth of the participant's concept network. The participant's own response is used as the next cue to increase the depth of the map. For example, if the stimulus cue is *cholesterol* and the person responds with *heart attack*, the next stimulus cue is *heart attack*. By using each response as the next stimulus cue, the researcher traces concepts from the most top-of-mind concepts to the less salient underlying concepts as the interview progresses. New stimulus cues are used to increase the breadth of the map. Continuing the example, a new stimulus cue that could broaden the map would be *sugar*.

Theoretically, concept maps can be used to tailor new messages that assimilate easily into a fundamental concept network that already exists in the minds of the target audience. For example, concept maps from the target audience may reveal a pattern where the concept of *fruit* has a closer association with the concept of *pesticides* than it has with the concept of *health*. In that case, the nutrition message should address the benefits of eating fruit in relation to the risks of pesticide exposure from fruits, emphasize the extent to which risk of exposure is reduced through careful washing, and provide tips for careful washing.

Cognitive response tasks involve the use of stimulus cues, often in the form of persuasive messages, to elicit thoughts. These thoughts are labeled *cognitive responses* and are presumed to mediate the persuasive impact of the message (25). The difference between cognitive response tasks and concept mapping is that the former focuses on cognitive processes, whereas the latter focuses on the content and structure of memory.

Shepherd and Sims (26) used the cognitive response task to explore women's mental reactions to a brochure encouraging the moderation of dietary fat and cholesterol. Rayner and coworkers (27) used a similar approach to investigate subjects' thoughts as they shopped "normally" and as they shopped "healthily" for foods on a predetermined list.

Group Interviews

Group interviews include the focus group interview, nominal group process, and Delphi process. Focus group interviews are designed to stimulate and facilitate topic- or product-relevant discussion among small groups of representatives of the target audience (28). Group dynamism is used to help draw out information about behaviors, attitudes, and opinions that may not be divulged as readily in one-to-one interviews (29). Participants can build on one another's comments and views, help clarify them, and contrast them with their own (30). Group interviews help reveal the words and phrases participants use to describe a phenomenon when discussing it among themselves, which may differ from the words and phrases used in one-to-one talks with an interviewer who does not share their vocabulary or terminology. For example, one-to-one interviews between adolescents and adult researchers are likely to yield responses in a different "language" than group interviews where adolescents are invited to discuss topics among themselves.

In focus groups, interviewers ask questions or introduce topics related to the phenomenon of interest and encourage participants to discuss those questions and topics among themselves. The interview typically starts with activities to establish rapport, followed by broad questions or topics that orient participants to the subject and get them involved in a group discussion. As the interview proceeds and participants grow more comfortable expressing their views in the group, the researcher narrows and focuses the discussion by introducing more specific topics and questions in a progressive manner.

The role of the focus group interviewer is to facilitate, guide, and manage the group discussion. This management involves introducing issues, encouraging participants to discuss the issues among themselves, gently drawing out quiet participants and discouraging those who might dominate the conversation, introducing ex-

hibits and activities, and making sure all issues are covered in the time allotted. The goal is not to conduct one-to-one interviews simultaneously in a group setting but to foster discussion among group members around the topics of research interest.

The focus group interview is probably the most widely used qualitative research technique in dietetics. Typically, focus groups are used as a part of audience assessment in planning nutrition education materials and programs. Researchers conduct focus groups to develop insight into participants' perceived needs and preferences, and they then use that information to develop strategies for intervention. For example, Conners et al (31) conducted focus group interviews with elementary schoolchildren to explore cafeteria factors that influence their milk-drinking behavior. Other investigators have used focus group techniques to explore the views of adolescents in relation to the family meal (32), to conduct needs assessment and establish instructional goals for a multimedia nutrition education program for adults (33), and to elicit perspectives related to support of breastfeeding by low-income fathers (34). Focus group research may be conducted with one interview per group or repeated interviews with groups that serve as panels (35).

One especially creative application of focus groups is the work reported by Balch and coworkers (3). In laying the groundwork for the national 5 A Day for Better Health campaign to increase fruit and vegetable intake, Balch et al selected as their target audience "people who are trying to eat more fruit and vegetables and are currently eating two to three servings a day, but have not achieved the 5-A-Day minimum." They conducted conventional focus groups as described earlier. They also conducted "piggyback" focus group sessions with members of the target audience and members of a comparison group. The comparison group consisted of adults who ate five or more servings of fruits and vegetables daily.

In the piggyback approach, Balch and coworkers had the comparison group discuss the perceptions and benefits that made and kept them heavy users of fruits and vegetables, as well as how they overcome barriers related to fruit and vegetable consumption. The target group observed this interview from a separate room through a two-way mirror. Afterward, the comparison group left, and the target group discussed their reactions to what they observed and heard in the comparison group interview. Results were used to identify motives and habits that distinguished the two groups, to determine whether and how members of the comparison group could serve as models for members of the target group, and to help campaign planners avoid unrealistic efforts to convert the former to the latter.

Like individual interviews, group interviews may include activities designed to uncover specific information sought by researchers. An innovation recently introduced in focus group research is the use of projective techniques. Projective techniques are activities designed to reveal deep-seated emotions. They are based on the assumption that individuals asked to respond quickly to unstructured stimuli will organize or interpret those stimuli in ways that reflect their basic perceptions of the world (36).

Projective techniques may help circumvent barriers that often prevent people from honestly expressing their basic motives and drives. Examples of these barriers include the difficulty of articulating complex motives and drives related to food, subjects' desire to please researchers by saying what they think they want to hear, and individuals' fear of being perceived as irrational if they reveal deep emotions about food. Rational questions from researchers tend to elicit rational answers from subjects but often fail to get at broader, underlying emotions.

Researchers use projective techniques in an attempt to circumvent these barriers by introducing "highly ambiguous, novel tasks" and severely limiting the response time so participants have little chance to formulate rational responses or censor their thoughts as usual in public. For example, participants might be asked, "If this nutrition program were a shoe, what kind of shoe would it be, and why?" They would be given 1 minute to confer and make a list of their responses; then they would be given more time to discuss and expand on the responses (37). A projective technique was used by McCashion (38) to explore emotions underlying meal planning and preparation. Women in focus groups were asked to draw spontaneous pictures depicting what dinnertime meant to them. The resulting artwork reflected intense frustration, feelings of helplessness, and emotional exhaustion in relation to the chore of coming up with ideas for dinner, shopping for dinner, and preparing it. These insights were used to drive the development of computer software called Ready, Set, Dinner.

The nominal group process is a group method of soliciting and consolidating opinions in situations where decision making is hampered by insufficient information or an overload of contradictory information (39). It is a consensus-generating technique designed to determine the extent to which experts or nonexperts agree about a given issue. The nominal group technique involves a highly structured meeting where each participant expresses opinions in writing, shares opinions with the facilitator one by one, reacts individually to all suggestions grouped by the facilitator according to some common characteristic, privately reevaluates personal opinions in light of what others have said, discusses differences within the group, and repeats the cycle until agreement is reached (39).

The Delphi process, a similar technique, is conducted by mail rather than in a group meeting. It sometimes uses anonymous participants, with the facilitator orchestrating the process and providing written summaries of input for consideration in subsequent "rounds" (39). For examples of the Delphi process in action, see Gregoire and Sneed (40,41).

Content Analysis

Content analysis is a method in which the researcher systematically identifies and examines characteristics of written documents, audiotapes, or videotapes with the goal of making inferences (29). Examples include the work of Matheson and Spranger (42), who examined the use of fantasy, challenge, and curiosity in school-based nutrition education programs; Byrd-Bredbenner and Grasso (43), who analyzed the nutrition information conveyed by television commercials widely viewed by children; and Potter et al (44), who analyzed changes in infant feeding messages appearing in a Canadian women's magazine from 1945 to 1995.

Historical research employs content analysis to interpret past events, drawing data from documents such as diaries, letters, poetry, music, and prose created at the time of the event (1). An example of historical research in dietetics is a study conducted by Liquori (45). Liquori examined administrative reports, faculty writings, and dissertations from a large academic nutrition department to explore the changing dimensions of science and practice in the nutrition profession over a 55-year period. Individual interviews with subjects who taught or studied in the graduate program from 1937 to 1992 were used to complement the document analysis.

Narrative analysis is similar to content analysis but is usually more liberal in its interpretation because of the special nature of the data. Narratives are human expressions in the form of contemporary stories that describe and explain life processes, situations, and events. The goal of narrative analysis is to illuminate an event, object, idea, or lived experience in a holistic manner that exposes its relevance to professional practice (46). Data gathering involves collecting stories related to the phenomenon of interest from a carefully defined sample of respondents. Again, narrative analysis goes beyond simply identifying the characteristics of the stories (as would be the case in content analysis), and interpretation is typically more liberal.

Individual interviews, group interviews, and analysis of material culture (newspaper stories, reports, diaries, photographs, films, transcripts of speeches, stories, and other narratives) are basic qualitative research methods available to dietitians. An exhaustive list of methods and all their variations would fill this volume and many more. It would also be dated because new methods are always being developed. This review is intended to introduce readers to fundamental methods in the hopes of encouraging further exploration of qualitative strategies that can be used to inform the practice of dietetics.

PRELIMINARY CONSIDERATIONS RELATED TO QUALITATIVE DATA COLLECTION

Qualitative research requires thoughtful and informed consideration of a number of preliminary issues. Decisions made early in the planning process determine the quality of resulting data, findings, and conclusions, so it pays to consider each option carefully.

Formulating Research Questions

Research questions reflect the purpose of a study. Mason (47) outlines three broad purposes related to qualitative research: (1) describe, explain, or compare phenomena, processes, locations, or meanings; (2) trace the development of a phenomenon or process within its context; and (3) create theory. The formulation of research questions for qualitative studies should start with one or more of these broad purposes. The research question is then refined to reflect the target audience, phenomenon of interest, and specific issues of interest. For example, an initial research question might be to describe healthful eating as perceived by teenagers. The focus of this research question could be narrowed and refined as the research revealed specific issues of interest—for example, to com-

pare the meanings of healthful snacks as perceived by normal-weight versus overweight 16-year-olds.

Developing Observation Forms and Interview Protocols

Qualitative research is, by definition, open ended. During data collection, it is acknowledged and accepted that the researcher and respondents will interact with and affect each other. Although this interaction precludes the possibility that any two observations or interviews will be identical, it is acceptable as long as they converge enough to answer the research questions. Data from observations are typically recorded on written forms, on audiotape and/or videotape, and in field notes. Observation forms (Figure 10.1) can help multiple observers know what to look for (in person or on tapes), based on the research objectives. The forms can also help observers describe what they observe in common terms so that subsequent comparisons are possible (47).

Observation forms vary in the amount of structure imposed, depending on the circumstances. Highly structured observation forms may be used to collect data in studies where enough is known about the phenomenon of interest to develop forms before data collection begins. Less-structured observation forms may be required when exploring newer phenomena about which little is known at the outset.

Field notes are an observer's free-flowing, personal account of the context and actions observed (1). Observers should be familiar enough with study objectives to produce field notes that reflect those objectives; at the same time, restricting field notes to those that reflect specified objectives limits the opportunity to capture serendipitous insights that could prove fruitful in the investigation.

Like observation forms, interview scripts range from structured to unstructured, depending on the extent to which the phenomenon is already understood. The more structured an interview script, the more like a survey it becomes. Researchers considering highly structured interview scripts should consider whether a survey would be more appropriate. A semistructured interview script (Figure 10.2) provides a general guide that is uniform enough to generate comparable responses but flexible enough to accommodate the variety of people encountered in an interview setting. In other words, it provides a basic framework for covering all topics of

To describe shoppers' initial physical reactions to an educational exhibit on comparing food labels, observers are required to record observations for every tenth shopper who passes within 3 ft of the front of the exhibit. The 3-ft limit is marked on the floor with masking tape. Return shoppers (those who have passed by or have already stopped at the exhibit during the observation period) are not counted a second time.

Times 1, 2, 3, and 4 on the record form refer to repeat reactions within one stop at the exhibit. For example, if a shopper looking at the exhibit picks up cereal A and reads the label, puts it down, and then comes back to it before leaving the exhibit, the amount of time spent the first time cereal A is examined is recorded in the column labeled "Time 1." The amount of time spent the second time the label of cereal A is examined is recorded in the column labeled "Time 2."

Observer #____   Shopper #____

	Amount of Time Spent (sec)			
Physical Reaction	**Time 1**	**Time 2**	**Time 3**	**Time 4**
Passed by without stopping (check here____)	N/A	N/A	N/A	N/A
Examined textual panels				
Examined cereal label A				
Examined cereal label B				
Compared cereal labels				
Examined salad dressing label A				
Examined salad dressing label B				
Compared salad dressing labels				
Examined tip sheet				
Did the shopper take a tip sheet?_____ yes_____ no				

FIGURE 10.1   Sample observation form.

interest while allowing the interviewer the latitude needed to approach interviewees as individuals and to follow up on unanticipated questions and issues raised during the encounter.

Pilot testing of observation forms and interview scripts is extremely important. Pilot testing of an observation form can help ensure that the form is sufficiently detailed and comprehensive to capture the essence of the phenomenon observed without overburdening observers, so that the research objectives underlying observations can be met. Pilot testing of an interview script with representatives of the target audience can help ensure that the questions are mutually understood by respondents and interviewers, the terms used in formulating questions are not offensive to respondents, the time allocated for each interview is adequate, the protocol facilitates rapport, and the interview produces the desired quantity and quality of information.

Selecting, Training, and Monitoring Observers and Interviewers

In qualitative research, the researcher is the data collection instrument (13). The ability of the researcher to obtain information is critical to the success of the study. Selection of observers should be based on their ability to distinguish actions or elements of interest from the surrounding context, record observations accurately, and articulate unanticipated observations clearly. Interviewers should be selected based on their ability to project consideration and concern through their words and actions, actively engage in listening, prompt without seeming to interrogate, be patient and comfortable with silence, avoid jargon, and avoid counseling or leading the participant (1). One additional factor that should be considered during the selection of interviewers is gender. In some cases, cross-gender interviewing has been shown to help

This script is used to elicit reactions of focus group participants to a proposed set of nutrition print materials on fat, cholesterol, sodium, and fiber. This part of the discussion focuses on content.

Estimated Time: 30 Minutes

One of the booklets you received earlier looks like this. Do you need a few minutes to look it over before you discuss it as a group? [*Allow 5 minutes for review.*]

What did you think of it? [*If they try to respond to you directly, remind them that they are here to discuss it among themselves—that you are here only to suggest topics and distribute related materials.*]

Should more or less scientific evidence be presented (to support the recommendations about diet)? Why?

What did you like the best about this one? Why?

What did you like the least? Why?

What could or should be eliminated, if anything? Why or why not?

[*If the following topics did not emerge naturally, ask these questions.*]

How did you feel about the "Did You Knows," the quick facts highlighted in yellow and sprinkled throughout the booklet? [*Turn to a "Did You Know" in the material, and display it.*]

How did you feel about the "Food Choice Checkup" on page 6? [*If nobody responds right away, move on to the next topic.*]

How about the recipe?

Did you try the recipe? Why or why not?

Do you think you will try it? Why or why not?

[*If the participants hesitate a long time, ask if they ever use recipes from nutrition materials. If not, skip the remaining questions on recipes, and move on to the next subject area.*]

How do you use a recipe like this one? [*If examples are needed, use the following: Do you use it as is, or do you just get ideas from it, use it to make changes in your own recipes, or what?*]

How would you handle a recipe printed in a brochure like this? [*If examples are needed, use the following: Would you cut it out, hand copy it onto one of your own recipe cards, just remember it, just remember where it was, or what?*]

What would be the best way to present recipes in a brochure like this?

Do you have any other comments on this piece before we move on?

FIGURE 10.2   Excerpt from a semistructured interview script.

reduce bias (48); other researchers have shown that bias effects due to gender depend on the topic and context of the interview (49). Pilot testing may be needed to determine whether the gender of the interviewer appears to influence responses.

Interviewers must be thoroughly familiar with the topics and issues to be covered according to specified re-

search objectives. They should also have enough training and expertise in the subject matter to enable them to prompt respondents intelligently. In our field, this usually means that they should be dietitians or nutritionists. Safety issues also must be considered if observations and interviews are to take place outside the university or worksite environment. It is important to determine, in advance, how potential safety issues should be handled for both interviewers and study participants (50). A tour of unfamiliar neighborhoods where observations or interviews will take place can help researchers anticipate safety issues and devise ways to minimize them (51).

Selection of observers and interviewers is followed by training and ongoing assessment of competency. Formal training can help ensure that observation forms and interview scripts are used as intended and that the protocol is consistently followed. Training can also help ensure that observers and interviewers produce consistent, comparable data across subjects, times, and places. The amount of training required to achieve this quality may vary considerably with the circumstances, even when experienced personnel are employed.

Training should include four components: reading, discussions with experienced observers or interviewers, one-to-one supervised experiential instruction, and practice. Readings should include "how-to" articles on observing and interviewing, as well as a wide variety of completed observation forms or transcripts. It is helpful to analyze and discuss those forms and transcripts in detail with the original observer or interviewer, if possible, or with another person who has experience using similar protocols with similar target groups. Discussions are important sources of insight that novice observers and interviewers can draw on for solving future problems on the spot as they arise during data gathering.

Interviewer instruction for one-to-one or group interviews proceeds most efficiently when the trainee is videotaped while conducting an interview. The trainee and trainer together can review the tape immediately after the interview, stopping whenever it is appropriate to comment. The process can be repeated as many times as necessary, but dramatic improvements between interviews are commonplace with this method. No amount of training, however, can replace practice. The authors have found that 8 to 10 one-to-one interviews or 3 to 4 group interviews using the same interview guide with participants from a single target group are required for a consistent, relaxed performance. If interviews are to be conducted in participants' homes, Balsa (50) recommends rehearsals in the homes of nonparticipants from the same target audience.

After training, occasional quality control checks are advised. For example, the trainer may review every 5th completed observation or interview. In cases where an observation or interview is not up to standard, the problem can be addressed before further data collection occurs.

Morse and Field (1) outline common pitfalls of interviewing and how to avoid them or minimize their effects. Typical problems that arise include interruptions, competing distractions, stage fright, asking questions in an illogical order, counseling, presenting one's own perspective, superficial questioning, confidential information divulged by the interviewee "off the record," and subjects who miss their scheduled interviews (no-shows).

Berg (29) adds to this list the potential bias arising from the effects of the interviewer's attributes. The outward appearance, dress, social characteristics, demeanor, and actions of interviewers can influence the way people react when interviewed. One way to reduce this bias is to train members of the audience of interest to serve as peer observers or interviewers. Another way is to use a dramaturgical interview. The dramaturgical interview is designed to maneuver around evasion tactics and communication-avoidance rituals that are part and parcel of all communication (29). The researcher choreographs the interview in a way that involves other people in the natural environment as unknowing "actors." For example, a participant-observer dressed as a coworker might ask if she could join a lone diner in a crowded worksite cafeteria as an opening to a dramaturgical interview about the food, policies, or prices. The obvious advantage of the dramaturgical interview is that it reduces intrusiveness and the impact of the researcher's presence on data collection. One obvious drawback is the difficulty of getting informed consent from participants after the fact (52).

Using Electronic Recording Equipment

Advancing technology has fed the growth of qualitative research by providing smaller, more affordable, easier-to-use recording equipment often needed to capture comprehensive qualitative data reliably. Voice inflections, facial expressions, and other body language can easily slip by even the most meticulous observers and interviewers who are busy following the action or conversation content, attending to the observation form or interview script, monitoring the time, and so forth. Audiotaping and videotaping also allow the investigator to employ multiple observers and coders, thereby enhancing the potential for reliable data analysis.

The potential of electronic recording equipment to change the way subjects would normally react when observed or interviewed was acknowledged and addressed years ago (53–55). Collectively, researchers found that the obtrusiveness of taping equipment was not extensive; anxiety peaked very early in the session and stabilized within minutes. The general conclusion across the three studies was that taping procedures, in and of themselves, are not intrusive enough to warrant undue concern.

Niebuhr and associates (55) note, however, that one-way glass and adaptation periods can reduce intrusiveness in behavioral research. Other methods for reducing the intrusiveness of electronic recording equipment include the use of cordless, remote microphones sensitive enough to pick up very low voice levels so that respondents need not see the equipment or be asked to speak up. An audio consultant can be especially helpful in identifying specific equipment that meets these needs. Naturally, respondents are always asked to sign an informed consent form when they are to be electronically recorded. This procedure is especially important when equipment is hidden to reduce intrusiveness.

High-quality, easy-to-operate electronic recording equipment and tapes always should be used to avoid loss of valuable data. Ninety-minute audiocassettes (45 minutes per side) are recommended. Longer tapes tend to be thinner, risking poor quality and breakage. Shorter tapes require more frequent handling, which can result in irritating interruptions and increase the obtrusiveness of the recording (56). Fresh batteries are also recommended for each session. Additional tips include the following:

- When choosing audio- or video-recording equipment, consider such features as voice activation capability (as opposed to manual activation) and external jacks for microphones, earphones, and foot pedals. Earphones are critical for maintaining confidentiality of the data during review and transcription. A foot pedal (to start, pause, stop, fast-forward, or rewind the tape) frees the hands during transcription (1).
- When choosing a microphone, consider such features as size and appearance (potential obtrusiveness) and range and direction of pickup (sensitivity). Shepherd (57) employed a microphone cover called a *mouse* to reduce ambient noise in a clinic where interviews were conducted. The mouse also served to disguise the microphone to some extent.
- When selecting equipment to be used in a hospital, worksite, supermarket, university or other institutional setting, request that it be inspected by the institution's engineering department to ensure that it meets local regulations to reduce fire and other hazards (1).

Of course, new technologies appear on the market

regularly, so a periodic review of all available options is advised. One recent advance that might become particularly useful for expanding the geographic scope of qualitative studies is real-time audio/video capabilities of computers that allow participants in an exchange to view each other on-screen and communicate via voice. Methods are being developed for electronic interviewing (19) and for conducting other types of qualitative research online (58).

Eventually, tapes must be transcribed and coded. The following guidelines facilitate these procedures:

- Speak clearly toward the microphone, and encourage respondents to do so as well.
- Restate comments that may be difficult to hear on subsequent review of the tape because of ambient noise.
- Avoid rustling papers, which can easily drown out voices.
- Start and end each recorded interview with a taped message that identifies participants by code. Conclude with a statement confirming that the interview is complete, and note any informal observations or insights that might be helpful in evaluating and interpreting the data at a later date (for example, observations regarding contextual issues that might have influenced the session).

Sampling

In qualitative research, sampling may relate to people, settings, times, events, and processes (59). According to Morse and Field (1), two principles guide qualitative sampling to increase the trustworthiness of data. The first principle is appropriateness, or the extent to which the sample includes all perspectives (people, settings, times, and so on) that can inform the study. The second principle is adequacy, the extent to which enough data are available to provide a rich description of the phenomenon and the context in which it occurs from each relevant perspective. Adequacy is achieved when results get repetitive or redundant (60) and additional interviews fail to provide fresh insights.

Decisions regarding sample size in qualitative research often rest on a compromise between the scope of topics and perspectives covered versus the depth to which each topic or perspective is studied. Studies that encompass a broad number of topics and perspectives are not likely to afford researchers the opportunity to explore each topic or perspective in depth with each participant or group. In contrast, studies that address issues in depth with each participant or group may need to be limited in the number of topics or perspectives covered and the number of subjects involved because of the usual constraints of time and money.

Three types of qualitative sampling have been described by Coyne (61): selective, purposeful, and theoretical. Selective sampling occurs when the researcher identifies the people, times, and places to be sampled in advance of study commencement. Selection is based on preconceived notions of when, where, and from whom the most fruitful data might come.

Purposeful sampling is similar, but it occurs after data collection and analysis have begun (62). Purposeful sampling is an ongoing process based on analysis of data gathered to date. Results from one round of data gathering and analysis are used to determine when, where, and from whom to collect the next round of data based on the needs of the study. For example, ongoing analysis of incoming data may suggest key informants whose insights have not been tapped or alternative times and sites that may prove fruitful.

Theoretical sampling is purposeful in the sense that it occurs after data collection and analysis have commenced. It differs from purposeful sampling, though, in that its focus is on filling information gaps that hinder theory development. Subjects are selected solely on the basis of their ability to provide information needed to develop, expand, and refine nascent theory emerging from data already collected and analyzed. Theoretical sampling may be used to learn more about concepts discovered through ongoing data analysis. It may also be used to clarify the relationships among those concepts, explore the relative importance of each concept, or examine the overlap of concepts that together form the framework for a developing theory. Theoretical saturation occurs when the addition of subjects, times, or places fails to offer new insights on the theory undergoing construction (63).

In sampling for group interviews, additional considerations related to group dynamics may apply. For example, it is often advisable to assemble relatively homogeneous groups (homogeneous with respect to age, educational background, ethnic group, status, or income, for example) so that group members are comfortable expressing their views in front of other members of the group (28). If a variety of perspectives is required, additional groups may be formed, each representing a different perspective. By the same token, it may be best for group members to be strangers to one another so that the social liability of candid discussion is minimized (29).

All sampling decisions be must be adequately justified and made explicit in reporting qualitative research. Only then can reviewers judge whether the sample was appropriate and adequate to support valid conclusions.

Transcribing Electronically Recorded Data

In most cases where researcher-subject encounters are electronically recorded, a written transcript is subsequently produced. Transcripts are usually verbatim accounts designed to preserve, as much as possible, everything that was said during the encounter. Transcripts, however, do not preserve nonlinguistic data such as emphasis, mood, tone of voice, and other descriptive information that can be so crucial in elaborating meaning (56,64). Because of this problem, Jones (64) warns against the temptation to let reading transcripts become a substitute for listening to tapes.

Transcribing tapes is very time-consuming and therefore costly. Miles (65) estimates that a 60- to 90-minute tape takes approximately 6 hours to 8 hours to transcribe. Morton-Williams (56) offers a rule of thumb of 4 hours to 6 hours per transcript for individual in-depth interviews or group interviews. Our experience places transcription time somewhere within these same ranges.

Transcribers should be trained so that the product meets the researcher's expectations and needs. A written set of instructions can be used to establish the format of the transcript. Instructions might include a listing of abbreviations, signs, and symbols that can be used to indicate the source of words and passages, gaps in the transcript caused by ambient noise on the tape or overtalk (when several people from a group interview talk at once), audible expressions such as laughing or crying, and other details that help provide context in reviewing a transcript (66). The best way to determine what should be included in instructions to transcribers is for the researcher to thoroughly pilot test the transcription process. The experience is invaluable in establishing guidelines and in estimating the amount of time (and cost) that should be allotted per transcript.

It is critical that the original interviewer edit each typed transcript carefully to check for accuracy, to fill in the gaps using notes taken during and after the interview, and to annotate the transcript appropriately. For example, annotations may be needed to clarify ambiguous situations (for example, "the numerous, intermittent comments regarding this issue were provided by a single respondent who kept repeating her position, rather than several different respondents in consensus").

Voice recognition software, an automated form of dictation and transcription, is a relatively new technological tool that qualitative researchers might consider in their work. It converts verbalizations into text via automated dictation. The first generation of voice recognition software was cumbersome and expensive, but two recent developments have increased its potential usefulness for qualitative research: (1) continuous speech recognition capabilities that translate at a normal conversational speed and (2) falling prices driven by competition in the software industry.

ANALYSIS OF QUALITATIVE DATA

Despite the growing number of texts on qualitative research methods, advice on how to analyze data produced by these methods remains relatively scarce in the literature (67). The starting point for analyzing qualitative data is to return to the research question in its original or most recent form (47). As mentioned earlier, qualitative researchers sometimes modify the research question or questions as the study unfolds and incoming data steer them in unanticipated directions.

Qualitative data analysis can proceed both inductively (moving from particular cases to generalizations) and deductively (moving from general cases to the particular). This discussion of qualitative analysis rests on two basic premises outlined in Chapter 9: (1) qualitative data analysis may be theory driven, theory generating, or both, and (2) analysis lies on a continuum that ranges from purely qualitative (involving no numbers) to more quantitative (where a content analyst counts the number of times a certain issue arises in a document). It should also be understood that qualitative data include researcher-generated information (for example, field notes, annotations, study diaries, and other documents that make up the audit trail) as well as subject-generated information (62). These premises should serve as a foundation for understanding the following discussion of the basics of qualitative analysis.

Unitizing

Unitizing is the process whereby a recorded stream of verbalization (in the form of a transcript or document) is segmented into units of analysis that can be categorized (11,68). Units may be defined in terms of time (for example, 20-second units), speaker (for example, all statements made by one speaker while holding the floor), or content (for example, each word, phrase, statement, or group of statements that express a single, coherent thought). Pilot testing should help determine which type of unit is the most appropriate for a given project and how the units will be recorded. Recording of units should always include cross-references that trace each unit back to its original location in the transcript so that the surrounding context may be revisited as the need arises. Context is often needed to clarify the intent of ambiguous comments. Moreover, preserving and emphasizing context is a fundamental principle of qualitative research that makes it unique in its contribution to the body of knowledge. Unitizing is employed primarily in cases where qualitative data are destined for quantitative analysis (68). Intercoder agreement of unitizing and coding is discussed later in the section on coding.

Coding

Coding facilitates the organization, management, and retrieval of qualitative data. It is used to link fragments of the data that share some commonality (62) so that they can be viewed together in an effort to derive meaning. Coding helps the investigator extract meaning from qualitative data in a systematic way, uncovering patterns or themes that might otherwise be obscured by the sheer mass of information.

Order and structure may be imposed on qualitative data in a number of ways, depending on the researcher's philosophy and objectives. Coding schemes may be developed inductively from the data themselves or be driven by existing theory in a deductive manner. Potential frameworks for organizing or coding qualitative data include existing theories, research questions (56,69), policy questions posed by funding agents (64), and results from task analyses (for coding cognitive processes involved in problem-solving tasks) (68).

The mechanical aspects of organizing or coding data involve a creative process that varies from researcher to researcher and from project to project. There is no particular formula; however, pilot work is needed to refine the system and make sure that it works. An investigator may start with a very elaborate coding scheme, only to find it too cumbersome to be practical. In contrast, an investigator may begin with a very simple scheme but find that it fails to cover or describe certain types of data adequately (70). In either case, adjustment or refinement of the coding system is necessary.

One way to maximize objectivity in qualitative data analysis is to use two or more independent analysts who can serve as cross-checks for one another (29). A subset of the data might be subjected to analysis by multiple, independent coders when researchers need some indication of interrater agreement but cannot afford to use multiple coders for the entire data set. The important point is that researchers must have a firm rationale for coding or organizing data in the way that they do. By specifying the rationale underlying the coding system, the investigator fosters consistency in the coding process (68) and exposes the process to personal and peer scrutiny.

Once a coding system has been established, it may be judged according to two criteria outlined by Guba (71): internal homogeneity and external heterogeneity. The former refers to the extent to which all data within a category reflect the concept represented by that category. In other words, do the data within each category follow the rules of inclusion for that category? (11) The latter refers to the extent to which the categories are mutually exclusive. In other words, are the differences between categories consistent?

There is some disagreement in the literature with respect to the external heterogeneity criterion proposed by Guba. For example, Berg (29) states that when a passage mentions or relates to more than one theme, it should be shown under both themes. Codes or categories can be nested or may be overlapped (62). For example, in coding a transcript for misconceptions about the Food Guide Pyramid, the following comment was categorized as a misconception about the grain group and a misconception about the vegetable group: "Shouldn't potatoes be here with the other fatty starches in the bread group?" To classify the quotation as one or the other (a misconception about the grain group or a misconception about the vegetable group) would have resulted in a considerable loss of information. However, a redefinition of categories would have been unwarranted, especially given that each category had already been used extensively, and this verbalization was the only one that satisfied both. As always, the important point is that the researcher be explicit about the criteria for multiple coding and be consistent in applying that criteria.

Use of Context in Coding

One question that often arises in coding unitized verbalizations is whether the context surrounding a unit should be brought to bear on the coding or categorization of that unit. Oral prose is often choppy, ungrammatical, and littered with partial phrases or even single words (68). A fragment of normal speech may express a complete thought—and thus constitute a unit—but only if the surrounding text is used to derive its meaning. Suppose speaker 1 says, "I like the one with the pictures of food on the cover." Speaker 2 then says, "Yeah, me too." Speaker 2 has expressed a complete thought, but without the preceding text, its meaning would be lost. Context helps make coding less ambiguous, thereby promoting objectivity—a primary concern in using verbal reports as data (68).

Second-Tier Coding

In some cases, a second round of coding may be advisable to describe the data further or to help determine the relative confidence the investigator has in the various units of data. Bogdan and Taylor (72) suggest a second-tier coding process that may help the investigator determine the relative confidence placed in various units of data once they are categorized. This coding scheme may differentiate verbal reports according to whether they are solicited or volunteered; made in a group or in a private, one-to-one situation; and made in an interview where rapport was good versus an interview in which the subjects appeared to be very guarded.

Shepherd (57) used a second-tier coding scheme to describe the magnitude of certainty expressed by subjects in their cognitive responses. It was accomplished by identifying specific words and phrases representing "weak" versus "strong" expressions. According to this scheme, a strong response would be, "I really love the one with pictures of food on the cover." A weak response would be, "I kind of like the one with pictures of food on the cover." Data may also be differentiated according to whether they are direct statements or indirect inferences derived by coders from fragmentary verbalizations. As mentioned earlier, qualitative data may be researcher generated as well as subject generated. Indirect inferences can provide valuable insight, but analysts may invest greater confidence in direct statements.

Intercoder Reliability

The unitizing and coding of qualitative data can be a very subjective process requiring considerable judgment on the part of coders unless specific steps are taken to minimize this potential problem. For this reason, extensive pilot testing of the process is recommended to generate a well-defined set of instructions that can increase the reliability of the processes.

When the units of analysis are to be counted, ranked, subjected to statistical analyses, or all three, reliability of the coding process should be firmly established. There are several methods for assessing intercoder agreement among multiple unitizers (73) and coders (74). A summary of various strategies used to determine intercoder reliability or agreement of subjective judgments is offered by Tinsley and Weiss (75). When the units of analysis will not be counted, ranked, or subjected to statistical analysis, consensus strategies are often used to code data. Members of the research team work together to assign codes to observations or verbalizations. In this case, intercoder reliability is not an issue.

Computer Analysis of Qualitative Data

The use of computers to manage qualitative data has become commonplace (76). Commercial software is available, as is dedicated software created by researchers for specific purposes. Examples of dedicated software include ATLAS/ti, NUD*IST, and The Ethnograph (77). Researchers share dedicated software, along with support and information on the use of commercial software, through a networking project commonly referred to as CAQDAS (Computer Assisted Qualitative Data Analysis Software). For more information on CAQDAS, see http://caqdas.soc.surrey.ac.uk or *Current Sociology* 1996;44:191–205.

The use of computer software in qualitative data analysis can reduce the time needed for manual tasks (such as cutting and pasting, or sorting and filing) so that more time can be spent on conceptual work. Software can also make it easier for researchers to experiment with coding schemes and share data with others on a research team (78). Good qualitative data analysis software should facilitate file management, on-screen coding, and easy searching for codes and strings of words with search results displayed in full context. The software also should provide multiple options for data display and offer ways to annotate text, search for annotations, and link annotations to each other (77).

Computer-assisted analysis also has its drawbacks. It is easy to overestimate what computer programs can do. Computers are data managers, not data analyzers (1). The computer does not code data; the researcher does. The computer just merges data and codes them into the same file to facilitate analysis. It is also easy to be distracted from the data and coding by the mechanics of using computer programs. Therefore, researchers with medium to small data sets might be well served

with a standard word-processing program or manual analysis.

Other potential drawbacks of computer-assisted qualitative analysis include the possibility that available analytic programs will dictate research goals and design, as well as the potential risk of violating confidentiality of data stored in systems accessible to others (78). It is recommended that novice researchers sort a small data set manually first to experience the process up close and personally. By going through the process manually once, researchers learn which attributes of a computer program could be helpful. They also may find that handling data in its physical form (as they pile, file, sort, shuffle, cut, and paste quotations from transcripts) can make them feel more in tune with the data than manipulating it electronically on a computer (1).

Displaying Data Visually

Data display is a way to summarize data in a visual fashion to facilitate analysis and reporting (79). Some examples of data displays are matrixes, diagrams, flowcharts, and concept maps. Data displays can help researchers spot connections and relationships that might otherwise be obscured (47). They can also help researchers report data in ways that enhance understanding (62).

Data displays have been proposed as a major strategy for improving qualitative data analysis and reporting, but they are subject to drawbacks. The amount of information that may be included in a visual display is limited by available space (79). In developing displays, it is often necessary to summarize raw data or restrict the display to especially illustrative examples. These requirements call for subjective judgment on the part of the researcher, who must take care that displays represent the bulk of the data accurately and adequately. For example, it is tempting to select quotations that are particularly colorful, but selection on this basis alone can be misleading if the quotations reflect the views of only one participant. As with coding, investigators working on data displays are advised to record and report decision rules used to selectively display data so that the process remains open to review.

Interpreting Data and Verifying Interpretation

This chapter has separated data analysis from interpretation for the sake of discussion. In reality, however, the two often proceed simultaneously to some extent. For example, investigators involved in organizing and categorizing data will almost always find themselves discovering insights, coming up with hunches, and developing preliminary interpretations of the data. Indeed, preliminary interpretation may provide direction for further data collection and analysis. It is important, however, to remember that this interpretation is merely preliminary. The final interpretation must rest on a comprehensive evaluation of all the data.

One way to keep interpretation credible is by working with a research team whose members serve as devil's advocates for one another, helping to identify potential biases that can influence interpretation (11,29). All researchers have biases resulting from the personal and professional experiences that make up their lives. For example, in a study of food insecurity, a team member who has experienced food insecurity in the past may have biases that differ from team members who have not, but all members will be biased in some way. It is human nature.

Interpretation of results is valid to the extent that it accurately reflects the reality represented by data (80). Interpretations are verified by actively scrutinizing the data for evidence of disconfirmation (rather than confirmation). Miles (65) and Miles and Huberman (79) provide some tactics for applying this scrutiny that remain useful today:

- Look for concomitant variation, and assess conditions that create greater or lesser concomitant variation. Does the pattern of variation observed in one part of the data hold true across all the data and/or across data reported by other researchers? If not, what are the circumstances (for example, settings, sources, or occasions) under which the pattern of variation seems to hold most consistently? What are the circumstances under which the pattern of variation is weaker or not observed?

- Look for negative cases. Are there data that seem to contradict a conclusion? If so, what is the extent and relative trustworthiness of these data?

- Rule out spurious or confounding factors. What are possible alternative explanations for the data? Are the alternative explanations supported by the data in part or in whole?

- Look for intervening variables. Are there potential intervening variables without which patterns of concomitant variation would evaporate?

- Make predictions and search for violations. What else would be true if this prediction were correct?

Is the prediction true according to the data? What would not be true if this prediction were correct? Is it "not true" according to the data?

- Get feedback from informants. Does the interpretation ring true to the people who provided the data? According to Maykut and Morehouse (11[p176]), "The validity of . . . findings ultimately rests on whether the participants or people who know them will see a recognizable reality" in the results. The key question as posed by Greenhalgh and Taylor (81[p742]) is, "How comprehensible would this explanation be to a thoughtful participant in the setting?"

Verification of interpretation is considerably easier if a variety of data collection strategies and analytic techniques have been used and yield convergent conclusions. This concept is known as *triangulation* (assuming the use of at least three different techniques), and it is probably the best defense against criticism of investigator bias or subjectivity in qualitative research (82). As is the case with all processes described in this chapter, the methods used to interpret data and verify interpretation should be reported. Keeping a record of the route by which interpretations are arrived at and verified can help expose the process to fellow researchers and improve confidence in the conclusions (47).

EVALUATING QUALITATIVE RESEARCH

The merit of qualitative research depends on the trustworthiness of its results and conclusions. Four distinct aspects of trustworthiness defined in the literature are dependability, credibility, confirmability, and transferability (83,84). Dependability is the extent to which participant's meanings are accurately understood by the researchers. Dependability can be strengthened by the judicious use of follow-up questions and probes to clarify and confirm the meaning of what an interviewee says. Dependability can also be strengthened by member checks, in which participants are asked to review data summaries to see if they ring true from the insider perspective.

Credibility is the extent to which the phenomenon of interest has been adequately described. Data are credible when they provide a rich description of the phenomenon from a variety of perspectives rather than merely describing its surface features from a limited number of critical vantage points.

Confirmability is the extent to which findings and conclusions are supported by evidence from the data. Confirmability can be enhanced by documenting the emergence and evolution of concepts and linking them with the data from which they are derived at each stage of the evolution. This process may be facilitated by the use of study diaries.

Transferability is the extent to which findings from a qualitative study are useful in understanding how people experience the target phenomenon in other settings or under other conditions. Transferability of findings is determined after the fact by subsequent research with different audiences in different circumstances.

In quantitative research, the confidence placed in results and conclusions rests largely on the validity and reliability of measurement instruments used to collect data. In qualitative research, confidence rests on trustworthiness. The use of different terminology to characterize the merits of quantitative versus qualitative research reflects differences in underlying philosophies, as reviewed in Chapter 9. The concept of trustworthiness in qualitative research continues to be refined, along with the terminology used to articulate it, the criteria used to judge it, and the strategies used to increase it (52). Efforts to improve the trustworthiness of qualitative research are fundamental to maximizing its usefulness in dietetics.

REFERENCES

1. Morse JM, Field PA. *Qualitative Research Methods for Health Professionals.* 2nd ed. Thousand Oaks, Calif: Sage Publications; 1995.
2. Denzin NK, Lincoln YS, eds. *Handbook of Qualitative Research.* 2nd ed. Thousand Oaks, Calif: Sage Publications; 2000.
3. Balch GI, Loughrey K, Weinberg L, Lurie D, Eisner E. Probing consumer benefits and barriers for the national 5-A-Day campaign: focus group findings. *J Nutr Educ.* 1997;29:178–183.
4. Satia JA, Patterson RE, Taylor VM, et al. Use of qualitative methods to study diet, acculturation, and health in Chinese-American women. *J Am Diet Assoc.* 2000;100:934–940.
5. Gittelsohn J, Toporoff EG, Story M, et al. Food perceptions and dietary behavior of American-Indian children, their caregivers, and educators: formative assessment findings from Pathways. *J Nutr Educ.* 1999;31:2–13.
6. Janas BG, Bisogni CA, Sobal J. Cardiac patients' mental representations of diet. *J Nutr Educ.* 1996;28:223–229.
7. Keenan DP, AbuSabha R, Sigman-Grant M, Achterberg C,

Ruffing J. Factors perceived to influence dietary fat reduction behaviors. *J Nutr Educ.* 1999;31:134–144.
8. Alaimo K, Olson CM, Frongillo EA. Importance of cognitive testing for survey items: an example from food security questionnaires. *J Nutr Educ.* 1999;31:269–275.
9. Derrickson J, Anderson J. Face validity of the Core Food Security Module with Asians and Pacific Islanders. *J Nutr Educ.* 1999;31:21–30.
10. Sandelowski M. Using qualitative methods in intervention studies. *Res Nurs Health.* 1996;19:359–364.
11. Maykut P, Morehouse R. *Beginning Qualitative Research: A Philosophic and Practical Guide.* Washington, DC: The Falmer Press; 1994.
12. Evans JF. Changing the lens: a position paper on the value of qualitative research methodology as a mode of inquiry in the education of the deaf. *Am Ann Deaf.* 1998;143:246–254.
13. Marshall C, Rossman GB. *Designing Qualitative Research.* Newbury Park, Calif: Sage Publications; 1989.
14. Mays N, Pope C. Observational methods in health care settings. In: Mays N, Pope C, eds. *Qualitative Research in Health Care.* London, England: BMJ Publishing Group; 1996:20–27.
15. Weber CD, Dalton A. A case study: the food habits of three terminally ill men. *Top Clin Nutr.* 1992;7:30–36.
16. Matheson D, Achterberg C. Ecologic study of children's use of a computer nutrition education program. *J Nutr Educ.* 2001;33:2–9.
17. Lipchik E. *Interviewing.* Rockville, Md: Aspen; 1988.
18. Sobal J. Sample extensiveness in qualitative nutrition education research. *J Nutr Educ.* 2001;33:184–192.
19. Fontana A, Frey JH. The interview: from structured questions to negotiated text. In: Denzin NK, Lincoln YS, eds. *Handbook of Qualitative Research.* 2nd ed. Thousand Oaks, Calif: Sage Publications; 2000:645–672.
20. Neumark-Sztainer D, Story M, Faibisch L, Ohlson J, Adamiak M. Issues of self-image among overweight African-American and Caucasian adolescent girls: a qualitative study. *J Nutr Educ.* 1999;31:311–320.
21. Gans KM, Lovell HJ, Fortunet R, McMahon C, Carton-Lopez S, Lasater TM. Implications of qualitative research for nutrition education geared to selected Hispanic audiences. *J Nutr Educ.* 1999;31:331–338.
22. Harnack L, Story M, Rock BH, Neumark-Sztainer D, Jerrery R, French S. Nutrition beliefs and weight loss practices of Lakota Indian adults. *J Nutr Educ.* 1999;31:10–15.
23. Paquette M, Devine CM. Dietary trajectories in the menopause transition among Quebec women. *J Nutr Educ.* 2000;32:320–328.
24. Daley BJ. Concept maps: linking nursing theory to clinical nursing practice. *J Contin Educ Nurs.* 1996;27:17–27.
25. Wright P. Message-evoked thoughts: persuasion research using thought verbalizations. *J Consumer Res.* 1980;7:151.

26. Shepherd SK, Sims LS. Employing cognitive response analysis to examine message acceptance in nutrition education. *J Nutr Educ.* 1990;22:215.

27. Rayner M, Boaz A, Higginson C. Consumer use of health-related endorsements on food labels in the United Kingdom and Australia. *J Nutr Educ.* 2001;33:24–30.

28. Krueger RA, Casey M. *Focus Groups.* 3rd ed. Thousand Oaks, Calif: Sage; 2000.

29. Berg BL. *Qualitative Research Methods for the Social Sciences.* 3rd ed. Boston, Mass: Allyn and Bacon; 1998.

30. Betts NM, Baranowski T, Hoess SL. Recommendations for planning and reporting focus group research. *J Nutr Educ.* 1996;28:279–281.

31. Conners P, Bednar C, Klammer S. Cafeteria factors that influence milk-drinking behaviors of elementary school children: grounded theory approach. *J Nutr Educ.* 2001;33:31–36.

32. Neumark-Sztainer D, Story M, Ackard D, Moe J, Perry C. The family meal: views of adolescents. *J Nutr Educ.* 2000;32:329–334.

33. Carlton DJ, Kicklighter JR, Jonnalagadda SS, Shoffner MB. Design, development, and formative evaluation of "Put Nutrition Into Practice," a multimedia nutrition education program for adults. *J Am Diet Assoc.* 2000;100:555–563.

34. Schmidt MM, Sigman-Grant M. Perspectives of low-income fathers' support of breastfeeding: an exploratory study. *J Nutr Educ.* 1999;31:31–37.

35. Shepherd SK, Sims LS, Davis CA, Shaw A, Cronin FJ. Panel versus novice focus groups: reactions to content and design features of print materials. *J Nutr Educ.* 1994;26:10–14.

36. Walker R. *Applied Qualitative Research.* London: Gower Publishing Company; 1985.

37. Braithwaite A, Lunn T. Projective techniques in social and market research. In: Walker R, ed. *Applied Qualitative Research.* London: Gower Publishing Company; 1985.

38. McCashion L. Ready, set, dinner: how the National Potato Promotion Board leveraged its nutrition education program for maximum results. *J Nutr Educ.* 1996;28:47D.

39. Jones J, Hunter D. Consensus methods for medical and health services research. In: Mays N, Pope C, eds. *Qualitative Research in Health Care.* London, England: BMJ Publishing Group; 1996:46–58.

40. Gregoire MB, Sneed J. Barriers and needs related to procurement and implementation of dietary guidelines. *Sch Food Serv Res Rev.* 1993;17:46–49.

41. Gregoire MB, Sneed J. Standards for nutrition integrity. *Sch Food Serv Res Rev.* 1994;18:106–111.

42. Matheson D, Spranger K. Content analysis of the use of fantasy, challenge, and curiosity in school-based nutrition education programs. *J Nutr Educ.* 2001;33:10–16.

43. Byrd-Bredbenner C, Grasso D. What is television trying to make children swallow? Content analysis of the nutri-tion information in prime-time advertisements. *J Nutr Educ.* 2000;32:187–195.

44. Potter B, Sheeshka J, Valaitis R. Content analysis of infant feeding messages in a Canadian women's magazine, 1945–1995. *J Nutr Educ.* 2000;32:196–203.

45. Liquori T. Food matters: changing dimensions of science and practice in the nutrition profession. *J Nutr Educ.* 2001;33:234–246.

46. Parse RR. Building knowledge through qualitative research: the road less traveled. *Nurs Sci Q.* 1996;9:10–16.

47. Mason J. *Qualitative Researching.* Thousand Oaks, Calif: Sage Publications; 1996.

48. Bailey KD. *Methods of Social Research.* 2nd ed. New York, NY: Collier Macmillan; 1982.

49. Riessman CK. When gender is not enough: women interviewing women. *Gender Soc.* 1987;1:172.

50. Belza B. Conducting research in respondents' homes: benefits, problems, and strategies. *Appl Nurs Res.* 1996;9:37–40.

51. McCausland M, Burgess A. The home visit for data collection. *Appl Nurs Res.* 1989;2:54–55.

52. Ambert A, Adler PA, Adler P, Detzner DF. Understanding and evaluating qualitative research. *J Marriage Fam.* 1995;57:879–893.

53. Weick KE. Systematic observational methods. In: Lindzey G, Aronson E, eds. *The Handbook of Social Psychology.* 2nd ed. Reading, Mass: Addison-Wesley; 1968.

54. Wiemann JM. Effects of laboratory videotaping procedures on selected conversation behaviors. *Hum Comm Res.* 1981;7:302.

55. Niebuhr RE, Manz CC, Davis KR Jr. Using videotape technology: innovations in behavioral research. *J Manage.* 1981;7:43.

56. Morton-Williams J. Making qualitative research work: aspects of administration. In: Walker R, ed. *Applied Qualitative Research.* Bookfield, Vt: Gower Publishing Company; 1985.

57. Shepherd SK. *An Information Processing Approach to the Evaluation of Nutrition Education Materials* [dissertation]. University Park, Pa: The Pennsylvania State University; 1987.

58. Mann C, Steward F. *Internet Communication and Qualitative Research: A Handbook for Researching Online.* Thousand Oaks, Calif: Sage; 2000.

59. Johnson JC. Research design and research strategies. In: Bernard HR, ed. *Handbook of Methods in Cultural Anthropology.* Walnut Creek, Calif: Altamira Press; 1998:131–153.

60. Lincoln YS, Guba EG. *Naturalistic Inquiry.* Beverly Hills, Calif: Sage; 1985.

61. Coyne IT. Sampling in qualitative research. Purposeful and theoretical sampling; merging or clear boundaries? *J Adv Nurs.* 1997;26:623–630.

62. Coffey A, Atkinson P. *Making Sense of Qualitative Data:*

Complementary Research Strategies. Thousand Oaks, Calif: Sage Publications; 1996.

63. Glaser BG, Strauss AL. *The Discovery of Grounded Theory: Strategies for Qualitative Research.* New York, NY: Aldine de Gruyter; 1967.

64. Jones S. The analysis of depth interviews. In: Walker R, ed. *Applied Qualitative Research.* Brookfield, Vt: Gower Publishing Company; 1985:56.

65. Miles MB. Qualitative data as an attractive nuisance: the problem of analysis. *Adm Sci Q.* 1979;4:590.

66. Silverman D. *Qualitative Research: Theory, Method and Practice.* Thousand Oaks, Calif: Sage Publications; 1997.

67. Morse JM. Validity by committee. *Qual Health Res.* 1998;8(4):443–445.

68. Ericsson KA, Simon HA. *Protocol Analysis: Verbal Reports as Data.* Cambridge, Mass: MIT Press; 1984.

69. Patton MQ. *How to Use Qualitative Methods in Evaluation.* Beverly Hills, Calif: Sage Publications; 1987.

70. Atkinson P, Coffey A. Analysing documentary realities. In: Silverman D, ed. *Qualitative Research: Theory, Method, and Practice.* Thousand Oaks, Calif: Sage Publications; 1997:45–62.

71. Guba EG. *Toward a Methodology of Naturalistic Inquiry in Educational Evaluation.* Los Angeles, Calif: UCLA Center for the study of Evaluation; 1978.

72. Bogdan R, Taylor SJ. *Introduction to Qualitative Research Methods.* New York, NY: John Wiley and Sons; 1975.

73. Geutzkow H. Unitizing and categorizing problems in coding qualitative data. *J Clin Psychol.* 1950;6:47–51.

74. Folger JP, Hewes DE, Poole MS. Coding social interaction. In: Dervin B, Voight M, eds. *Progress in Communi-*

cation Sciences. Norwood, NJ: Ablex Publishers; 1984:4.

75. Tinsley HEA, Weiss DJ. Interrater reliability and agreement of subjective judgments. *J Couns Psychol.* 1975;22:358.

76. Miles MB, Huberman AM. *Qualitative Data Analysis: An Expanded Sourcebook.* Thousand Oaks, Calif: Sage Publications; 1994.

77. Miles MB, Weitzman EA. 1996 The state of qualitative data analysis software: what do we need? *Curr Sociol.* 1996;44:207–224.

78. Conrad P, Reinharz S. Computers and qualitative data: editors' introductory essay. *Qual Sociol.* 1984;7:3.

79. Miles MB, Huberman AM. Drawing valid meaning from qualitative data: toward a shared craft. In: Fetterman DM, ed. *Qualitative Approaches to Evaluation in Education: The Silent Scientific Revolution.* New York, NY: Praeger; 1988:222.

80. Hirschman EC. Humanistic inquiry in marketing research: philosophy, method, and criteria. *J Marketing Res.* 1986;23:237.

81. Greenhalgh T, Taylor R. Papers that go beyond numbers (qualitative research). *Br Med J.* 1997;315:740–743.

82. Achterberg CL. Qualitative methods in nutrition education evaluation research. *J Nutr Educ.* 1988;20:244.

83. DePoy E, Gitlin LN. *Introduction to Research.* London, England: Mosby; 1994.

84. Leininger M. Evaluation criteria and critique of qualitative research studies. In: Morse JM. *Critical Issues in Qualitative Research Methods.* Thousand Oaks, Calif: Sage Publications; 1994:95–115.

Part 5

—∽—

Integrative and Translational Research

Integrative research is a relatively new term intended to encompass research that brings together multiple research studies or extends prior research, as in meta-analysis (Chapter 11) or the evaluation of existing large databases (Chapter 13). As such, integrative research extends available data through careful and constructive assimilation. Chapter 11 describes the steps of meta-analysis: constructing selection inclusion criteria, making a comprehensive search of existing studies that meet the criteria, and combining and assessing the data from the qualifying studies. Meta-analysis allows data from many empirical studies that meet the specified inclusion criteria of the researchers to be united into a larger unit that may yield more objective conclusions. The uses of well-designed meta-analyses are many, including the formation of public policy and the development of recommendations for evidence-based practice (Chapter 12).

Another example of integrative research is presented in the interpretation and use of national databases, such as the National Nutrition Monitoring System and Related Research Program(s) (Chapter 13). Surveillance data are based on self-selected populations—for example, women and children participating in pub-

licly funded nutrition and health programs. Population surveys, because of inherent sampling and design complexities, require adjustments for sample weights and design effects. Survey and surveillance data have multiple applications, including nutrition status monitoring, program planning, and market segment identification.

Translational research is a new and promising type of research whose goal is to translate new science to patient care. Upon this base rests evidence-based practice (Chapter 12). Medical nutrition therapy evolves from thoughtful evaluation of the beneficial effects of controlled laboratory studies and clinical investigations. The American Dietetic Association's *Medical Nutrition Therapy Evidence-Based Guides for Practice* provide recommendations for practice based on careful evaluation of scientific evidence. Translational research, as exemplified in evidence-based practice, is a strong link between research and practice. The support of the National Institutes of Health (NIH) for the strong application of research to practice is evident in the NIH fund for translational research related to the prevention and control of diabetes.

ERM, Editor

11

—⁓—

Meta-analysis in Nutrition Research

Lisa Brown, M.P.H., D.Sc., and Anne Dattilo, Ph.D., R.D., C.D.E.

This chapter introduces the topic of meta-analysis with a focus on the practical application of this procedure using examples of nutrition-related meta-analyses of randomized controlled trials. Assessment of the strengths and limitations of meta-analysis are presented, along with implications for the use of meta-analysis in nutrition policy.

Meta-analysis uses the results of many empirical studies to answer specific, quantitative questions (1). Glass (2) was the first to define the term as "the statistical analysis of a large collection of analysis results from individual studies for the purpose of integrating the findings." Glass and associates (3) more recently defined meta-analysis as "data analysis applied to quantitative summaries of individual experiments." They further explained that "meta-analysis is not a technique, rather it is a perspective that uses many techniques of measurement and statistical analysis."

Meta-analysis has become a popular and acceptable way to summarize results of different studies, and many meta-analyses have been published in health care research. A well-conducted meta-analysis (1) allows a more objective (quantitative) appraisal of the evidence than traditional narrative reviews, (2) provides a more precise estimate of a treatment effect or epidemiologic association, (3) may explain heterogeneity between the results of individual studies, and (4) may help answer new questions that individual studies cannot answer because of a lack of sufficient precision or power (4,5).

There have been several recent meta-analyses published in nutrition research, including analyses to study the relationship between blood lipid response and dietary fat (6), fiber (7,8), protein (9), fish oil (10), and weight reduction (11). Some applications have aimed at examining the effects of sodium (12), potassium (13), and garlic (14) on blood pressure. Others have used meta-analytic methods to describe the role of nutrition education as an effective strategy to control diabetes and to manage coronary disease (15,16). Meta-analytic techniques also have been applied to help determine the relationship of alcohol consumption to risk of breast (17) and colon (18) cancer, define the relationship of breast-feeding to the development of atopic disease in infants (19), assess the effectiveness of perioperative total parenteral nutrition (20), and describe trends in dietary consumption (21). The utility of meta-analyses in formulating Recommended Dietary Allowances also has been considered (22). These examples typify the broad range of applications for meta-analysis in nutrition.

BASIC STEPS FOR CONDUCTING A META-ANALYSIS

Prior to initiating a meta-analysis, a detailed research protocol should be written that clearly states the objectives, hypothesis to be tested, subgroups of interest, and proposed methods and criteria for identifying and selecting relevant studies and extracting and analyzing information. Thus, the basic steps for conducting a meta-analysis include (1) formulating goals for the analysis, (2) locating and evaluating relevant studies, (3) choosing an outcome measure, (4) data extraction, (5) calculating a summary measure of the study-specific results, (6) presenting the results, and (7) evaluating the statistical heterogeneity of the data.

Formulating Goals for the Analysis

There are several possible objectives for a meta-analysis. The process of developing a specific hypothesis that can be tested using meta-analytic techniques can be complex and requires understanding of the scientific literature. A meta-analysis may be used to help determine the effectiveness of specific medical or dietary therapies on health outcome. For example, does increased intake of dietary fiber decrease blood cholesterol levels? Specific objectives must be listed and primary and secondary objectives should be delineated before obtaining the data.

Locating and Evaluating Relevant Studies

A variety of useful electronic databases can be used to locate published studies, but they may miss a substantial proportion of relevant studies (23). Some investigators reported that only about 25 percent of the final studies included in their meta-analyses were located by database searches (1,24). Therefore, in addition to searching automated bibliographic systems, the researcher should scrutinize citation indexes and the bibliographies of review articles, monographs, and the located studies for relevant studies. Nevertheless, every study performed in a given area probably will not be uncovered.

Some of the considerations for inclusion and exclusion in a meta-analysis involve study design, type of experimental and control therapies, length of the study, outcomes of interest, and the overall study quality. Nonrandomized studies have a great potential for bias and therefore may be considered undesirable for inclusion in a meta-analysis. Also, it should be determined whether the search will be extended to include unpublished studies, as the results may be systematically different from the results of published trials. As will be discussed later, a meta-analysis that is restricted to published evidence may produce distorted results due to publication bias. Abstracts presented at professional meetings or published in abstract form have been included in some meta-analyses. However, published abstracts that were not subsequently published as papers have been shown to report larger effects than studies that were published as papers (25). In addition, assessing the quality of a study published in abstract form can be a subjective process, especially because the information reported is often inadequate for this purpose (26). The decision and rationale for the inclusion criteria should be clearly indicated by the analyst.

Choosing an Outcome Measure

In a meta-analysis, each study gives numerical summaries of outcome that the investigator subjects to statistical analysis to draw inferences about the magnitude of the overall effects. The numerical summary of outcomes is known as an *outcome measure*. There are many possible outcome measures that may be appropriate for meta-analyses, including relative risks, odds ratios, change in proportions, probability levels, and differences in means (effect size).

The choice of the outcome measure may be determined largely by what can be summarized from the primary studies. Where possible, the measure that is most relevant for the problem should be selected first. For example, if prevention of death is the purpose of a medical intervention, then gain (or loss) in survival is the natural measure. If the purpose is to determine whether dietary fiber reduces blood cholesterol, then the differences in mean or the percentage change in blood cholesterol response between the high- and low-fiber groups is the most relevant. If the outcome is disease versus no disease or dead versus alive, the odds ratios or relative risks are often calculated.

Data Extraction

After locating all relevant studies for inclusion in the meta-analysis, the actual data for the meta-analysis must be extracted. In general, each primary research finding should be included only once in the final analyses, and in its highest scientific form (for example, a published manuscript over an abstract). It may be possible to contact authors of primary research papers and obtain the original data. In this way, estimates of treatment effects or epidemiologic associations can be computed directly from the original data for each study. However, this practice may be very labor intensive and unrealistic. Usually the data can be extracted from the published or unpublished reports. In addition to the data necessary for calculating the treatment effect or epidemiologic associations, data on the study characteristics, such as age, gender, racial characteristics, and severity of conditions, may also be extracted.

A standardized form is needed for data abstraction. It is useful if two independent observers extract the data in order to avoid errors. At this stage, the quality of the studies may be rated with several specifically designed scales, as will be discussed later in the chapter. Blinding reviewers to the names of the authors and their institutions, the names of the journals, sources of funding, and acknowledgments leads to more consistent scores (27).

Studies with multiple findings (for example, results for male and female subjects or values for 10 g and 20 g of added dietary fiber versus no added fiber) can have more weight if they are represented more than once in the analyses compared with studies with only one reported finding. A decrease in reliability of summary statistics can result if researchers do not address nonindependence of effects from the same study. One approach is to use the entire study as the unit of analyses (that is, use the average effect), but this method severely limits the use of available data. Another approach is to include the multiple findings in an analyses, for example, for a dose-response analysis. The use of this approach assumes that each of the findings is independent of the others. Inferential statistics (means, correlations, and regression coefficients) could be reported with a qualifying statement of this assumption. Other, more complex methods to address interdependencies in large data sets use Tukey's jackknife method (28), which allows the analyst to determine if a transformation of the data is necessary and suitable.

Calculating a Summary Measure of the Study-Specific Results

After the data have been extracted and the appropriate statistics (epidemiologic association or effect size) have been computed from each study, a summary measure is calculated and tested for significance, and a 95 percent confidence interval is estimated from it. The summary measure is most often calculated as a weighted average of the results in which the larger trials have more influence than the smaller ones. The choice of weights to be assigned to the studies and ways to deal with variability among study results depends on whether a "fixed" or "random" effects model is used. The fixed effects model considers that the variability between studies is exclusively due to random variation. Therefore, if all the stud-

ies were infinitely large, they would give identical results. The random effects model assumes a different underlying effect for each study and takes this into consideration as an additional source of variation, which leads to somewhat wider confidence intervals than the fixed effects model. Effects are assumed to be randomly distributed, and the central point of the distribution is the combined effect estimate. There are a variety of techniques for calculating a summary measure, as described in detail elsewhere (28–31).

Some approaches are not recommended, such as counting the number of significant effects (vote counting) using the sign test. This method treats all studies as if they were of equal merit. Study results are grouped into three distinct categories: significantly positive outcomes, negative outcomes, and non-significant outcomes. The number of studies in each category is tallied. The category with the most votes is assumed to provide the best estimate of direction for the relationship between independent and dependent variables (32). This is not a good way of summarizing the data in a meta-analysis, because large studies are likely to find significant results, whereas small ones are not so likely to do so. In addition to this bias, vote counting disregards the quality of studies and the practical importance of statistically significant findings (33). Finally, vote counting neglects important information about the strength of, magnitude of, and relationships among variables (2).

Presenting Results

A detailed summary of characteristics should be reported for each of the studies included in the analysis. These details may help assure the reader that the design, cohort characteristics, exposure dose, and other covariates do not contribute greatly to the between-study variation in results. Any covariates that may be important for explaining the between-study variation can be included in the analysis. Enumeration of the relevant trials excluded and the reasons for exclusions are just as important as describing the trials that were included. However, space restrictions often make it difficult to include all of the descriptive information in the published manuscript.

The results of a meta-analysis are typically presented in a graphic form that shows the point estimates and confidence intervals for the individual studies, as well as the pooled estimate. Figure 11.1 provides an example of a meta-analysis plot of the effect estimates and is described more fully as part of the example described later in this

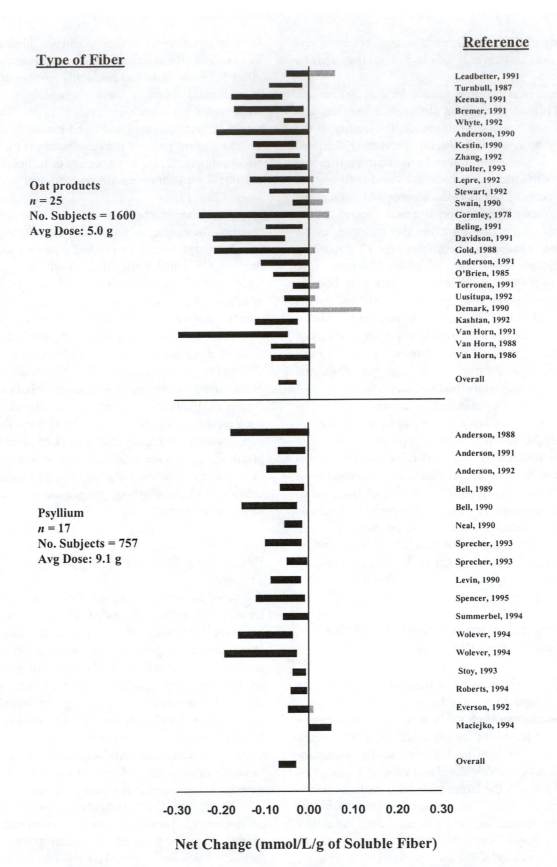

FIGURE 11.1 Net changes in total cholesterol. Reprinted from Brown LE, Rosner BR, Willett WC, Sacks FM. Cholesterol lowering effects of dietary fiber: a meta-analysis. *Am J Clin Nutr.* 1999;69:30–42. Reproduced with permission by the *American Journal of Clinical Nutrition.* © Am J Clin Nutr. American Society for Clinical Nutrition.

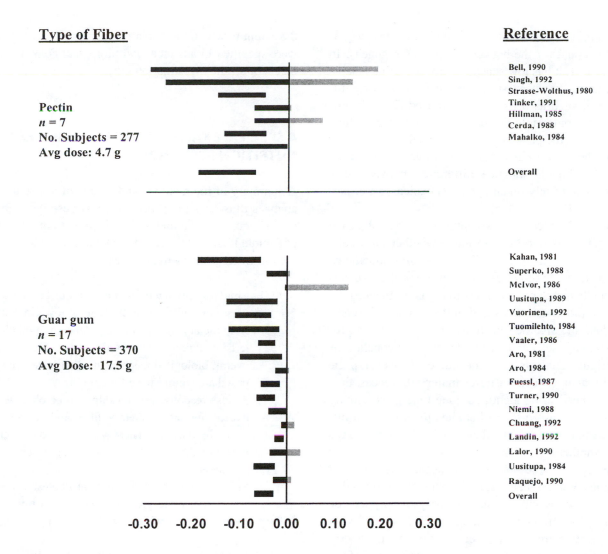

Net Change (mmol/L/g of Soluble Fiber)

FIGURE 11.1 (Continued)

chapter. It is also important to report results from subgroup analyses on key issues (average effects for crossover versus parallel design studies, males versus females, and so on).

Evaluating the Statistical Heterogeneity of the Data

Sometimes a group of studies is conducted in similar populations using similar protocols. More often, however, studies use different eligibility criteria for participants, different definitions of disease, different methods of defining or measuring exposure, or variations in treatments. The results from these similar studies may differ widely, possibly because of variation in study design or other factors. This disagreement of results can be termed *heterogeneity* (23). Regression models can be applied to a meta-analysis when relevant covariate information is available from the studies to examine sources of heterogeneity.

The test commonly used to assess the statistical significance of between-study heterogeneity is based on the chi-square distribution (29). It provides a measure of the sum of the squared differences between the results observed and the results expected in each study, under the assumption that each study estimates the same common treatment effect. A large total deviation (and corresponding significant P value) indicates that a single common treatment effect is unlikely. Any pooled estimate calculated must account for the between-study heterogeneity. In practice, this test has low sensitivity for detecting heterogeneity, and it has been suggested that a liberal significance level, such as 0.10, should be used (29). Heterogeneity in epidemiologic data is usual rather than exceptional. In the presence of heterogeneity, the guiding principle should be to investigate the influences of specific clinical and methodological differences between studies rather than to rely on an overall statistical test of heterogeneity (34).

Because a meta-analysis involves some subjective components, it is important to judge whether the results are sensitive to changes in the procedures undertaken (35). Sensitivity or subgroup analyses are useful to determine whether the common estimate is influenced by changes in the assumptions and in the protocol for combining data. Ideally, the sensitivity analyses will not produce different results and thus will justify the conclusions of the original analysis of all the studies. However, if the sensitivity analysis demonstrates major differences, then the causes need to be identified. One type of sensitivity analysis is to analyze first all studies together, then just the published studies, and then solely the unpublished studies. Another type of sensitivity analysis is to perform separate meta-analyses using other subsets of studies that have some common features, such as the background diet or length of follow-up. Sensitivity analyses may include examining the effect of deleting specific studies with comparatively extreme results or questionable methodology. Deleting studies from a meta-analysis because of extreme published results may substantially bias the mean estimate and underestimate the true variance. Often, studies that appear to be outliers can be explained by some difference in study design, patient characteristics, or treatment regimen. For this reason, eliminating studies without cause is generally dangerous for inference and is discouraged (36).

Discussion of heterogeneity in meta-analyses affects whether it is reasonable to believe one overall estimate that applies to all the studies included. Even after exploratory analyses have been performed, residual heterogeneity may remain because of unreported or unexplained study characteristics. Random-effects models, which take into account such heterogeneity in the summary estimate, may be useful but cannot completely solve the problem when heterogeneity is large. Guidelines for deciding whether to believe results from an investigation of heterogeneity depend on the magnitude and statistical significance of the differences identified, the extent to which the potential sources of heterogeneity were specified in advance, and biological considerations that support the investigation (35).

A SPECIFIC EXAMPLE OF META-ANALYSES IN NUTRITION RESEARCH

A summary of the methods and results of a recent meta-analysis illustrates the procedures just described. Brown et al (7) conducted a meta-analysis to examine the effect of soluble fiber on lowering blood cholesterol levels with the following primary hypotheses:

1. Lipid responses will be similar for different sources of soluble fiber. The cholesterol-lowering effects from dietary fibers will vary, depending on characteristics unique to the study design. However, the overall biological mechanisms that have been proposed are similar for different fibers.
2. A dose-response relationship will be observed between amount of dietary fiber and reduction in serum lipid levels. (There will be a greater decrease in serum cholesterol with increasing doses of soluble fibers.)
3. Subjects with high initial total cholesterol levels will demonstrate greater reductions in lipid levels compared with subjects with lower initial levels.

The investigators also examined the blood lipid changes with concurrent changes in dietary fat and cholesterol, as well as other aspects of study design such as length of follow-up and type of control. The analysis included primary sources of fiber, for which there were more than five trials per type: oat products, pectin, psyllium, and guar gum.

Methods

Trials of the effects of dietary fiber on blood cholesterol levels in adults were identified by a computerized literature search (MEDLINE, National Library of Medicine, Bethesda, Md) and examination of the cited reference sources. Only trials published in English were considered; however, one unpublished trial by Beling et al (1991, provided by Quaker Oats) had been previously referenced in the literature (8) and thus was included in the analysis. As will be discussed, the inclusion of only published trials can produce distorted results through publication bias. However, the investigators considered that the practical limitations of soliciting unpublished trials and issues related to study quality favored the inclusion of only trials published in peer-reviewed journals.

The following criteria were used to evaluate trials for inclusion in the meta-analysis:

- Controlled trials (insoluble-fiber or low-fiber diet for comparison with a high-fiber diet, or a placebo for comparison with a pure-fiber supplement) with either a randomized crossover or parallel design.
- Available data to calculate lipid changes (total cholesterol, low-density lipoprotein cholesterol [LDL-C], high-density lipoprotein cholesterol [HDL-C], and triglyceride concentrations) in the high-fiber and control groups.
- An intervention period of at least 14 days to allow the effect of dietary fiber on blood lipid levels to become manifested.
- The use of soluble fiber from a single source to permit analysis of differences among fiber types.
- Known amount of soluble fiber used daily. If the amount was not explicitly stated, trials were included if there was sufficient information provided to estimate the daily amount of soluble fiber from the published literature.
- Minimum lead-in period of 14 days for studies administering the fiber with a low-fat, low-cholesterol diet to eliminate possible effects on plasma lipids due to overall dietary changes.
- Any dietary changes for both the fiber and control groups made under isocaloric conditions to eliminate possible effects on plasma lipids due to uncontrolled dietary changes.

In all, 162 clinical studies reporting the effects of oat products, psyllium, pectin, or guar gum on blood cholesterol were reviewed. A description of the individual trials considered for this meta-analysis was too lengthy for inclusion in the published manuscript and may be requested by contacting the corresponding author (7). Ninety-two studies were excluded: 81 studies were not sufficiently controlled, 8 studies had insufficient information, and 3 studies had a treatment period shorter than 14 days. Seventy published reports were identified for a quantitative analysis. Three of these studies were included only in the dose-response analysis, because they did not use a true low-fiber control but rather compared a high versus lower dose of the same intervention fiber.

Data were abstracted from the published reports by the primary investigator and reviewed by the other investigators for accuracy and consistency. Most published reports did not provide a detailed description of the background diet or dietary changes; however, trials that indicated careful consideration of the possible confounding by dietary changes were included. For example, published reports indicating that the test diet was administered under isocaloric conditions without additional information were accepted for analysis. When published reports lacked information on variance measures and other key details, the investigators queried the authors for additional information. This process was time-consuming and yielded limited results.

Net changes in blood lipid levels were presented in millimoles per liter per gram of soluble fiber. For parallel group designs, lipid effects were calculated by subtracting the mean change among the controls (low-soluble-fiber group) from the mean change in the treatment group (high-soluble-fiber group). In crossover studies, the estimate represents the difference in the posttreatment lipid levels for the periods of high soluble fiber and low soluble fiber. The net change was divided by the daily dose of soluble fiber. Individual studies were weighted by the inverse of the variance of the fiber effect.

Summary estimates (effect sizes) of the net lipid changes were computed by combining the mean effect sizes reported by individual studies weighted by the inverse of the individual and between-study variance according to a random effects model (29). Summary estimates were computed for each type of soluble fiber separately and for all fibers combined.

Results

Results are presented for total cholesterol levels only here; however, additional findings for LDL-C, HDL-C, and triglyceride concentrations are presented in Brown et al (7). The 67 trials included in the analysis are summarized in Table 11.1 and include 25 trials of oat products, 17 trials of psyllium, 7 trials of pectin and, 18 trials of guar gum. Not all trials from different fiber sources provided total cholesterol, LDL-C, HDL-C, and triglyceride concentrations. The meta-analyses included 3,004 subjects, (1,725 men, 1,011 women, and 268 sex not specified), and the average age of the subjects was 50 years. The average daily dose of 9.5 g was administered over a mean treatment period of 49 days. Fifty-seven of the 67 studies (85 percent) included in the meta-analyses used a

TABLE 11.1 Summary of Trials Included in the Meta-Analysis[a]

Fiber Source	No. of Trials	No. of Subjects	Average Dose Soluble Fiber[d] (g)	Average Length on Treatment[d] (d)	Type of Control (no. of trials)	Subject Type (no. of trials)	Mean Age[d] (y)	Background Diet (no. of trials)	Mean Initial Lipid Levels (mmol/L)[b]
Oat products	25: 13 P, 12 X	1,600: 817M, 598F[c]; Parallel: 703T, 552C; Crossover: 345T, 345C	5.0 (1.5–13.0)	39 (14–84)	18 low-fiber control, 7 diet only	10 healthy, 13 hyperlipidemic, 1 DM + hyperlipidemic, 1 other	48 (26–61)	12 LFLC, 13 usual	TC: 6.31 ± 0.84; LDL: 4.40 ± 0.69; HDL: 1.28 ± 0.15; TG: 1.82 ± 1.98
Psyllium	17: 11 P, X	757: 515M, 242F; Parallel: 279T, 276C; Crossover: 202T, 202C	9.1 (4.7–16.2)	53 (14–112)	16 low-fiber control, 1 diet only	5 healthy, 12 hyperlipidemic	51 (44–59)	13 LFLC, 4 usual	TC: 6.41 ± 0.68; LDL: 4.37 ± 0.70; HDL: 1.23 ± 0.32; TG: 1.79 ± 0.72
Pectin	7: 3 P, 4 X	277: 216M, 61F; Parallel: 95T, 94C; Crossover: 88T, 88C	4.7 (2.2–9.0)	34 (28–42)	5 low-fiber control, 2 diet-only	4 healthy, 1 hyperlipidemic, 1 DM, 1 other	50 (31–65)	1 LFLC, 6 usual	TC: 5.62 ± 0.73; LDL: 4.0 ± 0.59; HDL: 1.48 ± 0.36; TG: 1.45 ± 0.44
Guar gum	18: 5 P, 13 X	356: 185M, 110F; Parallel: 69T, 59C; Crossover: 242T, 242C	17.5 (6.6–30.0)	66 (28–168)	18 low-fiber control	2 healthy, 4 hyperlipidemic, 8 DM, 4 DM + hyperlipidemic	52 (27–63)	3 LFLC, 15 usual	TC: 6.49 ± 0.88; LDL: 4.12 ± 0.72; HDL: 1.27 ± 0.21; TG: 1.76 ± 0.64
Total[e]	67: 32 P, 35 X	2,990: 1,725M, 1,011F[c]; Parallel: 1146T, 981C; Crossover: 877T, 877C	9.5 (1.5–30.0)	49 (14–168)	57 low-fiber control, 10 diet only	21 healthy, 30 hyperlipidemic, 9 DM, 5 DM + hyperlipidemic, 2 other	50 (26–65)	29 LFLC, 38 usual	TC: 6.23 ± 0.88; LDL: 4.25 ± 0.72; HDL: 1.27 ± 0.21; TG: 1.76 ± 0.64

[a]P, parallel; X, crossover; T, treated group; C, control group; hyperlipidemic, initial cholesterol >6.2 mmol/L (240 mg/dL); DM, diabetes mellitus; LFLC, low-fat, low-cholesterol diet (typically 30% calories from fat, ≤10% each from saturated, polyunsaturated, and monounsaturated fats; and <300 mg cholesterol); TC, total cholesterol, TG, triacylglycerol.

[b]To convert values for cholesterol to mg/dL, divide by 0.02586; to convert values for TG to mg/dL, divide by 0.01129. Not all studies of different fiber sources provided total-, LDL-, HDL-cholesterol and triacylglycerol concentrations.

[c]The number of male and female subjects does not equal the total number of subjects because some studies did not specify the sex of the subjects.

[d]Range in parentheses.

[e]Meta-analysis included 67 trials; however, studies did not necessarily report measurements of all 4 lipid changes (total cholesterol, LDL cholesterol, HDL cholesterol, and triacylglycerol).

Reprinted from Brown LE, Rosner BR, Willett WC, Sacks FM. Cholesterol lowering effects of dietary fiber: a meta-analysis. *Am J Clin Nutr.* 1999;69:30–42. Reproduced with permission by the *American Journal of Clinical Nutrition.* © Am J Clin Nutr. American Society for Clinical Nutrition.

control fiber that was low in soluble fiber, such as wheat bran, a cellulose-based placebo, or cornflakes. The remaining 10 trials (15 percent) compared the fiber intervention with a diet that excluded the fiber intervention (diet only). In 38 studies, the background diets were the subjects' "usual" diets, which were most often similar to conventional Western diets in fat and cholesterol content. In 29 studies, the diets were low in fat and cholesterol (less than 30 percent of energy from fat and less than 300 mg cholesterol per day).

Figure 11.1 represents the net change in total cholesterol based on the meta-analysis of 66 trials. Each study is represented by a horizontal line, which corresponds to the 95 percent confidence interval of the effect estimate (mean change in total cholesterol, comparing the high- to the low-fiber diets). The solid vertical line corresponds to no effect of treatment (effect estimate = 0). If the confidence interval includes 0, then the difference in the effect of experimental and control treatment is not significant at the level of $P > .05$. The last point estimate closest to the x-axis represents the overall effect estimate. The overall effect estimate shows that soluble fiber (average = 9.5 g/day) lowers total cholesterol by 0.028 (95 percent confidence interval = $-035, -0.022$) mmol/L per gram of soluble fiber (-1.10 mg/dL [$-1.34, -0.87$]). The individual point estimates indicate that the studies were fairly heterogeneous and the test for heterogeneity was statistically significant ($X^2 = 85.31, P < .001$).

As noted in the original paper, the trials differed in several aspects, including baseline lipid levels, type and dose of soluble fiber, background diet, and dietary assessment methodology. Therefore, it was not surprising that there was extensive heterogeneity. This indicates that the lipid changes may be better characterized by separate estimates for studies similar in design or by subject characteristics such as type of soluble fiber.

Subgroup analyses were performed using weighted least squares regression analyses to test for differences in lipid changes (without dividing by the dose of soluble fiber) using the independent variables; amount of soluble fiber; initial cholesterol level; type of dietary fiber; study design (parallel or crossover); health status of the study population (healthy, hyperlipidemic, or diabetic); mean age; background diet (low-fat, low-cholesterol diet versus usual diet); dietary changes (net change from the high-minus low-fiber period) in total fat, saturated fat, and dietary cholesterol; type of control (low-fiber control product versus diet only); and treatment length.

To study the relationship between dose of soluble fiber and mean total cholesterol changes, the net change

in total cholesterol level was plotted against the mean daily dose of soluble fiber (Figure 11.2). For each study, the net change in total cholesterol level (expressed as the change [millimoles per liter per gram] during the high-soluble-fiber diet minus the change during the low-soluble-fiber period) is plotted against the mean daily dose of soluble fiber. Individual studies with the smallest variance in the meta-analysis are denoted with circles around the point estimates. The plot shows an inverse association between dose of soluble fiber and mean changes in total cholesterol level ($P < .001$). It also suggests a nonlinear dose response. To test for nonlinearity, an exponential term for dose (natural log of the amount of soluble fiber) was used in weighted least squares regression models. There was significant nonlinearity with doses above 10 g/day for total cholesterol. The meta-analyses were repeated for the practical dose range (up to 10 g/day). The overall effects of fiber were greater compared with the results using the total dose range: 1 g of soluble fiber per day reduced total cholesterol by -0.045 mmol/L (-1.73 mg/dL)].

Initial total cholesterol was not a significant predictor of lipid changes after adjustment for dose when entered into the models as either a continuous variable ($P = .18$) or categorical (above versus below 6.20 mmol/L) variable ($P = .91$).

Soluble fiber from oat products, psyllium, pectin, and guar gum each significantly lowered total cholesterol levels (Figure 11.1) by about the same amount. One gram of soluble fiber from oats, psyllium, pectin, and guar gum lowered the total cholesterol level by $-0.037, -0.028, -0.070$, and -0.028 mmol/L ($-1.42, -1.10, -2.69$, and -1.10 mg/dL), respectively. These values were slightly higher when the meta-analysis was repeated for the practical dose range. Type of soluble fiber was not a significant predictor of lipid changes after controlling for initial lipid level using linear regression. However, the cholesterol-lowering effect of pectin appeared to be higher compared with other fibers. This finding was primarily due to two studies (Bell, 1990, and Singh, 1992, in Figure 11.1) that appeared to have greater cholesterol-lowering effects than the other five pectin studies included in the analysis. When we excluded these two trials, there was less of a difference in pectin, suggesting that these two trials were atypical. When we performed secondary analyses relaxing some of the inclusion criteria, the average estimated cholesterol-lowering effect of pectin was similar to that of other fibers, making it appear even less likely that type of fiber could have accounted for a significant amount of heterogeneity among the different fibers. However, it is possible

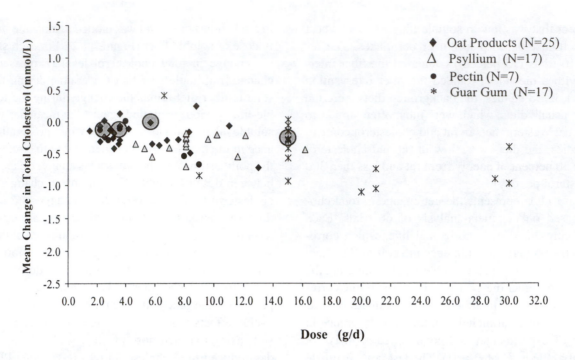

FIGURE 11.2 Relation between dose of soluble fiber and mean lipid changes. For each study, the net change in total cholesterol and LDL cholesterol (expressed as the change during the high-soluble-fiber period minus the change during the low-soluble fiber period) is plotted against the mean daily dose of soluble fiber. All models were weighted by using the inverse of the variance of each effect size and forcing the intercept through zero. Plots show an inverse association between dose of soluble fiber and mean changes in total and LDL cholesterol (*P* < 0.001). Individual studies with variance in the meta-analysis are denoted with circles around the point estimates. Reprinted from Brown LE, Rosner BR, Willett WC, Sacks FM. Cholesterol lowering effects of dietary fiber: a meta-analysis. *Am J Clin Nutr.* 1999;69:30–42. Reproduced with permission by the *American Journal of Clinical Nutrition.* © Am J Clin Nutr. American Society for Clinical Nutrition.

that small differences in response to cholesterol (−0.02 mmol/L to −0.03 mmol/L per gram of dietary fiber) for different fibers may not be detectable (37).

Several other subgroup analyses were conducted to examine the influence on blood lipids of type of study design, type of control, and treatment. None of the following factors turned out to be a significant predictor of the changes in blood lipids: length, background diet, type of subject, weight change, or changes of dietary intake of fat and cholesterol. We also performed analyses to included trials in which the background diet was not well characterized or controlled. The results from these analyses were not materially different from the primary analysis.

Summary

This analysis of 67 controlled clinical trials indicated that diets high in various soluble fibers decrease total cholesterol by similar amounts. The effect is small within the practical range of intake. These findings are generally

consistent with the individual published reports, because high intake of soluble fiber was associated with significant decreases in total cholesterol levels in 60 percent to 70 percent of the trials. There was substantial heterogeneity among individual studies, suggesting that effects of fiber are not uniform. Differences in the dose of soluble fiber account for some variability in study results. Neither initial cholesterol level nor type of fiber apparently accounted for a significant amount of variability in study results; however, it is possible that small differences of −0.07 mmol/L to −0.02 mmol/L between fibers could not be detected.

ASSESSING POTENTIAL FOR BIAS

The assessment of potential bias is a necessary part of a meta-analysis. Two major sources of bias are the failure to find all of the studies performed in the clinical domain and the uncertain reliability of poor-quality studies.

Publication Bias

One criticism of meta-analysis is that there may be some unpublished studies that would contradict the results of published studies. Studies with negative or contradictory results are more likely to remain unpublished, because investigators or the peer reviewers and editors are not enthusiastic about publishing "negative" information (38,39). The chances of not being published are probably greater if the negative study is small and nonrandomized (40).

Some meta-analysts choose to supplement their published data with unpublished trial data because of the potential for publication bias. However, unpublished results may be less reliable, because they have not been found acceptable by peer reviewers and may not be collected with the same rigor or accuracy as published results (41). This consideration makes it unclear whether both published and unpublished data should be given equal weight in the analysis.

Publication bias is difficult to eliminate, but some statistical procedures may help detect its presence. Light and Pillemer (33) proposed using a "funnel plot" to estimate whether publication bias exists, given a set of articles to be included in a meta-analysis. This method uses a scatter plot of studies that relates the magnitude of the treatment effect to the weight of the study (inverse of the variance). An inverted, funnel-shaped, symmetrical appearance of dots suggests that no study has been left out,

whereas an asymmetrical appearance suggests the presence of publication bias. This method is limited to meta-analyses with large enough numbers of studies to allow visualization of a funnel shape for the data.

In a recent meta-analysis by Midgley et al (12) to study the effect of reduced dietary sodium intake on blood pressure, a funnel plot was presented to explore publication bias (Figure 11.3). The vertical axis represents the effect size (between group difference in systolic blood pressure change), and the horizontal axis represents the sample size (weight). Data from the trials included in this analysis indicate a somewhat asymmetrical appearance, suggesting that there is an absence of small studies with large positive association with blood pressure change in contrast to those showing a large negative association. This finding might suggest that relatively fewer studies not supporting the current hypothesis were published. Similar results were found by Brown et al (unpublished data, 1999) in the meta-analysis of the effect of soluble fiber on lipid changes.

Some meta-analysts might suggest that unpublished work should be solicited for inclusion in the analysis. However, there may be a strong impetus not to publish negative trials when the research is supported by industry. In these instances it would perhaps be unlikely that the estimates could be improved upon. In the example of the fiber meta-analysis described above, if publication bias existed, the small effect estimates associated

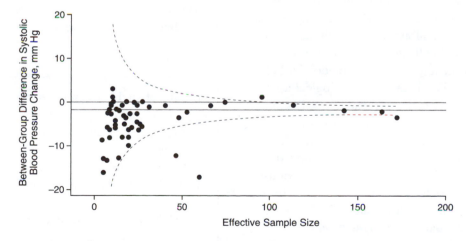

FIGURE 11.3 Funnel plot to explore publication bias in a meta-analysis studying the effect of reduced dietary intake of sodium on blood pressure. The vertical axis represents outcome systolic blood pressure minus baseline systolic blood pressure in the high-sodium group subtracted from the low-sodium group; horizontal lines are at zero and at the fixed-effects mean. The upper and lower dotted lines are twice the median variance divided by the effective sample size. Data from all trials were included in this analysis. Reprinted with permission from Midgley JP et al. Effect of reduced dietary sodium on blood pressure: a meta-analysis of randomized controlled trials. *JAMA.* 1996;275:1590–1597. Copyrighted 1996, American Medical Association.

with intake of dietary soluble fiber would have been further attenuated.

Formal computational approaches to test for, assess the extent of, and correct publication bias also have been described (42–45). None of the available methods is entirely satisfactory for dealing with publication bias, however. In the presence of publication bias, caution should be used in interpreting the pooled estimate. Currently, there is a movement to register all initiated clinical trials in the clinical trials field (46) and also, more specifically, in nutrition research (47). Registration at the time of initiation would obviate the need for searching for unpublished studies.

Study Quality

Variation in study quality can result in biased and imprecise effect estimates because of random and systematic errors in the measurement of exposure and outcome variables (48). The challenge is to identify the parameters that represent the quality of the study most adequately, recognizing that these parameters may differ across different exposure-disease relationships. Although quality assessments are vulnerable to criticism because they are subjective, several approaches have been suggested for measuring the quality of randomized controlled trials and observational studies (49–54). These suggestions have ranged from a simple approach (49) that considers quality assessment as part of a sensitivity analysis to a complex approach (50) using a fine scale of quality assessment that considers several aspects of study design and conduct. Chalmers and colleagues (51) have proposed a greatly simplified system for evaluating randomized clinical trials that is based on major methodological aspects of the studies, including method of randomization, handling of withdrawals in the analysis, and use of blinding of people assessing outcomes.

Quality assessment scores can be incorporated into meta-analyses in several ways. As mentioned previously, the quality score may be used as one of the criteria for selecting studies for inclusion in the analysis. The quality score could also be used as a weight when estimating overall summary statistics. However, if the study results are weighted by the quality score, a bias in evaluating the quality of studies could influence the results (55). In addition, regression analysis could be used to examine whether the estimated summary effect is associated with the quality score. Using the quality score as a covariate in regression models to explain heterogeneity of study effects, rather than as a weight in the analysis, is preferable to minimize the influence of quality-scoring bias (56).

Effects of important quality items are confounded within strata of the quality score, often to the point that no quality effects are apparent in the meta-analysis (26). For example, Emerson and coauthors (57) reviewed seven meta-analyses that used quality scores and found that in nearly all of the studies, the scores showed almost no relation to the study estimates. It has thus been argued that quality scoring should be replaced by direct regression or stratification on objective quality-related study characteristics, such as study design (controlled trial, cohort, case-control, and so on) and data collection methods that could influence the accuracy and precision of the effect estimates (26). Figure 11.4 lists design and data collection parameters to consider in evaluating study quality.

META-ANALYSIS FOR OBSERVATIONAL STUDIES

There is considerable debate as to whether meta-analysis should be considered for observational studies. Although randomization in clinical trials assures the investigator that bias is minimized, in observational studies bias and unmeasured confounding always remain as concerns. No amount of careful combining of data from studies can overcome inherent deficiencies in the original data. Based on this concern, Shapiro (58) argues that we should not proceed with meta-analysis of observational data. However, others argue that the systematic review of the literature may delineate some important features that may account

---

1. Type of study design (randomized controlled trial vs case-control, cohort, or other design).
2. Availability of data on potential confounders and known risk factors.
3. Representativeness of study sample.
4. Availability of information on possible sources of bias.
5. Validity and reliability of exposure (eg, specific nutrient of interest) assessment.
6. Type of exposure assessment (eg, direct interview, self-administered questionnaire, or medical record to assess intake of specific nutrients of interest).

FIGURE 11.4 Quality-related study characteristics to be evaluated in a meta-analysis.

for the variation in results and so explain the heterogeneity among studies (26). These features could be missed with a more traditional narrative review (59).

The principles for conducting a meta-analysis using observational study data are the same as the principles described for randomized data. However, greater care is needed in the conduct of the analysis and the interpretation of the results when nonrandomized and uncontrolled data are used, because these data are likely to be biased.

META-ANALYSIS FOR SETTING POLICY

The popularity of meta-analysis may partly come from the fact that it makes life simpler and easier for reviewers as well as readers. Increasing numbers of meta-analyses of diet and health have been conducted; however, it is not always clear to what extent they should influence nutrition policy, particularly because recent studies have brought into question disparities between large trials and meta-analyses (60–63).

A large randomized controlled trial is generally considered the gold standard for evaluating the efficacy of therapeutic interventions. Large trials, however, are often not simple to implement and potentially sacrifice rigor of protocol implementation for apparent statistical benefits from huge numbers and thoughtful designs. Therefore, in exploring the question of whether meta-analyses can substitute for large trials, it is important to evaluate the utility of meta-analyses in clinical practice and to understand the sources of discrepancies. Two recent studies addressing this issue reported moderate agreement between meta-analyses and large trials (60,61). However, other studies have concluded that results from meta-analyses do not agree with the results of large trials (62,63). For example, LeLorier et al (62) concluded that the meta-analysis failed to accurately predict the results of a subsequent large trial 35 percent of the time. Comparisons of large trials with meta-analyses may reach different conclusions, depending on how trials and meta-analyses are selected and how end points are defined.

Both large studies and meta-analyses of smaller studies add value to clinical decision making. Large studies may produce a more precise point estimate when the treatment effect is not large but is clinically important (64). In the absence of large trials, a well-conducted meta-analysis may provide the best summary of the evidence, but it is important to carefully consider the studies that were included and evaluate the consistency of their results. When the results are mostly in the same direction, the meta-analysis merits more confidence (65).

There are several reasons why meta-analyses are likely to have a role in the development of nutrition policy. First, meta-analyses are much less expensive to conduct then large randomized trials or observational studies. Also, as discussed earlier, meta-analysis may provide a more systematic method for summarizing the literature compared with the traditional review process, and it provides a way to combine the effects of many studies that are too small to have adequate statistical power to detect important effects. In addition, trials that involve changes in dietary patterns or behaviors may be difficult to conduct or may be ruled out by ethical considerations. For example, there was much controversy regarding the influence of alcohol and on the risk of breast cancer. Our knowledge of the effect of alcohol is based on observational studies, and it is unlikely that randomized trials could be conducted to examine the effect of alcohol use on breast cancer in human beings. In addition, it is unclear whether trials of sufficient size, duration, and degree of compliance can be conducted to evaluate hypotheses that involve major changes in eating patterns, such as reduction in fat intake (66). Meta-analyses also can be conducted fairly efficiently to provide information expeditiously to health policymakers.

By quantitatively summarizing the results from many clinical studies, meta-analysis provides information of a kind that no individual study can offer. Conducting a meta-analysis requires rigorous quantitative methods, and the results of such analysis should be interpreted with appropriate caution. Understanding the limitations of the data collection process is critical in performing and interpreting meta-analyses. In the future, meta-analysis could play a major role in the understanding and predicting of discrepancies and in planning clinical trials (67).

REFERENCES

1. Louis T. Finding for public health from meta-analyses. *Annu Rev Public Health.* 1985;6:1–20.
2. Glass GV. Primary, secondary and meta-analysis of research. *Educ Res.* 1976;5:3–8.
3. Glass G, McGaw B, Smith M. *Meta-analysis of Social Research.* Beverly Hills, Calif: Sage Publications; 1981.
4. D'Agostino RB, Weintraub M. Meta-analysis: A method for synthesizing research. *Clin Pharmacol Ther.* 1995;58:605–616.
5. Egger M, Smith GD, Phillips AN. Meta-analysis: principles and procedures. *BMJ.* 1997;315:1533–1537.

6. Mensink RP, Katan MB. Effect of dietary fatty acids on serum lipids and lipoproteins. A meta-analysis of 27 trials. *Arterioscl Thromb.* 1992;12:911–919.

7. Brown LE, Rosner BR, Willett WC, Sacks FM. Cholesterol lowering effects of dietary fiber: a meta-analysis. *Am J Clin Nutr.* 1999;69:1:30–42.

8. Ripsin CM, Keenan JM, Jacobs DR, et al. Oat products and lipid lowering. A meta-analysis. *JAMA.* 1992;267:3317–3325.

9. Anderson JW, Johnstone BM, Cook-Newell ME. Meta-analysis of the effects of soy protein intake on serum lipids. *New Engl J Med.* 1995;333:276–282.

10. Morris MC, Sacks F, Rosner B. Does fish oil lower blood pressure? A meta-analysis of controlled trials. *Circulation.* 1993;88:523–533.

11. Dattilo AM, Kris-Etherton PM. Effects of weight reduction on blood lipids and lip-proteins: a meta-analysis. *Am J Clin Nutr.* 1992;56:320–328.

12. Midgley JP, Matthew AG, Greenwood CMT, Logan AG. Effect of reduced dietary sodium on blood pressure. A meta-analysis of randomized controlled trials. *JAMA.* 1996;275;1590–1597.

13. Cappuccio FP, MacGregor GA. Does potassium supplementation lower blood pressure? A meta analysis of published trials. *J Hypertens.* 1991;9:465–473.

14. Silagy CA, Neil AW. A meta-analysis of the effects of garlic on blood pressure. *J Hypertens.* 1994;12:463–468.

15. Brown SA. Studies of education intervention and outcomes in diabetic adults: a meta-analysis revisited. *Patient Educ Couns.* 1990;16:189–215.

16. Mullen PD, Mains DA, Velez R. A meta-analysis of controlled trials of cardiac patient education. *Patient Educ Couns.* 1992;19:143–162.

17. Longnecker M, Berlin J, Orza M, Chalmers T. A meta-analysis of alcohol consumption in relation to risk of breast cancer. *JAMA.* 1988;260:652–656.

18. Longnecker MP, Orza MJ, Adams ME, et al. A meta-analysis of alcoholic beverage consumption in relation to risk of colorectal cancer. *Cancer Causes Control.* 1990;1:59–68.

19. Kramer M. Does breast feeding help protect against atopic disease? Biology, methodology, and a golden jubilee of controversy. *J Pediatr.* 1988;112:181–190.

20. Detsky A, Baker J, O'Rourke K, Goel V. Perioperative parenteral nutrition: a meta-analysis. *Ann Intern Med.* 1987;107:195–203.

21. Stephen A, Wald N. Trends in individual consumption of dietary fat in the United States, 1920–1984. *Am J Clin Nutr.* 1990;52:457–469.

22. Tucker K. The use of epidemiologic approaches and meta-analysis to determine mineral element requirements. *J Nutr.* 1996:126(suppl):2365–2372.

23. Dickersin K, Berlin JA. Meta-analysis: state-of-the-science. *Epidemiol Rev.* 1992;14:154–176.

24. Louis T. Findings for public health from meta-analyses. *Annu Rev Public Health.* 1985;6:1–20.

25. L'abbe K, Detsky A, O'Rourke K. Meta-analysis in clinical research. *Ann Intern Med.* 1987;107:224–233.

26. Greenland S. Invited Commentary: a critical look at some popular meta-analytic methods. *Am J Epidemiol.* 1994;140(3):290–296.

27. Glass G, McGaw B, Smith M. *Meta-analysis of Social Research.* Beverly Hills, Calif: Sage Publications; 1981.

28. Mosteller F, Tukey J. Data analysis, including statistics. In: Lindzey G, Aronson E, eds. *Handbook of Social Psychology.* Reading, Mass: Addison-Wesley; 1968.

29. Laird NM, Mosteller F. Some statistical methods for combining experimental results. *Int J Technol Assess Health Care.* 1990;6:5–30.

30. Greenland S. Quantitative methods in the review of epidemiologic literature. *Epidemiol Rev.* 1987;9:1–30.

31. Fleiss JL, Gross AJ. Meta-analysis in epidemiology, with special reference to studies of the association between exposure to environmental tobacco smoke and lung cancer: a critique. *J Clin Epidemiol.* 1991;44:127–139.

32. Light R, Smith P. Accumulating evidence: procedures for resolving contradictions among different studies. *Harvard Educ Rev.* 1981;41:429–471.

33. Light R, Pillemer D. *Summing Up: The Science of Reviewing Research.* Cambridge, Mass: Harvard University Press; 1984.

34. Thompson SG. Why sources of heterogeneity in meta-analysis should be investigated. *BMJ.* 1994;309:1351–1355.

35. Oxman AD, Guyatt GH. A consumer's guide to subgroup analyses. *Ann Intern Med.* 1992;116:78–84.

36. Mosteller F, Colditz GA. Understanding research synthesis (meta-analysis). *Annu Rev Public Health.* 1996;17:1–23.

37. Brown L, Rosner B, Willett W, Sacks FM. Reply to AS Truswell. *Am J Clin Nutr.* 1999;70:943.

38. Dickersin K, Chan S, Chalmers TC, Sacks HS, Smith H Jr. Publication bias and clinical trials. *Control Clin Trials.* 1987;8:343–353.

39. Dickersin K. The existence of publication bias and risk factors for its occurrence. *JAMA.* 1990;263;1385–1389.

40. Esterbrook PJ, Berlin JA, Gopalan R, Matthews DR. Publication bias in clinical research. *Lancet.* 1991;337:867–872.

41. Relman AS. News reports of medical meetings: how reliable are abstracts? *N Engl J Med.* 1980;303:277–278.

42. Begg CB, Mazumdar M. Operating characteristics of a rank correlation test for publication bias. *Biometrics.* 1994;50:1099–1101.

43. Dear KB, Begg CB. An approach for assessing publication bias prior to performing a meta-analysis. *Stat Sci.* 1992;7:237–245.

44. Hedges LV. Modeling publication selection effects in ran-

dom effects models in meta-analysis. *Stat Sci.* 1992;7:246–255.

45. Vevea JL, Hedges LV. A general linear model for estimating effect size in the presence of publication bias. Psychometrika. 1995:60:419–435.

46. Dickersin K. Report from the Panel on the Case for Registers of Clinical Trials at the Eighth Annual Meeting of the Society for Clinical Trials. *Control Clin Trials.* 1988;9:76–81.

47. Garrow JS. Would clinical nutrition benefit from meta-analyses and trials registers? *Eur J Clin Nutr.* 1992;46:843–845.

48. Detsky AS, Naylor CD, O'Rourke K, McGreer AJ, L'Abbe KA. Incorporating variations in the quality of individual randomized trials into meta-analysis. *J Clin Epidemiol.* 1992;45:255–265.

49. Sacks HS, Berrier J, Reitman D, Ancona-Berk VA, Chalmers TC. Meta-analyses of randomized controlled trials. *N Engl J Med.* 1987;316:450–455.

50. Chalmers TC, Smith H Jr, Backburn B, et al. A method for assessing the quality of a randomized control trial. *Control Clin Trials.* 1981;2:31–49.

51. Chalmers I, Hetherington J, Elbourne D, et al. Methods used in synthesizing evidence to evaluate the effects of care during pregnancy and childbirth. In: Chalmers I, Enkin M, Keirse MJNC, eds. *Effective Care in Pregnancy and Childbirth.* New York, NY: Oxford University Press; 1989:39–65.

52. Lichtenstein MJ, Mulrow CD, Elwood PC. Guidelines for reading case-control studies. *J Chronic Dis.* 1981;40:893–903.

53. Feinstein AR. Twenty scientific principles for trohoc research. In: *Clinical Epidemiology: The Architecture of Clinical Research.* Philadelphia: WB Saunders; 1985:543–546.

54. Moher D, Jadad AR, Nichol G, Penman M, Tugwell P, Walsh S. Assessing the quality of randomized controlled trials: an annotated bibliography of scales and checklists. *Control Clin Trials.* 1995;16:62–73.

55. Felson DT. Bias in meta-analytic research. *J Clin Epidemiol.* 1992;45:885–892.

56. Friedenreich CM. Methods for pooled analyses of epidemiologic studies. *Epidemiol.* 1993;4:295–302.

57. Emerson JD, Burdick E, Mosteller F, et al. An empirical study of the possible relation of treatment differences to quality scores in controlled randomized clinical trials. *Control Clin Trials.* 1990:11:339–352.

58. Shapiro S. Meta-analysis/Shmeta-analysis. *Am J Epidemiol.* 1994;140:771–778.

59. Petitti DB. Of babies and bathwater. *Am J Epidemiol.* 1994;140:779–782.

60. Villar J, Carroli G, Belizan JM. Predictive ability of meta-analyses of randomised controlled trials. *Lancet.* 1995;345:772–776.

61. Cappelleri JC, Ioannidis JPA, Schmid CH, et al. Large trials vs meta-analysis of smaller trials: How do their results compare? *JAMA.* 1996;276:1332–1338.

62. LeLorier J, Gregoire G, Benhaddad A, Lapierre J, Derderian F. Discrepancies between meta-analyses and subsequent large randomized controlled trials. *N Engl J Med.* 1997;337:536–542.

63. DerSimonian R, Levine RJ. Resolving discrepancies between a meta-analysis and a subsequent large controlled trial. *JAMA.* 1999;282:664–670.

64. Yusuf S, Collins R, Peto R. Why do we need some large, simple randomized trials? *Stat Med.* 1984;3:409–420.

65. Cook DJ, Guyatt GH, Laupacis A, Sackett DL, Goldbert RJ. Clinical recommendations using levels of evidence for antithrombotic agents. *Chest.* 1995;108(suppl):227–230.

66. Willett WC. Nutritional Epidemiology. 2nd ed. New York, NY: Oxford University Press; 1998.

67. Chalmers TC, Lau J. Changes in clinical trails mandated by the advent of meta-analysis. *Stat Med.* 1996;15:1263–1268.

12

Research in Evidence-Based Practice

Esther F. Myers, Ph.D., R.D., F.A.D.A., and Patricia L. Splett, Ph.D., R.D., F.A.D.A

The relationship between research and dietetics practice is a two-way interaction. Research findings are translated into dietetics practice, and dietetics practice identifies questions that need to be researched. This dynamic relationship has become even more evident with the widespread adoption of evidence-based medicine (EBM), also called evidence-based health care (EBHC). EBM uses the best available evidence to guide practice recommendations. Relevant evidence is brought together through the process of systematic review that includes searching for, critically reviewing, grading and summarizing the research reports and evidence. The resulting document represents a summary of the best available data, which is then used to develop evidence-based recommendations and to aid practice decisions. Documents summarizing evidence-based reviews are intended to inform and guide choices made by health care practitioners. The procedures used in the process must be explicit, transparent, and rigorous in terms of scientific methodology.

The American Dietetic Association (ADA) has embraced the concept of grading the evidence for medical nutrition therapy (MNT) protocols, practice guidelines, and other guides for dietetics practice. The ADA now uses a specific process to prepare the guides for clinical practice as *Medical Nutrition Therapy Evidence-Based Guides for Practice* and has created a tool kit to help practitioners develop and validate evidence-based guides for practice (1,2). Both practitioners and researchers make critical contributions to EBM by knowing what questions are faced in daily clinical practice, having

knowledge of a relevant body of research, developing the ability to critically assess published research and other data sources, and producing summary documents.

This chapter provides an overview of EBM and the systematic review process used to evaluate and present evidence. It includes examples of worksheets and the resulting summary document. The final section describes how various associations of health professionals and institutions use EBM.

EVIDENCE-BASED MEDICINE: AN OVERVIEW

In the 1980s, EBM began appearing in the medical literature; it became common terminology in the 1990s and is an expectation of practice today (3). Two major applications of EBM are especially relevant to dietetics practice: (1) review and synthesis of the best available evidence to create recommendations for a defined area of practice (guidelines development and health policy making), and (2) the search for scientific evidence to answer a specific question related to care for a specific patient or subgroup of patients (clinical decision-making). In 1996 Sackett et al defined EBM as the conscientious, explicit, and judicious use of current best evidence in making decisions about the care of individual patients (3). A later publication emphasized two fundamental principles of EBM. First there is a hierarchy of strength of evidence behind recommendations and second, the clinician uses judgment when weighing the tradeoffs associated with alternative management strategies, including consideration of patient values and preferences as well as societal values (4,5).

The methodology for accessing, reviewing, and summarizing research has evolved, and several distinct methods are now acknowledged in the medical literature and widely used (4–13). Many associations of health professionals, expert panels, and institutions have established mechanisms for conducting evidence reviews and producing clinical practice guidelines based on those reviews (6–8,14,15). Some critics of EBM consider it impossible to fully implement because of time demands and the lack of strong research in many areas of practice. Other critics feel EBM is a dangerous innovation perpetrated to serve those desiring to cut costs and suppress clinical decision-making freedom (16–20). Proponents have addressed these concerns and have clarified that evidence used in EBM is not limited to randomized trials and meta-analyses. Although there are limitations to the current practice of grading the evidence used to develop recommendations for practice, and the ultimate impact of the resulting clinical practice guidelines is not fully documented; the terminology and concepts of EBM are widely accepted and integrated into health care policy and academic curriculums (14,21–23). Currently, evidence-based reviews are being conducted by clinicians in response to specific questions they face in practice. Groups of practitioners and researchers also conduct systematic reviews in important areas of practice and make the summary documents available. Practitioners and policymakers can then turn to these preprocessed reviews for information to guide decisions.

SYSTEMATIC REVIEWS USED IN EVIDENCE-BASED MEDICINE

EBM relies on systematic reviews of the best available evidence. The key to this process is critical review of available published research studies and other sources of data. The following are the essential steps of this review process:

1. Identifying a specific problem or area of uncertainty.
2. Formulating the problem as a question.
3. Searching for and finding evidence.
4. Selecting relevant evidence.
5. Evaluating the reports and grading the evidence.

6. Forming recommendations or making decisions using the best available evidence.
7. Summarizing and disseminating the findings.

Various groups have organized the process of EBM into four to eight steps or components (7,24,25). However, all descriptions incorporate the seven listed steps, which will be discussed in this chapter. A basic requirement of the systematic review process used in EBM is that a protocol—the methodology—must be articulated prior to beginning the evidence search, review, and synthesis. In establishing the protocol, the reviewers must balance several objectives, some of which may conflict.

When developing their protocol, for example, the US Preventive Services Task Force identified several objectives:

- To obtain and use the best available empirical evidence to support decision making.
- To set standards that will improve the availability and quality of evidence over time.
- To make recommendations without requiring unobtainable research.
- To balance the need for a consistent approach with a need to have an evaluation approach that is appropriate and feasible across topics.
- To cope with constraints of time and resources (11).

Identifying a Specific Problem or Area of Uncertainty

The process begins by identifying an area to be explored. This step is commonly driven by questions and uncertainties identified by practitioners or raised by other parties, such as payers. It could involve a question about what nutrition services to offer (for example, What is the most effective approach to MNT for clients with hyperlipidemia?) or a question about treatment for an individual patient (for example, Should dietary intervention be recommended for this elderly woman with hyperlipidemia?). Chapter 31, which discusses research in practice, explores the question of application to individual patients in more depth.

Formulating the Question

In EBM, attention focuses on the art of asking specific questions that can be answered using existing data and that are relevant to clinical decision making. Questions about basic biological processes or background questions are not appropriate for EBM and would be better answered by appropriate texts on the topics (26). Craig et al provide a method for framing questions dealing with diagnosis, harm/etiology, prognosis, and intervention, all of which have a slightly different format for designing the question (26). Most questions in dietetics will deal with intervention and should include the following four components: a population with the specific clinical problem; an intervention, procedure, or approach (for example, the type, amount, or timing of MNT); the comparator intervention (other approaches to care); and the outcome of interest.

Table 12.1 illustrates how to use these components to frame dietetics questions and begin to plan the search strategy (26,27). One of the resulting questions from Table 12.1 could be as follows: For asymptomatic adults, what is the preferred intervention for reducing serum low-density lipoprotein cholesterol (LDL-C) and mortality—MNT for hyperlipidemia provided by a registered dietitian or physician-provided dietary advice? Another question might be, For patients with previous myocardial infarction, what is the preferred nutrition intervention for reducing serum LDL-C and mortality—nutrition education for the US Dietary Guidelines provided by a registered dietitian, MNT for hyperlipidemia provided by a registered dietitian, or dietary advice provided by the physician or other health care provider?

Finding the Evidence

After formulating the question that is the basis for the review, a search strategy must be identified for locating evidence in relevant research studies and other reports. Explicit a priori criteria are defined to guide decisions regarding types of evidence to be considered. Criteria should include the definition of the levels of evidence accepted for purposes of the review, as shown in second column of Table 12.2. Figure 12.1 shows the types of studies used to make treatment decisions, in a hierarchy according to strength of evidence. Although most reviews rely on published peer-reviewed research and desire evidence toward the top of the hierarchy, some institutions take a more liberal approach. Goode reported that the University of Colorado model includes nine nonresearch sources of evidence in the multidisciplinary practice model: benchmarking data; clinical expertise; cost-effective analysis; pathophysiology; retrospective or concurrent chart review; quality improvement and risk data; international, national, and local standards; infection control data; and patient preferences (28). Decisions about the types of data allowed must be explicitly defined in the protocol, implemented as defined, documented, and described in the final summary document.

The search strategy usually starts with electronic databases but can also include hand searching of relevant journals. For example, the search strategy reported by the Cochrane Collaborative for nutrition supplementation after hip fracture included studies found using electronic databases (BIOSYS, CABNAR, CINAHL, EMBASE, HEALTHSTAR, and MEDLINE), reference lists in clinical trial reports and other relevant articles, investigators and experts, and a hand search of four nutrition journals. The search strategy should also specify whether the keyword must be in the title or the text when using electronic databases, as well as the hand search methodology. Avenell et al concluded that if a researcher relied on just one of the most popular electronic databases, such as

TABLE 12.1 Asking Answerable Clinical Intervention Questions

Patient Population of Concern	Intervention	Outcome	Comparator	Best Feasible Primary Study Design	Best MEDLINE Search
Asymptomatic people	Medical nutrition therapy for hyperlipidemia	Reduced serum LDL cholesterol mortality	Usual care with assumption of prevention advice by physician	Randomized controlled clinical trial	"Clinical trials," if no hits with term for study type
Patients with previous myocardial infarction	Medical nutrition therapy for hyperlipidemia	Reduced serum LDL and cholesterol and mortality	Advice by physicians or other health care provider	Randomized controlled clinical trial	"Randomized controlled trial"

Adapted from Craig JC, Irwig LM, Stockler MR. Evidence-based medicine: useful tools for decision making. *Med J Aust.* 2001;174:248–253. © 2001. *The Medical Journal of Australia.* Reproduced with permission.

TABLE 12.2   Levels of Evidence and Grades of Recommendation[a]

Grade of Recommendation	Level of Evidence	Therapy/Prevention, Etiology, Harm	Economic Analysis
A	1a	SR (with homogeneity of RCTs)	SR (with homogeneity of Level 1 economic studies)
	1b	Individual RCT (with narrow Confidence Interval)	Analysis comparing critically validated alternate outcomes against appropriate cost measurement, and including sensitivity variations in important variables
B	2a	SR (with homogeneity) of cohort studies	SR (with homogeneity) of ≥ Level 2 economic studies
	2b	Individual cohort study including low-quality RCT; e.g. <80% follow up)	Analysis comparing a limited number of alternative outcomes against appropriate cost measurement, and including a sensitivity analysis incorporating clinically sensible variations in important variables
	2c	"Outcomes research"	
	3a	SR (with homogeneity) of case-control studies	
	3b	Individual case-control	Analysis without study's accurate cost measurement, but including a sensitivity analysis incorporating clinically sensible variations in important variables
C	4	Case series (and poor-quality cohort and case-control studies)	Analysis with no sensitivity analysis
D	5	Expert opinion without explicit critical appraisal, or based on physiology, bench research or "first principles"	Expert opinion without explicit, critical appraisal, or based on economic theory.

[a]RCT, randomized clinical controlled trials; SR, systematic review.
Adapted from Evidence based medicine tool kit. Available at: http://www.med.ualberta.ca/ebm. Accessed April 13, 2001. Used with permission.

MEDLINE, only approximately half the studies would have been identified. Avenell and coworkers showed that only 30 percent of the total study participants would have been identified using a single electronic database (29).

Selecting the Evidence

After locating articles and reports with potential evidence, each one must be carefully read to determine if it meets established criteria for inclusion (as defined in the protocol) and provides evidence related to the question. The US Preventive Services Task Force defined its criteria for inclusion as evidence as follows:

- Information that is appropriate for answering questions about an intervention's effectiveness.

- Data that are applicable (for example, thought to apply to additional populations and settings).
- Articles that identify all of the intervention's other effects—intended and nonintended.
- Data on economic impact.
- Articles that identify barriers that have been observed when implementing the intervention (11).

The reports being reviewed may be limited to Randomized Controlled Trials (RCT) or may include other types of studies. In some cases, a protocol may indicate that the review will include only a specific number (for example, six) of the most important studies relevant to the question rather than listing all available studies (13). However, the research selected must reflect the breadth of findings (including the range of positive and negative results), regardless of the number of studies selected for inclusion. Following are two examples of selection criteria

N of 1 RCT[a]

Systematic review of randomized trials

Single randomized trial

Systematic review of observational studies addressing patient-important outcomes

Single observational study addressing patient-important outcomes

Physiologic studies

Unsystematic clinical observations

[a]N of 1 RCT refers to a study design for a randomized clinical controlled trial where patients undertake pairs of treatment periods in which they receive a target treatment in one period of each pair and a placebo or alternative in the other period. Both patients and clients are blinded, the order of target and control treatment are randomized, and study is continued until both patient and clinician conclude the benefit or lack of benefit of the target intervention. There are limited circumstances when this study design is feasible (23).

FIGURE 12.1   Hierarchy of strength of evidence for treatment decisions. Adapted from Guyatt GH, Haynes RB, Jaeschke RZ, et al. Users' Guides to the Medical Literature: XXV. Evidence-based medicine: principles for applying the Users' Guides to patient care. Evidence-Based Medicine Working Group. *JAMA*. 2000;284:1290–1296. Used with permission from American Medical Association. Copyright 2000; American Medical Association.

for nutrition-related studies defined by the Cochrane Collaborative.

Selection Criteria for Study of Hyperlipidemia (30)

Randomized trials of dietary advice given by a dietitian were compared with advice given by another health professional or self-help resources. The main outcome was difference in serum cholesterol levels between groups receiving dietitian advice and each of the other intervention groups. The following selection criteria were used:

- *Age.* Studies of individuals at least 18 years old.
- *Gender.* Both males and females.
- *Health.* Studies of patients with or without existing heart disease or previous myocardial infarction.
- *Setting.* Free-living subjects recruited from primary care settings, workplaces, out-patient clinics, and other community settings. Studies of patients who

are hospitalized or living in institutions will be excluded.

- *Follow-up.* At least 6 weeks from the baseline visit.
- *Types of interventions.* Dietary advice primarily related to food intake rather than dietary supplements will be included. Advice may be about food preparation, shopping, and what foods to eat or avoid. Interventions are provided by health professionals. Self-help forms of dietary education will be included. Studies that include provision of meals and trials of lipid-lowering drugs where drugs are given to the intervention group only will not be included.
- Primary outcomes will be net change in serum cholesterol level. Secondary outcomes will be change in LDL-C, HDL-C, body mass index, and blood pressure. Data on patient satisfaction will also be examined.

Selection Criteria for Study of Energy/Protein Supplementation in Pregnancy (31)

The study examined acceptable controlled trials of energy/protein supplementation for pregnant women in which the protein content of the supplement was "balanced" (the protein content was less than 25 percent of the total energy content). The selection criteria were as follows:

- Pregnant women.
- Dietary supplementation as dietary intervention.
- Pregnancy outcome and infant outcomes.

Evaluating the Evidence

Up until the evaluation of the evidence, the EBM process is very similar to meta-analysis. However, instead of combining the results statistically, as is done in meta-analysis, evidence grading is used to determine the strength of the evidence. Then the body of literature is summarized in a table of evidence that can be used to formulate a recommendation. To do so, data from each of the selected studies are extracted according to the protocol. Some methodologies suggest that the abstraction process and criteria should vary depending on the question to be answered: prognosis, diagnoses, treatment, or economic (7,32). The following types of data are usually extracted: author and date, methodology/type of study, participants, intervention, outcome, and quality of the study (design and execution).

Various methods are used to characterize the hierarchy of evidence. Most are based on the type/design of the study. Within the hierarchy, studies are evaluated using criteria relevant to the particular study design. The qualities of using sound study design and execution are addressed other chapters of this book. In 1979 the Canadian Task Force on the Periodic Health Examination proposed one of the first hierarchics for rating or grading levels of evidence. It has been refined and has evolved over the years into Table 12.2 (7). The Institute for Clinical Systems Improvement (ICSI) developed an alternative and less complex system for classifying and grading studies (13). Table 12.3 shows the ICSI hierarchy of classes of research reports, and Figure 12.2 illustrates the a plus/minus/neutral scoring scheme for grading the quality of primary research reports that is being used by the American Dietetic Association.

Evaluation of the quality of a study also includes an assessment of the relevance of the report to practice and a critique of the study's validity. The questions asked in this two-step assessment differ somewhat depending on whether the study or report being considered is a single study or a systematic review of several studies. This is shown in Figure 12.3. The process of evaluating the quality of the evidence should have all the rigor of other scientific methods to ensure solid recommendations for clinical practice (25).

TABLE 12.3 Institute for Clinical Systems Improvement Classes of Research Reports

Primary Reports of New Data Collection	
Class	Type of Research
A	Randomized controlled trial
B	Cohort study
C	Nonrandomized trial with concurrent or historical controls Case-control study Study of sensitivity and specificity of diagnostic test Population-based descriptive study
D	Cross-sectional study Case series Case report

Reports That Synthesize or Reflect Upon Collections of Primary Reports	
Class	Type of Research
M	Meta-analysis Systematic review Decision analysis Cost-benefit analysis Cost-effectiveness study
R	Narrative review Consensus statement Consensus report
X	Medical opinion

Adapted from Greer N, Mosser G, Logan G, Halaas GW. A practical approach to evidence grading. *Jt Comm J Qual Improv.* 2000;26:700–712. Used with permission.

Formulating Recommendations

Over the past 20 years, information on the science of synthesizing research results has expanded. However, methods for linking evidence to recommendations are less well developed than methods for synthesizing evidence. A logical approach to identifying and mapping out a chain of hypothesized causal relationships among the determinants, interventions, and intermediate and ultimate health outcomes—is very helpful in formulating recommendations based on the evidence (11,33). When formulating the recommendation statements, it is helpful to "grade" or indicate the strength of the recommendation. Tables 12.4 and 12.5 show two methods of characterizing the strength of the recommendations that can be made from a body of evidence (11,13).

Summarizing and Disseminating Results

The process and findings of a systematic review are reported as in any research effort. Evidence tables are the "results" of a systematic review. The tables are presented along with a description of the protocol used.

Gallagher proposes a standard annotated outline format for published systematic reviews similar to CONsolidated Standard of Reporting Trials (CONSORT) (34). The outline of the preferred format for systematic reviews[a] is as follows:

I. Structured Abstract (including Objective, Methods, Results, and Conclusions)
II. Body of manuscript
   A. Introduction (purpose and objectives)
   B. Methods (search strategy, selection criteria, application of selection criteria, criteria for assessment of study quality, and method of data synthesis)
   C. Results (tables of included and excluded reports, description of studies)
   D. Methodological quality of selected studies
   E. Discussion
   F. Limitations and Future Questions
   G. Conclusions

[a]Outline reprinted from Gallagher EJ. Systematic reviews: a logical methodological extension of evidence-based medicine. *Acad Emerg Med.* 1999;6:1255–1260. Copyright 1999 by Hanley & Belfus Inc. Reproduced with permission of Hanley & Belfus Inc in the format Copy via Copyright Clearance Center.

RELEVANCE QUESTIONS		
1. Would implementing the studied intervention or procedure (if found successful) result in improved outcomes for the patients/clients/population group? (N/A for some Epi studies)	Yes	No
2. Did the authors study an outcome (dependent variable) or topic which the patients/clients/population group would care about?	Yes	No
3. Is the focus of the intervention or procedure (independent variable) or topic of study a common issue of concern to dietetics practice?	Yes	No
4. Is the intervention or procedure feasible? (N/A for some Epidemiological studies)	Yes	No
If the answers to all of the above Relevance Questions are "Yes," the report may be eligible for designation with a plus (+) on the Evidence Quality Worksheet, depending on answers to the following Validity Questions.		
VALIDITY QUESTIONS		

1. Was the *research question* clearly stated?
   a. Was the specific intervention(s) or procedure (independent variable(s) identified?
   b. Was the outcome(s) (dependent variable(s) clearly indicated?
   c. Were the target population and setting specified?
	Yes	No

2. Was the *selection* of study subjects/patients free from bias?
   a. Were inclusion/exclusion criteria specified (e.g., risk, point in disease progression, diagnostic or prognosis criteria), and with sufficient detail and without omitting criteria critical to the study?
   b. Were criteria applied equally to all study groups?
   c. Were health, demographics, and other characteristics of subjects described?
   d. Were the subjects/patients a representative sample of the relevant population?
	Yes	No

3. Were *study groups comparable*?
   a. Was the method of assigning subjects/patients to groups described and unbiased? (Method of randomization identified if RCT)
   b. Were distribution of disease status, prognostic factors, and other factors (e.g., demographics) similar across study groups at baseline?
   c. Were concurrent controls used? (Concurrent preferred over historical controls.)
   d. If a cohort study or cross-sectional study, were groups comparable on important confounding factors and/or were preexisting differences accounted for by using appropriate adjustments in statistical analysis?
   e. If a case control study, were potential confounding factors comparable for cases and controls?
   f. If a case series or trial with subjects serving as own control, this criterion is not applicable. Criterion may not be applicable in some cross-sectional studies.
   g. If a diagnostic test, was there an independent blind comparison with an appropriate reference standard (e.g., "gold standard")?
	Yes	No

4. Was method of handling *withdrawals* described?
   a. Were follow-up methods described and the same for all groups?
   b. Was the number, characteristics of withdrawals (i.e., dropouts, lost to follow-up, attrition rate) and/or response rate (cross-sectional studies) described for each group? (Follow-up goal for a strong study is 80%.)
   c. Were all enrolled subjects/patients (in the original sample) accounted for?
   d. Were reasons for withdrawals similar across groups?
   e. If a diagnostic test, was decision to perform reference test not dependent on results of test under study?
	Yes	No

5. Was *blinding* used to prevent introduction of bias?
   a. In an intervention study, were subjects, clinicians/practitioners, and investigators blinded to treatment group, as appropriate?
   b. Were data collectors blinded for outcomes assessment? (If outcome is measured using an objective test, such as a lab value, this criterion is assumed to be met)
   c. In a cohort study or cross-sectional study, were measurements of outcomes and risk factors blinded?
	Yes	No

FIGURE 12.2   American Dietetic Association's Evidence Analysis Process: Quality criteria checklist for primary research. N/A indicates not applicable.

d. In a case control study, was case definition explicit and case ascertainment not influenced by exposure status? e. In a diagnostic study, were test results blinded to patient history and other test results?			
6. Were *intervention*/therapeutic regimens/exposure factor or procedure and any comparison(s) described in detail? Were *intervening factors* described? a. In an RCT or other intervention trial, were protocols described for all regimens studied? b. In an observational study, were interventions, study settings, and clinicians/provider described? c. Was the intensity and duration of the intervention or exposure factor sufficient to produce a meaningful effect? d. Was the amount of exposure and, if relevant, subject/patient compliance measured? e. Were co-interventions (e.g., ancillary treatments, other therapies) described? f. Were extra or unplanned treatments described? g. Was the information for 6d, 6e, and 6f assessed the same way for all groups? h. In diagnostic study, were details of test administration and replication sufficient?	Yes	No	
7. Were *outcomes* clearly defined and the *measurements valid and reliable*? a. Were primary and secondary endpoints described and relevant to the question? b. Were nutrition measures appropriate to question and outcomes of concern? c. Was the period of follow-up long enough for important outcome(s) to occur? d. Were the observations and measurements based on standard, valid and reliable data collection instruments/tests/procedures? e. Was the measurement of effect at an appropriate level of precision? f. Were other factors accounted for (measured) that could affect outcomes? g. Were the measurements conducted consistently across groups?	Yes	No	
8. Was the *statistical analysis* appropriate for the study design and type of outcome indicators? a. Were statistical analyses adequately described the results reported appropriately? b. Were correct statistical tests used and assumptions of test not violated? c. Were statistics reported with levels of significance and/or confidence intervals? d. Was "intent to treat" analysis of outcomes done (and as appropriate, was there an analysis of outcomes for those maximally exposed or a dose-response analysis)? e. Were adequate adjustments made for effects of confounding factors that might have affected the outcomes (e.g., multivariate analyses)? f. Was clinical significance as well as statistical significance reported? g. If negative findings, was a power calculation reported to address the possibility of type 2 error?	Yes	No	
9. Are *conclusions supported by results* with biases and limitations taken into consideration? a. Is there a discussion of findings? b. Are biases and study limitations identified and discussed?	Yes	No	
10. Is bias due to study's *funding or sponsorship* unlikely? a. Were sources of funding and investigators' affiliations described? b. Was there no apparent conflict of interest?	Yes	No	

MINUS/NEGATIVE (–)

If most (six or more) of the answers to the above validity questions are "No," the report should be designated with a minus (–) symbol on the Evidence Quality Worksheet.

NEUTRAL (∅)

If the answers to validity criteria questions 2, 3, 6 and 7 do not indicate that the study is exceptionally strong, the report should be designated with a neutral (∅) symbol on the Evidence Quality Worksheet.

PLUS/POSITIVE (+)

If most of the answers to the above validity questions are "Yes" (must include criteria 2, 3, 6, 7 and at least one additional "Yes"); the report should be designated with a plus symbol (+) on the Evidence Quality Worksheet.

FIGURE 12.2 (continued)

RELEVANCE QUESTIONS		
1. Will the answer, if true, have a direct bearing on the health of patients?	Yes	No
2. Is the outcome or topic something which patients/clients/population groups would care about?	Yes	No
3. Is the problem addressed in the review one that is relevant to dietetics practice?	Yes	No
4. Will the information, if true, require a change in practice?	Yes	No
If the answers to all of the above Relevance Questions are "Yes," the report may be eligible for designation with a plus (+) on the Evidence Quality Worksheet, depending on answers to the following Validity Questions.		
VALIDITY QUESTIONS		
1. Was the *research question* clearly focused and appropriate?	Yes	No
2. Was the *search strategy* used to locate relevant studies comprehensive? Were the databases searched and the search terms used described?	Yes	No
3. Were explicit *methods used to select studies* to include in the review? Were inclusion/exclusion criteria specified and appropriate? Were selection methods unbiased?	Yes	No
4. Was there an *appraisal of the quality and validity of studies* included in the review? Were appraisal methods specified, appropriate and reproducible?	Yes	No
5. Were *specific treatments/interventions/exposures* described? Were treatments similar enough to be combined?	Yes	No
6. Was the *outcome* of interest clearly indicated? Were other potential harms and benefits considered?	Yes	No
7. Were processes for *data abstraction, synthesis and analysis* described? Were they applied consistently across studies and groups? Was there appropriate use of qualitative and/or quantitative synthesis? Was variation in findings among studies analyzed? Were heterogeneity issued considered? If data from studies were aggregated for meta-analysis, was the procedure described?	Yes	No
8. Are the *results* clearly presented in narrative and/or quantitative terms? If summary statistics are used, are levels of significance and/or confidence intervals included?	Yes	No
9. Are *conclusions supported by results* with biases and limitations taken into consideration? Are limitations of the review identified and discussed?	Yes	No
10. Was bias due to the review's *funding or sponsorship* unlikely?	Yes	No
MINUS/NEGATIVE (–) *If most (six or more) of the answers to the above validity questions are "No," the review should be designated with a minus (–) symbol on the Evidence Quality Worksheet.*		
NEUTRAL (() *If the answer to any of the first four validity questions (1–4) is "No," but other criteria indicate strengths, the review should be designated with a neutral (() symbol on the Evidence Quality Worksheet.*		
PLUS/POSITIVE (+) *If most of the answers to the above validity questions are "Yes," (must include criteria 1, 2, 3, and 4) the report should be designated with a plus symbol (+) on the Evidence Quality Worksheet.*		

FIGURE 12.3 American Dietetic Association's Evidence Analysis Process: Quality criteria checklist for review articles.

III. Tables and figures (tables of included and excluded studies, tables of evidence, and figures of abstracted data and comparisons)

IV. References

Evidence tables are often included as attachments to evidence-based clinical practice guidelines or published as a review article. The tables of evidence parallel the level of evidence criteria identified in the protocol. Table 12.6 and Table 12.7 illustrate examples of tables of evidence from the Cochrane Collaborative and from the American Dietetic Association guides (30,35). Some clinical practice guidelines include "Levels of Evidence" and "Grades of Recommendations" throughout the document after

TABLE 12.4 Conclusion Grades

Conclusion Grade	Description
Grade I: The conclusion is supported by good evidence.	The evidence consists of studies of strong design for answering the question addressed. The results are both clinically important and consistent, with minor exceptions at most. The results are free of any significant doubts about generalizability, bias, or flaws in research design. Studies with negative results have sufficiently large samples to have adequate statistical power.
Grade II: The conclusion is supported by fair evidence.	The evidence consists of results from studies of strong design for answering the question addressed, but there is some uncertainty attached to the conclusion because of inconsistencies among the results from the studies or because of minor doubts about generalizability, bias, research design flaws, or adequacy of sample size. Alternatively, the evidence consists solely of results from weaker designs for the question addressed, but the results have been confirmed in separate studies and are consistent, with minor exceptions at most.
Grade III: The conclusion is supported by limited evidence	The evidence consists of results from studies of strong design for answering the question addressed, but there is a substantial uncertainty attached to the conclusion because of inconsistencies among the results from different studies or because of serious doubts about generalizability, bias, research design flaws, or adequacy of sample size. Alternatively, the evidence consists solely of results from a limited number of studies of weak design for answering the question addressed.
Grade IV: The conclusion is supported only by commentators based on opinion.	The support for the conclusion consists solely of the statements of informed medical commentators about their clinical experience, unsubstantiated by the results of any research studies.

Adapted from Greer N, Mosser G, Logan G, Halaas GW. A practical approach to evidence grading. *Jt Comm J Qual Improv.* 2000;26:700–712. Used with permission.

each recommendation is presented. Figure 12.4 shows an example of a recommendation with evidence grading included in the text of the practice guideline (see page 180).

STRENGTHS AND LIMITATIONS OF EVIDENCE-BASED MEDICINE

The systematic review process results in consideration of the breadth of the evidence. It also enables objective assessment of the levels of evidence and the strength of support for specific recommendations or intervention alternatives. The use of EBM promotes the use of effective intervention alternatives and the reduction of ineffective ones. It pushes the profession forward as practitioners make practice decisions that are supported by empirical data and recognize where uncertainties exist. When these uncertainties are formulated into answerable questions, available data can be gathered and graded. When the level of evidence is low or the grading of evidence is neutral, additional studies are warranted. The identification of unanswered problems and uncertainties can stimulate research to fill gaps in important areas.

The systematic reviews used in EBM are subject to many of the same limitations as other types of research, including publication bias, timeliness of data publication,

and methodological issues. Several limitations of systematic reviews are of particular concern: practitioner skill in conducting the search and evidence review, amount of time required to complete a thorough evidence review, lack of relevant research, and applicability of RCT results to routine clinical settings (3,16–19,36).

Conducting evidence-based reviews requires practitioners to have skills to precisely define a patient problem needing "evidence" to resolve, conduct an efficient search of the literature, select the best of the relevant studies, apply rules of evidence to determine validity, and extract the clinical message and apply it to a patient problem. These skills must be tempered with an understanding of how the patient's values affect treatment decisions and the ability to involve the patient in the decision-making process. The rigor of the assessment of selected research is compromised if the practitioner lacks knowledge of research principles or is inexperienced in the area of investigation. To overcome this limitation, researchers familiar with the topic area can be included in the process.

A major barrier to the concept of EBM is the time required for conducting a thorough systematic review. To address this barrier, some institutions have created mechanisms for easy computer access to medical literature and preprocessed reviews and guidelines (for example, terminals at the hospital unit or clinic and wireless portable computers). At some institutions, especially academic

TABLE 12.5   Assessing the Strength of a Body of Evidence on Effectiveness of Population-Based Interventions in the *Guide to Community Preventive Services*

Evidence of Effectiveness[a]	Execution: Good or Fair[b]	Design Suitability: Greatest, Moderate, or Least	No. of Studies	Consistent[c]	Effect Size[d]	Expert Opinion[e]
Strong	Good	Greatest	At least 2	Yes	Sufficient	Not used
	Good	Greatest or moderate	At least 5	Yes	Sufficient	
	Good or fair	Greatest	At least 5	Yes	Sufficient	
Sufficient but not strong	Meets same criteria as above	Meets same criteria as above	Meets same criteria as above	Yes	Large	Not used
Sufficient	Good	Greatest	1	Not applicable	Sufficient	Not used
	Good or fair	Greatest or moderate	At least 3	Yes	Sufficient	Not used
	Good or fair	Greatest, moderate, or least	At least 5	Yes	Sufficient	Not used
Expert opinion	Varies	Varies	Varies	Varies	Sufficient	Supports a recommendation
Insufficient[f]	A. Insufficient execution	A. Insufficient design	B. Too few studies	C. Inconsistent	D. Small	E. Not used

[a]The categories are not mutually exclusive; a body of evidence meeting criteria for more than one of these should be categorized in the highest possible category.

[b]Studies with limited execution are not used to assess effectiveness.

[c]Generally consistent in direction and size.

[d]Sufficient and large effect sizes are defined on a case-by-case basis and are based on Task Force opinion.

[e]Expert opinion will not be routinely used in the *Guide* but can affect the classification of a body of evidence as shown.

[f]Reasons for determination that evidence is insufficient will be described as follows: A. Insufficient designs or executions. B. Too few studies. C. Inconsistent. D. Effect size too small. E. Expert opinion not used. These categories are not mutually exclusive and one or more of these will occur when a body of evidence fails to meet the criteria for strong or sufficient evidence.

Adapted by permission from Elsevier Science from Briss PA, Zaza S, Pappaioanou M, Fielding J, et al. Developing an evidence-based Guide to Community Preventive Services—methods. The Task Force on Community Preventive Services. *Am J Prev Med.* 2000;18(1 Suppl):35–43.

health centers, medical librarians are making rounds with the team so searches to resolve uncertainties can be quickly completed.

Another major limitation of EBM is the premise that published research and evidence already has been, or can be, conducted to answer important clinical questions. It is virtually impossible to create or find research to answer all important clinical questions because of the high cost involved in research, time required for research, and difficulty in conducting the research (21). Furthermore, the gold standard for studies to determine if a treatment is safe and effective is the RCT, which can be complex and costly to conduct. However, it is erroneous to conclude that a lack of research is evidence that a treatment is not warranted. An example of this illogical conclusion would be decision makers who attempted to rely on RCT to decide whether the use of insulin should continue in the treatment of persons with diabetes. Because insulin is considered standard practice, it would be unethical to deny patients the treatment to prove its efficacy. The same dilemma might exist when considering the question of whether MNT was beneficial to persons with other conditions.

Another barrier to the use of EBM is debate about the applicability of RCT to patient populations (16–19, 21,36). With tightly defined criteria for subject inclusion and the high commitment to compliance needed for valid clinical trials, the sample studied in the trial may not reflect the range of patients that practitioners are likely to encounter in routine practice.

USES OF PREPROCESSED EVIDENCE

The primary use of systematic reviews of evidence is to provide the basis for clinical decision making, either

TABLE 12.6 Example of Cochrane Collaborative Evidence Table (Table of included studies)

Study		Methods	Participants	Interventions	Outcomes	Notes	Quality
Barratt	1994	RCT Randomization concealment: NOT CLEAR	n (dietitian): 114	The study aim was to examine the feasibility of conducting a large work-site cholesterol screening project and to evaluate by randomized controlled trial two dietary interventions to lower cholesterol. The aim of the dietary interventions was to reduce total and saturated fat and increase fiber intake.	Blood cholesterol, HDLc, body weight	Authors concluded that there was no benefit from interventions in reducing blood cholesterol. Strategies are required to maintain high ongoing participation rates.	B
		Follow-up:	n (self-help methods): 310				
		Dietitian: NOT DONE	Inclusion criteria: blood pressure above 140/90 mmHg				
		Self-help: NOT DONE					
		Blinded assessment: DONE	Baseline blood cholesterol: Dt 6.2; SH 6.0 mmol/L				
		Baseline: NOT DONE	Setting: Workplace				
		Reliable outcomes: DONE	Country: Australia	1. Dietitian-led nutrition course (five 1-hour sessions) included demonstrations and discussions			
		Protection against contamination: NOT DONE		2. Self-help package (workbook with similar education content to nutrition course and quizzes, shopping guides, video and recipes)			
		Unit of allocation: participant		Other interventions: diet alone			
		Unit of analysis: participant		No lipid lowering drugs documented			
				Duration of study: 26 weeks			

Adapted with permission from Thompson RL, Summerbell CD, Higgins JPT, Little PS, Talbor D, Ebrahim S. Dietary advice given by a dietitian versus other health professional or self-help methods to reduce blood cholesterol (Cochrane Review). In: *The Cochrane Library.* Oxford, England: Update Software; 2003: Issue 1. Available at: http://www.cochrane.de.

TABLE 12.7 Example of American Dietetic Association Conclusion Conclusion Grading Worksheet for Hyperlipidemia Practice Guide

Stanols/Sterols ADA Conclusion Grading Worksheet for Research Articles

Work Group's Conclusions: *Plant stanol esters are effective in lowering serum total cholesterol and LDL cholesterol in healthy adults and in women with CA. A reduction of up to 10% total cholesterol is observed when 2–3 g of plant stanol/sterol esters are consumed daily. There is a dose response in serum cholesterol with a daily consumption of 1.6 to 3.2 g plant stanol/sterol esters*

Conclusion Grade: II. The conclusion is supported by fair evidence.

Evidence: RCT (feeding studies) demonstrate significant reductions in serum total and LDL cholesterol. No clinical outcome studies have been done.

Author / Year	Design Type	Class	Quality +,−,∅	Population Studied / Sample Size	Primary Outcome Measure(s) / Results (e.g., p value, confidence interval, relative risk, odds ratio, likelihood ratio, number needed to treat)	Authors' Conclusions / Work Group's Comments (italicized)*
Gylling H, et al. *Circulation.* 1997;96:4226–4231.	RCT	A	+	2 groups of postmenopausal women with CAD, 48 to 56 years of age in Finland 1. Group 1: women who had received angiography, 8 had CABG, 11 had angioplasty a. Women randomly assigned to 21 g rapeseed oil margarine without (*n* = 11) or with sitostanol ester (3 g) (*n* = 11) for 7 weeks, then switched to the other margarine for 7 weeks. 2. Group 2: 10 women receiving 10-20 mg/d of simvastatin over 1 year. a. Women replaced 21 g of daily fat intake with sitostanol ester margarine for 12 weeks. **Inclusion criteria:** Documented CAD disease ≥ 3 months: MI, angioplasty, or CABG **Exclusion criteria:** 1. Thyroid, liver, or renal disease. 2. ERT 3. On lipid (medications **Outcome measures:** 1. Total cholesterol 2. LDL cholesterol 3. HDL cholesterol 4. TG 5. Serum sterols 6. Dietary cholesterol absorption	**Group 1: no lipid lowering meds** Sitostanol ester margarine low-ered serum total cholesterol 13% (P <0.05) LDL cholesterol 20% (P <0.01) Sitostanol ester margarine ↓ serum total cholesterol in all women, LDL cholesterol (<100 mg/dL) in 32% and (<133 mg/dL) in 73% vs. none and 27% during the basal diet (P <0.01). **Group 2: on 10-20 mg simvastatin** Sitostanol ester margarine ↓ Total cholesterol 11 ± 3% (P <0.01) LDL cholesterol 16 ± 5% (P <0.01) The effects of sitostanol on cholesterol metabolism: ↓ absorption (−45%) ↑ Fecal elimination (+45% as neutral sterols) ↑ Synthesis (+39%)	Dietary use of sitostanol ester margarine normalizes LDL cholesterol in ~1/3 of women with previous MI, especially in those with ↑ baseline absorption and ↓ synthesis of cholesterol and when combined with statins ↓ the needed drug dose. High cholesterol and plant sterol (↑ cholesterol absorption) and low baseline precursor sterol proportions (low cholesterol synthesis) predicted high ↓ in serum cholesterol. *Use of sitostanol ester margarine can reduce the need for statins or reduce the amount of statins needed in women with hypercholesterolemia.* *Well-designed RCT, blinded crossover trial.*

| Miettinen TA, et al. *NEJM.* 1995; 333:1308–1312. | RCT | A | + | Subjects recruited from a random population sample from North Karelia, Finland as part of the Finnish 1992 study.

Inclusion criteria:
1. 25–64 years of age
2. BMI <30
3. Serum chol ≥216 mg/dL
4. TG <265 mg/dL
5. Stable meds for hpt, diabetes mellitus, or CHD

Exclusion criteria:
1. Absence of renal, alcohol, liver, or thyroid disease

Subjects randomly assigned to study diets for 6 months. a. 51 to margarine without sitostanol ester (control) b. 102 to margarine containing sitostanol ester (3g sitostanol/d). For the second 6 mos, the subjects on sitostanol were randomly assigned to the same amount of sitostanol or to (intake to 2 g/d

Outcome measures: Serum lipids | 153 subjects, 42% men participated in the study.

The differences in serum cholesterol between the control and experimental groups after 1 year:

Tchol -24 mg/dL (95% CI, -17 to 32. (*P* <0.001)

LDL chol -21 mg/dl (95% CI, -14 to -29) (*P* <0.001).

Serum campesterol (a dietary plant sterol whose levels reflect cholesterol absorption) was (by 36% in the sitostanol group that was directly correlated with the ↓ in total cholesterol. (r = 0.57, *P* <0.001) | Substituting sitostanol-ester margarine for part of the daily fat intake in subjects with mild hypercholesterolemia was effective in ↓ serum total cholesterol and LDL cholesterol.

Well-designed study. |

(continued)

TABLE 12.7 Example of American Dietetic Association Conclusion Grading Worksheet for Hyperlipidemia Practice Guide (continued)

Stanols/Sterols ADA Conclusion Grading Worksheet for Research Articles

Work Group's Conclusions: *Plant stanol esters are effective in lowering serum total cholesterol and LDL cholesterol in healthy adults and in women with CA. A reduction of up to 10% total cholesterol is observed when 2-3 g of plant stanol/sterol esters are consumed daily. There is a dose response in serum cholesterol with a daily consumption of 1.6 to 3.2 g plant stanol/sterol esters*

Conclusion Grade: II. The conclusion is supported by fair evidence.

Evidence: RCT (feeding studies) demonstrate significant reductions in serum total and LDL cholesterol. No clinical outcome studies have been done.

Author / Year	Design Type	Class	Quality +-, ∅	Population Studied / Sample Size	Primary Outcome Measure(s) / Results (e.g., p value, confidence interval, relative risk, odds ratio, likelihood ratio, number needed to treat)	Authors' Conclusions / Work Group's Comments (italicized)*
Hallikainen MA. *J Nutrition.* 2000;130:767–776.	RCT Single-blinded Repeated measures	A	+	26 subjects recruited from former studies carried out at the Department of Clinical Nutrition, U of Kuopio and from the local society of Finnish Heart Association **Inclusion criteria:** T chol: 5.0-8.5 mmol/L TG: <3.5 mmol/L Age: 25–65 years Willingness to participate **Exclusion criteria:** 1. Abnormal liver, kidney, or thyroid function 2. On lipid lowering meds 3. Unstable CHD 4. Alcohol abuse (>45 g ethanol/d) 5. Irregular eating habits **Study Design:** 1. 1 wk trial period, followed by assignment in random order to different levels of plant stanol ester in rapeseed oil-based margarine: 2.4, 3.2, 1.6, 0 (control), or 0.8 g/d each for a 4 wk period. 2. Subjects were instructed to follow a diet 34% fat, 12% saturated fat, 14% MUFA, 8% PUFA,.; subjects kept food records (3 days during pretrial and 4 days during each 4-week period). 3. Fasting blood lipid samples, during the pretrial period and at the beginning, middle and end of each study period. **Outcome measures:** Serum lipids, serum stanols	22 subjects completed the study (8 men, 14 women) Changes in serum lipids compared to controls on different doses of stanol: Stanol g/d |	0.8	1.6	2.4	3.2
T chol (%Δ)	2.8	6.8	10.3	11.3
(P value)	0.38	<0.001	<0.00	<0.001
LDL chol (%Δ)	1.7	5.6	9.7	10.4
(P value)	0.89	<0.05	<0.001	<0.001	 Although the ↓ were greater with 2.4 and 3.2 g/d doses of stanol, the differences were not significant (P <0.054 to 0.516) Apolipoprotein B concentration ↓ significantly at 0.8 g/d dose of stanol (P <0.001). Apolipoprotein E genotype did not affect the lipid responses.	Significant ↓ of serum total and LDL cholesterol is reached with 1.6 g stanol/day; ↑ the dose from 2.4 to 3.2 g does not provide a clinically important additional effect. *Well-controlled diet in free-living individuals.*

| Lichtenstein AH, Deckelbaum RJ. *Circulation.* 2001:103:1177–1179 | Narrative review | R | – | Since Stanol/Sterol esters do not occur in nature in foods commonly eaten, all studies to evaluate these have been clinical trials and the majority have been RCT. | **Benefits of Stanol/Sterol Ester containing fats:**

1. Sitostanol ester (3.4 g/d) in canola oil-based margarine lowers LDL cholesterol ~10% in modestly hypercholesterolemic subjects and in individuals with apo E4 alleles (previously reported to have the highest efficiency of cholesterol absorption).

2. Maximal efficacy with respect to total and LDL cholesterol lowering is achieved at ~2 g/d and that there is little effect on HDL cholesterol or triglycerides.

3. Consumption of sterol esters is efficacious in both normolipidemic and dyslipidemic individuals including those being treated with HMG-CoA reductase inhibitors or other lipid lowering medications.

4. Ingestion of 1.8 to 3 g/d of stanol esters in hypercholesterolemic children resulted in lower LDL cholesterol similar to that of adults (9% to 20%).

Possible adverse effects of consuming stanol ester foods:

1. Lower plasma alpha and beta carotenes, alpha-tocopherol, and/or lycopene especially in children and pregnant women | Stanol/Sterol Ester-containing fats should be reserved for adults requiring lowering of total and LDL cholesterol because of hypercholesterolemia or secondary prevention after an atherosclerotic event.

More long-term studies are needed before these products can be recommended for the general population to prevent CHD or for children with hypercholesterolemia, because of the possible side effects related to malabsorption of fat-soluble vitamins.

No details of the studies were given in this review. This was strictly a narrative review.

Data from RCT are available to demonstrate the efficacy of stanol/sterol ester containing foods in ↓ total and LDL cholesterol. |

Nutrition practice guidelines for hyperlipidemia. *Medical Nutrition Therapy Evidence-based Guides for Practice* [CD-ROM]. Chicago, Ill: American Dietetic Association; 2001.

Protein

Conclusion statement

What research evidence supports this conclusion?

Review Worksheets:

Level of Evidence: I

The recommended dietary allowance for protein is an additional 10 g per day in pregnancy, based on balance studies that show 1.3 to 2.1 g nitrogen (8.1 to 13 g protein) retention during pregnancy with the greater amount retained during the third trimester.

Inclusion of protein in meals and snacks does not significantly affect blood glucose excursions, and thus can be added for additional calories in place of carbohydrate foods.

Restriction or control of carbohydrate intake in women with GDM implies that the protein and fat intake may be increased to maintain adequate calories.

The level of protein needed during pregnancy is an additional 10 grams above the RDA of 0.8 g/kg DBW (1,2). The RDA for protein is easily met in meal plans for GDM when the carbohydrate is controlled to 40–45%. Protein generally comprises 20 –25% of calories. However, excessive protein should be avoided. The national WIC Evaluation (3), a population based study, showed an increase in birthweight for intakes of protein up to 69.5 g/day and a decrease in birthweight with protein intakes > 85 g/day.

What is the effect of protein on blood glucose? Research has shown that peripheral glucose levels do not increase after protein ingestion (4). Protein is often added to increase calories without affecting blood glucose levels (4–6).

1. Food and Nutrition Board. *Recommended Dietary Allowances.* 10th ed. Washington, DC: National Academy of Sciences; 1989:33–34.
2. King JC. Physiology of pregnancy and nutrient metabolism. *Am J Clin Nutr.* 2000;71(suppl): 1218S–1225S.
3. Sloan NL, Lederman SA, Leighton J, Himes JH, Rush D. The effect of prenatal dietary protein intake on birth weight. *Nutrition Research.* 2001;21:129–139.
4. Nuttall FQ, Gannon MC. Plasma glucose and insulin response to macronutrients in non-diabetic and NIDDM subjects. *Diabetes Care.* 1991;14:814–838.
5. Nuttall FQ, Mooradian AD, Gannon MC, Billington CJ, Krezowski PA. Effect of protein ingestion on glucose and insulin response to a standardized oral glucose load. *Diabetes Care.* 1998; 21:16–22.
6. Gannon MC, Nuttall JA, Damberg G, Gupta V, Nuttall FQ. Effect of protein ingestion on the glucose appearance rate in people with type 2 diabetes. *J Clin Endocrinol Metab.* 2001;86:1040–1047.

FIGURE 12.4 Example of recommendation statement from American Dietetic Association. Nutrition practice guidelines for gestational diabetes mellitus. *Medical Nutrition Therapy Evidence-based Guides for Practice* [CD-ROM]. Chicago, Ill: American Dietetic Association; 2001. DBW indicates desired birth weight; GDM, gestational diabetes mellitus; RDA, Recommended Dietary Allowance.

through the development of profession-wide or institution-based clinical practice guidelines, MNT protocols, or clinical pathways or by aiding practitioner decision making for individual patients. Evidence summaries are often the basis behind policies regarding the types and amount of care that will be covered by health plans. Evidence summaries are also tremendously helpful in identifying gaps in research and focusing future research to answer important practice questions. Table 12.8 classifies and describes the types of evidence reports that are now available (5).

Reviews and the recommendations and guidelines developed from them can become obsolete as new research becomes available and new procedures and therapies are introduced. Splett developed a checklist to determine when it is necessary to update an evidence-based guide (37). In most areas of dietetics practice, updates of reviews should be considered in at least 2-year intervals (38). The Cochrane Collaborative Web site maintains a listing showing the schedule for updating reviews (39).

FUTURE RESEARCH

In addition to identifying research gaps in the topic of the review, evidence is needed to determine the effect of var-

TABLE 12.8 Hierarchy of Preprocessed Evidence

Type of Evidence	Description of Evidence
Primary studies	Preprocessing involves selecting only studies that both are highly relevant and have study designs that minimize bias and thus permit a high strength of inference.
Summaries	Systematic reviews provide clinicians with an overview of all the evidence addressing a focused clinical question.
Synopses	Synopses of individual studies or of systemic reviews encapsulate the key methodological details and results required to apply the evidence to individual patient care.
Systems	Practice guidelines, clinical pathways or evidence-based textbook summaries of a clinical area provide the clinician with much of the information needed to guide the care of individual patients.

ious methods of presenting and disseminating EBM reviews on use in clinical decision making and policy formation (33,40,41). Questions include the desirability and impact of automated decision guides for practitioner implementation of evidence in daily practice.

APPROACHES TO EVIDENCE GRADING

Several entities conduct systematic reviews of evidence and make the summaries available in electronic or print format. The groups use somewhat different approaches, depending on the purpose of the review, the topic being studied, and the extent of available research. The methodology used, especially the criteria for inclusion of evidence and the method for evidence grading, should be explicitly described for the user. Applications of EBM by a range of organizations are briefly described below.

US Preventive Services Task Force

A series of articles describe the process developed and used by the 15-member US Preventive Services Task Force to evaluate the evidence for preventive services. Zaza and coworkers describe the lengthy data collection instrument for each research study included in the review (10). The assessment is based on 26 content questions and 23 questions about the quality of execution of the study. Researchers estimate that it takes 2 hours to 3 hours to review and abstract each study. Carande-Kulis and associates report the task force's procedure to collect,

abstract, adjust, and summarize results from various types of economic evaluations that are missing from many other review protocols (9).

Cochrane Collaborative Reviews

The Cochrane Collaborative maintains a database of structured reviews (39). The goal of the collaborative is to create, maintain, and disseminate a high-quality, systematic review of RCTs. Reviews involve the development of a detailed protocol with exhaustive searches for all published and unpublished RCTs on a particular topic. The analysis is based on a standardized methodology and meta-analysis summarized in an extensive handbook describing information on forming review groups, search methodology, and contacting existing groups. In April 2001 the database included 932 completed reviews and approximately 774 reviews in various stages of development. There were approximately 68 reviews identified using the keywords *nutrition, diet, diet therapy, dietary advice, nutritional therapy,* and *dietary therapy,* although many of these reviews include only a mention of the subject (that is, it is not the focus of the review).

Agency for Healthcare Research and Quality

The Agency for Healthcare Research and Quality (AHRQ), formerly called the Agency for Health Care Policy and Research (AHCPR), began funding comprehensive reviews of research in priority health conditions in the early 1990s (6). These reviews were initiated to define current practice and evidence for the effectiveness of those practices. The reviews identified many uncertainties in practice recommendations and gaps in research that became the foundation for several outcomes research agendas. Included in this effort was the critical appraisal of research on the effectiveness and cost-effectiveness of dietetics services (42). In its reviews, AHCPR recognized the role of experts, including researchers, experienced practitioners, and patients, as judges of clinical practices when research was lacking. AHRQ views research as the foundation for health care policies that affect clinical practice and, ultimately, health outcomes.

Institute for Clinical Systems Improvement

The ICSI developed a modified method of evaluating the evidence that attempts to address the limitations of the more restricted method employed by the public health community and national organizations (13). Its goal was to produce shorter, simpler guidelines that would be easily developed and employed by the practitioners who would use them. The ICSI goals were as follows:

- Increase the systematic use of evidence by work groups by providing a framework and step-by-step process for reaching key conclusions.
- Provide a method for reaching evidence-based conclusions that busy practicing clinicians accept as practical.
- Provide a reliable method for grading conclusions based on the strength of the underlying evidence.
- Convey to readers and users of the documents the strength of the underlying evidence.

The methodology is used in technology assessment reports focusing on safety and efficacy of technology and in practice guidelines recommending care for a specific health problem. The grading worksheet presented in Table 12.7 provides the basis for formulating a conclusion statement based on the body of evidence as summarized by design type, class of research report, quality score, information about the population studies, results of the study, and the author's conclusions. Conclusion grading worksheets are provided as the basis of all guidelines produced after 1998, with the intent that the worksheets can be updated with the publication of additional pertinent research.

ROLES OF PROFESSIONAL SOCIETIES

Criteria for Guidelines by Professional Societies

Grilli et al developed minimum criteria for published guidelines prepared by professional societies: (1) description of the type of professionals involved in the guidelines development, (2) strategy used to search for the primary evidence, and (3) explicit grading of recommendations according to the quality of supporting evidence. A total of 431 guidelines from 1988 to 1998 were evaluated according to these criteria. Only 33 percent described the type of professionals involved in development, 13 percent reported search strategy, and 18 percent used explicit criteria to grade the strength of the evidence to support their recommendations. Over half (54 percent) did not meet any of the three criteria, 34 percent met one criteria, and 7 percent met two of the three criteria. Forty-one percent of the guidelines were published from 1996 to 1998 (14).

American Medical Association *Users' Guides to the Medical Literature*

From 1993 to the present, The American Medical Association has produced and published a series entitled *Users Guides to the Medical Literature* (4,5,27,43–54). The first topic, in 1993, introduced the Evidence-Based Medicine Working Group members and provided the basics of evaluating literature to support medical practice (52). Users' guides have included articles on how to use systematic reviews, decision analyses, practice guidelines, and economic analysis, along with articles that make treatment recommendations (4,5,27,43–53).

American Academy of Family Practice

The American Academy of Family Practice systematically reviews research journals to select articles focused on Patient-Oriented Evidence that Matters (POEM) (55). These selected articles address a clinical problem or clinical question that primary care physicians will encounter in their practice, use patient-oriented outcomes, and have the potential to change our practice if the results are valid and applicable (56).

American Dietetic Association

The ADA began the development of profession-wide protocols with the publication of the first edition of *Medical Nutrition Therapy Across the Continuum of Care* (1,2). The latest versions of the MNT protocols are called "guides for practice" and include tables of evidence to support recommendations for care. The tables of evidence use the ICSI methodology (Tables 12.3 and 12.4) and a modification of their criteria for evaluating the quality of primary and review articles (Figures 12.2 and 12.3). Some ADA practice guides are supported by published validation studies, and studies are under way to validate other guides (57,58). A toolkit was published in 2000 to aid practitioners in developing and maintaining evidence-based guides (37).

REFERENCES

1. Myers EF, Pritchett E, Johnson, E. Evidence-based practice guides vs. protocols: What's the difference? *J Am Diet Assoc.* 2001;101:1085–1090.
2. Splett P. *Developing and Validating Evidence-Based Guides for Practice: A Tool Kit for Dietetics Profession-*

als. Chicago, Ill: The American Dietetic Association; 2000.

3. Sackett, DL, Straus, SE, Richardson, WS, Rosenberg, W, Haynes RB. *Evidence-Based Medicine: How to Practice and Teach EBM.* St Louis, Mo: Churchill Livingstone; 2000.

4. Guyatt GH, Haynes RB, Jaeschke RZ, et al. Users' Guides to the Medical Literature: XXV. Evidence-based medicine: principles for applying the Users' Guides to patient care. Evidence-Based Medicine Working Group. *JAMA.* 2000;284:1290–1296.

5. Guyatt GH. *Users' Guide to the Medical Literature: Essentials of Evidence-Based Clinical Practice.* Chicago, Ill: The American Medical Association; 2002.

6. The outcome of outcomes research at AHCPR: final report. Available at: http://www.ahcpr.gov/clinic/out2res/out2res/outfig1.htm. Accessed June 18, 2000.

7. Evidence based medicine tool kit. Available at: http://www.med.ualberta.ca/ebm. Accessed April 13, 2001.

8. Evidence-based medicine: finding the best clinical literature. Available at: http://www.uic.edu/lib/health/ebm.html. Accessed October 10, 2001.

9. Carande-Kulis VG, Maciosek MV, Briss PA, Teutsch SM, Zaza S, Truman BI, Messonier ML, Pappaioanou M, Harris JR, Fielding J. Methods for systematic reviews of economic evaluations for the Guide to Community Preventive Services. Task Force on Community Preventive Services. *Am J Prev Med.* 2000;18(1 Suppl):75–91.

10. Zaza S, Wright-De Aguero LK, Briss PA, Truman BI, Hopkins DP, Hennessy MH, Sosin DM, Anderson L, Carande-Kulis VG, Teutsch SM, Pappaioanou M. Data collection instrument and procedure for systematic reviews in the Guide to Community Preventive Services. Task Force on Community Preventive Services. *Am J Prev Med.* 2000;18(1 Suppl):44–74.

11. Briss PA, Zaza S, Pappaioanou M, Fielding J, et al. Developing an evidence-based Guide to Community Preventive Services—methods. The Task Force on Community Preventive Services. *Am J Prev Med.* 2000;18(1 Suppl): 35–43.

12. Truman BI, Smith-Akin CK, Hinman AR, Gebbie KM, Brownson R, Novic LF, Lawrence RD, Pappaioanou M, Fielding J, Evans CA, Guerra FA, Vogel-Taylor M, Mahan CS, Fullilove M, Zaza S. Developing the Guide to Community Preventive Services—overview and rationale. The Task Force on Community Preventive Services. *Am J Prev Med.* 2000;18(1 Suppl):18–26.

13. Greer N, Mosser G, Logan G, Halaas GW. A practical approach to evidence grading. *Jt Comm J Qual Improv.* 2000;26:700–712.

14. Grilli R, Magrini N, Penna A, Mura G, Liberati A. Practice guidelines developed by specialty societies: the need for a critical appraisal. *Lancet.* 2000;355:103–106.

15. Shaughnessy AF, Slawson DC. POEMs: patient-oriented evidence that matters. *Ann Intern Med.* 1997;126:667.

16. Bigby M. Challenges to the hierarchy of evidence: does the emperor have no clothes? *Arch Dermatol.* 2001;137:345–346.

17. Benson K, Hartz AJ. A comparison of observational studies and randomized, controlled trials. *N Engl J Med.* 2000;342:1878–1886.

18. Concato J, Shah N, Horwitz RI. Randomized, controlled trials, observational studies, and the hierarchy of research designs. *N Engl J Med.* 2000;342:1887–1892.

19. Ernst E, Pittler MH. Systematic reviews neglect safety issues. *Arch Intern Med.* 2001;161(1):125–126.

20. Grahame-Smith D. Evidence based medicine: Socratic dissent. *BMJ.* 1995;310:1126–1127.

21. Celermajer DS. Evidence-based medicine: how good is the evidence? *Med J Aust.* 2001;174:293–295.

22. Wolf FM, Shea JA, Albanese MA. Toward setting a research agenda for systematic reviews of evidence of the effects of medical education. *Teach Learn Med.* 2001;13:54–60.

23. Woolf SH, George JN. Evidence-based medicine. Interpreting studies and setting policy. *Hematol Oncol Clin North Am.* 2000;14:761–784.

24. Bannigan K, Droogan J, Entwistle V. Systematic reviews: what do they involve? *Nurs Times.* 1997;93:52–53.

25. Evans D. Systematic reviews of nursing research. *Intensive Crit Care Nurs.* 2001;17:51–57.

26. Craig JC, Irwig LM, Stockler MR. Evidence-based medicine: useful tools for decision making. *Med J Aust.* 2001;174:248–253.

27. Richardson WS, Wilson MC, Guyatt GH, Cook DJ, Nishikawa J. Users' Guides to the Medical Literature: XV. How to use an article about disease probability for differential diagnosis. Evidence-Based Medicine Working Group. *JAMA.* 1999;281:1214–1219.

28. Goode CJ. What constitutes the "evidence" in evidence-based practice? *Appl Nurs Res.* 2000;13:222–225.

29. Avenell A, Handoll HH, Grant AM. Lessons for search strategies from a systematic review, in The Cochrane Library, of nutritional supplementation trials in patients after hip fracture. *Am J Clin Nutr.* 2001;73:505–510.

30. Thompson RL, Summerbell CD, Higgins JPT, Little PS, Talbor D, Ebrahim S. Dietary advice given by a dietitian versus other health professional or self-help methods to reduce blood cholesterol (Cochrane Review). In: *The Cochrane Library.* Oxford, England: Update Software; 2003: Issue 1. Available at: http://www.cochrane.de.

31. Kramer M. Balanced protein/energy supplementation in pregnancy. [Cochrane Database of Systematic Reviews Web site]. Available at: http://biomedsearch.lib.umn.edu. Accessed August 10, 2000.

32. Levels of Evidence and Grades of Recommendations. Available at: http://cebm.jr2.ox.ac.uk/docs/levels.html. Accessed April 13, 2001.

33. Splett P. *Cost Outcomes of Nutrition Intervention: Part I Outcomes Research, Part II Measuring Effectiveness of Nutrition Interventions, Part III Economic and Cost Analysis.* Evansville, In: Mead Johnson & Company; 1996.

34. Gallagher EJ. Systematic reviews: a logical methodological extension of evidence-based medicine. *Acad Emerg Med.* 1999;6:1255–1260.

35. American Dietetic Association. *Medical Nutrition Therapy Evidence-based Guides for Practice* [CD-ROMs]. Chicago, Ill: American Dietetic Association.

36. Rubin GL, Frommer MS. Evidence-based medicine—time for a reality check. *Med J Aust.* 2001;174:214–215.

37. Hahn S, Garner P, Williamson P. Are systematic reviews taking heterogeneity into account? An analysis from the Infectious Diseases Module of the Cochrane Library. *J Eval Clin Pract.* 2000;6(2):231–233.

38. Thomas L, Cullum N, McColl E, Rousseau N, Soutter J, Steen N. Guidelines in professions allied to medicine [Cochrane Database of Systematic Reviews Web site]. Available at: http://www.cochrane.de. Accessed April 17, 2001

39. The Cochrane Database of Systematic Reviews. Available at: http://www.cochrane.de/. Accessed May 13, 2001.

40. Niessen LW, Grijseels EW, Rutten FF. The evidence-based approach in health policy and health care delivery. *Soc Sci Med.* 2000;51:859–869.

41. Macintyre S, Chalmers I, Horton R, Smith R. Using evidence to inform health policy: case study. *BMJ.* 2001;322:222–225.

42. Barr, JT. *Critical Literature Review: Clinical Effectiveness in Allied Health Practices.* Agency for Health Care Policy and Research: US Government Printing Office; 1993.

43. Archibald S, Bhandari M, Thoma A. Users' Guides to the Surgical Literature: how to use an article about a diagnostic test. Evidence-Based Surgery Working Group. *Can J Surg.* 2001;44:17–23.

44. Dans AL, Dans LF, Guyatt GH, Richardson S. Users' Guides to the Medical Literature: XIV. How to decide on the applicability of clinical trial results to your patient. Evidence-Based Medicine Working Group. *JAMA.* 1998;279:545–549.

45. Guyatt GH, Sackett DL, Cook DJ. Users' Guides to the Medical Literature. II. How to use an article about therapy or prevention. A. Are the results of the study valid? Evidence-Based Medicine Working Group. *JAMA.* 1993;270:2598–2601.

46. Guyatt GH, Sackett DL, Cook DJ. Users' Guides to the Medical Literature. II. How to use an article about therapy or prevention. B. What were the results and will they help me in caring for my patients? Evidence-Based Medicine Working Group. *JAMA.* 1994;271:59–63.

47. Guyatt GH, Sackett DL, Sinclair JC, Hayward R, Cook DJ, Cook RJ. Users' Guides to the Medical Literature. IX. A method for grading health care recommendations. Evidence-Based Medicine Working Group. *JAMA.* 1995;274:1800–1804.

48. Hayward RS, Wilson MC, Tunis SR, Bass EB, Guyatt G. Users' Guides to the Medical Literature. VIII. How to use clinical practice guidelines. A. Are the recommendations valid? The Evidence- Based Medicine Working Group. *JAMA.* 1995;274:570–574.

49. Jaeschke R, Guyatt GH, Sackett DL. Users' Guides to the Medical Literature. III. How to use an article about a diagnostic test. B. What are the results and will they help me in caring for my patients? The Evidence-Based Medicine Working Group. *JAMA.* 1994;271:703–707.

50. McAlister FA, Straus SE, Guyatt GH, Haynes RB. Users' Guides to the Medical Literature: XX. Integrating research evidence with the care of the individual patient. Evidence-Based Medicine Working Group. *JAMA.* 2000;283:2829–2836.

51. McGinn TG, Guyatt GH, Wyer PC, Naylor CD, Stiell IG, Richardson WS. Users' Guides to the Medical Literature: XXII: how to use articles about clinical decision rules. Evidence-Based Medicine Working Group. *JAMA.* 2000;284:79–84.

52. Oxman AD, Sackett DL, Guyatt GH. Users' Guides to the Medical Literature. I. How to get started. The Evidence-Based Medicine Working Group. *JAMA.* 1993;270:2093–2095.

53. Randolph AG, Haynes RB, Wyatt JC, Cook DJ, Guyatt GH. Users' Guides to the Medical Literature: XVIII. How to use an article evaluating the clinical impact of a computer-based clinical decision support system. *JAMA.* 1999;282:67–74.

54. Wilson MC, Hayward RS, Tunis SR, Bass EB, Guyatt G. Users' Guides to the Medical Literature. VIII. How to use clinical practice guidelines. B. what are the recommendations and will they help you in caring for your patients? The Evidence-Based Medicine Working Group. *JAMA.* 1995;274:1630–1632.

55. Shaughnessy AF, Slawson DC, Becker L. Clinical jazz: harmonizing clinical experience and evidence-based medicine. *J Fam Pract.* 1998;47:425–428.

56. Slawson DC, Shaughnessy AF, Ebell MH, Barry HC. Mastering medical information and the role of POEMs—Patient-Oriented Evidence that Matters. *J Fam Pract.* 1997;45:195–196.

57. Kulkarni K, Castle G, Gregory R, et al. Nutrition Practice Guidelines for type 1 diabetes mellitus positively affect decision practices and patient outcomes. *J Am Diet Assoc.* 1998;98:62–70.

58. Franz M, Splett P, Monk A, et al. Cost-effectiveness of medical nutrition therapy provided by dietitians for persons with non-insulin-dependent diabetes mellitus. *J Am Diet Assoc.* 1995;95:1018–1024.

13

Interpretation and Utilization of Data from the National Nutrition Monitoring and Related Research Program

Ronette R. Briefel, Dr.P.H., R.D., and Karil Bialostosky, M.S.

The National Nutrition Monitoring and Related Research Program (NNMRRP), previously referred to as the National Nutrition Monitoring System, is composed of interconnected federal and state activities that provide information about the dietary and nutrition status of the U.S. population, U.S. conditions that affect the dietary and nutrition status of individuals, and relationships between diet and health (1–4). *Nutrition monitoring* has been defined as "an ongoing description of nutrition conditions in the population, with particular attention to subgroups defined in socioeconomic terms, for purposes of planning, analyzing the effects of policies and programs on nutrition problems, and predicting future trends" (5). This chapter provides an overview of the uses of nutrition-monitoring data, the program's surveys and surveillance systems, research activities, and the resources available to dietitians and nutritionists. These resources include published reports, data sets for secondary data analysis, and applied research methodologies. The chapter also provides information on uses and limitations of nutrition-monitoring data, tips for the proper interpretation of the data, and sources of further information.

The NNMRRP is considered one of the best nutrition-monitoring systems in the world. A complete history of the program has been described elsewhere (1–4). The National Nutrition Monitoring and Related Research Act of 1990 (3) called for the development of a Ten-Year Comprehensive Plan, which was published for public comment in 1991 (6). Representatives of state and local agencies, along with public and private organiza-

tions, provided recommendations for their specific needs for nutrition-monitoring data and research (7). Representatives in the areas of maternal and child health, chronic disease prevention, hunger advocacy, and the food industry also provided recommendations for prioritizing activities (7). Public input was also solicited through presentations at professional meetings, including the 1991 annual meeting of the American Dietetic Association. The act established several mechanisms to ensure the collaboration and coordination of federal agencies, as well as state and local governments involved in nutrition monitoring. The plan was finalized in 1993 (8) and included three primary goals: (1) to provide for a comprehensive NNMRRP through continuous and coordinated data collection, (2) to improve the comparability and quality of data across the NNMRRP, and (3) to improve the research base for nutrition monitoring. These national goals are complemented by state and local objectives to strengthen data collection capacity; to improve the quality of state and local data; and to improve methodologies to enhance the comparability of NNMRRP data across national, state, and local levels. State and local government agencies collect state surveillance system data (for example, in clinics that house the Special Supplemental Nutrition Program for Women, Infants, and Children [WIC]) and use available information to plan programs for target populations (7,9).

The program aims to study the relationship between food and health through data collection in five measurement component areas: (1) nutrition and related health measurements; (2) food and nutrient consumption; (3) knowledge, attitudes, and behavior assessments; (4) food composition and nutrient databases; and (5) food supply determinations. Nutrition-monitoring data collected at the national, state, and local levels are used directly and indirectly to assess the contributions that diet and nutrition status make to the health of the American people, and to learn about the factors affecting dietary and nutrition status.

PURPOSES AND RESEARCH USES OF NUTRITION-MONITORING DATA

Nutrition monitoring is vital to policy making and research (see Figure 13.1) (4,5,8–12). The nutrition-monitoring measurement components also provide information to help establish research priorities. Nutrition research provides data for policy making and for identifying nutrition-monitoring needs (8,11,12). Figure 13.2 provides examples of uses of nutrition-monitoring data in public policy and scientific research. For example, nutrition-monitoring data have been used to evaluate progress toward achievement of the *Healthy People 2000: National Health Promotion and Disease Prevention Objectives* (13); to establish *Healthy People 2010* (14); to develop guidelines for prevention, detection, and management of nutrition conditions (15–17); and to evaluate the impact of nutrition initiatives for military feeding systems (18).

National data are used to develop reference standards for nutrition status. One important example is the use of the National Health and Nutrition Examination Survey (NHANES) data to produce the Centers for Disease and Control and Prevention (CDC) Growth Charts (19). The newly revised charts include charts for infants through adolescents 19 years of age, as well as a new chart for body mass index by age. The charts are included in the Anthro module of the computer software package EpiInfo; both z scores and percentiles are provided for each chart (20).

Monitoring provides information for public policy decisions related to nutrition education programs, such as 5-A-Day for Better Health (21); U.S. Dietary Guidelines for Americans (22); public health programs, such as the National Cholesterol Education Program (23) and the National High Blood Pressure Education Program (24); federally supported foodservice and food assistance programs, such as the Food Stamp Program and WIC (9,25–27); and the Thrifty Food Plan (28).

Nutrition-monitoring data are also used to make public policy decisions related to the regulation of fortification, safety, and labeling of the food supply (29,30); food production and marketing, such as the development of reduced -fat food products; and food safety programs (31,32). Data have been used by regulatory agencies to provide dietary exposure estimates for nutrient and non-nutrient food components (31–33) and to examine U.S. food fortification policies (29). For example, nutrition-monitoring data collected between 1988 and 1994 in the NHANES III were used to assess folate status and the relationship between serum determinations, diet, and other nutrition and health variables prior to folate food fortification rule-making by the Food and Drug Administration (FDA) (34).

In the early 1990s the U.S. president's science adviser identified the need for human nutrition research "that is ultimately aimed at promoting health, preventing disease, and reducing health care costs" (35). The NNM-RRP supports research on the nutrient requirements throughout the life cycle and the development of the Dietary Reference Intakes (36–38) and their applications (39), research on food composition and nutrient content and bioavailability (40–42), nutrition education research (12,21,43), research on the relationship of knowledge and attitudes to dietary and health behavior (43–45), and research on the economic aspects of food consumption (46). Data have also provided information about the role of nutrition in the etiology, prevention, and treatment of chronic diseases and conditions (47,48), and have been used to identify food and nutrition research priorities of significance to public health (10–14,35).

Applied nutrition research is conducted to improve survey methods (1,8,11,49,50), to interpret dietary intake and nutrition status (51–53), to measure food security (54–56), and to increase the capability to capture state and local nutrition information (7–9,56,57). For example, the Federal Interagency Working Group for Food Security Measurement developed an 18-item scale that allows households to be classified as *food secure, food insecure with no hunger, food insecure with moderate hunger,* and *food insecure with severe hunger* (54–56). A comparable 6-item scale was developed for use in state and local monitoring efforts (57).

COMPONENTS OF NUTRITION-MONITORING MEASUREMENT

The first national dietary surveys were carried out in the 1930s. Since then, more than 40 surveys and surveillance

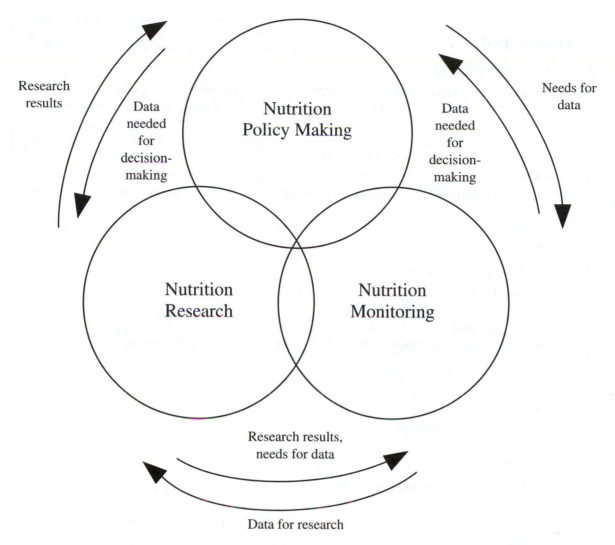

FIGURE 13.1   Relationship among nutrition policy making, nutrition research, and nutrition monitoring. Adapted from U.S. Department of Health and Human Services and U.S. Department of Agriculture. *Ten-year Comprehensive Plan for the National Nutrition Monitoring and Related Research Program.* Washington, DC: U.S. Government Printing Office; 1993. Publication 58:32752-32806.

systems have evolved in response to the information needs of federal agencies and other nutrition-monitoring data users. Chronological listings of past nutrition-monitoring surveys and activities have been published (1,2,6,8). Table 13.1 lists the major survey and surveillance activities, sponsoring agencies, dates conducted, and coverage of target populations since the 1990 legislation, organized by the five measurement component areas. These data collection activities are briefly summarized in the following sections. More detailed descriptions can be found in *Nutrition Monitoring in the United States: The Directory of Federal and State Nutrition Monitoring and Related Research Activities* (50) and previous publications (1,8,49,58,59). The *Directory* is part

of an effort to improve the dissemination of information about nutrition-monitoring data and activities by periodically providing updated information and contacts for nutrition monitoring on the Internet (50). The *Directory* also includes a section on nutrition-monitoring research activities.

Nutrition and Related Health Measurements

Nutrition and related health data have a wide variety of applications to policy making, research, health and nutrition education, medical care practices, and reference

PUBLIC POLICY

Monitoring and Surveillance

- Identify high-risk groups and geographic areas with nutrition-related problems to facilitate the implementation of public health intervention programs and food assistance programs.
- Evaluate changes in agricultural policy that may affect the nutrition quality and healthfulness of the U.S. food supply. ASsess progress toward achieving the nutrition objectives in *Healthy People 2000* and *Healthy People 2010*.
- Evaluate the effectiveness of nutrition initiatives for military feeding systems.
- Recommend guidelines for the prevention, detection, and management of nutrition and health conditions.
- Develop reference standards for nutrition status.
- Monitor food production and marketing.

Nutrition-Related Programs

- Develop nutrition education and dietary guidance (e.g., U.S. Dietary Guidelines for Americans and 5 A Day for Better Health).
- Plan and evaluate food assistance programs.
- Plan and assess nutrition intervention programs and public health programs.

Regulatory Activities

- Develop food-labeling policies.
- Document the need for, and monitor, food fortification policies.
- Establish food safety guidelines.

SCIENTIFIC RESEARCH

- Help establish nutrient requirements throughout the life cycle (e.g., Dietary Reference Intakes).
- Study diet-health relationships and the relationship of knowledge and attitudes to dietary and health behavior.
- Foster and conduct both national and international nutrition-monitoring research.
- Conduct food composition analysis.
- Study the economic aspects of food consumption.

FIGURE 13.2   Uses of nutrition-monitoring data. Adapted from references 1 and 8.

standards. The cornerstone of this NNMRRP measurement component, the NHANES, provides national data on the nutrition status, dietary intake, and numerous health indexes of the U.S. population (1–3,8,11,59–61). It also provides national population reference distributions, national prevalences of diseases and risk factors, and trends in nutrition and health status over time. The design for the third NHANES (1988 to 1994) emphasized producing reliable national estimates for the total U.S. non-institutionalized population, as well as Mexican Americans, African Americans, older persons, and children younger than 6 years (60). Physical measurements, such as body measurements, blood pressure, findings of dental examinations, and results of biochemical and hematologic tests, allow for studying the relationships among diet, nutrition, and health.

A special study conducted from 1982 to 1984, the Hispanic Health and Nutrition Examination Survey, aimed to collect data on the health and nutrition status of the three largest Hispanic subgroups in the United States: Mexican Americans, Cubans, and Puerto Ricans in certain parts of the country, for whom national estimates cannot be made. NHANES follow-up studies allow epidemiologic investigations of the relationships of nutrition and health to risk of death and disability. Beginning in 1999, the NHANES had a continuous, annual design and an oversampling of Mexican Americans, African Americans, older persons, adolescents, and pregnant females in the first 3 years (61). Oversampling of low-income persons in the NHANES was instituted in 2000 (62).

The National Health Interview Survey annually provides information about self-reported health conditions; it periodically provides information about special nutrition and health topics, such as vitamin/mineral supplement use, youth risk behavior, aging, food program participation, diet and nutrition knowledge, cancer, disabilities, and food preparation. Other special supplements relate to the tracking of U.S. health and nutrition objectives.

A number of record-based surveys recently were merged and expanded into one integrated survey of health care providers, called the National Health Care Survey. Data on alternative health care settings—such as ambulatory surgical centers, hospital outpatient departments, emergency rooms, hospices, and home health agencies—are being provided through this system. The survey provides information on the availability and utilization of dietary and nutrition services in these types of agencies. For hospital outpatient department visits, nutrition-related information also includes physician-reported hypertension and obesity, as well as counseling services for diet, weight reduction, and cholesterol reduction. The survey also provides information on hospitalizations resulting from nutrition-related diseases.

A number of other surveys and surveillance systems, primarily conducted by the CDC, also contribute nutrition-related health information, particularly for low-income pregnant women, infants, and children who participate in publicly funded health, nutrition, and food assistance programs (9,50). These surveillance systems provide data representative of the participating populations in participating states and include physical measurements such as height, weight, hemoglobin levels, and hematocrit levels.

The Pediatric Nutrition Surveillance System (PedNSS), sponsored since 1973, is used to monitor simple key indicators of nutrition status among low-income, high-risk infants and children who participate in publicly funded health, nutrition, and food assistance programs (9,50,63). The coverage of PedNSS reflects the number of clinic visits in participating programs from more than 43 states plus the District of Columbia, Puerto Rico, and six Indian reservations. Data can be analyzed at individual, clinic, county, state, and national levels. The Pregnancy Nutrition Surveillance System (PNSS), sponsored

since 1973, and in continuous operation since 1978, tracks nutrition-related problems and behavioral risk factors associated with low birth weight among high-risk prenatal populations (9,50,64). The PNSS is used to identify preventable nutrition-related problems and behavioral risk factors in order to target interventions. The coverage of PNSS reflects the number of pregnant women who participate in the programs contributing to the surveillance system.

Food and Nutrient Consumption

Food and nutrient consumption measurements include estimates of individuals' intakes of foods and beverages (nonalcoholic and alcoholic) and nutrition supplements, as well as levels of nonessential nutrients, such as dietary fiber. The Continuing Survey of Food Intakes by Individuals (CSFII) of the U.S. Department of Agriculture (USDA) and the NHANES of the U.S. Department of Health and Human Services, the two cornerstone NNM-RRP surveys, were established to provide national estimates of food and nutrient intakes in the general U.S. population and subgroups. The CSFII (which was integrated within the NHANES in 2002) emphasized the food and nutrient intake of the general population and the low-income population (65,66). It collected data on dietary intake on two independent days and captured information on economic variables such as where food was purchased and where food was eaten. The NHANES collects information on one day of intake and on a second day on a subsample. Prior to their integration, both surveys covered intake for all days of the week and all the seasons. In the NHANES, dietary intake is related to health status in the same individuals; in addition, there is an emphasis on racial-ethnic determinants of health. These surveys also provide the ability to compare intake with Food Guide Pyramid food groups. In addition to, and together with, the U.S. Food and Drug Administration's Total Diet Study (67), these studies provide the potential to assess levels of additives and pesticides in diets consumed. NHANES III data were used to prepare methylmercury intake estimates for the 1997 U.S. Environmental Protection Agency *Mercury Study Report to Congress,* which looked at human exposure to mercury from fish and shellfish intake (33).

As noted above, in 2002 the NHANES and the CSFII were integrated within the continuous NHANES framework. The U.S. Department of Health and Human Services and the USDA have jointly implemented

TABLE 13.1 Federal Nutrition Monitoring Surveys and Surveillance Activities Since 1990[a, b]

Date Initiated	Department	Agency	Survey	Target U.S. Population	Sample Size and Type	Response Rate[c]	Comments
			Nutrition and related health measurements				
Continuous (1915)	HHS	CDC/NCHS	National Vital Registration System	Total U.S. population	All births and deaths in the U.S.	—	Complete coverage
Annual (1957)	HHS	CDC/NCHS	National Health Interview Survey (NHIS)	Civilian, noninstitutionalized household population	103,477 individuals, 39,832 households	92%	1997 survey
1985, 1990, 1998	HHS	CDC/NCHS	National Health Interview Survey on Health Promotion and Disease Prevention	Civilian, noninstitutionalized household population in the U.S., ages 18+ y	41,104 households	83%	1990 survey
1987, 1992, 2000	HHS	CDC/NCHS	National Health Interview Survey on Cancer Epidemiology and Cancer Control	Civilian, noninstitutionalized household population ages 18+ y in the U.S.	12,000 households	86%	1992 survey
1991	HHS	CDC/NCHS	1991 National Health Interview Survey on Health Promotion and Disease Prevention	Civilian, noninstitutionalized, household population of the United States, ages 18+ y	43,732 households	88%	
1992–93	HHS	CDC/NCHS	National Health Interview Survey on Youth Behavior Supplement	Youth ages 12–21 y	10,645 households	77%	Administered to one adult per household
1994	HHS	ASPE, SSA, HRSA	National Health Interview Survey on Disability	Civilian, noninstitutionalized household population	107,469 individuals	87%	
1993, 1995	HHS	CDC/NCHS	National Health Interview Survey Year 2000 Objectives Supplement	Civilian, noninstitutionalized household population in U.S., ages 18+ y	17,317 households	81%	1995 survey; administered to one adult per family
1990, 1995 (1973)	HHS	CDC/NCHS	National Survey of Family Growth	Women, ages 15–44 y	10,847 households	79%	1995 survey
Continuous (1973)	HHS	CDC/NCCDPHP	Pregnancy Nutrition Surveillance System (PNSS)	Low-income, high-risk pregnant women	599,000 records	—	1995; coverage reflects no. of women participating in programs in a given year in 18 states, the Navajo Nation, and the Intertribal Council of AZ

Period	Dept	Agency	Survey	Population	Sample	Response rate	Comments
Continuous (1973; continuous since 1978)	HHS	CDC/ NCCDPHP	Pediatric Nutrition Surveillance System (PedNSS)	Low-income, high-risk children, birth-17 y of age	8,800,000 records	—	1995; coverage reflects the no. of clinic visits in participating programs in 43 states and DC, Puerto Rico, and 6 Indian reservations
1988–90	HHS	CDC/NCHS	National Maternal and Infant Health Survey	Women, hospitals, and prenatal care providers associated with live births, still births, and infant deaths	9,953 live births / 3,309 fetal deaths / 5,332 infant deaths	74% / 69% / 65%	
1988–94	HHS	CDC/NCHS	Third National Health and Nutrition Examination Survey (NHANES III). Includes Follow-Up Study.	U.S. noninstitutionalized, civilian population, ages 2+ mo; Oversampling of blacks and Mexican-Americans, children ages 0–5 y, and individuals ages 60+ y	33,994 interviewed / 31,311 examined	86% / 79%	
1989–1993	HHS	CDC; NIH	National Health and Nutrition Examination III Supplemental Nutrition Survey of Older Americans	NHANES III (1988–91) examinees ages 50+ years.	2,602 completed NHANES III dietary recall (DR) and 1st SNS interview / 2,519 completed NHANES III DR and 2nd SNS interview / 2,261 completed NHANES III DR and 2 SNS interviews	75% / 72% / 65%	
1990–91	HHS	IHS	Survey of Heights and Weights of American Indian School Children	American Indian school children, ages 5–18 y	9,464	NA	1990–91 school year records
1991–92	HHS	IHS	Navajo Health and Nutrition Survey	Persons ages 12+ y residing on or near the Navajo reservation in AZ, NM, and CO	985 individuals examined	58%	
1991–92	HHS	CDC/NCHS	Longitudinal Followup to the National Maternal and Infant Health Survey	Participants of the 1988 NMIHS	9,400 mothers of 3-yr-olds / 1,000 women who had infant deaths / 1,000 women who had late fetal deaths in 1988	89% / 82% / 82%	

(continued)

TABLE 13.1 Federal Nutrition Monitoring Surveys and Surveillance Activities Since 1990[a,b] (continued)

Date Initiated	Department	Agency	Survey	Target U.S. Population	Sample Size and Type	Response Rate[c]	Comments
1992	HHS	CDC/NCHS	NHANES I Epidemiologic Followup Study	Individuals examined in NHANES I, ages 25–74 y at baseline (1971–74)	9,281	92%	1992 cohort
Continuous (1992)	HHS	CDC/NCHS	NHANES II Mortality Followup Survey	Individuals examined in NHANES II, ages 30–74 y at baseline (1976–80)	9,252	—	
Continuous (1992)	HHS	CDC/NCHS	Hispanic HANES (HHANES) Mortality Followup Survey	Individuals interviewed in HHANES, 20–74 y at baseline (1982–84)	NA	—	
Annual (1992)	HHS	CDC/NCHS	National Health Care Survey (integrates: National Home and Hospice Care Survey (1992–94, 1996), National Nursing Home Survey (since 1973–74) and Follow-up (1995, 1997), National Hospital Discharge Survey (since 1965), National Ambulatory Medical Care Survey (since 1973), National Hospital Ambulatory Medical Care Survey (1992), and National Survey of Ambulatory Surgery (1994–96)	Record-based health care provider surveys including: visits to hospital emergency and outpatients departments of non-federal, short-stay, general and specialty hospitals and ambulatory surgical centers; office visits to non-federal, office-based physicians; and home health agencies and nursing homes	1,200 1996 NHHCS facilities, 5,438 current patients, 4,758 discharged patients; 1,500 1995 NNHS nursing homes, 8,056 current residents; 525 1995 NHDS hospitals, approx 282,000 discharges; 3,173 1996 NAMCS physicians, 29,805 office visits; 486 1996 NHAMCS hospitals, 21,902 ER visits, 29,806 outpatient visits; 418 1996 NSAS hospitals, 333 freestanding ambulatory surgery centers, approx 125,000 surgical visits	96% 85% 82% 97% 93% 95% NA 70% NA 95% NA NA 91% 70%	

Frequency	Department	Agency	Survey	Population	Sample size	Response rate	Notes
Continuous (1992)	HHS	CDC/NCHS	NHANES III Mortality Follow-up Survey	Individuals interviewed and examined in NHANES III, ages 20+ y at baseline (1988–94)	NA	—	
1996–99	HHS	CDC/NCHS	Demonstration Project for PedNSS and PNSS	Low-income, high-risk women, infants, and children that participate in government food assistance programs and participate in PedNSS and PNSS	Minimum of 1,000 children enrolled in WIC (for PedNSS) / Minimum of 300 women enrolled in WIC (for PNSS)	NA / NA	
1999–	HHS	CDC/NCHS	National Health and Nutrition Examination Survey	Civilian, noninstitutionalized individuals. In the first 3 years, oversampling of blacks, Mexican-Americans, adolescents, older persons, and pregnant women.	NA	NA	
Food and nutrient consumption							
Continuous (1917)	DOD	USARIEM	Nutritional Evaluation of Military Feeding Systems and Military Populations	Enlisted personnel of the Army, Navy, Marine Corps, and Air Force; limited cadet population	20–240 individuals, depending on study focus	90–99%	
Annual supplement (Annually since 1995)	BLS, CB, USDA	FNS, ERS	Current Population Survey (CPS), Supplement on Food Security	Civilian, noninstitutionalized U.S. population	Approx 59,500 for CPS	86–96%	Response rate is for supplement
Continuous (1980)	DOL	BLS	Consumer Expenditure Survey	Civilian, noninstitutionalized, population and a portion of the institutionalized population	5,000/quarter for quarterly interview survey of consumer units / 6,000/year for diary survey of consumer units kept for 2 consecutive 1-week periods	85% / 87%	

(continued)

TABLE 13.1 Federal Nutrition Monitoring Surveys and Surveillance Activities Since 1990[a, b] (continued)

Date Initiated	Department	Agency	Survey	Target U.S. Population	Sample Size and Type	Response Rate[c]	Comments
Continuous (1983)	DOC	Census	Survey of Income and Program Participation (SIPP)	Civilian, noninstitutionalized population of the U.S.	11,600–36,800 households	NA	Continuous series of panels
1994, 1996 (1984)	USDA	FNS	Study of WIC Participants and Program Characteristics	WIC participants using mail surveys of State and local WIC agencies, record abstractions at local WIC service sites and, in 1988, interviews with participants	7,000,000+	—	1996 Near census of WIC participants
1988–94	HHS	CDC/NCHS	NHANES III and Supplemental Nutrition Survey of Older Americans	See NHANES III listing above. Individuals ages 50+ y examined in NHANES III with telephones	See listing above.		
1989–91, annual 1994–96, annual (1985–86)	USDA	HNIS ARS[d]	Continuing Survey of Food Intakes by Individuals (CSFII) (Intake of Pyramid Servings and Servings database, 1994–96)	Females ages 19–50 y and their children ages 1–5 y and males ages 19–50 y residing in households in 48 conterminous states in 1985–86; individuals of all ages residing in households in 48 conterminous states in 1989–91, and nationwide in 1994–96; oversampling of individuals in low-income households; individuals ages 2+ y from CSFII 1994–96	15,303	76%	1994–96 CSFII Two days of dietary intake
1989–91	HHS	IHS	Strong Heart Dietary Survey	American Indian adults ages 45–74 y in SD, OK, and AZ	888	NA	275 from SD; 316 from OK; 297 from AZ
1991–92	DOC	NOAA/NMFS	Development of a National Seafood Consumption Survey Model	Individuals residing in eligible households and recreational/subsistence fishermen	—	—	

Year	Agency	Sub-agency	Study	Sample description	Sample size	Response rate	Data source
1992	USDA	FNS	School Nutrition Dietary Assessment Study	School-age children in grades 1–12 in 48 conterminous states and D.C.	380 school districts, 607 schools, 4,489 students	90% 88% 75%	
1992	USDA	FNS	Adult Day Care Program Study	Adult day care centers and adults participating in the Child and Adult Care Food Program	282 CACFP Centers, 282 non-CACFP centers, 942 participating adults	78% 83% 68%	
1994–95	USDA	FNS	WIC Infant Feeding Practices Study	Nationally representative sample of WIC mothers and infants living in the 48 contiguous states, the District of Columbia and the 33 WIC agencies on Indian reservations.	971	89%	
1995	USDA	FNS	Early Childhood and Child Care Study	Child care sponsors, providers, and children participating in the CACFP	566 sponsors, 1,962 providers, 1,951 households, 2,174 child-day observations	74% 87% 82% 59%	
1997–98	USDA	ARS[d]	Supplemental Children's Survey	Noninstitutionalized children ages 0–9 y in households in the U.S.; oversampling of low-income households	Approx 5,000	NA	
1998	USDA	FNS	School Nutrition Dietary Assessment Study II	School-age children in grades 1–12 in 48 conterminous states and D.C.	Approx 1,152 schools	NA	
1999–	HHS	CDC/NCHS	National Health and Nutrition Examination Survey	Civilian, noninstitutionalized individuals. In the first 3 years, oversampling of blacks, Mexican-Americans, adolescents, older persons, and pregnant women.	Approx 3,200	NA	
Knowledge, attitudes, and behavior assessments							
Continuous (1984)	HHS	CDC/NCCDPHP	Behavioral Risk Factor Surveillance System (BRFSS)	Individuals ages 18+ y residing in households with telephones in participating states	2,039 (median state sample size) 50 states	80%	1995 BRFSS
1990, 1994 (1982)	HHS	FDA;NIH/NHLBI	Health and Diet Survey	Civilian, noninstitutionalized individuals in households w/telephones, 18+ y	5,005	57%	1995 survey

(continued)

TABLE 13.1 Federal Nutrition Monitoring Surveys and Surveillance Activities Since 1990[a, b] (continued)

Date Initiated	Department	Agency	Survey	Target U.S. Population	Sample Size and Type	Response Rate[c]	Comments
1989–91 1994–96	USDA	HNIS ARS[d]	Diet and Health Knowledge Survey	Main meal-planners/preparers in households participating in 1989–91 and 1994–96 CSFII	5,765	74%	1994–96 survey
Annual (1990)	HHS	CDC/NCCDPHP	Youth Risk Behavior Survey (YRBS)	Youths attending school in grades 9–12 and ages 12–21 y in households in 50 states, D.C., Puerto Rico, and Virgin Islands	Avg 12,000 (national surveys) Avg 2,000 (and local surveys)	60% 60%	
1990	HHS	NIH/NHLBI	Cholesterol Awareness Survey—Physicians' Survey	Physicians practicing in the conterminous U.S.	1,604	68%	
1990–91	HHS	NIH/NHLBI	Nationwide Survey of Nurses' and Dietitians' Knowledge, Attitudes, and Behavior Regarding Cardiovascular Risk Factors	Registered nurses and registered dietitians currently active in their professions	7,200 registered nurses 1,621 occupational health nurses 1,782 registered dietitians	63% — 76%	Oversample of occupational health nurses (part of 7,200)
1990–91	HHS	FDA	Nutrition Label Format Studies	Primary food shoppers, ages 18+ y	2,676	NA	
1991	HHS	FDA, NIH/NHLBI	Weight Loss Practices Survey	Individuals currently trying to lose weight, ages 18+ y, in households with telephones	1,232 current dieters 205 African Americans 218 nondieting controls	58% 68% NA	Oversample of African Americans
1991	HHS	NIH/NCI	5 A Day for Better Health Baseline Survey	Individuals ages 18+ y with telephones	2,059	43%	Estimated response rate for random digit dial sample
1992–93, 1998	HHS	FDA	Consumer Food Handling Practices and Awareness of Microbiological Hazards Screener	Individuals ages 18+ y in households w/telephones	1,620	65%	
1993–94	HHS	FDA	Infant Feeding Practices Survey	New mothers and healthy, full-term infants ages 0–1 y	1,200	NA	
1994–95	USDA	FNS	WIC Infant Feeding Practices Survey	Prenatal and postnatal women and their infants participating in the WIC program	971	89%	

Food composition and nutrient data bases[e]

Continuous (1892)	USDA	ARS[d]	National Nutrient Data Bank Food Composition Laboratory	—	—	—
Annual (1961)	HHS	FDA	Total Diet Study	Representative diets of specific age-sex groups	—	—
1991–93, 1993–94, 1995–96 (1977)	HHS	FDA	Food Label and Package Survey	1,250 food brands	—	
Continuous (1977)	USDA	ARS[d]	Survey Nutrient Data Base for CSFII 1989–91, 1994–96; NHANES III (1988–94)	—	—	
1988–94	HHS	CDC/NCHS	Technical Support Information for the NHANES III, 1988–94 Dietary Interview Data Files	—	—	
1994–96	USDA	ARS[d]	CSFII 1994–96 Technical Support Files: Food Coding Database, Recipe Database, Survey Nutrient Database, and related files	—	—	

Food supply determinations[f]

Annual (1909)	DOC	NOAA/NMFS	Fisheries of the United States	—	—	
Annual (1909)	USDA	ERS, ARS[d]	U.S. Food and Nutrition Supply Series: Estimates of Food Available, Estimates of Nutrients	—	—	
Continuous (1985)	USDA	ERS, FCS	A.C. Nielsen SCANTRACK	—	3,000	supermarkets (Since 1988)

[a] Note that reference is made to a few surveys that took place before 1990. Dates for these appear in parenthesis.

[b] ARS, Agricultural Research Service; ASPE, Assistant Secretary for Planning and Evaluation; BLS, Bureau of Labor Statistics; CACFP, Child and Adult Care Food Program; CB, Census Bureau; CDC, Centers for Disease Control and Prevention; DOC, Department of Commerce; DOD, Department of Defense; DOL, Department of Labor; FDA, Food and Drug Administration; ERS, Economic Research Service; FNS, Food and Nutrition Service; HHS, Department of Health and Human Services; HNIS, Human Nutrition Information Service; HRSA, Health Resources Services Administration; IHS, Indian Health Service; NA, not available; NCCDPHP, National Center for Chronic Disease Prevention and Health Promotion; NCHS, National Center for Health Statistics; NCI, National Cancer Institute; NHLBI, National Heart, Lung, and Blood Institute; NIH, National Institutes of Health; NMFS, National Marine Fisheries Service; NOAA, National Oceanic and Atmospheric Administration; SSA, Social Security Administration; USARIEM, U.S. Army Research Institute of Environmental Medicine; USDA, U.S. Department of Agriculture.

— = Not applicable.

[c] Percentage of sample population that responded.

[d] HNIS was integrated into ARS in 1994.

[e] See Directory of Federal and State Nutrition Monitoring Activities for additional information on the various food composition databases (http://www.cdc.gov/nchs/data/nutrimon.pdf).

[f] See Directory of Federal and State Nutrition Monitoring Activities for additional information on food supply determinations (http://www.cdc.gov/nchs/data/nutrimon.pdf).

improvements in sample design, dietary methodologies, and related survey questionnaires. The ARS has the lead responsibility for developing the 24-hour dietary recall methodology, maintaining and updating the food composition database, and processing dietary recall data. The ARS has developed a computerized dietary intake interview system and tested the accuracy and response rates of administering dietary recall interviews by telephone. The NCHS has been evaluating telephone and in-person modes of administering 24-hour recall interviews within the NHANES survey environment (1,62).

The survey now includes a nationally representative annual sample of African American, white, and Mexican American persons for all-income and low-income households, as well as a common dietary data collection and processing system. Federal agencies, including the Agricultural Research Service (ARS) and the National Center for Health Statistics (NCHS), have conducted sample design and dietary survey methodology research, evaluated the extent of seasonal and geographic coverage with the combined annual survey, and designed and implemented the survey to better meet the needs of nutrition-monitoring data.

Periodic assessments of food and nutrient consumption for specific subgroups of the population that were not adequately covered in national surveys have been conducted for military populations, American Indians, children, and low-income populations (18,50). A Supplemental Children's Survey was conduced by the USDA from 1997 to 1998 specifically to assess pesticide exposure in the diets of infants and young children. Since 1995 a special yearly supplement to the Current Population Survey (CPS) conducted by the U.S. Bureau of the Census has been devoted to measuring the extent of food insecurity and hunger among people living in U.S. households (54–56). In addition, the NHANES (beginning in 1999), the Survey of Program Dynamics, and the U.S. Department of Education's Early Childhood Longitudinal Study (kindergarten cohort in 1998 and birth cohort in 2000) have begun to incorporate the measure.

Evaluations of the USDA nutrition and food assistance programs are routinely conducted. For example, the Adult Day Care Program Study and the Early Childhood and Child Care Study each determined the characteristics and dietary intakes of their participants and of the day-care centers participating in the Child and Adult Care Food Program. A number of studies have been conducted to evaluate the nutrition and health effects of participating in WIC; to provide current participant and program char-

acteristics of the WIC program; and to describe the infant feeding practices of WIC participants, including breast-feeding initiation and duration, formula feeding, and the introduction of supplementary foods (25,50). The School Nutrition Dietary Assessment Study assessed the diets of American schoolchildren and the contribution of the National School Lunch Program to overall nutrient intake (27). A follow-up study was conducted to compare changes over time.

Knowledge, Attitude, and Behavior Assessments

National surveys that measure knowledge, attitudes, and behavior about diet and nutrition and how they relate to health were added to the nutrition-monitoring program from 1985 through the 1990s. In general, the Health and Diet Survey, sponsored by numerous agencies, focuses on people's awareness of relationships between diet and risk for chronic disease, and on health-related knowledge (specifically on hypertension, hypercholesterolemia, coronary heart disease, and cancer) and attitudes. The survey also determines consumer use of food labels and has been used to assess the effectiveness of the National Cholesterol Education Program and to compare consumer awareness and practices related to cholesterol with those of physicians. Weight-loss practices were studied in 1991 (68,69). The focus of the Diet and Health Knowledge Survey initiated by the USDA in 1989 is on the relationship of individuals' knowledge and attitudes about dietary guidance and food safety to their food choices and nutrient intakes (65,66).

Surveys addressing specific topics, such as infant feeding practices, weight-loss practices and progress toward achieving related national health objectives, and cholesterol awareness of health professionals, have been periodically conducted to meet specific data needs. The National Cancer Institute conducted the 5 A Day for Better Health Baseline Survey in collaboration with the food industry to assess knowledge, behavior, and attitudes about fruits and vegetables (21). The institute also conducted the Cancer Prevention Awareness Survey and the National Knowledge, Attitudes, and Behavior Survey to measure progress on knowledge, attitudes, and behaviors regarding lifestyle and cancer prevention and risk factors (50). The FDA conducted a study to assess consumer food-handling practices and awareness of microbiological hazards and also conducted a number of studies to evaluate the features and usability by consumers of the Nutrition Facts Label (70).

The focus of the Behavioral Risk Factor Surveillance System, initiated in 1984, is on personal behavior and its relationship to nutrition and health status. It has been used by state health departments to plan, initiate, and guide health promotion and disease prevention programs, as well as to monitor their progress over time (71,72). The Youth Risk Behavior Survey monitors priority health risk behaviors among adolescents through national, state, and local surveys (73,74).

Food Composition and Nutrient Databases

Since 1892 the USDA has operated the National Nutrient Data Bank to derive representative nutrient values for more than 6,000 foods and as many as 80 components consumed in the United States. Data are obtained from the food industry, USDA-initiated analytical contracts, and the scientific literature. Values from the data bank are released in *Agriculture Handbook No. 8* and as part of the USDA Nutrient Data Base for Standard Reference, which is updated annually to reflect changes in the food supply and in analytical methodology. These values are used as the core of most nutrient databases developed in the United States for special purposes, such as databases used in the commercially available dietary analysis programs (40–42). The USDA's Survey Nutrient Data Base contains data for 28 food components and energy for each food item for analysis of the NHANES and the CSFII. The USDA has a system to periodically update this database with the most current information available from National Nutrient Data Bank.

The FDA's Total Diet Study (67) provides annual food composition analysis based on the foods consumed most frequently in the CSFII and the NHANES. Representative foods are collected from retail markets, prepared for consumption, and analyzed individually for nutrients and other food components at the Total Diet Laboratory to estimate consumption of selected nutrients, minerals, and organic and elemental contaminants.

The Food Label and Package Survey, sponsored by the FDA, was conducted to monitor labeling practices of U.S. food manufacturers (75,76). The survey also includes a surveillance program to identify levels of accuracy of selected nutrient declarations compared with values obtained from nutrient analyses of products.

Food Supply Determinations

Since 1909 U.S. food supply estimates have indicated levels of foods and nutrients available for consumption. These data, updated and published annually by USDA as the U.S. Food and Nutrient Supply Series, are used to assess the potential of the U.S. food supply to meet the nutrition needs of the population and changes in the food supply over time. The data are also used to evaluate the effects of technological alterations and marketing changes on the food supply over time; to study the relationships between food and nutrient availability and nutrient-disease associations; and to facilitate the management of federal marketing, food assistance, nutrition education, food enrichment, and fortification policy. Conducted annually by the National Marine Fisheries Service since 1909, the Fisheries of the United States survey provides annual estimates of fish and shellfish disappearance in the distribution system (50).

NUTRITION-MONITORING RESOURCES AVAILABLE TO RESEARCHERS

Published Scientific and Technical Reports

A number of scientific and technical reports have been periodically produced under the guidance of the Interagency Board for Nutrition Monitoring and Related Research (1,50,58,59). Scientific reports were designed to provide summary statistics on the dietary and nutrition status of the American population, as well as to provide recommendations to improve the program. Research summaries and full reference citations can be found in *Nutrition Monitoring in the United States: The Directory of Federal and State Nutrition Monitoring and Related Research Activities* (50) and the *Third Report on Nutrition Monitoring in the United States* (59). The *Directory* provides information on the multitude of surveys, surveillance systems, and selected research activities completed or under way at the federal level, as well as some state-level surveys. The on-line publication provides hypertext links to Web sites that describe each activity in more detail (50).

Technical reports on applied research methods have been published to standardize the data collection and reporting of data from the program. Examples include reports on sociodemographic indicators (77) and dietary assessment methods (52,78,79). These reports have improved the coordination of nutrition-monitoring and research activities across the program and have documented national survey methods so that state and local researchers can use common data collection methods to compare state and local data with national data.

Progress has been made in using electronic bulletin boards to announce or distribute survey data, survey reports, and nutrition-monitoring publications and to distribute data in various electronic forms, such as tapes, diskettes, and CD-ROMs. In addition to preparing, promoting, and distributing survey reports and data tapes, increased efforts are being directed toward instructing users on how to access, process, and interpret data appropriately via the provision of training manuals, survey documentation on methods and quality control procedures, and data user conferences at national and regional levels. One widely used training tool is the *NHANES III Anthropometric Procedures Video,* a resource to enable nutritionists and dietitians to collect data comparable to national data (80). This product demonstrates the standardized anthropometric procedures that were used to collect body measurements in the NHANES III. The procedures shown in the videotape allow others to follow the NHANES III anthropometric methodology and enable researchers to compare data collected in local clinics and other population-based studies with national reference data.

Other Sources of Information on Nutrition Research

The Internet has greatly facilitated access to information. Research abstracts and, in many cases, the actual reports of findings can be found on-line. For example, an excellent source of research information is the federal Human Nutrition Research and Information Management system database, which includes national nutrition-monitoring research and applied methodologies supported in whole or in part by the federal government. Each participating agency submits data, which are then combined in the main system database. The database contains approximately 4,000 projects for each fiscal year beginning in 1985, and it includes information on the sponsoring organization, the project title and name of the principal investigator, and a project abstract. The database is maintained at the National Institutes of Health (NIH) under the auspices of the Interagency Committee on Human Nutrition

Research. Further information is available on the World Wide Web at http://hnrim.nih.gov.

A useful guide on NIH research activities is found in a periodic report entitled *National Institutes of Health Program in Biomedical and Behavioral Nutrition Research and Training.* The report is prepared by the Division of Nutrition Research Coordination at the NIH. Other health resources at the NIH (such as consumer health publications, information on clinical trials, health hotlines, Grateful Med, and the NIH Health Information Index) can be found at http://www.nih.gov/health. The NIH Health Information Index is a subject-word guide to diseases and conditions under investigation at NIH and helps users find the NIH institute that supports research related to a given health concern. Research on dietary supplements, for example, can be found at the Web page of the NIH Office of Dietary Supplements (http://dietary-supplements.info. nih.gov).

A listing of research and other publications conducted at the CDC can be obtained at http://www.cdc. gov/publications.htm. The most relevant sources for nutrition research include the NCHS, the National Center for Chronic Disease Prevention and Health Promotion, and the National Center for Environmental Health. NCHS data systems include data on vital statistics, as well as information on health status, lifestyle, exposure to unhealthy influences, the onset and diagnosis of illness and disability, and the use of health care. The National Center for Chronic Disease Prevention and Health Promotion carries out surveillance and behavioral research and demonstration projects on maternal and child health, as well as chronic disease prevention. More information about the CDC National Prevention Research Network can be obtained at http://www.cdc.gov/nccdphp/aag/aag_ prc.htm. Program review and recent research activities at the National Center for Environmental Health (NCEH), a part of the CDC, can be reviewed at http://www.cdc.gov/ nceh. Areas of coverage include public health surveillance and applied research (epidemiologic studies, laboratory analyses, statistical analyses, and behavioral interventions).

A compilation of the approximately 186 Center for Food Safety and Applied Nutrition publications pertaining to scientific research and regulatory programs can be found on the FDA's Web site. Many of the published studies have had a direct impact on consumer protection, such as the development of methods for monitoring contaminants in foods. Other published studies include information used in the development of regulatory policy (http://vm.cfsan.fda.gov). Information about the surveys conducted by the National Marine Fisheries Service can be accessed at http://www.nmfs.noaa.gov.

The USDA Food and Nutrition Service research page (http://www.fns.usda.gov/oane) provides information on published reports and ongoing research in the areas of child nutrition programs, the Food Stamp Program, food security, and WIC. Information that links policy with research conducted by the USDA Center for Nutrition Policy and Promotion is found at http://www.usda.gov/cnpp/center.htm. The center publishes the *Family Economics and Nutrition Review* each quarter. A link to Economic Research Service (ERS) food and nutrition assistance programs, through which you can download research reports and information on research-funding opportunities, can be found on-line at http://www.ers.usda.gov/briefing. A great deal of ERS research is published in an in-house journal, *Food Review*. A description of the Agricultural Research Service's research and quarterly reports from 1994 to 1998 is found at http://www.ars.usda.gov/is/qtr, and information about the service's Food Survey's Research Group can be accessed at http://www.barc.usda.gov/bhnrc/foodsurvey/home.htm.

Thousands of scientific journals contain information on federal and nonfederal nutrition research. To find the most current listing of journals, researchers are encouraged to use the Internet to search MEDLINE and AGRICOLA (AGRICultural OnLine Access), bibliographic databases that include information about food and nutrition. AGRICOLA consists of citations for journal articles, monographs, theses, audiovisual materials, and technical reports relating to all aspects of agriculture, whereas MEDLINE is a biomedical database consisting of citations from journal articles only. AGRICOLA and MEDLINE can be used to retrieve journal abstracts. MEDLINE/PubMed and other related databases can be accessed through MEDLARS, a free service provided by the National Library of Medicine. The service can be accessed through the Internet (http://www.ncbi.nlm.nih.gov/PubMed). MEDLINE and AGRICOLA on CD-ROM are produced by SilverPlatter, Inc., and are available at many libraries. On-line access to both AGRICOLA and MEDLINE is available through commercial vendors, including the Dialog Corporation and DIMDI (Germany). AGRICOLA is also available through the National Agricultural Library's Web site (http://www.nal.usda.gov). For more information about how to use AGRICOLA or MEDLINE to locate nutrition-monitoring research articles, see *Nutrition Monitoring in the United States: The*

Directory of Federal and State Nutrition Monitoring and Related Research Activities (50).

The use of a database requires the development of a search strategy. A search strategy contains the key words, phrases, or terms of interest; synonyms for these terms; and how they should be combined. This chapter includes a section on ways to obtain data sets and federal research information.

Data Sets for Secondary Data Analysis

The surveys of the National Nutrition Monitoring Program generate a large amount of data. For selected surveys, agencies produce data sets for public use and publish survey findings in government and peer-reviewed reports. Many agencies offer information on CD-ROMs and are phasing out the more expensive public-use data tapes. In addition, many agencies are making data sets accessible through the Internet. In other cases, agencies provide data for a cost. Some agencies make data sets available through the National Technical Information Service (http://www.ntis.gov). Still other reports and documents are available from the U.S. Government Printing Office.

The Federal Electronic Research and Review Extraction Tool (FERRET), a computer search tool developed by the U.S. Department of Commerce's Census Bureau and the U.S. Department of Labor's Bureau of Labor Statistics, enables users to access and manipulate large demographic and economic data sets over the Internet (http://ferret.bls.census.gov/cgi-bin/ferret). FERRET was developed to provide one-stop access to statistics from the CPS and the Survey of Income and Program Participation (SIPP). FERRET allows users to quickly locate current and historical information from these sources, get tabulations for specific information they need, make comparisons between different data sets, create simple tables, and download large amounts of data from the Internet to desktop and larger computers for custom reports. For agency-specific information on ways to obtain data sets, consult the *Directory* (50). A PDF file can be downloaded from the Internet at http://www.cdc.gov/nchs/products/pubs/pubd/other/miscpub/miscpub.htm.

Many agencies that conduct national nutrition surveys, such as the NHANES, maintain lists of peer-reviewed research articles or bibliographies of survey findings. These references can be found by visiting the surveys' home pages. Many other agencies that use national survey data also list publications or links to publications on their Web sites.

Limitations and Other Factors in Survey and Surveillance Data Analysis

When analyzing survey and surveillance data, one must consider whether the data are suitable for the questions being asked. The design of the survey, the appropriateness of the methods used, and the introduction of bias must be considered. Bias is a consistent error that can be introduced in a number of ways and can take many forms. Researchers must learn to evaluate surveys and surveillance data to assess whether or not bias has been introduced.

Sampling Bias

Examples of sampling bias include frame bias and consistent sampling bias. A *frame* is the sampling list used when the listing of the sampling units in the population is too difficult or tedious. Frame bias can be caused by the use of an incomplete list, for example, a listing of telephone numbers for a particular city or geographic area. Such a sample would include only those households that have telephones or telephone numbers in a directory. The sample would therefore be biased in two directions: neither households without telephones nor households with unlisted numbers would be represented. The sample would likely underrepresent low-income households and people who prefer unlisted numbers.

Consistent sampling bias can be introduced by the mechanical procedures used to select units from the frame into the sample. In the telephone survey example, a consistent sampling bias could arise if the sample of telephone numbers were contacted from 9 AM to 5 PM on weekdays. Employed persons and students would be unlikely to be at home during those hours.

Sometimes decisions are made to narrow the areas covered in area probability samples to reduce the costs associated with collecting the data. These decisions can lead to noncoverage bias, that is, the failure to include elements in the sample that would properly belong in the sample. An example is the exclusion of areas with a low Hispanic population from the Hispanic Health and Nutrition Examination Survey, which resulted in a slight underrepresentation of more affluent Hispanics in the sample (49).

Nonsampling Bias

Nonsampling bias arises from systematic errors related to nonresponse, measurement, or data processing. Nonresponse bias results from the failure to obtain observations on some elements selected and designated for the sample. This bias occurs because people are not at home despite repeated attempts to contact them, they refuse to participate, or they are incapacitated and unable to participate. This bias also occurs because of lost data, such as lost interviews and laboratory accidents. Incomplete reporting is a potential for bias in survey and surveillance data. Missing data elements should be excluded from analyses.

Statisticians frequently use the survey response rate as an overall indicator of the quality of a survey. When a substantial proportion of the sample selected for a survey does not participate, a potential for bias exists if the nonrespondents differ from the respondents in some systematic way. The greater the nonresponse, the greater the potential for bias. The *Third Report on Nutrition Monitoring in the United States* (59) and *Nutrition Monitoring in the United States: The Directory of Federal and State Nutrition Monitoring and Related Research Activities* (50) include summary information on response rates for recent surveys and surveillance systems.

Even when a substantial proportion of the original sample does not participate in the survey, the sample may not be biased, and studies of nonresponse bias can be performed. These types of studies have been performed for some of the national surveys (59). Nonresponse bias analyses to examine whether there were systematic differences between samples interviewed but not examined and the examined samples were performed for the NHANES I, II, and III and found no evidence of bias (81–83).

Measurement bias refers to consistent errors arising in the interview or laboratory method used to obtain the data. In 24-hour dietary recalls, measurement bias can be introduced through the interview methods (for example, when probing for amounts of fat or alcoholic beverage consumption), coding assumptions (for example, rules for assigning default codes), errors in the food composition database used to estimate nutrient levels, or selection of days of the week to conduct the interviews. Systematic bias with respect to underreporting energy intake with the 24-hour recall method is well-established (84), and its impact on the interpretation of national dietary intakes has been studied (52).

Sample Weights and Design Effects

The statistical technique used to identify survey samples introduces complexities into the analysis of the data. In area probability sampling, some trade-offs are made in the randomness of the sample to minimize the costs of the survey. The technique is multistage, and at each stage, sample elements with a known probability are selected. In the NHANES, the stages of selection are defined as counties, areas within counties (called *segments*), households, and household members. To produce the estimates for the nation based on observations from individuals, the data for individuals must be inflated by their probability of selection, adjusted for nonresponse, and then poststratified to bring the population estimate into close agreement with the U.S. Census Bureau estimates. To make these procedures easier for the users of the survey data, sample weights incorporating the three levels of adjustments appear on the public use data files. For weighted analyses, analysts can work with special computer software packages that use an appropriate method for estimating variances for complex samples, such as SUDAAN (85), WesVarPC (86), and STATA (87).

Area probability samples are not simple random samples, and the assumptions of simple random sampling do not apply when hypothesis testing is performed with survey data. Data CD-ROMs distributed by the National Center for Health Statistics and other sources describe special computer programs that take into account the complex nature of the sample in the calculation of test statistics (60). The design effect can be used to adjust estimates and statistics computed by using assumptions of simple random sampling for the complexities in the sample design (88).

Determining whether a subsample is free of bias involves comparing the subsample with the overall sample for characteristics related to the subject of inquiry. Whenever analyses of this type are performed, it is essential that the analytic subsample be examined for bias and that the sample weights and design effects be used in the analysis.

Program Participation Data

Surveillance data collected on women and children participating in publicly funded food assistance, nutrition, or health programs involve a self-selected population and thus are not representative of the community at large.

Factors that differentiate members of this group from the general population include their meeting the income eligibility level, having a nutrition or health risk, and having the personal initiative or knowledge to participate in available programs (89). The PedNSS and PNSS involve primarily low-income populations and have overrepresentation by racial and ethnic minority populations in comparison with the general population. Although the surveillance population does not represent all women and children in the state, the data can be representative of program participants and thus be very useful for planning public health and nutrition programs and evaluating the impact of these programs on the nutrition and health status of the target populations (9). Eligibility criteria can vary from state to state and over time, making comparisons across states and time difficult. Knowledge of program enrollment criteria and changes in criteria over time is important for appropriately interpreting nutrition surveillance data.

Quality of Data

Nutrition surveillance data are collected in over 4,000 public health clinics across the country, and each data set has its own quality issues. Clinic staff members have a wide range of expertise in nutrition assessment and data collection. Calibrated equipment, periodic training of staff, and quality control and assurance programs are important aspects of maintaining high-quality surveillance data. Consultation, training, and written protocols are available from the CDC (9,89). In recent years, emphasis has been placed on improving the quality control of data collected in the surveillance systems.

National surveys that collect physical measurements, such as the NHANES, have extensive quality control and assurance programs, as well as well-documented data collection and laboratory protocols (50,60); however, data quality may also be a concern with national survey methods. Researchers should review the survey methods and quality control procedures and data prior to their analysis and interpretation of the data.

Survey and surveillance data collected through personal or proxy interviews are self-reported data, and thus subject to error. Inaccuracy may be related to poor recall; sensitivity to, or lack of understanding of, the question; or lack of knowledge to answer the question. For example, it has been shown that self-reported heights and weights are biased; men report being taller than they are, and women report weighing less than they actually do (90). Parents' reporting of their children's heights and weights have also been shown to be inaccurate (91); however, maternal recall of infant birth weight has been validated and shown to be accurate (92). Interviewer training on how to ask sensitive questions and elicit responses can improve the quality of self-reported data.

GETTING STARTED ON YOUR OWN RESEARCH

What Is Your Area of Interest, and How Will Your Research Be Put to Use?

Before you begin your research, it is important to ask yourself certain questions: What is my outcome of interest? Is it, for example, nutrition and food security of people who participate in one of the food assistance programs? Is it how well knowledge and attitudes about nutrition translate into action? Is the purpose of the study to determine whether or not an intervention has had an impact on health status (for example, has it lowered blood cholesterol levels or blood pressure)? The purpose could also be to determine whether participation in a given program has saved health care dollars or lives. Perhaps you are interested in the general population, children, older Americans, a particular racial or ethnic group, people with low incomes, or pregnant women.

Nutrition-monitoring information may be used in several ways to suit your needs: for analysis of raw survey data to answer your research questions about trends in diet and nutrition status or about national incidences or estimates, to study relationships of diet and health, to investigate the contribution of diet and supplements to total nutrient intake, to cite published findings or reference data, or to use national methods in your own research study. If you are designing your own study, you may want to use national data collection and survey tools to allow data comparisons.

Before starting your research, it is important to decide what practical applications it will have. In other words, will you be enhancing the pool of knowledge, and will the findings be useful to you and others? Perhaps the research will be used to develop educational programs. Alternatively, it might be used to develop a tool to evaluate a program or to evaluate an intervention. Research you conduct might be used to develop new food products or test their attributes. It might be used to set reference standards or to promulgate policy.

Where Should You Turn Next?

Once you decide in what nutrition-monitoring measurement area your interests lie, it is useful to go to key sources, such as *Nutrition Monitoring in the United States: The Directory of Federal and State Nutrition Monitoring and Related Research Activities* (50), journals, and reference reports (58,59), and determine whether or not a certain survey or surveillance system may include variables of interest. *Directory* entries, for example, include a section on "key variables of interest," which may be a useful guide. Journal articles and federal agency Web sites provide information on recent studies that may be pertinent to your area of research. Reference materials provide information on normal values or targets to which your findings can be compared.

Remember, too, that there are benefits and trade-offs when using a public-access data set, as opposed to collecting your own data. Surveys such as the NHANES, for example, provide a nationally representative sample, do not require that you spend time and money collecting data, and are recognized as credible sources of data. However, in using these survey results you might be limited to the use of variables that did not exactly meet your needs, and you might not get information about your particular population of interest.

Who Is Your Audience?

Before beginning your research, you will need to decide whether it can be translated for use by its intended audience. Therefore, knowledge of your beneficiaries is important. Perhaps your research will benefit consumers who are looking for information to make decisions about their nutrition and health. Public and private policy makers might use research findings as a basis for creating dietary guidance materials and programs to enhance the nutrition quality of food supplies, provide food assistance, and evaluate policies. Health educators might make use of your findings to develop a framework for population subgroups and disease prevention guidelines. Physicians and other health professionals might use your research to keep abreast of current knowledge or to provide dietary recommendations to patients. Food, nutrition, and health associations may use knowledge gleaned from your study to set policy or to educate their constituencies. The media may use your research as an educational tool or for background information. Finally, trade associations and people in industry may use it to develop guidelines for product development and improvement.

What Are Your Resources and Level of Expertise?

Before embarking on your research project, it is important to know your financial and staffing resources and constraints. Do not underestimate the financial, human, and labor resources that are required to conduct research. You will need to determine if your staff has the expertise and ability to analyze survey data that use a complex design. Depending on resources and appropriateness, you may decide to conduct one of the different types of studies described in Chapters 1, 2, and 8, or you may decide to analyze data from one of the surveys or surveillance activities described in this chapter and further elaborated upon in *Nutrition Monitoring in the United States: The Directory of Federal and State Nutrition Monitoring and Related Research Activities* (50). Another consideration is the sample size required to obtain estimates of interest. The length of time you have to conduct your research might also influence your study design and other options. If you are collecting dietary intake data, the 1994 report of the Consensus Workshop on Dietary Assessment includes guidelines and considerations for selecting a dietary method to meet your data needs (78). Other publications can help you apply the Dietary Reference Intakes (DRIs) to group dietary data (39).

REFERENCES

1. Briefel RR. Nutrition monitoring in the United States. In: Bowman B, Russell R, eds. *Present Knowledge in Nutrition*. 8th ed. Washington, DC: ILSI Press; 2001:615633.
2. Kuczmarski MF, Moshfegh AJ, Briefel RR. Update on nutrition monitoring activities in the United States. *J Am Diet Assoc*. 1994;94:753–760.
3. U.S. Congress. *National Nutrition Monitoring and Related Research Act of 1990*. Washington, DC: 101st Congress; 1990. Pub L 101–445.
4. Ostenso GL. National Nutrition Monitoring System: a historical perspective. *J Am Diet Assoc*. 1984;84:1181–1185.
5. Mason JB, Habicht J-P, Tabatabai H, Valverde V. *Nutritional Surveillance*. Geneva, Switzerland: World Health Organization; 1984.
6. U.S. Department of Health and Human Services and Department of Agriculture. *Proposed Ten-Year Comprehensive Plan for the National Nutrition Monitoring and Re-

lated Research Program*. Washington, DC: U.S. Government Printing Office; 1991. Publication 91–25967:SS 716–55767.
7. Division of Nutrition, National Center for Chronic Disease Prevention and Health Promotion. *Report of the State and Local Input Meeting. National Nutrition Monitoring and Related Research Plan*. Atlanta, Ga: U.S. Department of Health and Human Services; 1991.
8. U.S. Department of Health and Human Services and U.S. Department of Agriculture. *Ten-year Comprehensive Plan for the National Nutrition Monitoring and Related Research Program*. Washington, DC: U.S. Government Printing Office; 1993. Publication 58:32752–32806.
9. Wilcox LS, Marks JS, eds. *From Data to Action: CDC's Public Health Surveillance for Women, Infants, and Children*. Washington, DC: Public Health Service; 1994.
10. Food and Agriculture Organization of the United Nations, World Health Organization Joint Secretariat for the Conference. *The International Conference on Nutrition: World Declaration and Plan of Action for Nutrition*. Rome, Italy: FAO/WHO; 1992.
11. Woteki CE. Nutrition monitoring research. The Research Agenda for Dietetics, Conference Proceedings. *J Am Dietetic Assoc*. 1993;93:39–48.
12. Sims LS. Research aspects of public policy in nutrition generating research questions to determine the impact of nutritional, agricultural, and health care policy and regulations on the health and nutritional status of the public. The Research Agenda for Dietetics, Conference Proceedings. *J Am Diet Assoc*. 1992;92:25–38.
13. U.S. Department of Health and Human Services. *Healthy People 2000: National Health Promotion and Disease Prevention Objectives*. Washington, DC: U.S. Government Printing Office; 1991. DHHS publication (PHS) 91–50212.
14. U.S. Department of Health and Human Services. *Healthy People 2010: Understanding and Improving Health*. 2nd ed. Washington, DC: U.S. Government Printing Office; 2000. Also available at: http://www.health.gov/healthypeople. Accessed June 9, 2001.
15. Earl R, Woteki CE, eds. *Iron Deficiency Anemia: Recommended Guidelines for the Prevention, Detection, and Management Among U.S. Children and Women of Childbearing Age*. Washington, DC: National Academy Press; 1993.
16. Centers for Disease Control and Prevention. Recommendations to prevent and control iron deficiency in the United States. *MMWR Morb Mortal Wkly Rep*. 1998;47(RR-3):1–29.
17. National Institutes of Health. *NIH Consensus Statement: Optimal Calcium Intake*. Bethesda, Md: National Institutes of Health; 1994.
18. Committee on Military Nutrition Research, Food and Nutrition Board, Institute of Medicine. *Military Nutrition Ini-

tiatives. Washington, DC: U.S. Government Printing Office; 1991. Report 91–05.

19. Kuczmarksi RJ, Ogden CL, Grummer-Strawn LM, et al. *CDC Growth Charts: United States.* Washington, DC: National Center for Health Statistics; 2000.

20. Centers for Disease Control and Prevention. Epi Info-Epi Map. Available at: http://www.cdc.gov/epiinfo. Accessed June 9, 2001.

21. Heimendinger J, Van Duyn MA, Chapelsky D, Foerster S, Stables G. The national 5-A-Day for Better Health Program: a large-scale nutrition intervention. *J Public Health Manage Pract.* 1996;2(2):27–35.

22. U.S. Department of Agriculture and Department of Health and Human Services. *Nutrition and Your Health: Dietary Guidelines for Americans.* 5th ed. Washington, DC: U.S. Government Printing Office; 2000. USDA Home and Garden Bulletin No. 232.

23. National Cholesterol Education Program. Executive summary of the third report of the National Cholesterol Education Program (NCEP) expert panel on detection, evaluation, and treatment of high blood cholesterol in adults (Adult Treatment Panel III). *JAMA.* 2001;285(19):2486–2497.

24. National Heart, Lung, and Blood Institute. Sixth report of the Joint National Committee on Detection, Evaluation, and Treatment of High Blood Pressure. Washington, DC: U.S. Department of Health and Human Services; 1997. DHHS Publication 98–4080.

25. Randall B, Bartlett S, Kennedy S. *Study of WIC Participant and Program Characteristics, 1996.* Alexandria, Va: U.S. Department of Agriculture, Food, and Nutrition Service; 1998.

26. Devaney B, Fraker TM. Cashing out food stamps: impacts on food expenditures and diet quality. *J Policy Analysis Manage.* 1986;5(4):725–741.

27. Burghardt JA, Devaney BL, Gordon AR. The School Nutrition Dietary Assessment Study: summary and discussion. *Am J Clin Nutr.* 1995;61(suppl):252–257.

28. U.S. Department of Agriculture, Center for Nutrition Policy and Promotion. *The Thrifty Food Plan, 1999: Executive Summary.* CNPP-7A. Available at: http://www.usda.gov/cnpp/FoodPlans/TFP99. Accessed June 9, 2001.

29. Forbes AL, Stephenson MG. National Nutrition Monitoring System: implications for public health policy at Food and Drug Administration. *J Am Diet Assoc.* 1984;84:1189–1193.

30. U.S. Department of Health and Human Services, Food and Drug Administration. Notice of final rule: food labeling: health claims and label statements; dietary fiber and cardiovascular disease; dietary fiber and cancer. *Federal Register.* January 5, 1993;2552–2605, 2537–2552.

31. Anderson SA, ed. *Estimation of Exposure to Substances in the Food Supply.* Bethesda, Md: Life Sciences Research Office; 1988.

32. Institute of Medicine. *Estimating Consumer Exposure to Food Additives and Monitoring Trends in Use.* Washington, DC: National Academy Press; 1992.

33. U.S. Environmental Protection Agency, Office of Air Quality Planning & Standards and Office of Research and Development. *Mercury Study Report to Congress.* Washington, DC: Environmental Protection Agency; 1997. EPA-452/R-97–003.

34. Wright JW, Bialostosky K, Gunter EW, et al. *Blood Folate and Vitamin B12: United States, 1988–94.* Washington, DC: National Center for Health Statistics; 1998. Vital Health Stat 11(243).

35. Office of Science and Technology Policy, Executive Office of the President. *Meeting the Challenge. A Research Agenda for America's Health, Safety, and Food.* Washington, DC: U.S. Government Printing Office; 1996.

36. Institute of Medicine, Food and Nutrition Board. *Dietary Reference Intakes for Calcium, Phosphorus, Magnesium, Vitamin D, and Fluoride.* Washington, DC: National Academy Press; 1997.

37. Institute of Medicine, Food and Nutrition Board. *Dietary Reference Intakes for Thiamin, Riboflavin, Niacin, Vitamin B6, Folate, Vitamin B12, Pantothenic Acid, Biotin, and Choline.* Washington, DC: National Academy Press; 1998.

38. Institute of Medicine, Food and Nutrition Board. *Dietary Reference Intakes for Vitamin C, Vitamin E, Selenium, and Carotenoids.* Washington, DC: National Academy Press; 2000.

39. Institute of Medicine, Food and Nutrition Board. *Dietary Reference Intakes: Applications in Dietary Assessment.* Washington, DC: National Academy Press; 2001.

40. Haytowitz DB, Pehrsson PR, Smith J, Gebhardt SE, Matthews RH, Anderson BA. Key foods: setting priorities for nutrient analyses. *J Food Comp Analysis.* 1996;9(4):331–364.

41. Schakel SF, Buzzard IM, Gebhardt SE. Procedures for estimating nutrient values for food composition databases. *J Food Comp Analysis.* 1997;10:102–114.

42. Holden JM, Davis CS. Strategies for sampling: the assurance of representative values. In: Greenfield H, ed. *Quality and Accessibility of Food-related Data: Proceedings of the First International Food Data Base Conference.* Arlington, Va: AOAC International; 1995:105–117.

43. Trudeau E, Kristal AR, Li S, Patterson RE. Demographic and psychosocial predictors of fruit and vegetable intakes differ: implications for dietary interventions. *J Am Diet Assoc.* 1998; 98(12):1412–1417.

44. Patterson RE, Satia JA, Kristal AR, Neuhouser ML, Drewnowski A. Is there a consumer backlash against the diet and health message? *J Am Diet Assoc.* 2001;101(1):37–41.

45. Edmundson E, Parcel GS, Feldman HA, et al. The effects of the Child and Adolescent Trial for Cardiovascular Health upon psychosocial determinants of diet and physical activity behavior. *Prev Med.* 1996;25(4):442–454.

46. Putnam JJ, Allshouse JE. *Food Consumption, Prices, and Expenditures, 1970–97.* Washington, DC: U.S. Department of Agriculture; 1999. Statistical Bulletin No. 965.

47. U.S. Department of Health and Human Services. *The Surgeon General's Report on Nutrition and Health.* Washington, DC: U.S. Government Printing Office; 1988. PHS publication 88–50210.

48. National Research Council. *Diet and Health. Implications for Reducing Chronic Disease Risk.* Washington, DC: National Academy Press; 1989.

49. Woteki CE, Wong FL. Interpretation and utilization of data from the National Nutrition Monitoring System. In: Monsen ER, ed. *Research. Successful Approaches.* Chicago, Ill: American Dietetic Association; 1992:204–219.

50. Bialostosky K, ed. *Nutrition Monitoring in the United States: The Directory of Federal and State Nutrition Monitoring and Related Research Activities.* Hyattsville, Md: National Center for Health Statistics; 2000. DHHS publication 00–1255. Also available at: http://www.cdc.gov/nchs/data/nutrimon.pdf. Accessed June 9, 2001.

51. Briefel RR. Assessment of the U.S. diet in national nutrition surveys: National collaborative efforts and NHANES. *Am J Clin Nutr.* 1994;59(suppl):164–167.

52. Briefel RR, Sempos CT, McDowell MA, Chien S, Alaimo K. Dietary methods research in the third National Health and Nutrition Examination Survey: under reporting of energy intake. *Am J Clin Nutr.* 1997;65(suppl):1203–1209.

53. Yetley E, Johnson C. Nutritional applications of the Health and Nutrition Examination Surveys (HANES). *Annu Rev Nutr.* 1987;7:441–463.

54. Hamilton WL, Cook JT, Thompson WW, et al. *Household Food Security in the United States in 1995: Summary Report of the Food Security Measurement Project.* Alexandria, Va: U.S. Department of Agriculture, Food, and Consumer Service; 1997.

55. Hamilton WL, Cook JT, Thompson WW, et al. *Measures of Food Security, Food Insecurity, and Hunger in the United States in 1995: Technical Report of the Food Security Measurement Study.* Alexandria, Va: U.S. Department of Agriculture, Food, and Consumer Service; 1997.

56. Economic Research Service. Food security in the United States. Available at: http://www.ers.usda.gov/briefing/foodsecurity. Accessed June 9, 2001.

57. Blumberg SJ, Bialostosky K, Hamilton WL, Briefel RR. The effectiveness of a short form of the Household Food Security Scale. *Am J Public Health.* 1999;89:1231–1234.

58. Ervin B, Reed D, eds. *Nutrition Monitoring in the United States. Chartbook I: Selected Findings from the National Nutrition Monitoring and Related Research Program.* Hyattsville, Md: Public Health Service; 1993. DHHS publication (PHS) 93–1255–2.

59. Life Sciences Research Office, Federation of American Societies for Experimental Biology. *Third Report on Nutrition Monitoring in the United States: Volumes 1 and 2.Prepared for the Interagency Board for Nutrition Monitoring and Related Research.* Washington, DC: U.S. Government Printing Office; 1995.

60. U.S. Department of Health and Human Services, National Center for Health Statistics. Third National Health and Nutrition Examination Survey, 1988–94, Reference Manuals and Reports [survey on CD-ROM]. Hyattsville, Md: Centers for Disease Control and Prevention; 1996.

61. National Center for Health Statistics. National Health and Nutrition Examination Survey, Background. Available at: http://www.cdc.gov/nchs/nhanes.htm. Accessed June 9, 2001.

62. National Center for Health Statistics. Current NHANES on into the 21st century. Available at: http://www.cdc.gov/nchs/nhanes.htm. Accessed June 9, 2001.

63. Centers for Disease Control and Prevention. *Pediatric Nutrition Surveillance: 1997 Full Report.* Atlanta, Ga: U.S. Department of Health and Human Services; 1998.

64. Centers for Disease Control and Prevention. *Pregnancy Nutrition Surveillance:1996 Full Report.* Atlanta, Ga: U.S. Department of Health and Human Services; 1998.

65. Agricultural Research Service, Food Surveys Research Group. What we eat in America. Available at: http://www.barc.usda.gov/bhnrc/foodsurvey/home.htm. Accessed June 9, 2001.

66. Tippett KS, Enns CW, Moshfegh AM. Food consumption surveys in the U.S. Department of Agriculture. *Nutr Today.* 1999;34(1):33–46.

67. Pennington JAT, Capar SC, Parfitt CH, Edwards CW. History of the Total Diet Study (Part II). *J AOAC Int.* 1996;79:163–170.

68. Heaton AW, Levy AS. Information sources of U.S. adults trying to lose weight. *J Nutr Educ.* 1995;27:182–190.

69. Levy AS, Heaton AW. Weight control practices of U.S. adults trying to lose weight. *Ann Intern Med.* 1993;119:661–666.

70. Schucker RE, Levy AS, Tenney JE, Mathews O. Nutrition shelf-labeling and consumer purchase behavior. *J Nutr Educ.* 1992;24(2):75–81.

71. Figgs LW, Bloom Y, Dugbatey K, Stanwyck CA, Nelson DE, Brownson RC. Uses of Behavioral Risk Factor Surveillance System data, 1993–1997. *Am J Public Health.* 2000;90:774–776.

72. Centers for Disease Control and Prevention. Behavioral Risk Factor Surveillance System. Available at: http://www.cdc.gov/nccdphp/behavior.htm. Accessed June 9, 2001.

73. Centers for Disease Control and Prevention. Youth Risk Behavior Surveillance System. Available at: http://www.cdc.gov/nccdphp/youthris.htm. Accessed June 9, 2001.

74. Kann L, Kinchen SA, Williams BI, et al. Youth Risk Be-

havior Surveillance—United States, 1997. State and Local YRBS Coordinators. *J Sch Health.* 1998;68:355–369.

75. O'Brien T. *Office of Food Labeling, Center for Food Safety and Applied Nutrition, Food and Drug Administration. Status of Nutrition Labeling of Processed Foods: 1995 Food Label and Package Survey (FLAPS).* Washington, DC: Food and Drug Administration; 1996.

76. Brecher S. *Office of Food Labeling, Center for Food Safety and Applied Nutrition, Food and Drug Administration. Status of Serving Size in the Nutrition Labeling of Processed Foods: Food Label and Package Survey (FLAPS).* Washington, DC: Food and Drug Administration; 1997.

77. Survey Comparability Working Group. *Improving Comparability in the National Nutrition Monitoring and Related Research Program: Population Descriptors.* Hyattsville, Md: National Center for Health Statistics; 1992.

78. Wright J, Ervin B, Briefel R, eds. *Nutrition Monitoring and Tracking the Year 2000 Objectives.* Hyattsville, Md: National Center for Health Statistics; 1994.

79. Briefel RR. Assessment of the U.S. diet in national nutrition surveys: national collaborative efforts and NHANES. *Am J Clin Nutr.* 1994;59(suppl):164–167.

80. National Center for Health Statistics. *NHANES III Anthropometric Procedures* [videotape] Washington, DC: U.S. Government Printing Office; 1996. Stock Number 017–022–01335–5.

81. Landis JR, Lepkowski JM, Eklund SA, Stehouwer SA. *A Statistical Methodology for Analyzing Data from a Complex Survey: The First National Health and Nutrition Examination Survey.* Washington, DC: U.S. Government Printing Office; 1992. DHHS publication 82–1366. Vital and Health Statistics, Series 2, No. 92.

82. Forthover RN. Investigation of nonresponse bias in NHANES II. *Am J Epidemiol.* 1983;117:507–515.

83. Khare M, Mohadjer LK, Ezzati-Rice TM, Waksberg J. An evaluation of nonresponse bias in NHANES III (1988–91). *1994 Proceedings of the Section on Survey Research Methods, American Statistical Association.* 1995;2:949–954.

84. Bingham SA. The dietary assessment of individuals: methods, accuracy, new techniques, and recommendations. *Nutr Abst Rev.* 1987;57:705–742.

85. Shah BV, Barnwell BG, Bieler GS. *SUDAAN User's Manual: Software for Analysis of Correlated Data. Release 6.04.* Research Triangle Park, NC: Research Triangle Institute; 1995.

86. Westat Inc. *A User's Guide to WesVarPC.* Rockville, Md: Westat, Inc; 1996.

87. Stata Corporation. *STATA Statistical Software.* Available at: http://www.stata.com. Accessed June 10, 2001.

88. Rust KF, Rao JN. Variance estimation for complex surveys using replication techniques. *Stat Methods Med Res.* 1996;5:283–310.

89. Trowbridge FL, Wong FL, Byers TE, Serdula MK. Methodological issues in nutrition surveillance. *J Nutr.* 1990;120(suppl 11):1512–1518.

90. Rowland ML. Self-reported weight and height. *Am J Clin Nutr.* 1990;52:1125–1133.

91. Davis H, Gergen PJ. Mexican-American mothers' reports of the weights and heights of children 6 months through 11 years old. *J Am Diet Assoc.* 1994;94:512–516.

92. Gayle HD, Yip R, Frank MJ, Nieburg P, Binkin NJ. Validation of maternally reported birthweights among 46,637 Tennessee WIC program participants. *Public Health Rep.* 1988;103:143–147.

Part 6

—\\\\—

Evaluation Methods in Research

Methods to evaluate food and its intake are a cornerstone of nutrition and diabetes research. To assess intake, specialized questionnaires are commonly developed and evaluated for validity and reliability. Food composition data are critical to translate food intake to intake of specific nutrients and other food components, and biomarkers can validate intake. Underlying all, of course, is food choice, which is strongly influenced by the sensory properties of food.

Questionnaires are ubiquitous research instruments. They are used extensively in qualitative and epidemiologic research. When a new client is asked to fill out a form, it is usually a type of questionnaire. The design and construction of questionnaires are critical to their successful use. Chapter 4 discussed research errors that have a high degree of association with questionnaire formation and use. Chapter 14 presents critical issues to consider in developing, formatting, and validating questionnaires. Securing approval by the appropriate institutional review board is necessary before a questionnaire is used. Pretesting and pilot tests are invaluable because they encourage refinements in language and response options that can increase the reliability and validity of the instrument and its applicability to the specific research setting. Suggestions for administering the questionnaire and procedures to increase response rate will enhance effectiveness. Future research will likely emphasize enhanced reliability and

validity, computer questionnaire administration, incorporation of video technology, and expansion of questionnaire use to a broader range of settings.

Dietary intake data may be categorized as group data (such as national food availability data), individual data, or pooled individual data. Precision must be higher when the data are collected to characterize an individual (for example, when data are to be used to customize nutrition counseling or in correlating an individual client's intake with a serum value) than when the data will be pooled to characterize a group (for example, vegans versus omnivores). Various methods for estimating the dietary intake of individuals are clearly presented and discussed in Chapter 15. The authors point out that biomarkers, such as doubly labeled water, can be used to validate dietary intake. The important issue of underreporting is also addressed: who underreports, why underreporting occurs, and how to handle the problem. These issues are critical in collecting reliable data.

Chapter 16 delineates the wide uses of food composition data and the extensive development of databases, including several compilations of new databases for food components such as the carotenoids, flavonoids, and food contaminants. Researchers using any nutrient database are cautioned to ascertain how missing values are handled: Are they imputed, left blank, or designated as zero? The chapter provides excellent guidance on selecting a nutrient database or database system.

The emerging role of biomarkers in research is discussed in Chapter 17. Biological processes can be identified and monitored by biomarkers; thus, biomarkers can serve as indicators of dietary intake and aid in validating dietary intake assessment methods. In addition, biomarkers can quantify cellular exposure to products and by-products of dietary constituents. Biomarkers for phytochemical intake and oxidative stress are of particular interest today. Researchers will find the discussion of quality assurance for biomarker assessment of great value.

The taste, odor, and physical stimuli of food are among its great pleasures. Chapter 18 discusses evaluative methods for research on the human sensory system. In addition, critical concerns about subject selection are delineated; topics include genetic traits, smoking status, and medication use. Chemosensory function can be assessed in several ways, including threshold measurements by paired comparisons, the duo-trio test, the triangle test, and a staircase procedure. In addition, several intensity scales have been developed, including a pictorial scale of pleasure/displeasure. Research in human sensory systems has wide-ranging benefits extending from product development through food selection to clinical nutrition protocols.

ERM, Editor

14

Design and Use of Questionnaires in Research

Judy E. Perkin, Dr.P.H., R.D.

The questionnaire is an important tool in dietetics survey research, just as it is in other areas often studied using survey research techniques, such as marketing and political science. Aday (1), citing a publication of the American Statistical Association (2), has noted that the survey method of gathering data is characterized by the existence of multiple characteristics: (1) a clear focus on a topic of interest, (2) the use of questions to obtain information from individuals, (3) a defined system of data gathering, (4) a purpose related to the production of statistics summarizing and/or analyzing population responses to questions, and (5) the generation of results that can be used to make inferences or statements about populations. Questionnaires are key to survey research. Defined by Berdie et al (3[p1]) as a "series of predetermined questions," a questionnaire can provide important information about knowledge, behaviors, attitudes, beliefs, and characteristics of populations.

Survey studies using questionnaires can be either descriptive or analytic (4) and may use several design types, among them cross-sectional, group comparison, longitudinal, or experimental designs (1). Questionnaires and survey research can be used to test or develop theories (4).

Some general considerations and suggestions may be applicable to all questionnaires, but there are no hard and fast rules that apply in every situation. Each questionnaire is a product of survey design and may be unique, depending on survey factors such as population

sample, objectives, methods, timetable, and budget. This chapter provides guidance to the dietitian who wishes to use the questionnaire as a tool in research, practice, or both.

As described in this chapter, the questionnaire design process consists of four steps: (1) conceptualization, (2) construction, (3) pretesting, and (4) administration. The use of a questionnaire also involves analysis of results. Once a questionnaire has been successfully designed, implemented, and analyzed, the results may be used to affect knowledge, action, or both.

Questions or questionnaires are also evaluated as research measures using the concepts of validity and reliability. Validity involves the ability of the question to measure specified concepts appropriately (5). Reliability is an assessment of how consistently the question performs (3,5). Berdie et al (3[p3]) define a reliable question as one "that consistently conveys the same meaning to all people in the population being surveyed."

STEPS IN THE QUESTIONNAIRE DESIGN PROCESS

Questionnaire design is not a linear process. The four steps of questionnaire design described in this chapter sometimes overlap. An attempt has been made to note these overlaps as the various steps are discussed.

Conceptualization

A common problem in the questionnaire design process is lack of attention paid to conceptualization. Conceptualization should encompass (1) defining the survey objectives, (2) visualizing the questionnaire instrument needed to achieve survey objectives, and (3) anticipating the implementation strategies most likely to elicit response. Thinking through the questionnaire process to visualize how the results will be analyzed, how they will look, and how they will be used is also very important. Although conceptualization may seem time-consuming at first, it actually can conserve time and resources in the overall study process. Aday (1[p17]) has noted that "good survey design is basically a matter of good planning."

Surveys using the questionnaire as an instrument should have defined, meaningful, and measurable objectives (1). The survey design should be appropriate to the survey's objectives and the overall research purpose (1,4). Issues addressed by the questionnaire should relate to the survey objectives (4,5). Kelly and Long (4) note that questionnaire conceptualization should include a literature review on the topic of interest and, if appropriate, an exploration of the theoretical framework being tested. It is also useful to ascertain if any other previously developed questionnaires on the survey's research topic exist (6). With permission and citation, questions from these instruments may be used. The researcher might also determine that an entire existing questionnaire would be most desirable to survey the population of interest. Readers are referred to *Measuring Health: A Guide to Rating Scales and Questionnaires* (7) for an excellent overview of tested health questionnaires. Using questions from previously developed instruments or previously tested instruments in their entirety may improve the ability to compare questionnaire results with other studies.

Thinking about how the questionnaire results will be used should be part of the conceptualization. The focus should be on answers the researcher "needs to know" rather than on answers that would be "nice to know" (3). The latter kinds of answers usually are only tangential to survey objectives and often are never analyzed. They have the further disadvantage of lengthening the questionnaire. In other words, the researcher must ensure that the questionnaire is asking questions that really need to be answered to increase knowledge or decide about action.

Will the right people be asked the questions? Determining the right people to answer questions in the conceptualization stage usually involves defining respondents on the basis of one or more characteristics, such as age, gender, race, location, health status, occupation, socioeconomic status, and/or educational level. The knowledge and ability of potential respondents to answer questions should be determined (8). Assessment of ability to answer questions should take into consideration education level; literacy status; ability to recall information; language or languages spoken; and the physical ability to hear, see, speak, and write. Environmental factors related to ability are also important. Does the proposed respondent population receive mail; have telephones; have fax machines; and/or have access to, and familiarity with, computer hardware and software? Can the respondents be interviewed in their homes or at another site? What is the extent of respondent motivation to complete the questionnaire, and how can this motivation be increased? (4)

The mode of questionnaire administration (interviewer administration versus respondent self-administration) and questionnaire administration location (in person, by phone, by mail, by fax, or by computer) are just two examples of design considerations that are influenced by knowledge of respondent abilities. These and other respondent population considerations relevant to ability will be discussed later as they relate to questionnaire construction.

The number of people to survey also must be determined. Will the survey have a budget such that the entire population can be surveyed and sampling will not be necessary? If the entire population cannot be surveyed, will survey sampling be such that respondents are representative of the population of interest? (4,5,9) Sampling is addressed further in the discussion of questionnaire administration.

The conceptualization process also should include a consideration of findings concerning how people think about answering questions and ways that answers might be biased (4,9). The ideal process by which survey respondents answer questions has been described by Krosnick and others as "optimizing" (9–11). Optimizing, as outlined by Krosnick (9), broadly involves four steps: (1) question interpretation, (2) memory scanning relevant to the question, (3) integration of memory information into a single thought or "judgment," and (4) conversion of the thought into a response appropriate to the question response format and questionnaire design.

This portrayal of the steps in an ideal response scenario brings to mind steps in which the process may be compromised with less-than-desirable responses being received. For example, failure to interpret a question properly or memory lapse can lead to answers that are not desirable. Also, questionnaire respondents may "satisfice," which is defined as going through the previously described optimizing steps in a superficial manner or skipping some of the steps (9).

Questionnaire design and implementation should encourage respondents to optimize. One factor related to the promotion of optimizing is being aware of, and capitalizing on, what has been described as the potential questionnaire respondent's "need for cognition" (9,12). The need for cognition refers to an individual's desire to think, problem solve, and participate in knowledge generation (12). It is also helpful if the respondent perceives questions as being useful and important (9). Respondents who are rested and not under pressure are also more likely to optimize (9).

In addition to satisficing, other factors may contribute to responses that are not complete or accurate. These factors are frequently referred to as *response biases* (13). Response bias may be intentional or unintentional (13). Response biases include (1) answering questions in a way perceived as being socially acceptable or perhaps acceptable to a health professional, (2) answering questions in an aberrant or socially deviant fashion, and (3) answering questions by choosing responses in a random manner (13). Another much discussed response bias is acquiescence (9,13)—the term used to describe a respondent's "tendency to give positive responses . . . to a question" (13[p78]). One way to counteract this possible bias is to have an equal number of questions where responses are worded such that *yes* and *no* both have positive meanings (13). For example, on a dietary questionnaire, one could first ask a yes/no question to see if at least five servings of fruits and vegetables are eaten each day. This question could be followed by a question asking if salt is added to at least one food at most meals. In this example, *yes* is positive for a response to the first question, whereas *no* is a positive response to the second question.

In responding to questions posed as scales, another type of bias, described as "end-aversion" or "central tendency," has been described (13). Respondents exhibiting this bias tend to mark the midpoints of scale questions and avoid the scale extremes (13). One way to deal with this bias is to have the researcher put the extremes of interest within a wider scale where the extremes represent options unlikely to be chosen and the expected extremes are visually closer to the scale's middle (13). Another strategy to minimize this type of bias is to soften the wording of the labels on the end of scales. For example, Streiner and Norman (13) suggest using the term *almost always* instead of *always*.

McClendon and O'Brien (14) also suggest two principles related to respondent ability that should be considered in questionnaire design: recency and cognitive accessibility. Their recency principle states that in terms of more accurate respondent recall, recent use or thought about a piece of information is more important than when the information was acquired (14). In other words, recency of thought about a topic is more important than the time when it was first learned in terms of recall ability. The principle of cognitive accessibility states that respondents will respond with the most easily accessed information they have on a topic (14). Applying these principles in assessment of ability has definite implications for questionnaire design.

Loftus et al (15) have studied the ability of persons to remember health-related events. These researchers found that people tend to report having had more specific procedures than can be documented by a medical record check but report fewer visits to a health clinic than actually occurred (15). These researchers found that asking patients to recall information starting with the most recent time and then recalling back in time progressively (most recent to earliest) was helpful in reducing errors (15).

Conceptualization involves general thoughts about (1) the scope and content of relevant survey questions, (2) the appropriate population to be asked these questions, (3) the best means of asking the questions to minimize bias, and (4) ways to ask questions that obtain accurate and thoughtful responses. Conceptualization also involves thought about how to achieve a high response rate. The process involves thinking about the survey and its questionnaire prior to the questionnaire construction.

Construction

The construction step in questionnaire design is complex and involves consideration of numerous factors, including mode of questionnaire administration and receiving responses, question development, response formats and options, question order and placement, questionnaire length, questionnaire format and appearance, identification of questionnaire respondents, methods of answer tabulation and questionnaire analysis, procedures for increasing response rate, and review by the relevant institutional review board or boards. The budget and timetable for a survey research project will have considerable influence on questionnaire construction.

Mode of Questionnaire Administration and Receiving Responses

An important initial design consideration is whether the questionnaire is to be administered by an interviewer or completed by the respondent (5). Decisions also need to be made regarding the questionnaire administration technologies to be used by interviewers or respondents. These technologies could range from paper and pencil to computers or facsimile machines. If the respondent is to complete the questionnaire, decisions also need to be made regarding the mode of response. The response mode is often, but not always, the same mode employed in administration (16). For example, respondents could receive a questionnaire by mail but be requested to return it via mail or fax (16). The use of multiple technologies may permit more respondents to be reached, and response may be facilitated by allowing respondents to use the technology perceived as most convenient. Wilkins et al (17) reported an increased response rate by using telephone interviews to follow up on nonrespondents to a questionnaire first sent by mail.

Interviews offer the following advantages, as described by Bailey (5): (1) flexibility, or the ability to repeat, probe, and make on-site distinctions about question appropriateness; (2) higher response rate; (3) the ability to standardize and control the environment (including the ability to record the time of the answer); (4) the ability to control question order; (5) the ability to observe nonverbal behavior; (6) the ability to record the first answer of a respondent; (7) the assurance that only the designated respondent answers the questions; and (8) an enhanced ability to ensure that all questions are answered. Bailey (5) also suggests that a more complex questionnaire (one with detailed instructions, multiple areas to be skipped, and many charts) may be better handled by interview. Interviews also may be the only option for questionnaire administration if a respondent population is illiterate, semiliterate, or physically disabled to the extent that questionnaire self-administration is difficult or impossible.

The option of completion of the questionnaire by the respondent also has its own advantages, among them (1) cost (the interview format entails more labor costs); (2) speed (enhanced ability to administer questionnaires simultaneously to large numbers of subjects); (3) greater convenience for the respondent; (4) potential ability for respondents to remain anonymous; (5) ability to standardize wording completely; (6) ability to allow for the respondent to consult, review records, or conduct research as part of the answer process; and (7) greater accessibility to respondents with regard to both numbers and location (5). A further advantage of the self-administered questionnaire is that it excludes the possibility of interviewer bias or error (5). Bailey (5) includes a full discussion of considerations involved in making the decision related to interviewer or respondent questionnaire completion.

Computers are increasingly becoming involved in both questionnaires completed by an interviewer and questionnaires completed by the respondent Computer involvement may take many forms, including computer-assisted personal interviews (CAPI), computer-assisted telephone interviews (CATI), and computer-assisted self-administered interviewing (CASAI) (1). CAPI involves the use of computer-programmed interview questions so that an interviewer can transport and use a computer to complete a face-to-face interview (1). CATI involves having a program for the telephone interviewer to input answers (1). In CASAI, the respondents themselves enter answers into the computer (1). One study has noted that CASAI may be particularly helpful in trying to obtain sensitive information from members of populations who may feel more comfortable with computers, such as adolescents (18).

Computer questionnaire administration may also be more cost-effective and less restrictive in terms of hours available for subject response (5). Other cited advantages of using a computerized questionnaire are fewer skipped questions and more responses being given within stated ranges (5). Computerized questionnaires, however, may not be appropriate if the technology is inaccessible or if persons expected to use the computer are not computer literate (5). Also, some individuals may feel that computers are less private and may be less willing to reveal sensitive information in answering a questionnaire on the computer.

Survey research and questionnaire administration can also be accomplished using e-mail or the World Wide Web (19–28). These forms of administration have the advantage of speed of delivery and may allow respondent replies to come back more quickly (20,26). One study found that e-mail questionnaire responses were more quickly received than responses to mailed questionnaires (26). Fischbacher et al (20), however, note that although individuals may respond more quickly by e-mail, the total time period needed to achieve a desirable response rate may not differ from the time required for questionnaires to be returned by mail. It has been found that e-mail may not yield more total responses than mailed surveys (21,22,26). In populations who frequently use e-mail, however, response rates via e-mail might be higher (26). Eley and Lean (19) used an e-mail questionnaire to survey university students about their eating habits. Taulois-Braga and Marcenes (25) used an e-mail questionnaire to collect information from students related to their attitudes toward, and knowledge about, sugar (7). Schaefer and Dillman (23) and Dillman (28) outline a recommended methodology for e-mail questionnaires that includes sending individual, personalized e-mails; using a short cover letter; and making the questionnaire column width 70 characters or less (23,28).

E-mail questionnaires have potential problems. For some surveys, the desired respondents may not have access to e-mail (28). Fischbacher et al (20) note that researchers must be extremely carefully to ensure that e-mail addresses are correct to avoid an excessive number of nondeliverable messages. It may be desirable to program e-mail software to confirm e-mail receipt (20). E-mail usually provides limited design options, particularly if the researchers send the questionnaire as part of the text of an e-mail message (20). Incompatible word-processing software may also make e-mail questionnaire attachments impossible for the respondent to read (20).

E-mail text and attachments can be easily forwarded and may lead to response by individuals not in the original sample population (20). Lack of confidentiality in e-mail response may also be a problem, because e-mail typically identifies the sender. Fischbacher et al (20) and Dillman (28) report that confidentiality can be maintained if respondents remove identifiers from an e-mail survey and then return the survey by another means, such as mail or fax. Researchers using an e-mail questionnaire should keep an accurate listing of all e-mail addresses to which questionnaires were sent and from which they were received to have an appropriate denominator for response rate calculation (20).

Some studies have placed questionnaires on the World Wide Web (20,21,24,28). This practice can potentially generate a large number of responses (27). Web surveys may also be cost-effective (24). One study found that the cost of a Web-based survey was 38 percent less than a comparable mail survey (24).

Just as with other survey modes, there are disadvantages associated with use of the World Wide Web. A major concern to date has been the fact that only those individuals with Internet access can be reached (27). Differences in computer hardware and software may make it difficult for a potential respondent to view the questionnaire (28). Calculation of response rate is also a concern (20). The response rate for Web questionnaires

may be impossible to calculate unless access to the questionnaire is given to only a defined population via the use of passwords (28). Some researchers have also calculated Web-based questionnaire response rates using an approximated number of potential respondents based on review of what were viewed as appropriate databases (20). The use of one-time passwords for Web-based surveys may be important (27). Wyatt (27) notes that if this type of control is not in place, there is a potential for an individual respondent to complete the questionnaire numerous times.

One study examining health practices of employees compared return rates and costs associated with a mail survey, an e-mail survey, and use of the World Wide Web (21). Mail surveys yielded the highest response (72 percent) when compared with e-mail (34 percent) and the World Wide Web (19 percent) (21). Use of regular mail, however, was associated with the greatest cost (21). Refinement of technology and increased access to the Internet are likely to make electronic methods of surveying more popular in the future.

Question Development

Once the mode of administration has been chosen, the dietetics researcher or practitioner can make decisions about the language or languages to be used. These considerations should include not only the use of foreign languages along with or instead of English, but also the need to use Braille, sign language, or other language forms appropriate to the defined respondent population. Another important consideration in question development involves the selection of appropriate reading levels for all questionnaire words, particularly for health-related terms. For example, given the defined respondent population, would *bedsores* or *decubitus ulcers* be the most appropriate term? Will respondents understand the meaning of words such as *delineate* or *verify?* Readability (or comprehension level) can be estimated through a variety of formulas, including the SMOG formula (29,30), the FOG index (31), the Lorge and Flesch readability formula (32), the Cloze procedure (33), and the Flesch-Kincaid formula (34). Computer programs that assess readability may also be available (34).

It is important to remember that questions should be relevant to the research objectives and to respondents (5). Once drafted, questions should be referenced to research objectives. Ideas for research-appropriate questions may come directly from the researcher or the research team or may come from ideas generated by content experts, focus groups, or persons knowledgeable about the respondent population (1,6,13).

Dillman (28) recommends phrasing questions as complete sentences rather than as words or sentence fragments. If appropriate and necessary, multiple questionnaires can be tailored to specific characteristics of the respondent population (for example, male/female, patient/caregiver, vegetarian/omnivore) (5). Another commonly used technique to make questions relevant is to construct contingency or skip questions, such as "If you answer no, proceed to Question 4" (5).

Care should be taken to avoid double-barreled questions (5,13,28). A double-barreled question is a question worded so that it includes two questions, such as "Do you like milk and ice cream?" If the respondent answers no, the researcher or practitioner might conclude that neither food is liked, when the respondent is actually answering that he or she does not like the combination or that he or she likes one food but not the other. The use of double-barreled questions is a common mistake (5,13,28) that poses problems for both the respondent and questionnaire analyst.

Another consideration in the construction of questions is the attempt to minimize ambiguity (3,5). One solution is to provide definitions of terms in the questionnaire instrument. For example, terms such as *rural, urban,* and *poor* are subjective and need to be defined. Sentences also may be ambiguous. A poorly written, ambiguous question composed by this author for a diet-related questionnaire was "Do you read food labels?" To dietitians, this question usually means reading the portions of the food label listing ingredients and nutrition information. Most respondents, however, interpreted this question to mean "Do you read the front of the label?" or "If you wish to purchase corn, do read the front of the label and check that it says *corn?*" The question is ambiguous.

Question length also needs to be considered (1). In the past, questionnaire writers have been advised to make questions as short as possible (1). This advice probably continues to be good in most circumstances, but some research indicates that in some cases a longer question may generate a better response (1). The postulated rationale for the better response is that the respondent may have more time to think and more information to think about if a question is longer (1).

Wording questions to avoid "leading" is a good general practice (5,35). Leading questions are ones that encourage or suggest an answer to a question and put the onus on the respondent if he or she wishes to deviate from the subtly prompted response. An example of a leading question that inappropriately suggests an answer is "You don't binge, do you?" (5) The respondent may hesitate to admit to this behavior, so the hidden suggested response is no. An alternative question that may be helpful is "How often do you binge?" (5) The respondent could respond with "never" but potentially would feel comfortable responding with a number.

Double negatives should be avoided in questions because they are confusing (8,28,35). An example of a question using a double negative is "Do you favor or oppose passage of a USDA regulation not allowing food stamps to be used to purchase peanut butter?"

Another rule of questionnaire construction is that in general, factual questions are better than abstract questions (5). For example, "How would you rate your overall diet—good, fair, poor?" is a difficult questions for a respondent to answer. The answer is also difficult for the investigator to interpret. The concept of "overall diet" is unclear: is this diet throughout the life span or for 1 year? The rating scale is also both abstract and subjective. One person's "fair" may be another person's "good."

If possible, questions that heavily rely on memory should be avoided. Responses may not be accurate, or respondents may choose to not answer the question at all (24). Dillman (28) also recommends that it is best if respondents are not asked to perform calculations. Again, such questions may lead to inaccurate responses through either miscalculations or poor estimates (28).

Two excellent resources for additional information on question construction can be found on the World Wide Web: *How to Write A Good Survey* (35) and *Questionnaire Design and Analysis: A Workbook by Alison Galloway* (36). Readers are also referred to Chapter 2 in Dillman's *Mail and Internet Surveys: The Tailored Design Format* (28). Aday (1) provides specific guidance related to formulating questions about health.

In some instances, dietitians may be faced with translating a questionnaire in one language to another language. If so, experts advise that the translated instrument achieve semantic, conceptual, and normative equivalence (37). Semantic equivalence involves the maintenance of question meaning (37). Conceptual equivalence involves ensuring that the question invokes thoughts about similar constructs in both languages (37). Normative equivalence means ensuring that the translation is accompanied by consideration of cultural norms (37). Attention to this latter concept should ensure that questions are perceived as both respectful and appropriate.

Response Formats and Options

The response format needs to be addressed when constructing questions. The two major response formats categorize questions as either open ended or closed ended (5,36). The response format to an open-ended question is not specified, whereas the response format to a close-ended question is specified (5,36). Some questionnaires include both types of response formats, whereas others use only one type. Study or survey goals, budget, analytic capabilities, and timetables all influence the choice of response format.

Both major response format types have advantages and disadvantages. Open-ended questions, for example, may be useful in preliminary survey work when the researcher does not know all possible answers or believes that all answers cannot be anticipated (11). Responses from an initial open-ended question may later give the researcher more confidence in constructing a closed-ended question on the topic (11). Another potential advantage to the use of open-ended questions is that they can be helpful when the number of potential responses is large (5). For example, asking "What vegetables do you eat more than three times per week?" and leaving a blank space for a response would be simpler than listing all potential vegetables that could be cited. In this case, the use of an open-ended question also shortens questionnaire response time for the respondent. Another advantage of the open-ended question is that it can allow for creativity, complexity, and clarity in response (5). Galloway (36) gives examples of creative ways that open-ended questions may be constructed. Two examples cited by Galloway (36) are asking respondents to associate words or asking respondents to tell a story based on provided information. Some respondents may feel more assured that they have answered a question more accurately and may appreciate the chance to express themselves in a way that is not structured by the researcher (5). In a recent review of survey research techniques, Krosnick (9) supports the usefulness, as well as the reliability and validity of, appropriately used open-ended questions.

One potential disadvantage of an open-ended question is that it may not truly reflect a response, because persons with better writing skills are at some advantage when faced with this type of question (5). Geer (38) states, however, that subject interest is a more important factor than writing ability in generating a good open-ended response. Other cited drawbacks of open-ended questions relate to potentially increased costs with use,

coding difficulties (38), and collection of irrelevant information (5). Open-ended responses may also be difficult to read (5). Open-ended questions may be perceived as too time-consuming or laborious by some potential respondents (5). Researchers choosing to use open-ended questions in dietetics research may wish to consult with a sociologist or statistician trained in techniques for coding open-ended questions. The use of specified procedures can increase the reliability of coding open-ended questions (39).

Closed-ended questions have their own set of advantages (5). Responses are in standard categories and are easier to code and analyze (5). Responses are usually relevant to the questions as defined by the intent of the persons constructing the questionnaire (5). Respondents may be able to ascertain question intent more easily if they see response categories (5). Another important advantage of the closed-ended question is that some respondents may perceive this question type as simpler to answer (5).

Disadvantages of closed-ended questions include possible guessing or random responses, inability or unwillingness of a respondent to answer within categories provided, and the possibility of forcing choices and therefore not describing or seeing the potential true level of response variation in the respondent population (5,36).

Open-ended questions usually are followed by a blank space for a response (5,36). The response formats for closed-ended questions fall into one of several types, depending on elicited response content: interval, ratio, nominal, and ordinal (1,5). An interval response is a response that is ordered and for which it is assumed that there is equality among all ranks and no set zero point (1,5). An example of an interval response is degrees measuring temperature (1). A ratio response is similar to an interval response, but there is a set zero point (1,5). An example is the number of beverages consumed per day (1). A nominal response is a response that is discrete (nonoverlapping) and nonnumerical (5). An example of a nominal response is "male" or "female" (1). An ordinal response format uses rank-ordered categories (such as "excellent," "good," "fair," and "poor") and therefore has a directional meaning (1,5). In constructing closed-ended responses, all potential answers should be included in an uncluttered fashion, and all potential answers should have a clear meaning (5).

For interval and ratio responses, all potential responses can be listed; for reasons of both space and utility, however, interval and ratio responses are more commonly grouped (5). An example is income response categories (5). Response categories should not overlap (5,28,36).

Nominal responses are generally formatted with a blank or box to be checked or crossed (5). Assigning a number to a nominal response and requesting that the number be circled is another option (5). Nominal response categories are most frequently listed one above another, but side-by-side placement can be used with appropriate spacing, dots, or parentheses (5). Berdie and associates (3) recommend vertical over horizontal placement, because respondents sometimes mark blanks incorrectly when they are not sure if they are to mark before or after their desired response. Dillman (28) recommends making nominal response categories mutually exclusive, if at all possible. It is important to list all possible nominal responses (5). If there are too many possible responses, respondents may be asked to check "other" and then write their response.

Some categories of responses are nonnumerical but potentially not mutually exclusive (3). Use of "other" or "none of the above" as responses or having the respondent check all that apply may be helpful in these instances (3). An example is asking about dietary supplement use, which is nonnumerical and not mutually exclusive because respondents may take more than one supplement at a time. It may be useful to mark all that apply in terms of questionnaire-listed supplements taken and then to have respondents list "others" if supplements are taken that are not on the questionnaire (40).

Ordinal response categories may be formatted similarly to nominal categories (boxes or blanks to be checked or numbers to be circled), but they also may be shown as a continuum labeled at each end (5). Care must be taken in designing the scoring or labeling system for a continuum. Too few categories may not distinguish these differences among respondents, but too many categories can be confusing (5). Berdie and associates (3) recommend that an equal number of options be placed on each side of the midpoint. Streiner and Norman (13) argue that both an even or odd number of options on a continuum may be appropriate. They indicate that an odd number may allow the respondent to state no opinion, but an even number forces the respondent to one side of the continuum (13). One example of an ordinal scale is the Likert scale, where the response continuum provides various levels of agreement and disagreement (7,36).

One issue pertinent to all categories of response is whether to include such options as "don't know," "no opinion," and "can't decide." Berdie et al (3) recommend

inclusion of the "don't know" option rather than risk the chance of obtaining incorrect information by forced choice. Poe and colleagues (41) recommend that "don't know" not be included as a potential response to factual questions. In analyzing pretest results from a mortality survey conducted under the auspices of the National Center for Health Statistics, these researchers found that the exclusion of the "don't know" option resulted in a greater number of usable responses without altering the substance of responses (41). They also noted that exclusion of the "don't know" option made their questionnaire less cluttered and slightly shorter (41).

Another issue to be considered when asking questions about frequency and magnitude of dietary intake is whether the options as constructed could lead to underreporting or overreporting (42). Research on questionnaire use with alcoholics, for example, indicates that providing response options indicative of greater intake and frequency than might be expected are most effective in avoiding the problem of underreporting (43). Chapter 13 includes a thorough discussion of the concepts and research related to reporting of dietary intake.

Question Order and Placement

Once questions and response categories have been formulated and formatted, the process of determining question placement or question ordering can begin. Potential respondent views on question placement should be assessed in the pretesting phase. Some groups may prefer placement of easy-to-answer demographic questions first, whereas other respondent populations may prefer to answer substantive research questions first and provide demographic information later (44). Respondents should perceive that questions are in a logical order (44). The following are some additional suggestions for question placement:

- Sensitive or difficult questions should be placed close to the end of the questionnaire. Respondents may be more likely to answer sensitive questions if they have already taken the time to complete other parts of the questionnaire (5).
- Transitional phases or visual distinctions should be provided between content sections (3).
- Important items should not be placed last on the questionnaire, as they may be overlooked or left unanswered (3).
- The question-numbering system should be clear (3).

Questionnaire Length

At this point, the investigator should assess the appropriateness of questionnaire length. Questions should be reviewed again for relevance to study objectives. In general, the longer the questionnaire, the more costly it will be in terms of supplies, resources, and time. It is thus important to ensure that all information requested is needed and will be used. Although the effect of questionnaire length on response rate is debatable (44), it seems reasonable that there would be a length limit beyond which persons would fail to respond. Interest value of a questionnaire (3) and maintaining respondent motivation (44) may be more important than questionnaire length in determining response.

Questionnaire Format and Appearance

Berdie and associates (3) make the following suggestions regarding visual appearance and enhancement of design for self-administered questionnaires:

- Instructions should be concise and clear. Better yet, if a change in question wording can eliminate the need for instructions, the question should be changed. (Galloway [36] suggests that instructions be presented in upper case.)
- The areas where answers are to be marked should be as close to the questions as possible.
- The term *questionnaire* should not appear on the form itself. The term may have a bad connotation if a respondent has previously received badly designed questionnaires.
- The word *over* should be included at the bottom of the front side of a two-sided form.
- Too many questions should not be placed on one page, as it would create a crowded appearance.
- If the questionnaire is to be mailed, a name and return address should be printed directly on the questionnaire. This advice is useful even when a self-addressed return envelope is included, because the envelope may be misplaced or lost.

Another design consideration for the self-administered questionnaire is paper color. The use of colored paper may be helpful in increasing response by making the questionnaire more noticeable to the respondent (44–46). Berdie et al (3) also recommend that printing and paper for questionnaires be of the best quality possible within the limits of the study budget. Investigators need

to convince respondents of the quality of their studies, and respondents may be influenced by these visual cues.

There are also design considerations unique to questionnaire forms that are to be used in an interview setting. Berdie and colleagues (3) suggest the following:

- Different type styles or some distinctive device should be used to separate parts of the questionnaire to be read to the respondent from parts not to be read to the respondent.
- Questions should be printed only on the front of pages.
- Sufficient instructions should be provided to interviewers to allow them to proceed in the desired question sequence. These instructions are particularly important if a questionnaire includes skip or contingency questions.
- Enough space should be allowed on the form so that the interviewer may record pertinent additional information.
- Response options should be limited to a number that the respondent can easily remember.
- The interview should end with a closed-ended, rather than an open-ended, question. This technique will help the interviewer close the interview.

Identification of Questionnaire Respondents

A design consideration for the self-administered questionnaire is whether respondents are to be anonymous or identified (36). Bailey (5) believes that unless knowledge of identity is important to ensure response clarity, allowing respondents to be anonymous is the best decision. Anonymity, as defined by Bailey (5[p168]), is when "the researcher is unable to link the respondent with the questionnaire he or she answered." If follow-up while assuring anonymity is desired, Bailey (5[p168]) states that a note worded as follows may be sent to all potential respondents: "If you have already mailed your questionnaire, please disregard this notice. We have no means of identifying respondents, as all replies are anonymous. Thus, we are sending this reminder to all, since we have no way of knowing whether or not you have responded already."

Another relatively inexpensive alternative is to instruct respondents to return a separate postcard listing their names and addresses after completing and returning the questionnaire (5). Both Bailey (5) and Berdie et al (3) advise against techniques such as writing identification numbers in invisible ink, because this attempt to hide responses that can be linked to specific respondents may be considered unethical (5).

Not all researchers in the area of questionnaire design have found that anonymity increases response rate or influences response. Fuller (47), for example, found little difference between respondent answers in anonymous versus identity-known situations. Identifying participants in some manner also helps readily identify those who need follow-up. Researchers should keep in mind that confidentiality can be maintained even if respondents are not anonymous to the researcher. A system of code numbers linked to name on only one document kept by the researcher is one method (5). Indication in a cover letter that only aggregate information will be used for publication or report purposes also aids in maintaining confidentiality for individual respondents (16).

Methods of Answer Tabulation and Questionnaire Analysis

It is important in the question construction phase to consider how results will be tabulated and analyzed. There are ways to construct questionnaires and collect answers that can make tabulation and analysis easier. An example would be to provide respondents with a written questionnaire but have answers recorded on a form that could be read by a scanning machine (16). Some questionnaires can be constructed so that answers on the questionnaire form itself can be scanned and then tabulated and analyzed by a software program (1). World Wide Web-based questionnaires and scanned questionnaires can also be constructed so that answers are immediately placed in a statistical analysis program (1,27). If the researcher has to read and translate answers into another format for tabulation and analysis, great care should to be taken to ensure that answers are not changed in the process. Electronic spreadsheets may be useful for initial tabulation prior to statistical analysis, but where there is a large amount of answer data, scanning technology or direct input of responses into a statistical analysis package may be more appropriate (1,16). Aday (1[p344]) provides a useful model for planning questionnaire analysis and gives excellent suggestions for identifying and correcting problems with questionnaire data prior to analysis. To summarize, attention to plans for tabulation and data analysis may influence questionnaire construction in ways that can save time and increase accuracy.

Procedures to Increase Response Rate

Achieving a good (or high) response rate is a major goal of questionnaires. Response rate calculation should be defined prior to questionnaire administration and when reporting results (48). Kviz (48) suggests that response rate is defined as C/E, where C is the number of completed questionnaires and E is the number of persons sampled by the questionnaire. Even this definition is problematic, however, because all questions on a questionnaire might not be answered, and how one defines the population sampled is not always clear (48). For instance, do questionnaires returned for incorrect addresses count as mailed questionnaires? The best course is for the researcher to both define and report response rate in research reports (48).

The definition of an adequate response rate to a questionnaire is not absolute. Obviously, the higher the response rate the better, because a greater representation of the population is achieved. Some researchers define a 50 percent response rate as adequate (5), whereas others seek a rate of more than 90 percent (5). Mailed surveys are more likely to have response rates in the 30 percent to 50 percent range, whereas interviews typically yield response rates of more than 70 percent (49). Informed consent may affect response rate if sensitive issues are being surveyed.

King et al (44) identify several factors that appear to increase response rate to mailed questionnaires: (1) inclusion of a stamped return envelope with first-class postage, (2) mentioning of a sponsor perceived positively by respondents, and (3) use of monetary or other incentives. The use of incentives to increase response rate has been extensively studied (44). It must always be examined in light of the cost versus benefit gained in increased response rate (44). King et al,(44) in reviewing numerous studies regarding the use of incentives, found that monetary incentives ranging from $0.25 to $40 have been reported to increase response rate from 7.3 percent to 33.3 percent. Parkes et al (50) have reported that a cash incentive was superior to the use of an enclosed information brochure. Baron et al (51) found that offering the chance to participate in a lottery increased the response rate by slightly more than 5 percent but yielded an increased cost of $16 (Canadian) per returned questionnaire.

Delivery of mailed questionnaires by overnight courier service may increase response rate (52). Kasprzyk et al (52) found that physicians were more likely respond to their survey on sexually transmitted diseases when overnight courier service delivery was combined with a $25 monetary incentive.

The effect of mailing variables on response rate has also been studied. Groves and Olsson (53) found that using an adhesive return address label for some populations may produce a more cost-effective response rate than using a stamped return envelope. Becker and colleagues (54) compared the effectiveness of sending a postcard versus a second questionnaire to nonrespondents. The second questionnaire strategy did increase response rate but also was more expensive (54). Follow-up letters, postcards, or calls can increase response rates to mailed questionnaires (28). A follow-up letter to a nonrespondent can include another copy of the questionnaire.

Review of the Questionnaire by an Institutional Review Board

Another consideration prior to questionnaire design administration is obtaining approval from the appropriate institutional review board dealing with human subjects. Some boards may require that participants sign a consent form before the questionnaire is administered. In some instances, boards may decide that completion of the questionnaire after the purpose is explained denotes implied consent. Use of a questionnaire is a form of human research and requires appropriate review. Researchers should also be aware that questionnaires mailed to another institution for distribution will most likely need to be reviewed again by the appropriate secondary institutional review board. Multiple institutional review is also usually needed if researchers are representatives of more than one institution (16).

Pretesting

The third step in the questionnaire process is the pretesting phase. Pretesting ideally should be conducted with persons typical of the respondent population in order to assess face validity, as well as with experts who are qualified to make assessments about content validity (7). These validity concepts will be discussed in more detail later in this chapter. Persons typical of the respondent population can provide information related to question wording and interpretation (28). Content experts can provide information about question comprehensiveness and appropriateness (28). They also can provide feedback on how survey questions might be better formulated to relate to the existing body of knowledge (28).

It may be helpful to have respondents or the interviewer record the amount of time taken to complete the questionnaire. An estimate of the time needed to complete the questionnaire can help provide respondents with knowledge needed to give informed consent (40). Questionnaires should be pretested using the mode of administration specified for the final questionnaire (5).

Krosnick (9) has reviewed additional types of pre-

testing, which may be considered. One is "cognitive pretesting," in which researchers listen as respondents verbalize their thoughts when answering questions (9). A method that may be used to pretest interviews involves an observer recording interactions between interviewers and respondents and noting any potential problems in question cognition or response (9).

Clues to problems in questionnaire design and construction that may become apparent in the pretesting phase include a large number of nonresponses not attributable to contingency or skip questions, a pattern of small variation in response, many responses given with qualifications, and responses perceived as meaningless (5). These clues need to be examined critically to determine if they are indicative of problem areas. Hunt and associates (55) report that pretests are particularly useful in detecting missing alternate responses.

Once the questionnaire has been pretested, the designer needs to review the results and make appropriate changes in question wording, response categories, question order, instructions (including definitions), and questionnaire length. If major changes are made at this point, the revised questionnaire also should be pretested to ensure that the appropriate changes were made (11,28).

Administration

Questionnaire Introduction

Respondents need to have an introduction to a questionnaire. In a mailed survey this is accomplished in a cover letter (5,28,44). Information can also be given to potential respondents verbally, in a written information sheet, in an e-mail message, or in a survey introduction placed on the World Wide Web (20,23,28).

The introduction should explain the survey objectives, as well as respondent benefits and risks relative to questionnaire completion (5). Information should also be given about institutional sponsorship and how the information will be used (44). Potential respondents need to be informed about whether their responses will be identifiable and if so, in what way (44). If responses are not collected anonymously, how respondent confidentiality will be maintained is important to address. Information concerning the desired timing of questionnaire response may be included in the introduction. The respondents should also be given the names of the researchers and researcher contact information, including mailing address, telephone number, fax number, and e-mail address.

Population Sampling

Another critical administration step, which has already been mentioned, is sampling or administering the survey to persons determined to be representative of the population. (In some instances, it may be possible to survey the entire population of interest, but this is usually not the case.) When the entire population cannot be surveyed, probability sampling methods, such as simple randomization, stratified randomization, systemic randomization, and cluster sampling, can be used (1). Krosnick (9) has noted that the use of probability sampling reduces the importance of response rate. He asserts that if probability sampling is used, even if a low response rate is achieved, the questionnaire results may still be representative of the population (9). Some researchers have used a sampling technique known as *snowballing* to administer questionnaires (5). This technique can be a method of probability or nonprobability sampling (5,56). It involves using initially selected respondents to identify other respondents. This process can continue until the desired number of respondents has been identified (5). Etter and Perneger (56) report success in using the snowballing technique in surveys concerning smoking attitudes and behaviors.

Considerations Unique to Modes of Administration

Special considerations involved in mail and electronic modes of administration of questionnaires (e-mail and the World Wide Web) have been addressed. A fax machine is another mode of administration. It can be used to send questionnaires, return questionnaires, or both and may be a good way to contact persons in businesses or organizations (1).

An interview format presents unique considerations in terms of administration. Completion of an interview questionnaire involves contacting the respondent and conducting the interview. The questionnaire designers must understand the respondent population in order to facilitate the contact process (3). For example, the questionnaire designer must be aware of the language of the target population as well its demographic, cultural, and socioeconomic profile. The purpose of the interview and other information that would be conveyed in a cover letter accompanying a mailed survey must be reviewed verbally upon respondent contact (3,57).

Using an interview questionnaire usually means selecting, training, and supervising interviewers (57). Detailed aspects of these processes are reviewed by van Kammen and Stouthamer-Loeber (57). Aspects they discuss include the establishment of training sessions and the development of a training manual (57). They also provide tips to ensure that interviewers understand and adhere to study protocols (57).

Frank and associates (58) recommend interviewer training when using the 24-hour dietary recall for research purposes. Their report emphasizes the importance of interviewers being familiar with, and consistent in, the use of criteria for naming foods, recording food quantities consumed, and coding foods (58). These researchers recommend conducting duplicate recalls as a quality assurance technique (58).

Telephone interviewing is a technique being explored for dietary questionnaire administration (59,60). Krantzler et al (60) report that the telephone interview can obtain dietary information similar in quality to the information obtained in a personal interview. Lyu et al (61) have also reported that telephone interviews can be effective for obtaining food frequency information. The use of premailed photographs showing portion sizes can help increase the accuracy of telephone food frequency interviews. A new development in the field of telephone surveying is the potential to use an automated system, which can administer surveys 24 hours a day via the use of a toll-free number (62). Computerized interviewing, which was discussed earlier in this chapter, is another option for interview administration (1).

Dietitians may administer questionnaires in a way not typically discussed in social science methodology texts. For example, questionnaires may be distributed in a clinic or educational setting to be completed by the respondents and returned on site. In these cases, the cover letter may be attached to the front of the questionnaire or read aloud to the respondent or respondents. This form of administration combines many of the advantages of the interview and the self-administered questionnaire. Knowledge of population literacy and vocabulary still remain important design issues. Having writing instruments on site will facilitate response.

Maintaining and Monitoring Responses

Unless responses are automatically entered into a database, consideration needs to be given to how responses will be recorded and maintained prior to analysis. For example, a file or location should be designated to store completed questionnaires, and returned questionnaires need to be noted on a listing of all questionnaires that have been sent.

EVALUATION OF QUESTIONS AND THE QUESTIONNAIRE

As mentioned previously, questionnaires are typically evaluated in terms of their validity, and they may also be evaluated for reliability. Assessment of validity is addressed in various phases of the questionnaire process. Question validity is usually approached according to face validity (6,7), content validity (1,6,7), criterion validity (1), and/or construct validity (1). Face validity is defined by research judgment and is an assessment of whether the question truly measures a behavior, attitude, or opinion (1,6,7). Stanton et al (6) report that face validity can be assessed via health professional review and focus groups.

Content validity determines whether the instrument measures content relative to study objectives (1). Content validity can be assessed in a variety of ways, such as literature review, researcher observation, health professional review, and focus group discussion with potential respondents (6).

Criterion validity involves measuring the question against "the truth" derived by an already accepted measure (1,7). Criterion validity is measured through computation of correlation coefficients and the measures of sensitivity and specificity (1).

Assessment of construct validity involves specifying a theory and examining how well a questionnaire instrument provides data that supports the theory and correlates or fits with data generated by other instruments that support the theory (5,7).

Reliability measures look at the consistency of questions in generating information (5). Assessment of reliability requires that the questionnaire be administered at least once, and in some instances more than once (5). Numerous statistical formulas can be used to test reliability, depending on data type (nominal, ordinal, or interval) (1). Examples include the Kuder-Richardson (1), Spearman rank correlation (ρ), Cronbach α, and κ statistic formulas (1).

ANALYSIS OF QUESTIONNAIRES AND USE OF RESULTS

The analysis of questionnaires involves consideration of how results are to be tabulated and then how information can be analyzed statistically. As discussed previously, both these aspects should be considered when the questionnaire is being conceptualized and constructed. Failure to specify tabulation and statistical methodology prior to data collection can lead to an inability to use or analyze information. Care should be taken in reporting questionnaire results to accurately reflect the results of analysis. Tables, charts, or graphs may be useful in reporting questionnaire results.

Questionnaire results can provide important information for policy makers and decision makers, as well as for researchers. Questionnaire results may provide knowledge that has an effect on the management of food-service operations (63,64), clinical nutrition practice (63,65,66), or community nutrition programming and service delivery (67,68). Questionnaire or survey research can set the stage for the development of nutrition laboratory research or clinical randomized trials (69). Questionnaires can also be useful in determining practice knowledge and attitudes related to nutrition education effects (70,71). Dietitians may also find questionnaires useful to measure other health-related measures, such as stage of change (72–74), locus of control (75,76), and self-efficacy (76,77). When appropriately constructed, administered, and analyzed, questionnaires can advance knowledge and provide the framework for constructive action.

REFERENCES

1. Aday LA. *Designing and Conducting Health Surveys: A Comprehensive Guide*. San Francisco, Calif: Jossey-Bass Publishers; 1996.
2. American Statistical Association. *What Is a Survey?* Washington, DC: American Statistical Association; 1995.
3. Berdie DR, Anderson JF, Niebuhr MA. *Questionnaires: Design and Use*. Metuchen, NJ: The Scarecrow Press; 1986.
4. Kelly B, Long A. The design and execution of social surveys. *Nurse Res*. 2000;8:69–83. Also available at: http://proquest.umi.com/pqdweb. Accessed April 24, 2001.
5. Bailey KD. *Methods of Social Research*. New York, NY: The Free Press; 1994.
6. Stanton WR, Willis M, Balanda KP. Development of an instrument for monitoring adolescent health issues. *Health Educ Res*. 2000;15: 181–190.
7. McDowell I, Newell C. *Measuring Health- A Guide to Rating Scales and Questionnaires*. New York, NY: Oxford University Press; 1996.
8. Sheatsley PB. Questionnaire construction and item writing. In: Rossi PH, Wright JD, Anderson AB, eds. *Handbook of Survey Research*. Orlando, Fla: Academic Press; 1983:195–230.

9. Krosnick JA. Survey research. *Annu Rev Psychol.* 1999;50:537–567.

10. Sudman S, Bradburn NM, Schwarz N. *Thinking about Answers: The Application of Cognitive Processes to Survey Methodology.* San Francisco, Calif: Jossey-Bass Publishers; 1996.

11. Tourangeau R, Rips L, Rasinski K. *The Psychology of Survey Response.* Cambridge, England: Cambridge University Press; 2000.

12. Cacioppo JT, Petty RE, Feinstein JA, Jarvis WBG. Dispositional differences in cognitive motivation: the life and times of individuals varying in need for cognition. *Psychol Bull.* 1996;119:197–253.

13. Streiner DL, Norman GR. *Health Measurement Scales: A Practical Guide to Their Development and Use.* 2nd ed. New York, NY: Oxford University Press; 1995.

14. McClendon MJ, O'Brien DJ. Question order effects on the determinants of subjective well-being. *Public Opinion Q.* 1988;52:351–364.

15. Loftus EF, Smith KD, Klinger MR, Fiedler J. Memory and mismemory for health events. In: Tanur JM, ed. *Questions About Questions: Inquiries into the Cognitive Bases of Surveys.* New York, NY: Russell Sage Foundation; 1992.

16. Perkin JE, Rahr RR, Kurial M. Health promotion and wellness in US physician assistant programs. *Perspect Physician Assistant Educ.* 2001;12:5–12.

17. Wilkins JR, Hueston WD, Crawford JM, Steele LL, Gerken DF. Mixed mode survey of female veterinarians yields high response rate. *Occup Med (Lond).* 1997;47:458–462.

18. Wright DL, Aquilino WS, Supple AJ. A comparison of computer-assisted and paper-and-pencil self-administered questionnaires in a survey on smoking, alcohol, and drug use. *Public Opinion Q.* 1998;62:331–353.

19. Eley S, Lean MEJ. Using electronic mail for monitoring compliance to Scottish dietary targets. *Proc Nutr Soc.* 1998;57:137A.

20. Fischbacher C, Chappel D, Edwards R, Summerton N. Health surveys via the Internet: quick and dirty or rapid and robust? *J R Soc Med.* 2000;93:356–359.

21. Jones R, Pitt N. Health surveys in the workplace: comparison of postal, email, and World Wide Web methods. *Occup Med (Lond).* 1999;49:556–558.

22. Mavis BE, Brocato JJ. Postal surveys versus electronic mail surveys—the tortoise and the hare revisited. *Eval Health Prof.* 1998;21:395–408.

23. Schaefer DR, Dillman DA. Development of a standard E-mail methodology: results of an experiment. *Public Opinion Q.* 1998;62:378–397.

24. Schleyer TKL, Forrest JL. Methods for the design and administration of web-based surveys. *J Am Med Inform Assoc.* 2000;7:416–425.

25. Taulois-Braga W, Marcenes W. Electronic-mail: a new tool for data collection in dental public health. *Community Dent Oral Epidemiol.* 1995;23:379–380.

26. Tse ACB. Comparing the response rate, response speed, and response quality of two methods of sending questionnaires: E-mail vs. mail. *J Market Res Soc.* 1998;4:353–361.

27. Wyatt JC. When to use web-based surveys. *J Am Med Inform Assoc.* 2000;7:426–430.

28. Dillman DA. *Mail and Internet Surveys: The Tailored Design Method.* New York, NY: John Wiley & Sons; 2000.

29. *Pretesting Health Communications: Methods, Examples, and Resources for Improving Health Messages and Materials.* Rev. ed. Bethesda, Md: US Dept of Health and Human Services, Public Health Service, National Institutes of Health, National Cancer Institute; 1982. NIH publication 83–1493.

30. McLaughlin GH. SMOG grading: a new readability formula. *J Reading.* 1969;12:639–646.

31. Gunning R. The fox index after twenty years. *J Business Commun.* 1968;6:3–13.

32. Lorge I. The Lorge and Flesch readability formulae: a correction. *SchSoc.* 1948;67:141–142.

33. Taylor WL. Cloze procedure: a new tool for measuring readability. *Journalism Q.* 1953;30:415–432.

34. Heidel JJ, Glazer-Waldman HR, Parker HJ, Hopkins KM. Readability and writing style analysis of allied health professional journals. *J Allied Health.* 1991;29:25–37.

35. Info Poll Online Technical Support. *How to Write a Good Survey.* Available at: http://www.infopoll.com/tips.htm. Accessed April 10, 2001.

36. Galloway A. *Questionnaire Design and Analysis: A Workbook by Alison Galloway.* Available at: http://www.tardis.ed.ac.uk/~kate/qmcweb/qcont.htm. Accessed April 10, 2001.

37. Behling O, Law KS. *Translating Questionnaires and Other Research Instruments: Problems and Solutions.* Thousand Oaks, Calif: Sage Publications; 2000.

38. Geer JG. What do open-ended questions measure? *Public Opinion Q.* 1988;52:365–371.

39. Montgomery AC, Crittenden KS. Improving coding reliability for open-ended questions. *Public Opinion Q.* 1977;41:235–243.

40. Perkin JE, Wilson WJ, Schuster K, Rodriguez J, Allen-Chabot A. Prevalence of nonvitamin, nonmineral supplement usage among university students. *J Am Diet Assoc.* 2002;102:412–414.

41. Poe GS, Seeman I, McLaughlin J, Mehl E, Dietz M. "Don't know" boxes in factual questions in a mail questionnaire: effects on level and quality of response. *Public Opinion Q.* 1988;52:212–222.

42. Kubena KS. Accuracy in dietary assessment: on the road to good science. *J Am Diet Assoc.* 2000;100:775–776.

43. Poikolainen K, Karkkainen P. Nature of questionnaire op-

tions affects estimates of alcohol intake. *J Stud Alcohol.* 1985;46:219–222.

44. King KA, Pealer LN, Bernard AL. Increasing response rates to mail questionnaires: a review of inducement strategies. *Am J Health Ed.* 2001;32:4–15.

45. Mangione TW. *Mail Questionnaires: Improving the Quality.* Thousand Oaks, Calif: Sage Publications; 1995.

46. Fox RJ, Crask MR, Kim J. Mail survey response rate: a meta-analysis of selected techniques for inducing response. *Public Opinion Q.* 1988;52:467–491.

47. Fuller C. Effect of anonymity on return rate and response bias in a mail survey. *J Appl Psychol.* 1974;59:292–296.

48. Kviz FJ. Toward a definition of a standard response rate. *Public Opinion Q.*1977;41:265–267.

49. Goyder J. Face-to-face interviews and mailed questionnaires: the net difference in response rate. *Public Opinion Q.*1985;49:234–252.

50. Parkes R, Kreiger N, James B, Johnson KC. Effects on subject response of information brochures and small cash incentives in a mail-based case-control study. *Ann Epidemiol.* 2000;10:117–124.

51. Baron G, DeWals P, Milozd F. Cost-effectiveness of a lottery for increasing physician's responses to a mail survey. *Eval Health Prof.* 2001;24:47–52.

52. Kasprzyk D, Montano DE, St. Lawrence JS, Phillips WR. The effects of variations in mode of delivery and monetary incentive on physicians' responses to a mailed survey assessing STD practice patterns. *Eval Health Prof.* 2001;24:3–17.

53. Groves BW, Olson RH. Response rates to surveys with self-addressed, stamped envelopes versus a self-addressed label. *Psychol Rep.* 2000;86:1226–1228.

54. Becker H, Cookson J, Kulberg V. Mailed survey follow-ups—are postcard reminders more cost-effective than second questionnaires? *West J Nurs Res.* 2000;22:642–647.

55. Hunt SD, Sparkman RD, Wilcox JB. The pretest in survey research: issues and preliminary findings. *J Marketing Res.* 1982;19:269–273.

56. Etter JF, Perneger TV. Snowball sampling by mail: application to a survey of smokers in the general population. *Int J Epidemiol.* 2000;29:43–48.

57. Bok Van Kammen W, Stouthamer-Loeber M. Practical aspects of interview data collection and data management. In: Bickman L, Rog DJ, eds. *Handbook of Applied Social Research Methods.* Thousand Oaks, Calif: Sage Publications; 1998;375–397.

58. Frank GC, Hollatz AT, Webber LS, Berenson GS. Effect of interviewer practices on nutrient intake: Bogalusa heart study. *J Am Diet Assoc.* 1984;84:1432–1439.

59. Schucker RE. Alternative approaches to classic food consumption measurement methods: telephone interviewing and market data bases. *Am J Clin Nutr.* 1982;35:1306–1309.

60. Krantzler NJ, Mullen BJ, Schulz HG, Grivetti LE, Holden CA, Meiselman HL. Validity of telephoned diet recalls and records for assessment of individual food intake. *Am J Clin Nutr.* 1982;36:1234–1242.

61. Lyu LC, Hankin JH, Lui LQ, et al. Telephone vs. face-to-face interviews for quantitative food frequency assessment. *J Am Diet Assoc.* 1998;98:44–48.

62. Apian Software Homepage. STAR for telephony surveys. Available at: http://www.apian.com/partners/start.htm. Accessed April 19, 2001.

63. Chong Y, Unklesbay N, Dowdy R. Clinical nutrition and food service personnel in teaching hospitals have different perceptions of total quality management performance. *J Am Diet Assoc.* 2000;100:1044–1049.

64. Johnson BC, Chambers MJ. Foodservice benchmarking: practices, attitudes, and beliefs of foodservice directors. *J Am Diet Assoc.* 2000;100:175–180.

65. Stapleton DR, Gurrin LC, Zubrick SR, Silburn SR, Sherriff JL, Sly PD. What do children with cystic fibrosis and their parents know about nutrition and pancreatic enzymes? *J Am Diet Assoc.* 2000;100:1494–1500.

66. Walker BH, Mattfeldt-Beman MK, Tomazic TJ, Sawicki MA. Provision of nutrition counseling, referrals to registered dietitians, and sources of nutrition information among practicing chiropractors in the United States. *J Am Diet Assoc.* 2000;100:928–933.

67. Houghton MD, Graybeal TE. Breast-feeding practices of Native American mothers participating in WIC. *J Am Diet Assoc.* 2001;101:245–247.

68. Anderson JV, Bybee DI, Brown RM, et al. 5-day fruit and vegetable intervention improves consumption in a low income population. *J Am Diet Assoc.* 2001;101:195–202.

69. Willett W. *Nutritional Epidemiology.* New York, NY: Oxford University Press; 1998.

70. Touger-Decker R, Barracoto JM, O'Sullivan-Maillet J. Nutrition education in health professions programs: a survey of dental, physician assistant, nurse practitioner, and nurse midwifery programs. *J Am Diet Assoc.* 2001;101:63–69.

71. Box S, Creswell B, Hagan DW. Alternative health care education in dietetic training programs: a survey of perceived needs. *J Am Diet Assoc.* 2001;101:108–110.

72. Rosal MC, Ebbeling CB, Lofgren I, Ockene JK, Ockene IS, Herbert JR. Facilitating dietary change: the patient-centered counseling model. *J Am Diet Assoc.* 2001;101:332–341.

73. Steptoe A, Kerry S, Rink E, Hilton S. The impact of behavioral counseling on stage of change in fat intake, physical activity, and cigarette smoking in adults at increased risk of coronary heart disease. *Am J Public Health.* 2001;91:265–269.

74. Siero FW, Broer J, Bemelmans WJ, Meyboom-deJong BM. Impact of group nutrition education and surplus value of Prochaska-based stage-matched information on

health-related cognitions and on Mediterranean nutrition behavior. *Health Educ Res.* 2000;15:635–647.

75. Murphy PA, Prewitt TE, Bote E, West B, Iber FL. Internal locus of control and social support associated with some dietary changes by elderly participants in a diet intervention trial. *J Am Diet Assoc.* 2001;101:203–208.

76. Kendall A, Olson CM, Frongillo EA Jr. Evaluation of psy-chosocial measures for understanding weight-related be-haviors in pregnant women. *Ann Behav Med.* 2001;23:50–58.

77. Thomas LK, Sargent RG, Michels PC, Richter DL, Valois RF, Moore CG. Identification of the factors associated with compliance to therapeutic diets in older adults with end-stage renal disease. *J Ren Nutr.* 2001;11:80–89.

15

Dietary Assessment and Validation

Rachel K. Johnson, Ph.D., M.P.H., R.D., and Jean H. Hankin, Dr.P.H., R.D.

For more than 50 years, diet has been recognized as a primary determinant of health and disease at all ages. Dietary assessment and validation of dietary intakes are increasingly incorporated into the design of national and international nutrition status and epidemiologic studies (1–4). There is no single dietary method or "gold standard" that is applicable to all clinical, community, or research activities. Differences exist according to the purpose of the study, necessary precision, particular population, time period of interest, and available resources.

The aim of this chapter is to review dietary methods appropriate for assessing individual intakes of nutrients, particular foods or food groups, or dietary patterns. The chapter also discusses the validation of dietary intake methodology. Methods for estimating national food availability or disappearance data are described in other publications (5–9). Their major use is to measure the adequacy of the food supply and to assess trends among and within countries. Nonetheless, Armstrong and Doll (8) correlated the per-capita food and nutrient intakes from selected countries with incidence or mortality rates of cancer to illustrate associations of diet and disease, such as the relationships of dietary fat and breast cancer and of meat and colon cancer. Such correlations provide leads for further research but cannot be used to demonstrate cause and effect or true associations, as discussed by Willett (4). Chapter 13 of this book reviews the U.S. Department of Agriculture (USDA) Nationwide Food Consumption Surveys conducted periodically among randomly selected households in the United States to identify dietary varia-

tions among U.S. regions. This method has also been used in other selected countries (10).

During the last 30 years, several papers (3,11–15), reports (16–18), and books (2,4) have been published concerning the selection of individual dietary methods for research investigations among large populations. Generally, these methods include the 24-hour dietary recall (or recent recalls of 3 to 7 days), food records or diaries, diet histories, and food frequency questionnaires. Often more than one method is used in a particular study, and the methods should be tested for reproducibility, comparability, and validity of the reported dietary intake data.

Thompson and Byers have compiled descriptions of several existing methods and illustrations of questionnaires in the *Dietary Assessment Resource Manual* (1). The aim of this chapter is to review the individual methods with their strengths and limitations and selected examples of their use. It also discusses studies that test the reproducibility of methods and techniques for cross-comparisons of different dietary methods, as well as validation of dietary methods using biomarkers.

24-HOUR DIETARY RECALL

In the 24-hour dietary recall, the interviewer (usually a dietitian, nutritionist, or nonnutritionist trained in the use of the method) obtains information on all food items consumed during the past 24 hours, the previous day, or a defined 24-hour period. The information may be recorded and coded in the traditional way or be recorded with the assistance of a computer (19–20). Interviewers should have knowledge of the foods available in the community, usual eating and cooking practices, and probing methods. Recalls may be administered face to face or by telephone with similar results (21–25). Visual aids, such as food models, geometric models, photographs, or household measuring utensils may be useful to help subjects estimate quantities consumed.

It is important to have a quality control system in place to minimize errors and increase reliability of interviewing. Training and retraining sessions for interviewers (for example, via group meetings or periodic conference calls) are essential to discuss problems among interviewers. Some investigators tape telephone interviews (with the concurrence of the subjects). This technique has improved quality control in a large multiethnic population study using 24-hour dietary recalls for calibration of a mailed quantitative food frequency questionnaire (26).

From 1965 to 1991, the USDA used the 24-hour dietary recall combined with 2 subsequent days of food records to derive average daily intakes of randomized samples of the American population in its nationwide food consumption surveys (7). After 1991, the USDA began using 2 days of 24-hour dietary recalls in its nationwide surveys (27). Similarly, the National Health and Nutrition Examination Survey (NHANES) has used 24-hour recalls, as well as frequencies of various food items, in its surveys of stratified national probability samples of the population (28–29).

The major strength of the 24-hour dietary recall is its ability to compare groups of people, as has been noted. For example, 24-hour recalls of random samples of four groups of Micronesians revealed differences in nutrient intakes and associations of diet with illness characteristics according to degree of westernization (30). Similarly 24-hour recalls among men of Japanese ancestry living in San Francisco, Hawaii, and Japan demonstrated a stepwise increase in dietary fat intake and a similar decrease in carbohydrate intake from Japan to Hawaii to California, which paralleled the increase in coronary heart disease mortality rates among these populations (31). The USDA has shown that individual intakes, based on 2- or 3-day means, differ between blacks and whites, socioeconomic groups, geographic regions, and other demographic characteristics (32). These differences have been repeated in subsequent surveys. The NHANES collects biological, anthropometric, and physiological measurements on subjects. Hence, the data have been useful for examining group differences in diet in relation to various health and disease characteristics (33).

There are many advantages of the 24-hour dietary recall. It places little burden on the subjects, and if unannounced, it is unlikely to alter eating behavior. Because of the short time interval, memory problems are usually minimal. In addition, participants are generally willing to respond to the interviewer, and thus refusals are less likely to occur than in other, more demanding requests for dietary information. For group averages, the method has been shown to be comparable to more cumbersome methods (34). In the past, the method was labor intensive, as nutrition professionals were usually involved directly or indirectly in data collection, review, and coding of the recalls. However, direct coding of the foods reported during the interview is now possible using automated software that specifies the information needed for clarifying and coding each response (20,35). This automated software is being used in several studies in the United States; however, this procedure has the potential effect of losing the subject's verbal description, which would be available in the written recall conducted by an interviewer. The automated method also may be difficult to use if interviews are being conducted among heterogeneous ethnic populations who prepare and consume foods that are unfamiliar to the interviewer and are not included in the food composition database.

The multiple-pass 24-hour dietary recall was originally developed by the USDA for use in its Nationwide Food Consumption Surveys (27). These surveys are conducted by the USDA approximately twice each decade and are designed to answer the question, What are Americans Eating? The multiple-pass 24-hour dietary recall was designed specifically to limit the extent of underreporting of food intake in the USDA surveys. This method differs from the traditional 24-hour dietary recall because the interviewer uses three distinct passes to gather information about a subject's food intake during the preceding 24 hours. These passes include the following:

1. *First pass—quick list.* The respondent is asked to recall everything he or she ate the previous day using any recall strategy the respondent chooses.
2. *Second pass—detailed description.* The respondent is asked to clarify any foods mentioned in the quick list. For example, if the respondent reported that he or she ate breakfast cereal, the interviewer would then ask whether milk was consumed with the cereal and if so, the type and amount.

3. *Third pass—review.* The interviewer reviews the list of foods mentioned and probes for additional eating occasions (for example, "Did you eat anything after dinner, before bedtime?") and clarifies portion sizes.

The major limitation of the 24-hour recall relates to the daily variation in food intakes of most persons. Because of the large intraindividual variability in food and nutrient intakes of most people, a single 24-hour recall is not appropriate for estimating the usual intakes of one person (36). However, multiple 24-hour recalls obtained on random days during a 1-year interval may provide a satisfactory picture of the usual diet. When group assessment is the objective, the interviews should be scheduled on various days of the week to account for daily variation in food choices, particularly between weekdays and weekends, as well as between weeks and seasons of the year.

FOOD RECORDS OR DIARIES

Food records or diaries require participants to weigh, measure, or estimate and record all foods consumed over a specified period of time, usually 3 to 7 consecutive days or multiple periods within a year. The method requires good instructions, demonstrations, and ideally some observations. Generally, persons who agree to participate are dedicated, highly motivated, literate subjects and thus may not be representative of the general population. Although subjects are asked to follow their usual dietary patterns, they may modify their eating practices to reduce their workload (for example, substituting a frozen dinner rather than preparing their usual recipe).

The most accurate method entails the weighing of all ingredients in recipes, the portion selected, and the plate waste. This detailed procedure is generally feasible only for persons familiar with using scales calibrated in grams and kilograms in food preparation or in the work setting (3,37). This procedure also has been used successfully among retired people who were motivated to participate in a scientific study (38). Because weighing foods may be difficult for some subjects, household-measuring utensils, such as cups and spoons, have been used more frequently than scales in food record studies in the United States (1). In both instances, directions should be included concerning methods of estimating and recording food items consumed away from home. Other methods of

quantifying consumption have been reported. For instance, in a dietary cross-comparison study among multiethnic groups in Hawaii, Hankin and coworkers (39) gave subjects a book of photographs showing three different typical portions of various food groups for use in estimating amounts consumed. This method was appropriate for this population, which included males and females of five ethnic groups, many of whom were not familiar with household scales or even measuring utensils.

A major strength of food records is that they do not rely on memory. Because of the difficulty in assessing a person's true usual intake, investigators in the past have used food records as a reference or standard for validating other dietary methods that are based on long-term recall (12). Although food records are not necessarily error-free, investigators often assumed that they approximated the truth. They were presumed to have greater face validity than a diet history or food frequency questionnaire. However, with the advent of biomarkers (an indicator that measures body fluids or tissues and can independently reflect individual nutrient intakes), it is now known that none of the dietary intake methods (weighed food records, 24-hour recalls, food frequency questionnaires, or diet history questionnaires) give accurate estimates of the usual energy intakes of individuals (40). Hence, there is a need to reevaluate the common philosophy that weighed dietary intakes provide a better indication of dietary intake than any other method.

Food records can provide helpful information for developing a structured food frequency questionnaire for a particular population. Food items that are important contributors to the intakes of particular dietary components (such as macronutrients and micronutrients, fiber, and phytoestrogens) can be identified, along with the range of expected portion sizes for each item. In addition, records are often used to motivate participants in dietary intervention studies, which may encourage weight loss (41).

Along with its strengths, the use of food records has serious limitations as well. First, the selected time period for collecting and recording intakes may be atypical for the subject, possibly because of illness, business obligations, or travel. Also, this method would not be appropriate for people who consume most of their meals in restaurants. Second, as noted previously, persons who agree to keep detailed food records may not be representative of the general population in the study. Immigrants whose primary language is not English also may find it very difficult to keep a food record or diary. However, Hankin and Huenemann (42) translated instructions for keeping 7-day food records into Japanese for first-generation immigrants in California and used trained bilingual persons to interpret and code the dietary intakes to reduce possible problems. Third, because of the labor-intensive methodology, food records are difficult to administer in large population studies and are costly in time and personnel. Fourth, food records provide data only on the current diet. If the investigator wishes to obtain dietary information on foods consumed 3 years in the past for an epidemiologic study, current intakes may be dissimilar. Fifth, food records covering a single series of 3 to 7 consecutive days most likely will not reflect the true variability in the diets of most individuals. Finally, the act of recording food intake may actually change people's dietary patterns. For example, people may choose to eat simpler meals or eliminate snacking to make the task easier.

INTRAINDIVIDUAL VARIABILITY OF DIET

Both the single 24-hour dietary recall and the food record are limited by their short time coverage. For most people today, eating patterns are characterized by large variations from day to day, week to week, and often season to season. This is particularly true in developed countries, with their wide choice of available foods, and it is increasingly true in developing countries as well. Food intakes during the weekend usually differ considerably from meals consumed on weekdays, and dietary patterns are also likely to vary by season of the year. Furthermore, people are consuming more of their meals away from home, adding further variability to their diets. The large variation in daily and even weekly diets suggests that no single day or week can be representative of long-term usual intake.

Variability of diet within a population may be divided into within-person (or intraindividual) variation and between-person variation. It has been reported that within-person variation, which represents day-to-day differences in intake, is generally as large as or larger than between-person variation (34,36,43–46). Consequently, a longer time period is needed to characterize the usual diet of an individual than the usual diet of a group of persons. Several investigators have analyzed the variability in multiple 24-hour dietary recalls and food records and determined the number of days needed to achieve reliable estimates of average nutrient intakes of individuals (10,34,36,45,47). For example, in a study among 29 adults who measured and recorded their food intakes for 1 year, Basiotis et al (36) found that 57 days were needed

to estimate the total fat intake within 10 percent of the true average individual intakes for males with 95 percent confidence, whereas 71 days were needed for females. For vitamin A, 390 days were needed for males and 474 days for females. When the objective was to estimate mean intakes of the group with precision, a smaller number of days of food records was needed—specifically, 6 days to estimate the fat intakes of both males and females and approximately 40 days to estimate the vitamin A intakes with 95 percent confidence.

Other investigators have defined *precision* as an estimate within 20 percent of the true usual intake (48). With this increased latitude, considerably fewer days would be needed to estimate individual average intakes. These findings indicate that the use of a short recall or food record for diet and disease studies could lead to considerable error, with misclassification on the distribution of individual intakes occurring along a continuum (48).

DIET HISTORIES

For research concerning the etiology of diseases, such as cancer and heart disease, investigators seek information on the usual diet consumed during a considerable period of time. The first and classic diet history to assess the usual diet was conceived by Burke (49), who developed a subjective interview administered by highly trained dietitians. The method included a 24-hour recall with typical variations (such as information on the different fruits that might be eaten at breakfast), a checklist of foods consumed over the preceding month (or the last 3 to 6 months), and a measured 3-day food record. From these data, the dietitians calculated the average daily intake of energy and nutrients. This method was used in research concerning diet and child growth (50,51) and was subsequently modified for use in epidemiologic studies of diet and heart disease (52,53). However, the subjective diet history was time-consuming and expensive, and a highly skilled professional was needed for both the collection and the processing of the information.

FOOD FREQUENCY QUESTIONNAIRES

The checklist used by Burke was the forerunner of the more structured dietary questionnaires being used today. During the 1950s and 1960s, nutritionists and epidemiologists in the United States and England (4) pioneered the development of the more structured food frequency questionnaires for use in large epidemiologic studies on diet and coronary heart disease (and later cancer, osteoporosis, and other chronic diseases).

The basic assumption of food frequency questionnaires is that the average long-term diet is the conceptually important exposure instead of dietary intakes during a few specific days. With this method, precision is sacrificed. The method is simple to administer by a trained interviewer or by the respondent directly using a mailed questionnaire. The questionnaire can be computerized and optically scanned for analysis. The method is objective, as it is based on lists of selected foods and groups of items with similar nutrient values used interchangeably in the diet. In the past, food items were often selected to test particular hypotheses concerning diet and disease, such as vitamin A or beta carotene and lung cancer (54–56). More recently, because of the uncertainty concerning the role of particular nutrients and other food components in the etiology of several chronic diseases, investigators have included sufficient foods to assess the total diet. It also is valuable to examine interactions between dietary components and to have adequate data for analysis of particular foods, food groups, and eating patterns in relationship to disease.

Selection of Food Items

It is preferable to select food items for the questionnaire based on the study population's eating patterns. General guidelines are to choose foods that are consumed by a sizable number of people, vary in frequency and quantity among the population, and provide significant amounts of all dietary components. These food items may be selected using various methods. For example, Willett et al (37) obtained an extensive list of food items using four 1-week weighed food records from a representative sample of the study population. Others have used population data, such as 24-hour recalls of adults participating in the NHANES II survey (57–59), for selecting particular food items for questionnaires. Some food frequency questionnaires have been modified or expanded periodically to account for additional foods on the market or to test particular hypotheses (4).

Semiquantitative Versus Quantitative Food Frequency Questionnaires

Some food frequency questionnaires solicit frequency responses only (37,60–62), although a usual serving size

may be listed with each item (37). These questionnaires are called semiquantitative food frequency questionnaires. The questionnaires developed for the Nurses Cohort Study (37) and the Male Health Professionals Cohort Study (63) illustrate this method. Frequencies are obtained by checking the appropriate column showing ranges per day, week, month, or year. The nutrient intakes are computed by multiplying the midpoint of the frequency interval by the nutrients in the specified portion of the food. This method may be satisfactory if all of the respondents generally consume similar amounts of the items—for example, 5 ounces of meat or a half-cup of vegetables—and if amounts are highly correlated with frequencies. A problem may occur if the usual portions of some subjects differ markedly from the portions specified and if the respondents do not adjust the frequencies accordingly. Marr (11), a distinguished pioneer in dietary methodology, indicated that a semiquantitative instrument could lead to a systematic bias toward either underestimates or overestimates of food and nutrient intakes. However, Willett et al (37) and Hunter et al (64) reported that specifications of quantities consumed provided little additional information to frequency data. These investigators concluded that the frequency of eating particular foods was a greater determinant of nutrient intakes than quantity and that the use of a single serving size did not introduce a large error in the individual estimates.

The alternative procedure assumes that amounts consumed are likely to vary among the population and that more valid data will be obtained if subjects choose their own portion size according to their usual habits. Cummings and coworkers (65), Chu et al (66), and the multiethnic cohort study in Hawaii and Los Angeles (67) found that if a standard portion size is used, misclassification and inconsistent results may occur when compared with studies allowing the subjects to choose their own serving size.

Various techniques have been employed to help subjects estimate amounts consumed. The directions for completing Block's questionnaire specify that a small portion is about one-half the specified medium serving size and a large portion is about one and a half times as much (59). Several epidemiologists in Europe, such as Pietinen et al (68), have developed booklets showing different portion sizes of each item in the questionnaire to assist subjects. Others have used geometric models printed on a foldout that accompanies the questionnaire (21–23). The Hawaii group (14) used color photographs of food items in three portion sizes in home interviews for several case-control studies (69–72). This technique was found to be highly satisfactory because of the wide variation in amounts consumed among the ethnic groups.

Food frequency questionnaires may be processed in two ways. If the information is obtained by personal interview, the frequency interval may be precise, for example, "three times a month" or "four times a day." However, food frequency questionnaires are often self-administered. In this case, the respondent chooses the appropriate frequency interval from the listed series, such as "one to three times a month," for each category of foods and the usual serving size. This format is designed for direct machine entry, such as optical scanning, and is generally preferable for the large population studies often administered by mail. Some investigators (1,4) also include a few answers to be written in. In this case, review of each questionnaire is needed prior to coding and processing.

Before using any dietary research instrument, it should be pretested extensively among representative samples of the population (73). When using a food frequency instrument, the pretesting should include a write-in section for recording other items usually eaten. Doing so will help improve the questionnaire by yielding the suggestions for the addition of particular foods or for clarifying instructions. In addition, if the questionnaire will be self-administered by mail or completed by telephone interview, trial runs should be conducted among representative samples of the study population. In some geographic areas with large immigrant populations, it may be desirable to translate the instrument into other languages to ensure its comprehension. Among particular groups, such as the elderly, videotapes may be used to obtain an accurate estimate of individual intakes. Brown et al (74) tested this technique among elderly women living in a retirement home and showed that its accuracy was superior to the 24-hour dietary recall.

POTENTIAL ERRORS OF INDIVIDUAL DIETARY INTAKE METHODS

It is clear that none of the individual methods of dietary assessment are free from error. Witschi (41) classified errors into three categories: respondent and recorder errors, interviewer and reviewer errors, and nutrient database errors. Briefly, in 24-hour dietary recalls and diet histories, subjects may fail to recall all foods and amounts consumed. Even for home-prepared meals, persons not involved in food preparation may not be aware of the components of mixed dishes or vegetables served with entrees. They may not know what kinds of fats and oils were used, whether butter or margarine was served, and if their portion of a mixed dish was 1 or 2 cups. Subjects also may want to please the interviewer and may be reluctant to admit consumption of an alcoholic beverage or an excessive intake of "sin foods," such as candy or desserts. In addition, some persons may believe that certain foods are good or bad for health and may either exaggerate or underestimate their intakes of them. Some investigators have found that large intakes tend to be underestimated and small intakes overestimated (75,76). This phenomenon has been called the *flat slope syndrome*.

The food composition databases are also not error-free. However, the values published by the USDA are carefully selected averages from various sources and are reviewed and revised periodically. Beginning in 1972 (77), these reviews and revisions incorporate new dietary components and updated analyses to the existing database. This database is an appropriate primary resource for studies in the United States, but it may need supplementation from other publications, such as Pennington (78) and McCance and Widdowson (79), as well as from subsequent additions, commercial tables, and laboratory analyses of local foods. Food composition tables may include imputed values for some nutrients. There is divided opinion from researchers concerning their use, and it is likely that either inclusion or exclusion will result in some error in the estimated intakes. If used, food composition tables should be based on the analyses of similar foods and should be updated as new analytic information becomes available. Other potential unavoidable errors include changes occurring during food preparation or food storage, as well as in the bioavailability of some nutrients. Although differences exist between calculated and analyzed values of food intake data (3,11–14), these errors cannot be eliminated in large population studies.

The errors in dietary methodology, along with the large, random within-person variability, generally decrease the strength of the statistical association of diet with another variables, such as a biochemical measurement or disease status, providing that the errors are distributed randomly among the comparison groups. In contrast, if errors are biased and not random, as occurs with underreporting, this bias can both remove or create associations (80).

Hence, failure to identify a relationship between a dietary variable and a disease does not necessarily mean the absence of an association. For example, there has been inconsistent evidence from epidemiologic studies on the relationship of dietary fat and breast cancer (81,82). This inconsistency may be due to the homogeneity of fat intakes within populations, to the substantial measurement error in dietary assessment (83), to the large intraindividual variation in dietary fat intakes (84), and to the selective underreporting of high-fat foods (80).

Measurement error may be a significant problem in large population or cohort studies that include subgroups for whom a single food frequency questionnaire may perform differently; this fact complicates comparisons between the groups (26). To provide an unbiased estimate, data from the dietary questionnaire may be compared with dietary information from a second source, such as multiple 24-hour recalls from representative samples of the population groups. These data can then be used for correction of risk estimates obtained from analysis of nutrition factors and incidences of particular diseases among the groups. For example, investigators conducted a calibration substudy among the multiethnic groups in the Hawaii-Los Angeles cohort study (26). The intakes from the quantitative food frequency questionnaires were compared with the intakes from three 24-hour telephone recalls of the previous day's diet to derive statistical equations for correcting measurement error in associations of diet and disease.

VALIDITY AND REPRODUCIBILITY OF DIETARY INTAKE DATA

To promote confidence in dietary data and diet-disease findings, the dietary method should be tested for both validity and reproducibility in a representative sample of the study population. Although it would be expedient to use a method evaluated in another population, the instrument is appropriate only if the eating patterns of the reference and study populations are similar. Structured quantitative food frequency questionnaires, in particular, should be tailored to the eating patterns of the study population. For example, a valid and reproducible questionnaire developed for nurses or health professionals in the United States would most likely not be appropriate for a multiethnic randomized population of Japanese Americans, Latinos, African Americans, Native Hawaiians, and whites living in Hawaii and Los Angeles (67).

Several studies and reviews have been reported on the evaluation of particular dietary methods. A succinct and comprehensive review is found in Thompson and Byer's *Dietary Assessment Resource Manual* (1). This chapter includes only a brief review to illustrate the objectives, general protocols, and relevant findings.

Dietary Validity or Comparability

Dietary validity is the ability of an instrument to measure what it purports to measure in regard to diet, such as the intake in a particular meal or day or the usual diet consumed during the past year. Validation requires that the truth be known, and the truth is difficult to obtain among free-living persons for extended periods. This problem is particularly relevant today because of the large variability in people's eating patterns. However, dietary validity for short time intervals has been assessed by surreptitiously weighing foods of people eating in an institutional setting and then asking the subjects the following day to recall what they ate (75,76,85,86). In the past, food frequency questionnaires were validated by measuring the relative validity of the new instrument by comparing it with a method that had evidence of greater accuracy or face validity (4,12). The choice was generally food records, either weighed, measured, or estimated and collected at multiple time periods during a year to reflect within-person variability among representative samples of the population. Some investigators have used repeated 24-hour dietary recalls collected by trained interviewers of the same ethnic group by personal interview or telephone (26) to obtain a second set of usual intakes for testing among the study population. Nonetheless, the reference data may underestimate the usual intakes of the individuals in the study. Investigators can now use biomarkers as independent markers of dietary intake to validate food intake measurements.

Willett et al (37) compared a 61-item food frequency questionnaire with 4 weeks of measured food intakes recorded at 3-month intervals during the year. Because the record keeping could sensitize the subjects and thus increase the accuracy of the questionnaire responses, the instrument was completed on two occasions—before the first set of food records and after the last set of records. The first questionnaire pertained to the previous year and would probably underestimate agreement, whereas the second questionnaire could overestimate agreement. The true relationship would likely fall between the two values. As expected, the results revealed higher values in the comparison of the second questionnaire with the records.

Food frequency questionnaires are being used in several large cohort studies on diet and disease in the United States, Europe, and Asia (1,67,68,87–89). In these investigations, participants (preferably randomly selected among subjects defined by age, gender, ethnicity, or profession) complete a dietary questionnaire at the start of the study. Several years later, the original dietary intakes are tested for associations with diseases that may have developed, such as cancer and heart disease. The aim is to identify dietary and other environmental or genetic factors that may be related to risk of disease. The findings, if confirmed among multiple populations and substantiated with biological research, may be used to identify potential risks and, it is hoped, to prevent these diseases. A major problem is that estimates of risk within cohorts can be substantially attenuated by measurement errors in assessing individual intakes (26). These problems are increased in cohort studies that include subgroups in which the questionnaire may perform differently. Consequently, the use of calibration substudies, in which data from the questionnaires are compared with a second source that is assumed to provide an unbiased estimate, allows for correction of risk estimates for measurement error. In these studies, investigators begin by assuming that there is error in food frequency questionnaires. Thus, rather than trying to validate the frequency data, statistical methods are used to adjust the dietary intakes of each participant within the subgroup. A recent calibration substudy conducted among the multiethnic cohort in Hawaii and Los Angeles illustrates the epidemiologic and statistical methods used (26).

Use of Biomarkers to Validate Dietary Intake Methods

All the traditional dietary intake methods (24-hour dietary recalls, food records, diet histories, and food frequency questionnaires) rely on information reported by the subjects themselves. In the past, there was a tacit assumption that this self-reported information was valid or correct. It is now believed that this assumption can only be verified by the use of external independent markers of intake (90). Hence, in recent years the search has begun for biomarkers that closely reflect dietary intake but do not rely on self-reports of food consumption (91). A biomarker is defined as a variable measured in body fluids or tissues that independently reflects the intake of a food component (92).

Doubly Labeled Water

Doubly labeled water (DLW) is currently the most widely used and well-accepted biomarker. DLW is an ideal measure of people's free-living total energy expenditure. The DLW method was originally described for use in small animals by Lifson and colleagues in the 1940s (93). It is based on the principle that carbon dioxide production can be estimated by the difference in elimination rates of body hydrogen and oxygen. Through observations, Lifson and coworkers concluded that the oxygen in expired carbon dioxide was derived from total body water (94). This results from the equilibrium between the oxygen in body water and the oxygen in respiratory carbon dioxide (93). With this finding, the researchers predicted that carbon dioxide production could be indirectly measured by separately labeling both the hydrogen and oxygen pool of the body water with naturally occurring, stable isotopes. In 1982 Schoeller and van Santen first used this technique to measure total energy expenditure in free-living humans (95).

The DLW method provides an accurate measure of the total energy expenditure in free-living subjects. Hence, it is now well accepted as a gold standard to determine the validity of tools designed to measure energy intake (90). Its use as a validation tool is based on the principle of energy balance; that is, if a person is in energy balance, then his or her energy expenditure, as measured by doubly labeled water, must be equal to his or her energy intake (96,97). It is important to point out that DLW can determine the accuracy of a dietary intake method only with respect to total energy. However, if a dietary assessment tool is accurate with respect to energy, there is a reasonable probability that it will also be accurate for specific macronutrients and micronutrients (98,99). In contrast, if a tool is not accurate with respect to energy, then it is not likely to provide an accurate measure of the absolute intake of other nutrients (98,99). Hence, it is accepted that when group estimates of energy intake are truly validated against a well-accepted criterion method (such as the DLW method), the coinciding estimates of macronutrient and micronutrient intakes can also be considered valid (100).

There are numerous advantages to the DLW technique, including the ease of administration and the ability of the subject to engage in free-living activities during the measurement period. This characteristic is extremely advantageous when the DLW method is used as an objective criterion measure to validate self-reported estimates of dietary intake, because the subject is not confined to a clinical research setting (such as a whole-room calorimeter) where usual activities are restricted. Most important, the method is accurate and has a precision of between 2 percent and 8 percent (101).

Although there are many advantages to the DLW technique, there are also drawbacks—namely, the expense of the stable isotopes (approximately $500 per dose for an adult of average weight) and the expertise required to operate the highly sophisticated and costly mass spectrometer for analysis of the isotopes. Thus, to date, the use of the DLW method has been confined to a few research laboratories around the world, and the method does not lend itself to routine use in large epidemiologic studies. It can be used, however, in a subsample from large cohort studies to validate energy intakes obtained from the dietary method of choice. This approach has been used by Bingham and colleagues in the European Prospective Study of Diet and Cancer (102). Currently, the USDA is conducting a DLW validation study with 400 volunteers to determine the accuracy of the multiple-pass 24-hour dietary recall. This method also was with the 2000 USDA Nationwide Food Consumption Survey—The Continuing Survey of Food Intakes of Individuals (NFCS-CSFII).

Other Biomarkers

In recent years several other biomarkers that reflect nutrient intake have attracted considerable attention in nutrition epidemiology (103) and are being introduced to validate dietary assessment methods (104).

The pattern of fatty acids in the blood has been used as a biomarker of fatty acid intake (105). Andersen and colleagues demonstrated that intakes of eicosapentaenoic acid and docosahexaenoic acid, as well as fish, were significantly related to concentrations of these fatty acids in plasma phospholipids (106). In this study, dietary intake data generated from a food frequency questionnaire were validated when both dietary and biomarker data classified people into similar groupings of intake. This type of analysis can increase confidence that the estimated intake actually reflects the intake of a nutrient or a food containing that nutrient (107). For example, a biomarker confirming the quintile distributions of fat intake would have added substantially to the credibility of reports suggesting that a diet providing 30 percent of energy as fat was unlikely to result in a substantial reduction in the risk of breast cancer (108) or that total dietary fat was not associated with coronary heart disease in women (109).

Bingham and Cummings pioneered the use of urinary nitrogen measurement to validate protein intake. For people in energy and nitrogen balance, urinary nitrogen level, as assessed from 8 days of complete 24-hour urine collections, is an independent measure of protein intake

(110). Bingham and colleagues have since used the 24-hour urinary nitrogen technique to validate reported protein intakes in 24-hour recalls, food frequency questionnaires, and food records (91,102,111).

Vegetables and fruits are the primary source of carotenoids in the diet (112), and circulating concentrations of carotenoids have been shown in feeding studies (113,114) to respond to dietary changes. Thus, serum carotenoid concentrations, as well as ascorbic acid levels, have been used as markers of fruit and vegetable consumption (115,116). Scott and colleagues examined the relationships between dietary intakes of lutein, lycopene, and beta carotene and their concentrations in blood and found that plasma carotenoid concentrations were indicative of dietary intake (117). Bingham used plasma carotenoids and vitamin C to validate dietary assessments for the European Prospective Study of Diet and Cancer (102). Murphy and colleagues used serum carotenoids to validate changes in fruit and vegetable consumption resulting from nutrition education intervention (118). Furthermore, Italian investigators determined that urinary fructose and sucrose can be used as a marker of sucrose intake (119).

In the future, the collection of biological samples to validate estimates of dietary intake should become routine in nutrition epidemiology and surveillance (104). However, it is important to recognize that biomarkers cannot substitute for collecting estimates of dietary intake. As Conner states, "food intake is the bottom line as people eat food, not nutrients" (107). Biomarkers can be used to validate, as well as to interpret, dietary intake data.

UNDERREPORTING DIETARY INTAKE

Based on data collected from a variety of volunteers, it is now well accepted that underreporting of food intake is pervasive (90). Underreporting occurs when people report food intakes so much lower than their measured total energy expenditure that the intakes are not biologically plausible. In other words, a person could not support fundamental physiological processes or survive over the long term on intakes so low.

Who Underreports?

It has been shown that underreporters constitute anywhere from 10 percent to 45 percent of the total, depending on the age, gender, and body composition of the sample.

Based on numerous papers published over the past decade, underreporting has been consistently shown to be more prevalent and more severe among obese in comparison with lean subjects (120,121). These studies and others found that obese subjects underreport their energy intake to a greater degree (ranging from 30 percent to 47 percent) than do lean subjects. Thus, it is now well accepted that obese subjects are inclined toward underreporting their dietary intake.

Underreporting is not just confined to obese people, however. In reviewing the findings from large nationwide surveys of both British and American adults, it is clear that women are at greater risk for underreporting than men (122–124). In addition, people of low socioeconomic status, characterized by low incomes and low education attainment, are more likely to report low energy intakes (122–124). These characteristics are also risk factors for a number of chronic diseases, which place these subgroups of the population at risk for lower health status. Thus, simply eliminating the subjects with questionable energy intake values from a sample would seriously alter the nature of most samples, specifically eliminating subjects who are frequently of most concern in terms of their health risk.

Why Do People Underreport?

It is not enough to just know who underreports. To fully understand the problem of underreporting, the reasons why people underreport their food intake need to be known. Obesity is not causing people to underreport; instead, the psychological and behavioral characteristics associated with obesity probably lead people to underreport.

Recently, a number of psychological characteristics have been associated with underreporting. Specifically, a high need for social acceptability, high levels of body dissatisfaction, and dietary restraint have been associated with underreporting (125–127).

What Foods and Nutrients Are Prone to Underreporting?

If underreporting occurred simply across the board—that is, all foods and nutrients were underreported to the same degree—the solution to the problem of underreporting would be relatively simple. A correction factor could be added to the dietary intake data of underreporters, which would bring their intake of all nutrients into line with that of the valid reporters. Unfortunately, the solution is not that simple. It has become clearer that underreporters often fail to report those foods that have a "bad" or even "sinful" connotation (99).

In a large U.S. nationwide survey, 1,224 out of 8,334 adults were found to be low energy reporters. In comparing the low energy reporters with those who were not low energy reporters, the following were among the foods most likely to be underreported: cake and pie, savory snacks, cheese, white potatoes, meat mixtures, regular soft drinks, fat-type spreads, and condiments (128). British investigators found that underreporters reported consuming significantly less cake, sugar, fat, and breakfast cereal. However, they found no discernible differences in reports of bread, potatoes, meat, or vegetable and fruit consumption between underreporters and other subjects (91).

At this time, there is no consensus in the literature as to whether or how much the macronutrients are differentially reported. Some research suggests that underreporters reported lower intakes of fat as a percentage of total energy, as well as higher intakes of protein and carbohydrate (124,129). Others have demonstrated that reported added sugar intake was significantly lower than measured, in part because of the omission of snack foods from the dietary record (130).

Effect of Underreporting on Conclusions About Diet and Health

In nutrition epidemiology, it is important to classify nutrient intakes correctly from low to high and then determine whether associations exist between nutrient intake and the occurrence of disease. As evidence of differential reporting of food and nutrients by underreporters continues to accumulate, the possibility of the misclassification of subjects' nutrient intakes in studies of diet and disease is very real.

This problem is exacerbated because the probability of underestimation of food intake, as well as differential reporting of foods and nutrients, increases with other known factors of health risk, such as obesity and low socioeconomic status. For example, because obesity is a known risk factor for a number of chronic diseases, such as coronary heart disease, people at higher risk of these diseases are more likely to differentially report foods and macronutrients. Because bias in measuring dietary intake can both remove and create associations, it can generate seriously misleading conclusions about the impact of diet on disease (80,131).

Identifying Underreporters with the Goldberg Cutoff

Ideally, all dietary studies should incorporate independent biomarkers of energy intake as measures of validity. Unfortunately, no biomarkers are currently available that can be used in the field on a routine basis. DLW is expensive, and its use requires sophisticated laboratory technology. However, researchers can apply the Goldberg cutoff, which has been extensively described by Goldberg and colleagues (132) and Black and colleagues (133). The Goldberg cutoff evaluates energy intake against estimated energy requirements and defines cutoff limits, which identify the most obviously implausible intake values. Briefly, height and weight measurements are used to predict basal metabolic rate from a standard formula (Goldberg et al recommend the Schofield equation [134]). A ratio of estimated energy intake (EI) to predicted basal metabolic rate (BMR) is calculated as EI/BMR. This ratio can then be compared with a study-specific cutoff value (provided in Goldberg et al [132]) that represents the lowest value of EI/BMR that could, within defined bounds of statistical probability, reflect the habitual energy expenditure, given a sedentary lifestyle. In a large study of British adults, 39 percent of the women (344 of 873) and 27 percent of the men (264 of 983) were classified as low energy reporters using a cutoff EI/BMR of 1.2 (123). In the NHANES III, Briefel and colleagues used the Goldberg cutoff and classified 18 percent of the men and 28 percent of the women as underreporters (124). These examples indicate of how the Goldberg cutoff has been used to provide some indication of whether estimates of dietary intake are biased.

There are limitations to the Goldberg cutoff, however. It underestimates the incidence of underreporting, as it is assumes all people have a sedentary physical activity level. For improved identification of individual underreporters, additional knowledge about lifestyle, occupation, and leisure physical activity is required to estimate subject-specific physical activity levels and calculate more subject-specific cutoffs (135,136).

Handling Underreporting in Dietary Intake Data

Researchers have not yet come up with good answers about what to do with study databases that contain large numbers of underreporters. Several approaches have been suggested to handle the bias, none of which are ideal. One obvious technique is to exclude from analyses those people who report energy intakes that are biologically implausible. This technique is problematic, however, because underreporting is known to be concentrated within specific subgroups of the population, such as the obese people, smokers, and less-educated people (122–124). Excluding these subjects would seriously alter the size and nature of the sample, eliminating people who might be of most concern in terms of health risk (122). Their removal could mask or distort important diet-disease associations. Some investigators have analyzed their data using all observations and then reanalyzed the data with the underreporters removed (137). If the findings remained consistent this analysis could improve confidence in the results and conclusions.

Upward adjustment of all nutrients equally to account for underreporting is another possible technique for handling underreporting, but it is only be acceptable if all nutrients are underreported. Unfortunately, across-the-board underreporting is not the case; research has shown that people may fail to report food items that have a "bad" connotation to a greater degree than foods that have a "healthy" connotation. Hence, underreporters tend to report diets that are micronutrient-rich in comparison with valid reporters (122). Adjusting all nutrients upward would create an artificial impression of the sample's nutrition status.

Epidemiologists recommend adjusting nutrient intakes for energy intake using the regression of nutrient versus energy (138). Again, this technique would be valid only when underreporting results from a systematic underestimation of portion sizes (across-the-board underestimation), but the actual foods are accurately reported. However, as stated earlier, it is likely that certain foods are underreported more than others (systematic omissions), so energy adjustment could make matters worse (139). For example, if fat-containing foods are more likely to be underreported and foods containing vitamin A are less likely to be underreported, energy adjustment would provide a lower-than-actual measure of fat intake and a higher-than-actual measure of vitamin A intake. Researchers have acknowledged that energy adjustment cannot eliminate bias caused by selective underreporting of certain foods (122,140).

REFERENCES

1. Thompson FE, Byers T. Dietary assessment resource manual. *J Nutr.* 1994;124 (suppl):2245–2317.
2. Cameron ME, van Staveren WA, eds. *Manual on*

Methodology for Food Consumption Studies. New York, NY: Oxford University Press; 1988.

3. Bingham SA. The dietary assessment of individuals; methods, accuracy, new techniques and recommendations. *Nutr Abst Rev.* 1987;57:705–742.

4. Willett W. *Nutritional Epidemiology.* 2nd ed. New York, NY: Oxford University Press; 1998.

5. Anderson SA, ed. *Guidelines for Use of Dietary Intake Data.* Washington, DC: Food and Drug Administration; 1986.

6. Peterkin BP, Rizek RL, Tippett KS. Nationwide food consumption survey, 1987. *Nutr Today.* 1988;23:18–24.

7. Pao EM, Sykes KE, Cypel YS. *USDA Methodological Research for Large-Scale Dietary Intake Surveys, 1975–1988.* Washington, DC: US Dept of Agriculture; 1989. Home Economics Research Report no. 49.

8. Armstrong B, Doll R. Environmental factors and cancer incidence and mortality in different countries, with special reference to dietary practices. *Int J Cancer.* 1975;15:617–631.

9. Jolliffe N, Archer M. Statistical associations between international coronary heart disease death rates and certain environmental factors. *J Chronic Dis.* 1959;9:636–652.

10. James WPT, Bingham SA, Cole TJ. Epidemiological assessment of dietary intake. *Nutr Cancer.* 1981;2:203–212.

11. Marr JW. Individual dietary surveys: purposes and methods. *World Rev Nutr Diet.* 1971;13:105–161.

12. Block G. A review of validations of dietary assessment methods. *Am J Epidemiol.* 1982;115:492–505.

13. Callmer E, Haraldsdottir J, Lokn EB, Seppanen R, Solvoll K. Selecting a method for a dietary survey. *Naringsforskning.* 1985;29:43–52.

14. Hankin JH. A diet history method for research, clinical, and community use. *J Am Diet Assoc.* 1986;86:868–875.

15. Lee-Han H, McGuire V, Boyd NF. A review of the methods used by studies of dietary measurement. *J Clin Epidemiol.* 1989;42:269–279.

16. Committee on Food Consumption Patterns, Food and Nutrition Board, National Research Council. *Assessing Changing Food Consumption Patterns.* Washington, DC: National Academy Press; 1981.

17. Subcommittee on Criteria for Dietary Evaluation, Food and Nutrition Board, National Research Council. *Nutrient Adequacy: Assessment Using Food Consumption Surveys.* Washington, DC: National Academy Press; 1986.

18. Den Hartog AP, van Staveren WA. *Manual for Social Surveys on Food Habits and Consumption in Developing Countries.* Wageningen, The Netherlands: Centre for Agricultural Publishing and Documentation; 1983.

19. *NHANES III Dietary Interviewer's Manual.* Rockville, Md: Westat Inc; 1989.

20. McDowell MA, Briefel RR, Warren RA, Buzzard IM, Feskanich D, Gardner SN. The dietary data collection system—an automated interview and coding system for NHANES III. In: *Proceedings of the Fourteenth National Nutrient Databank Conference in Iowa City, Iowa, June 19–21.* Ithaca, NY: The CBORD Group Inc; 1989:125–131.

21. Posner BM, Borman CL, Morgan JL, Borden WS, Ohls JC. The validity of a telephone-administered 24-hour dietary recall methodology. *Am J Clin Nutr.* 1982;36:546–553.

22. Krantzler NJ, Mullen BJ, Schutz HG, Grivetti LE, Holden CA, Meiselman HL. Validity of telephoned diet recalls and records for assessment of individual food intake. *Am J Clin Nutr.* 1982;36:1234–1242.

23. Morgan KJ, Johnson SR, Rizek RL, Reese R, Stampley GL. Collection of food intake data: an evaluation of methods. *J Am Diet Assoc.* 1987;87:888–896.

24. Lyu L-C, Hankin JH, Liu LQ, et al. Telephone versus face-to-face interviews for quantitative diet history assessment. *J Am Diet Assoc.* 1998;98:44–48.

25. Tran KM, Johnson RK, Soultanakis RP, Matthews DE. In-person versus telephone administered multiple-pass 24-hour recalls in women: validation with doubly labeled water. *J Am Diet Assoc.* 2000;100:777–783.

26. Stram DO, Hankin JH, Wilkens LR, et al. Calibration of the dietary questionnaire for a multiethnic cohort in Hawaii and Los Angeles. *Am J Epidemiol.* 2000;151:358–370.

27. Moshfegh A, Borrud L, Perloff B, LaComb R. Improved method for the 24-hour dietary recall for use in national surveys. *FASEB.* 1999;13(4):A603.

28. Woteki CE. Dietary survey data: sources and limits to interpretation. *Nutr Rev.* 1986;44 (suppl):204–213.

29. Welsh S. The joint nutrition monitoring evaluation committee. In: Food and Nutrition Board, National Research Council. *What Is America Eating?* Washington, DC: National Academy Press; 1986:7–20.

30. Hankin JH, Reed D, Labarthe D, Nichaman M, Stallones RA. Dietary and disease patterns among Micronesians. *Am J Clin Nutr.* 1970;23:346–357.

31. Kagan A, Harris BR, Winkelstein W. *Epidemiologic Studies of Coronary Heart Disease and Stroke in Japanese Men Living in Japan, Hawaii, and California.* Hiroshima, Japan: Atomic Bomb Casualty Commission; 1972.

32. Human Nutrition Information Service, US Department of Agriculture. *Food Consumption: Households in the United States, Spring 1977.* Washington, DC: US Government Printing Office; 1982. Publication H-1.

33. Woteki C, Johnson C, Murphy R. Nutritional status of the US population: iron, vitamin C, and zinc. In: Food and Nutrition Board, National Research Council. *What Is America Eating?* Washington, DC: National Academy Press; 1986:21–39.

34. Beaton GH, Milner J, McGuire V, Feather TE, Little JA.

Sources of variance in 24-hour dietary recall data: implications for nutrition study design and interpretation. Carbohydrate sources. Vitamins and minerals. *Am J Clin Nutr.* 1983;37:986–995.

35. Buzzard M. 24-hour dietary recall and food record methods. In: Willett W, ed. *Nutritional Epidemiology*. 2nd ed. New York, NY: Oxford University Press; 1998:50–73.

36. Basiotis PP, Welsh SO, Cronin FJ, Kelsay JL, Mertz W. Number of days of food intake records required to estimate individual and group nutrient intakes with defined confidence. *J Nutr.* 1987;117:1638–1641.

37. Willett WC, Sampson L, Stampfer MJ, et al. Reproducibility and validity of a semiquantitative food frequency questionnaire. *Am J Epidemiol.* 1985;122:51–65.

38. Garry P, Goodwin JS, Hunt WC, Hooper EM, Leonard AG. Nutritional status in a healthy elderly population: dietary and supplemental intakes. *Am J Clin Nutr.* 1982;36:319–331.

39. Hankin JH, Wilkens LR, Kolonel LN, Yoshizawa CN. Validation of a quantitative diet history method in Hawaii. *Am J Epidemiol.* 1991;133:616–628.

40. Sawaya AL, Tucker KT, Tsay R, et al. Evaluation of four methods for determining energy intake in young and older women: comparison with doubly labeled water measurements of total energy expenditure. *Am J Clin Nutr.* 1996;63:491–499.

41. Witschi JC. Short-term dietary recall and recording methods. In: Willett W, ed. *Nutritional Epidemiology*. 2nd ed. New York NY: Oxford University Press; 1990:52–68.

42. Hankin JH, Huenemann RL. A short dietary method for epidemiologic studies. I. Developing standard methods for interpreting seven-day measured food records. *J Am Diet Assoc.* 1967;50:487–492.

43. Hankin JH, Reynolds WE, Margen S. A short dietary method for epidemiologic studies. II. Variability of measured nutrient intakes. *Am J Clin Nutr.* 1967;20:935–945.

44. McGee D, Rhoads G, Hankin J, Yano K, Tillotson J. Within-person variability of nutrient intake in a group of Hawaiian men of Japanese ancestry. *Am J Clin Nutr.* 1982;36:657–663.

45. Hunt WC, Leonard AG, Garry PJ, Goodwin JS. Components of variance in dietary data for an elderly population. *Nutr Res.* 1983;3:433–444.

46. Sempos CT, Johnson NE, Smith EL, Gilligan C. Effects of intraindividual and interindividual variation in repeated dietary records. *Am J Epidemiol.* 1985;121:120–130.

47. Liu K, Stamler J, Dyer A, McKeever P. Statistical methods to assess and minimize the role of intraindividual variability in obscuring the relationship between dietary lipids and serum cholesterol. *J Chronic Dis.* 1978;31:399–418.

48. Block G, Hartman AM. Dietary assessment methods. In: Moon TE, Micozzi MS, eds. *Nutrition and Cancer Prevention. Investigating the Role of Micronutrients*. New York, NY: Marcel Dekker; 1989:159–180.

49. Burke BS. The dietary history as a tool in research. *J Am Diet Assoc.* 1947;23:1041–1046.

50. Reed RB, Burke BS. Collection and analysis of dietary intake data. *Am J Public Health.* 1954;44:1015–1026.

51. Beal VA. The nutritional history in longitudinal research. *J Am Diet Assoc.* 1967;51:426–432.

52. Mann GV, Pearson G, Gordon T, Dawber TR, Lyell L, Shurtleff D. Diet and cardiovascular disease in the Framingham study. I. Measurement of dietary intake. *Am J Clin Nutr.* 1962;11:200–225.

53. Paul O, Lepper MH, Phelan WH. A longitudinal study of coronary heart disease. *Circ.* 1963;28:20–31.

54. Samet JM, Skipper BJ, Humble CG, Pathak DR. Lung cancer risk and vitamin A consumption in New Mexico. *Am Rev Respir Dis.* 1985;131:198–202.

55. Ziegler RG, Mason TJ, Stemhagen A. Carotenoid intake, vegetables, and the risk of lung cancer among white men in New Jersey. *Am J Epidemiol.* 1986;123:1080–1093.

56. Hankin JH. Dietary methods for estimating vitamin A and carotene intakes in epidemiologic studies of cancer. *J Can Diet Assoc.* 1987;48:219–234.

57. Block G, Dresser CM, Hartman AM, Carroll MD. Nutrient sources in the American diet: quantitative data from the NHANES II survey. I. Vitamins and minerals. *Am J Epidemiol.* 1985;122:13–26.

58. Block G, Dresser CM, Hartman AM, Carroll MD. Nutrient sources in the American diet: quantitative data from the NHANES II survey. II. Macronutrients and fats. *Am J Epidemiol.* 1985;122:27–40.

59. Block G, Hartman AM, Dresser CM, Carroll MD, Gannon J, Gardner L. A data-based approach to diet questionnaire design and testing. *Am J Epidemiol.* 1986;124:453–469.

60. Stuff JE, Garza C, O'Brian Smith E, Nichols BL, Montandon CM. A comparison of dietary methods in nutritional studies. *Am J Clin Nutr.* 1983;37:300–306.

61. Gray GE, Paganini-Hill A, Ross RK, Henderson BE. Assessment of three brief methods of estimation of vitamin A and C intakes for a prospective study of cancer: comparison with dietary history. *Am J Epidemiol.* 1984;119:581–590.

62. Rohan TE, Potter JD. Retrospective assessment of dietary intake. *Am J Epidemiol.* 1984;120:876–887.

63. Rimm EB, Giovannucci EL, Stampfer MJ, Colditz GA, Litin LB, Willett WC. Reproducibility and validity of an expanded self-administered semiquantitative food frequency questionnaire among male health professionals. *Am J Epidemiol.* 1992;135:1114–1126.

64. Hunter DJ, Sampson L, Stampfer MJ, Colditz GA, Rosner B, Willett WC. Variability in portion sizes of commonly consumed foods among a population of women in the United States. *Am J Epidemiol.* 1988;127:1240–1249.

65. Cummings SR, Block G, McHenry K, Baron RB. Evaluation of two food frequency methods of measuring dietary calcium intake. *Am J Epidemiol.* 1987;126:796–802.

66. Chu SY, Kolonel LN, Hankin JH, Lee J. A comparison of frequency and quantitative dietary methods for epidemiologic studies of diet and disease. *Am J Epidemiol.* 1984;110:323–334.

67. Kolonel LN, Henderson BE, Hankin JH, et al. A multiethnic cohort in Hawaii and Los Angeles: baseline characteristics. *Am J Epidemiol.* 2000;151(4):346–357.

68. Pietinen P, Hartman AM, Haaoa E, et al. Reproducibility and validity of dietary assessment instruments. I. A self-administered food use questionnaire with a portion size picture booklet. *Am J Epidemiol.* 1988a;128:655–666.

69. Kolonel LN, Yoshizawa CN, Hankin JH. Diet and prostate cancer: a case-control study in Hawaii. *Am J Epidemiol.* 1988;127:999–1012.

70. LeMarchand L, Yoshizawa CN, Kolonel LN, Hankin JH, Goodman MT. Vegetable consumption and lung cancer risk: a population-based case-control study in Hawaii. *J Natl Cancer Inst.* 1989;81:1158–1164.

71. LeMarchand L, Wilkens LR, Hankin JH, Kolonel LN, Lyu LC. A case-control study of diet and colorectal cancer in a multiethnic population in Hawaii (United States): lipids and foods of animal origin. *Cancer Causes Control.* 1997;8:637–648.

72. Goodman MT, Wilkens LR, Hankin JH, Lyu LC, Wu AH, Kolonel LN. Association of soy and fiber consumption with the risk of endometrial cancer. *Am J Epidemiol.* 1997;146:294–306.

73. Hankin JH. Development of a diet history questionnaire for studies of older persons. *Am J Clin Nutr.* 1989;50:1121–1127.

74. Brown JE, Tharp TM, Dahlberg-Luby EM. Videotape dietary assessment: validity, reliability, and comparison of results with 24-hour dietary recalls from elderly women in a retirement home. *J Am Diet Assoc.* 1990;90:1675–1679.

75. Madden JP, Goodman SJ, Guthrie HA. Validity of the 24-hour recall. *J Am Diet Assoc.* 1976;68:143–147.

76. Gersovitz M, Madden JP, Smickilas-Wright H. Validity of the dietary recall and seven-day record for group comparisons. *J Am Diet Assoc.* 1978;73:48–56.

77. US Department of Agriculture. *Nutrient Data-base for Standard Reference, Release 11.* Bethesda, Md: USDA Human Nutrition Information Service; 1997.

78. Pennington JAT. *Bowes & Church's Food Values of Portions Commonly Used.* 17th ed. Philadelphia, Pa: JB Lippincott Co; 1998.

79. Holland B, Welch AA, Unwin ID, Buss DH, Paul AA, Southgate DAT. *McCance and Widdowson's The Composition of Foods.* 5th ed. Cambridge, England: Royal Society of Chemistry & Ministry of Agriculture, Fisheries and Food; 1991.

80. Johnson RK, Black AE, Cole TJ. Letter to the editor. *N Engl J Med.* 1998;338:917–919.

81. Willett WC, Reynolds RD, Cottrell-Hoehner S, Sampson L, Browne ML. Validation of a semi-quantitative food frequency questionnaire: comparison with a l-year diet record. *J Am Diet Assoc.* 1987;87:43–47.

82. Hankin JH. Role of nutrition in women's health: diet and breast cancer. *J Am Diet Assoc.* 1993;93:994–999.

83. Prentice RL, Pepe M, Self SG. Dietary fat and breast cancer: a quantitative assessment of the epidemiological literature and a discussion of methodological issues. *Cancer Res.* 1989;49:3147–3156.

84. Hegsted DM. Errors of measurement. *Nutr Cancer.* 1989;12:105–107.

85. Karvetti RL, Knuts LR. Validity of the 24-hour recall. *J Am Diet Assoc.* 1985;85:1437–1442.

86. Linusson EEI, Sanjur D, Erickson EC. Validating the 24-hour recall method as a dietary survey tool. *Arch Latinoam Nutr.* 1974;24:277–294.

87. Willett W. Dietary fat and breast cancer. In: Willett W, ed. *Nutritional Epidemiology.* 2nd ed. New York, NY: Oxford University Press; 1998:377–413.

88. Riboli E, Kaaks R. The EPIC project: rationale and study design. *Int J Epidemiol.* 1997;26(suppl 1):6–14.

89. Pietinen P, Hartman AM, Haapa E, et al. Reproducibility and validity of dietary assessment instruments II. A qualitative food frequency questionnaire. *Am J Epidemiol.* 1988b;128:667–676.

90. Black AE, Prentice AM, Goldberg GR, et al. Measurements of total energy expenditure provide insights into the validity of dietary measurements of energy intake. *J Am Diet Assoc.* 1993;33:572–579.

91. Bingham SA, Cassidy A, Cole TJ, et al. Validation of weighed records and other methods of dietary assessment using the 24 h urine nitrogen technique and other biological markers. *Br J Nutr.* 1995;73:531–550.

92. Katan MB. Biochemical indicators of dietary intake [abstract]. *Eur J Clin Nutr.* 1998;52:S5.

93. Lifson N, Gordon GB, Visscher MB, Nier AO. The fate of utilized molecular oxygen and the source of heavy oxygen of respiratory carbon dioxide, studied with the aid of heavy oxygen. *J Biol Chem.* 1949;180:803–811.

94. Lifson N, Gordon GB, McClintock R. Measurement of total carbon dioxide production by means of D_2O^{18}. *J Appl Physiol.* 1955;7:704–710.

95. Schoeller DA, van Santen E. Measurement of energy expenditure in humans by the doubly labeled water method. *J Appl Physiol.* 1982;53:955–995.

96. Poehlman ET. A review: exercise and its influence on resting energy metabolism in man. *Med Sci Sports Exerc.* 1989;21:515–525.

97. Poehlman ET. Energy expenditure and requirements in aging humans. *J Nutr.* 1992;122:2957–2965.

98. Schoeller DA. How accurate is self-reported dietary energy intake? *Nutr Rev.* 1990;48:373–379.

99. Mertz W. Food intake measurements: Is there a "gold standard"? *J Am Diet Assoc.* 1992;92:1463–1465.

100. Johnson RK, Driscoll P, Goran MI. Comparison of multiple-pass 24-hour recall estimates of energy intake with total energy expenditure determined by the doubly labeled water method in young children. *J Am Diet Assoc.* 1996;96:1140–1144.

101. Schoeller DA. Measurement of energy expenditure in free-living humans by using doubly-labeled water. *J Nutr.* 1988;1278–1289.

102. Bingham SA. Dietary assessments in the European prospective study of diet and cancer (EPIC). *Eur J Can Prev.* 1997;6:118–124.

103. Kok FJ, van't Veer P. *Biomarkers of Dietary Exposure: Proceedings of the 3rd Meeting on Nutritional Epidemiology.* London, England: Smith-Gordon & Co; 1991.

104. Bingham S. Challenges in dietary approaches [abstract]. *Eur J Clin Nutr.* 1998;52:S4.

105. Zock PL, Mensink RP, Harryvan J, de Vries JHM, Katan MB. Fatty acids in serum cholesteryl esters as quantitative biomarkers of dietary intake in humans. *Am J Epidemiol.* 1997;145:1114–1122.

106. Andersen LF, Solvoll K, Drevon DA. Very-long-chain n-3 fatty acids as biomarkers for intake of fish and n-3 fatty acid concentrates. *Am J Clin Nutr.* 1996;64:305–311.

107. Conner SL. Biomarkers and dietary intake data are mutually beneficial. *Am J Clin Nutr.* 1996;64:379–380.

108. Willet WC, Stampfer MJ, Colditz GA, Rosner BA, Hennekens CH, Speizer FE. Dietary fat and the risk of breast cancer. *N Engl J Med.* 1987;316:22–28.

109. Hu FB, Stampfer MJ, Manson JE, et al. Dietary fat intake and the risk of coronary heart disease in women. *N Engl J Med.* 1997;337:1491–1499.

110. Bingham SA, Cummings J. Urine nitrogen as an independent validatory measure of dietary intake: a study of nitrogen balance in individuals consuming their normal diet. *Am J Clin Nutr.* 1985;42:1276–1289.

111. Black AE. Under-reporting of energy intake at all levels of energy expenditure: evidence from doubly labeled water studies. *Proc Nutr Soc.* 1997;56:121A.

112. Chug-Ahuja JK, Holden JM, Forman MR, Mangels AR, Beecher GR. The development and application of a carotenoid database for fruits, vegetables, and selected multicomponent foods. *J Am Diet Assoc.* 1993;93:318–323.

113. Yeum KJ, Booth SL, Sadowski JA, Liu C, Tang G. Human plasma carotenoid response to the ingestion of controlled diets high in fruits and vegetables. *Am J Clin Nutr.* 1996;64:594–602.

114. Martini MC, Campbell DR, Gross MD, Grandits GA, Potter JD. Plasma carotenoids as biomarkers of vegetable intake: the University of Minnesota Cancer Prevention Research Unit Feeding Studies. *Cancer Epidemiol Biomarkers Prev.* 1995;4:491–496.

115. Le Marchand L, Hankin JH, Carter FS, et al. A pilot study on the use of plasma carotenoids and ascorbic acid as markers of compliance to a high fruit and vegetable dietary intervention. *Cancer Epidemiol Biomarkers Prev.* 1994;3(3):245–251.

116. Pierce JP, Faerber S, Wright FA, et al. Feasibility of a randomized trial of a high-vegetable diet to prevent breast cancer recurrence. *Nutr Cancer.* 1997;28(3):282–288.

117. Scott KJ, Thurnham DI, Hart DJ, Bingham SA, Day K. The correlation between the intake of lutein, lycopene, and beta-carotene from vegetables and fruits, and blood plasma concentrations in a group of women aged 50–65 years in the UK. *Br J Nutr.* 1996;75:409–418.

118. Murphy SP, Bunch SJ, Kaiser LL, Joy AB. A food behavior checklist can measure changes resulting from a nutrition education intervention. Abstract presented at: Advancing Nutrition Education—Moving Toward Healthful, Sustainable Diets, 31st Annual Meeting of the Society for Nutrition Education, Albuquerque, NM, July 18–22, 1998.

119. Luceri C, Caderni G, Lodovici M, et al. Urinary excretion of sucrose and fructose as a predictor of sucrose intake in dietary intervention studies. *Cancer Epidemiol Biomarker Prev.* 1996;65;165–171.

120. Prentice AM, Black AE, Coward WA, et al. High levels of energy expenditure in obese women. *Br Med J.* 1986;292:983–987.

121. Lichtman SW, Pisarska K, Berman ER, et al. Discrepancy between self-reported and actual caloric intake and exercise in obese subjects. *N Engl J Med.* 1992;327:1893–1898.

122. Price GM, Paul AA, Cole TJ, Wadsworth MEJ. Characteristics of the low-energy reporters in a longitudinal national dietary survey. *Br J Nutr.* 1997;77:833–851.

123. Pryer JA, Vrijheid M, Nichols R, Kiggins M, Elliot P. Who are the 'low energy reporters' in the dietary and nutritional survey of British adults? *Int J Epidemiol.* 1997;26:146–154.

124. Briefel RR, Sempos CT, McDowell MA, Chien SCY, Alaimo K. Dietary methods research in the third national health and nutrition examination survey: under-reporting of energy intake. *Am J Clin Nutr.* 1997;65(suppl):1203–1209.

125. Taren D, Tobar M, Hill A, et al. The association of energy intake bias with psychological scores of women. *Eur J Clin Nutr.* 1999;53:570–578.

126. Johnson RK, Soultanakis RP, Matthews DE. Psychologi-

cal factors and energy intake underreporting in women. *FASEB.* 1999;13(5):A695.

127. Kretsch MJ, Fong AKH, Green MW. Behavioral and body size correlates of energy intake underreporting by obese and normal-weight women. *J Am Diet Assoc.* 1999;99(3):300–306.

128. Krebs-Smith SM, Graubard B, Cleveland L, Subar A, Ballard-Barbash R, Kahle L. Low energy reporters vs others: a comparison of reported food intakes. *Eur J Clin Nutr.* 1998;52(2):S18.

129. Voss S, Kroke A, Lipstein-Grobusch K, Boeing H. Is macronutrient composition of dietary intake data affected by underreporting? Results from the EPIC-Potsdam study. *Eur J Clin Nutr.* 1998;52:119–126.

130. Poppitt SD, Swann D, Black AE, Prentice AM. Assessment of selective under-reporting of food intake by both obese and non-obese women in a metabolic facility. *Int J Obes.* 1998;22:303–311.

131. Livingstone MBE, Prentice AM, Strain JJ, et al. Accuracy of weighed dietary records in studies of diet and health. *Br Med J.* 1990;300:708–712.

132. Goldberg GR, Black AE, Jebb SA, et al. Critical evaluation of energy intake data using fundamental principles of energy physiology: 1. Derivation of cut-off limits to identify under-recording. *Eur J Clin Nutr.* 1991;45:569–581.

133. Black AE, Goldberg GR, Jebb SA, Livingstone MBE, Cole TJ, Prentice AM. Critical evaluation of energy intake data using fundamental principles of energy physiol-ogy: 2. Evaluating the results of published surveys. *Eur J Clin Nutr.* 1991;45:583–599.

134. Schofield WN, Schofield C, James WPT. Basal metabolic rate. *Hum Nutr Clin Nutr.* 1985;39C(suppl 1):1–96.

135. Black AE. Poor validity of dietary assessment: what have we learnt? *Eur J Clin Nutr.* 1998;52(2):S17.

136. Black AE. The sensitivity and specificity of the Goldberg cut-off for EI:BMR for identifying diet reports of poor validity. *Eur J Clin Nutr.* 2000;54(5):395–404.

137. Munoz K, Krebs-Smith S, Ballard-Barbash R, Cleveland L. Food intakes of US children and adolescents compared with recommendations. *Pediatrics.* 1997;100(3):323–329.

138. Willett W, Stampfer MJ. Total energy intake: implications for epidemiologic analyses. *Am J Epidemiol.* 1986;124(1):17–26.

139. Carter LM, Whiting SJ. Underreporting of energy intake, socioeconomic status, and expression of nutrient intake. *Nutr Rev.* 1998;56(6):179–182.

140. Stallone DD, Brunner EJ, Bingham SA, Marmot MG. Dietary assessment in Whitehall II: the influence of reporting bias on apparent socioeconomic variation in nutrient intakes. *Eur J Clin Nutr.* 1997;51:815–825.

The authors would like to thank Debra McKenzie, M.S., for her assistance with the preparation of this chapter.

16

Development and Use of Food Composition Data and Databases

Jean A.T. Pennington, Ph.D., R.D.

This chapter provides an overview of the generation, reporting, and compiling of food composition data and databases. It emphasizes the care that should be taken in using food composition data because of their inherent and acquired variability.

DATA USERS AND DATA USES

Food composition databases are used to assess the dietary status of patients, clients, students, and population groups with defined demographic characteristics; to plan and evaluate the dietary adequacy of meals and diets; and to discern relationships between diet, health, and disease from the results of clinical and epidemiologic studies. Food composition databases may be used to assess the nutrient content of individual foods or a group of similar foods for the purpose of developing food standards, formulating new food products, determining the potential use of a food in a therapeutic diet, establishing definitions for dietary claims, or determining whether foods meet such claims. Databases are also used to develop nutrition education materials and programs for students, foodservice workers, caregivers, homemakers, and the general public.

Dietitians and nutritionists may have a specific need or range of needs for food composition data, depending on their place of employment and job responsibilities. Dietitians working in hospitals, schools, prisons, and other institutions and dietitians in private practice may use databases to plan and evaluate meals and daily diets, develop therapeutic diets, and educate patients or residents. Within hospitals and clinics, databases may also be used to counsel patients and design diets for clinical trials. Academic nutritionists use databases for diet-disease epidemiologic research and for student education in nutrition, food science, and health courses. Government nutritionists at the Food and Drug Administration (FDA), the National Institutes of Health, and the U.S. Department of Agriculture (USDA) may use databases to develop policies concerning nutrient fortification, food standards, and label claims; to assess the safety and adequacy of the food supply; or to design and evaluate the results of epidemiologic studies and clinical trials. Nutritionists at food companies use databases for product development, nutrition labeling, and dietary claims. Grocery stores may use databases for shelf-labeling programs, and restaurants may use them to make nutrition claims about foods on their menus.

Because food composition databases are widely available, many of their users are not nutrition professionals. Some of these users may not understand or be aware of the appropriate uses or limitations of the data. The most frequent complaints from students and consumers regarding databases are that certain data are missing, that they cannot find the foods they are looking for, and that they need different serving portions than those listed. Consequently, common errors made by these users are selecting the wrong food (not making the best match between the food of interest and the foods listed in the database), assuming that missing values are zeros, and not adjusting serving portions (assuming that the portion listed in the database is the amount consumed). When data are missing from a database, it is usually because the analyses have not been performed or because the manufacturers are unable to release the data. Currently, data for many multi-ingredient foods are not available for inclusion in food composition databases; these foods include some homemade, frozen, and shelf-stable entrees and desserts; fast foods and carryout foods; and ethnic foods.

FOOD ANALYSTS AND FOOD ANALYSIS

Food composition data originate from the work of chemists in government, industry, academic, and private laboratories who analyze individual or composite samples (mixtures of individual samples) of foods to determine the levels of nutrients and other food components, such as pesticide residues, toxicants, heavy metals, radionuclides, and food additives. The procedures and accepted methods for collecting and analyzing foods for various nutrients are discussed in detail in *Food Composition Data: Production, Management and Use* (1).

Each food that is analyzed requires a unique sampling design to be sure that the samples that are analyzed are representative of the foods typically consumed. The sampling design should include variables that affect the composition of the food. Nationwide food sampling involves different variables than does local food sampling. The variables for raw fruits and vegetables may include season, geography, and cultivar (genetic strain or variety), whereas variables for processed foods may include the location of the processing plant and the market share of the brand-name products. If compositing methods are used for the foods, they should be appropriate for the intended purposes of the resulting data.

The analytic methods and laboratory practices should be specific for the analytes and approved by the Association of Official Analytical Chemists (2). Quality control procedures should include duplicate analyses and recoveries of reference standards, spiked/fortified samples, and standard reference materials. Spiked/fortified samples contain a known added amount of the nutrient and are used to determine if the analytic method accurately measures the amount present. Standard reference materials contain a government-certified amount of a nutrient in a food and are purchased and analyzed by laboratories to ascertain the accuracy of their analytic methods.

It is important for analysts to document how the foods are sampled, selected, collected, prepared, and analyzed, as well as how the results are verified and evaluated. If calculations are required to determine nutrient levels (such as protein content calculated from nitrogen content), they should be explained and documented. When many samples of the same food are analyzed individually to determine the concentration of a nutrient, the distribution of those concentrations is rarely normal (Gaussian). Statistical treatment of analytic data typically includes the calculation of means, standard deviations, coefficients of variation, and medians. Means may be weighted by variety, cultivar, species, market share, or year-round availability of the individual foods.

Much can be learned by evaluating the distribution of the analytic data points for each nutrient in a food. Outliers can be identified, and their treatment (that is, inclusion or omission from the evaluation) can be determined and documented. If bimodal or other modal distributions occur, it might be necessary to separate the samples into groups to obtain more useful data. For example, the distribution of the iron content of wheat flake breakfast cereals might show a bimodal distribution reflecting two different levels of iron fortification (for example, 18 mg/oz and 4.5 mg/oz). The overall mean concentration of iron would be an intermediate value that would not reflect either type of cereal. It would be best to list both types of cereal separately in a database, even if all the other nutrient values for the two types of cereal were similar.

DATA COMPILERS AND DATA COMPILATIONS

The data compiler gathers data from the available sources and organizes, evaluates, and aggregates the data into a useful database (3). Database compilers gather data from previous compilations, food companies, and scientific papers. They might also obtain data directly from laboratories; however, nutrient composition data resulting from laboratory analyses usually appear first in professional or trade journals. The data from the various sources are collected by database compilers and incorporated into the files of individual databases. The compiler cannot check the documentation for every nutrient value for every food with regard to sampling, number of samples, analytical method, and laboratory quality control. However, any data that appear to be clearly out of line should be questioned and either verified or omitted.

Compilers of food composition data may be employed by government agencies, food companies, academic institutions, private businesses, hospitals, clinics, foodservice institutions, or private companies. They may also be independent contractors hired by these organizations or be self-employed. Compilers should hold degrees in nutrition, dietetics, or food science and should be knowledgeable about food sampling, analysis, descriptions, and processing; culinary terms; and cuisines. Knowledge about computerized database systems and the retrieval of information from databases is also very important. It is best to have the compiler work directly with the person who designs the computer system so that the system performs the necessary operations accurately and efficiently.

Many compilations of food composition data are currently available in the United States and other countries. Many countries have a national food composition database that reflects foods that are available and most commonly consumed by their populations. Most food composition databases are stored and maintained as computer files, and their availability to users may be as hard copy and/or electronic files. The major database developed and used in the United States is the USDA Nutrient Database for Standard Reference (NDSR), available from the USDA Web site (4). (This database is no longer available in hard copy, and previous hard copies are now out of date.) The NDSR contains about 6,000 foods and includes data for 70 food components. It serves as the foundation for many of the food composition databases that have been developed in U.S. colleges, universities, hospitals, and clinics, as well as by private individuals and companies. The NDSR also serves as the foundation for databases in several other countries where resources for analyzing local foods are not available.

Compilers who use the NDSR as the foundation for their databases select the foods and nutrients that they need from this source and then add other foods and nutrients that they obtain from the literature, food companies, restaurants, and other sources. Database compilers may fill in missing values in the NDSR by imputation or calculation, and they may add foods to the database that have nutrient values determined by imputation or calculation. Some compilers may include nutrition-labeling values for some foods if the original data are not available to them from the food companies. The food composition data generated by food companies for the purpose of nutrition labeling is adjusted by the use of formulas and by rounding so that the resulting values are in compliance with FDA and USDA regulations. (The USDA regulates the nutrition labeling of meat and poultry and products containing meat and poultry; the FDA regulates the nutrition labeling of all other foods.)

In addition to the NDSR, the USDA also maintains the Survey Nutrient Database (5), which is used to assess the food and nutrient intake of participants in national food consumption surveys. The Survey Nutrient Database contains data on energy, dietary fiber, cholesterol, alcohol, moisture, protein, fat, carbohydrate, 10 vitamins, 8 minerals, total fatty acids, and 19 individual fatty acids for over 7,300 foods. There are no missing values in this database. Nutrient values that were not available from laboratory analysis were imputed or were calculated from recipes by the USDA. The foods in this database are generally in the "as-consumed" state, and the database is updated from survey to survey to keep pace with trends and changes in American eating patterns.

The challenge in using the Survey Nutrient Database and other databases for assessing diets is to appropriately match the foods described by study participants, students, patients, or clients to the foods listed in the databases (that is, to select the best fit). This challenge is one reason why food descriptions are so important. Because survey participants are not always able to provide accurate descriptions of the foods they eat, the Survey Nutrient Database includes some generic foods with the descriptor *not further specified* (NFS). The nutrient data for NFS foods are based on data for similar or representative foods. For example, an NFS sandwich might reflect the most commonly consumed sandwich in the survey (perhaps a baloney sandwich on white bread with mayonnaise), or it might be a composite sandwich with nutrient values calculated from weighted data from other sandwiches in the database.

Features of databases that may distinguish one database from another include the foods and nutrients contained, the form of the database (for example, hard copy or electronic file), periodicity of update, format on the page or computer screen, and intended use (for example, reference database, diet analyses, or product development). Some databases are updated routinely as new data become available; others are updated at specific intervals, such as every year or every few years. Foods in databases may appear alphabetically or alphabetically by food group. One common format for listing foods and nutrients is to have the foods listed in the left-hand column with the nutrient values listed in columns across the page or screen. An alternative format is one food per page or screen, with the nutrients in the left-hand column and the values per several serving portions in the columns across the page or screen. The computer system for a database may allow the user to select several alternative formats for data display and presentation.

Food Descriptions in a Database

Database compilers must give accurate and appropriate names to each food and sufficient descriptive terms to distinguish each food from all the other foods in the database. Foods that are poorly named or described or foods with inconsistent or ambiguous descriptive terms will cause confusion for the user and may lead to improper use of the data. Similarly, when food composition data are published in journals, the data should be accompanied by complete and accurate food descriptions.

Guidelines and methods for describing foods have been developed, and issues related to food descriptions and to the development of descriptive terms have been discussed (6–10). The luxuries of unlimited space for food names and open-ended food descriptors (as might be found in analytic reports or scientific papers) are not usually allowed in databases available in hard copy or as electronic files. Therefore, it is necessary to provide, in the allotted space, the food names and descriptive terms that will be most useful for the data user. The compiler should strive for uniformity in describing foods in a database by using a selected order of descriptors and standardized terms and abbreviations. For example, the compiler might use the order of descriptors shown in Table 16.1.

Not all of the descriptors shown in Table 16.1 are applicable or useful for each food. The information for "part of plant or animal" should indicate information on such things as whether peel or seeds are present for fruits and vegetables, whether fat is present on meat cuts or has been trimmed away, and whether rind is included or not for cheese. Redundant or commonly assumed information is not usually included (for example, that fruits and vegetables are rinsed before use, that ice cream is frozen, or that frozen entrees are heated before serving). Footnotes might be added to provide ingredients for mixed dishes (for example, a footnote might say that a tuna-noodle-vegetable casserole contains tuna canned in water; egg noodles; chopped, frozen broccoli; and condensed mushroom soup) but are not usually necessary for well-known items with quality control (for example, a Big Mac).

TABLE 16.1   Example of Order of Food Description Terms in a Database

Type of Term	Food with Descriptive Terms (italicized)
Color	Apple, *red*, Red Delicious, with peel, without core, raw
Flavor	Pudding, *vanilla*, prepared from instant mix, JELL-O
Part of plant or animal	Beet, *greens and root*, diced, boiled
Accompaniments	Ice cream, vanilla *with chocolate syrup*
Preservation, treatment methods, and containers	Fruit cocktail *in light syrup*, *canned*, Del Monte
Preparation or cooking method	Frankfurter, beef and pork, *boiled*
Brand name	Peas, green, with cream sauce, frozen, *Birds Eye*

A thorough index with cross-references is useful to locate foods in a hard copy database because of the many synonyms for some foods (Figure 16.1) and the many ways of describing and placing foods in alphabetical listings. Computerized systems can have similar cross-references within their alphabetical listing of food names.

Food Groupings in a Database

Database compilers often organize the foods into groups based on food source (for example, grains, fruit, nuts, or vegetables) or food use (for example, beverages, breakfast cereals, condiments, desserts, entrees, or snacks). Food groups may then be further organized into subgroup hierarchies. Food groups and subgroups in databases help users locate items and prevent redundancy in terms, such as *ready-to-eat cereal* or *candy bar*. Food use groupings

Fries; French fries; fried potatoes; home fries; cottage fries

Green beans; snap beans; string beans

Hamburger; ground beef; minced beef; ground round; ground chuck

Milkshake; malt; shake; malted

Pancakes; hotcakes; flapjacks

FIGURE 16.1   Examples of food name synonyms

have cultural significance that might make a database useful in its country or region of origin but less useful internationally. Therefore, databases designed specifically for international use may need an alphabetical organizational structure or food groups that are based on food source rather than food use.

Because there are many potential hierarchies for food subgroups, thought must go into constructing them so they will be most useful. Consider the potential subgroups and hierarchical structure for *pizza* (Figure 16.2). There may be subgroups according to crust (deep-dish, regular, thick, or thin), topping (cheese, mushroom, pepperoni, or sausage), source (frozen, carryout, homemade, or restaurant chain), or brand name. The resulting hierarchies are affected by the order in which the variables are selected. Likewise, cakes may be subgrouped by flavor (chocolate, cherry, pound, or yellow) or by source (bakery, homemade, box mix, or frozen). Ready-to-eat cereals may be grouped by grain type (corn, oat, rice, or wheat), listed alphabetically by cereal brand name (Trix, Froot Loops, Shredded Wheat), or subgrouped according to the manufacturer's name (General Mills, Kellogg's, Post). The decisions for grouping and subgrouping are made by the compiler and often depend on how many items are available under each subheading (that is, whether there are enough foods with nutrient values to make a subhead). The group and subgroup designations affect the usefulness of the compilation, so the compiler must make these decisions with care.

Data Aggregation by Database Compilers

After organizing foods into groups, subgroups, and hierarchies within the subgroups, compilers aggregate the data for individual foods to prevent duplicates. This aggregation requires that the data for foods that appear to have the same or similar name and descriptors be closely scrutinized to determine which foods and their corresponding nutrient values may be consolidated into a single food entry in the database. The compiler may also combine data for foods with similar descriptions that have identical (or nearly identical) nutrient composition data, such as different flavors for a brand name of reduced-fat yogurts or different cultivars of apples.

Aggregation of nutrient data for the same food from various sources requires that food descriptions be as similar as possible (for example, have the same processing or preparation methods) and that nutrients have the same specificity and units for measurements. For example, vi-

Crust (level 1)	Topping (level 2)	Location of Preparation (level 3)
Deep-dish	Cheese	Carryout
Regular	Mushroom	Frozen
Thick	Pepperoni	Homemade
Thin	Sausage	Restaurant

Pizza Hierarchy Example

Level 1	Deep-dish	
Level 2		Cheese
Level 3		Carryout
Level 3		Frozen
Level 3		Homemade
Level 3		Restaurant
Level 2		Mushroom
Level 3		Carryout
Level 3		Frozen
Level 3		Homemade
Level 3		Restaurant
Level 2		Pepperoni
Level 3		Carryout
Level 3		Frozen
Level 3		Homemade
Level 3		Restaurant
Level 2		Sausage
Level 3		Carryout
Level 3		Frozen
Level 3		Homemade
Level 3		Restaurant

Level 1   Regular crust
    Repeat above for levels 2 and 3.
Level 1   Thick crust
    Repeat above for levels 2 and 3.
Level 1   Thin crust
    Repeat above for levels 2 and 3.

FIGURE 16.2 Example of a subgroup hierarchy for pizza. This example uses only four descriptive terms from each of the three subgroups and shows only part of one hierarchical arrangement (crust first, topping second, and location of preparation third). Fifteen other hierarchical arrangements are possible with these three subgroups.

tamin E may be expressed as international units or as milligrams of individual tocopherols. Similarity of common nutrient values (for example, water, energy, protein, and fat) for information from several sources provides some basis for food name and data aggregation. Evaluation of major and minor nutrients might indicate that foods with slightly different names are basically the same food. Aggregation allows for summarizing the data for the same food (or very similar foods) and uses fewer lines in the database.

When data for the same food are aggregated from various sources, the challenge is usually to calculate representative values for the various nutrients using statistical models that weight the important factors contributing to variability. Data for aggregated foods may be averaged (that is, each data point carries the same value), or they may be weighted and averaged (for example, data for four brands of canned corn might be weighted and averaged by market share or averaged by the number of samples from each source). The data sources and data manipulation should be documented, but it is not usually possible to provide this documentation with the database. This information usually remains in the files of the data compiler.

Sometimes the aggregation of data from various sources allows for completion of the nutrient profile of a food, because some sources may provide nutrients that are not provided by other sources. For example, one source might have extensive trace mineral values for a food, and another source might provide individual carotenoid values for the same food. Before combining data from different sources, it is important to be sure the food names and descriptions indicate that the foods are the same and to check for comparability of data provided by the sources (for example, comparability of water, protein, fat, carbohydrate, and dietary fiber).

Missing Values in a Database

Reference databases contain data gathered from available sources and generally do not contain imputed or calculated data for missing values, whereas databases used to analyze dietary information from food consumption surveys and studies should have as few missing values as possible. If missing values are not imputed or calculated, estimates of daily intakes will be underestimated. Imputed or calculated values should be identified as such, and the process used for imputation should be documented.

Procedures used to impute values are found in Chapter 5 of *INFOODS Guidelines for Compiling Data for Food Composition Databases,* by Rand et al (3). Some blanks may be filled in with zeros (for example, cholesterol and vitamin B-12 for plant materials or dietary fiber for animal-based foods). Other data may be imputed from a different form of the same food (for ex-

ample, data for canned corn might be used for frozen corn with adjustment for the sodium content) or from similar foods (for example, data for pinto beans might be used for navy beans). Missing values for multi-ingredient foods may be filled in with data calculated from recipes. These calculations usually require corrections for refuse (for example, bone, shell, peel, or trimmed fat), loss or gain of moisture or fat with cooking, and nutrient loss or retention with cooking. Chapter 6 of *INFOODS Guidelines for Compiling Data for Food Composition Databases* (3) provides information on how to estimate nutrients for multi-ingredient foods.

Because so few data are available for some nutrients, such as vitamins D and K, chromium, and other trace minerals, these nutrients may not be included in large databases. It is difficult to estimate accurately intakes of these nutrients using large databases because of so many missing values. Supplemental tables for these nutrients, such as those found in *Bowes & Church's Food Values of Portions Commonly Used* (11), may be useful in printed databases to provide easy access to the values and prevent wasted space.

Database Checks

Computerized tools are available to help the compiler assess the validity and integrity of the compiled database (12). These tools include checks for weights of major nutrients compared with the total weight of the food, caloric sums of energy-yielding nutrients compared with the caloric value of the food, and limits of nutrient concentrations in various food groups. For example, 1/2 c of boiled mashed pumpkin weighs 122 g, and the sum of the weights of the values for water, protein, fat, and carbohydrate is 121 g. The energy value of this food is 24 kcal per half-cup, and the sum of the energy equivalents of the protein, fat, and carbohydrate (with a correction for dietary fiber) is 25 kcal. These checks indicate data comparability. The computer system can identify foods and nutrients with potential problems to allow the database compiler to evaluate them. Foods with missing values will generally be flagged with the database checks unless the system is designed to exclude them.

Database Inconsistencies

Inconsistencies in nutrient values among foods occur in databases. Some inconsistencies may be picked up with the database checks and may then be verified or corrected. Other inconsistencies may become apparent only when one compares nutrient values for foods with a group or subgroup. For example, one might expect higher values for vitamin C in fresh orange juice than in processed orange juice, but the aggregated data from different varieties, regions, and seasons may show somewhat higher average levels in canned or reconstituted frozen juice. Such apparent inconsistencies might reflect the fact that the data came from different sources and might be the result of differences in food storage and sampling, differences in laboratory analytic methods and techniques, or nonidentical samples.

Another example of an apparent inconsistency is that the cholesterol content of tuna canned in vegetable oil (26 mg cholesterol per 3-oz drained tuna) is less than that for tuna canned in water (35 mg cholesterol per 3-oz drained tuna). Because cholesterol is lipid soluble, some of it dissolves into the vegetable oil and thereby reduces the amount of cholesterol in the drained tuna. Tuna in vegetable oil therefore might appear to be a better choice for cholesterol-conscious individuals; however, the cholesterol difference (9 mg/oz of tuna) is not of practical significance. Tuna canned in water is still a better choice for people following diets low in total fat and energy. (Tuna canned in water contains 116 kcal and 2.1g fat per 3 oz, whereas tuna canned in oil contains 158 kcal and 6.9 g fat per 3 oz.)

Basis of Data in a Database

Nutrient data for foods in databases are presented on a wet weight basis, so data available on a dry weight basis should be converted to wet weight before being added to a database. (Dry weight basis means that all the water in the food has been removed by a dehydration process and that the food is in a powdered state.) Dry weight data should not be included in a database unless the product is available as a powder. It is important for analysts to include the percentage of water with the other nutrients for each food when they publish data in the scientific literature so that nutrient values can be converted from a dry weight to a wet weight basis.

In addition to the issue of wet versus dry weight, it should be clear whether the data are presented *as purchased* (with waste or refuse) or as *edible portion* and if the weight of the food includes or excludes possible waste or refuse (bone, peel, core, husk, or shell). For example, the data for an apple presented on a 100-g basis may or may not include the weight of the core and the peel. The data for a baked chicken breast may or may not include the weight of the bones and skin. It should also be

clear whether the foods are in a raw, cooked, or processed state, and the methods of cooking and processing should be indicated.

Dietitians are most likely to need nutrient values per weight of edible portion of *as-consumed* foods (for example, cooked meat without bones, popped popcorn, or apples without cores). The food weight in the database may be per typical serving portion or per 100 g. If a serving portion is given, it should be unambiguously described. Consistency in listing serving portions within each food group of a database is useful for comparative purposes (for example, so users can compare nutrient values for 8 fl oz of milks, 6 fl oz of fruit juices, 1 oz or 1 c of ready-to-eat cereals, 3.5 oz of meats, 1/2 c of cooked vegetables, 1/2 c of canned fruits, 1 oz of nuts, and 1 oz of cheeses).

SPECIAL DATABASES

Carotenoids, Flavonoids, Dietary Fiber Fractions, Trace Elements, and Dietary Supplements

Because there is interest in relating the intake of various carotenoids (13–18), flavonoids (19–21), dietary fiber fractions (22), trace elements (23,24), and dietary supplements (25,26) to health and disease (such as cancer, cardiovascular disease, and immune system diseases), food composition databases for these substances are needed. Data for some of these substances may be kept in separate databases rather than incorporated into the larger reference databases. This probably reflects how the data are obtained (by separate analysis rather than along with the complete nutrient profile) and the use of the data (special studies to determine relationships to cancer and other diseases). Eventually, data for more of these substances may be incorporated into the larger databases that contain the more complete nutrient profiles.

Carotenoids, flavonoids, and dietary fiber fractions exist in specific parts of the food supply, and there is much to be learned about their concentrations in foods and their biochemical functions in the body. The carotenoids (beta carotene, alpha carotene, lutein, and lycopene) occur primarily in green and yellow vegetables and in yellow and red fruits. There are about 5,000 flavonoid compounds; these substances are found primarily in vegetables, fruits, cereals, legumes, nuts, tea, coffee, wine, and beer (19). Dietary fiber fractions are found in plant foods (vegetables, fruits, and grains).

Dietary supplements (including pills, herbal preparations, and other dietary preparations) include thousands of different products with different brand names and potencies. There are also different potencies of the same compound with the same brand name. Data for dietary supplements are not currently available in most food composition databases. Databases for dietary supplements will likely evolve over the next decade as more research is conducted on the bioavailability of these substances and their relationship to health promotion, health maintenance, and disease prevention (27).

Food Contaminants

Data on the levels of contaminants in foods are not usually included in the same databases as nutrients. The development of food composition databases for food contaminants poses special challenges, because average levels are not generally reported and could be misleading if they were. The presence of pesticide residues, toxins, or other contaminants in foods is often a matter of chance. Experts in these areas speak of the number of *detections*, rather than average levels, and the residue levels are usually quite low compared with accepted standards. For example, an analysis of 200 samples of a food may reveal a pesticide residue in only 10 of the samples. The average level for these 10 samples may be measurable; however, the average for the 200 samples may have no significant figures. In addition, pesticide levels are considerably reduced in foods during rinsing, peeling, and processing.

Although much work has been done to determine pesticide residues and other contaminants in foods, it has been done to monitor the food supply (to assess safety by confirming that levels are below acceptable daily intakes) rather than to provide average values for databases. It might be more informative for these databases to provide a ratio of detected to nondetected contaminants and to provide reported values for the detected contaminants only, as well as for all samples analyzed. The databases for food contaminants are evolving, and the accepted format and standards for these databases will likely be developed.

IMPLICATIONS FOR DIETITIANS

The selection of a nutrient database or database system for use in a dietary department, educational facility, or research clinic requires consideration of the specific needs of the users and the features and limitations of the various database systems (28). The users should consider factors such as the number and types of foods included, the nutrients included and their units of measure, the sources of the data, the quality of the data, availability of data updates, and the desired software features, along with considerations for such items as initial cost, maintenance costs, and hardware concerns. It may be useful to talk with individuals who use different database systems and to ask specific questions of the database system developers. The choices are many and varied. Experimentation with database systems at conference exhibits may be helpful in making decisions.

Except perhaps for carefully formulated products (such as medical formulas and infant formulas), the nutrient data for foods in databases are not precise because of inherent and acquired variability. For example, the average vitamin C content of an orange may be 80 mg, but the actual vitamin C content of each orange depends on factors such as season, sunlight exposure, cultivar, species, variety, time of day of harvest, storage length and temperature, and ripeness at harvest. Average values for individual nutrients may have large standard deviations, and most food composition tables do not provide standard deviations, nor do they usually include the number of samples analyzed or the documentation for the data aggregation.

Considering the extent of nutrient variation, diet recommendations for patients and clients should not be rigid. One food should not be recommended over another as a better or worse source of a nutrient unless the difference between the nutrient values for the foods will be of practical importance for the patient or client. Small differences in average values for nutrients should not be used to make comparative selections for foods. Rigid dietary recommendations may override the dietary variety that dietitians try to encourage.

The many causes of nutrient variation are compounded in food composition databases because the data are aggregated from various sources. Variables within any one food include genetics; environmental conditions (climate, temperature, and soil type); and methods of preservation, processing, and preparation. Because multi-ingredient foods are made from mixtures of different foods, they have mixtures of these variables. Contributing further to nutrient variation are different analytic methods and techniques, use of different recipes to calculate nutrient values for a mixed dish, and the compiler's unique methods of aggregating foods and nutrient values.

We should try not to extend the uses of food composition databases beyond their limitations. Databases may be used for multiday individual dietary assessments or 1-day group dietary assessments, but they probably should not be used to assess the dietary adequacy or deficiency of 1-day diets of individual subjects. Databases are not accurate enough to use for planning or assessing diets for metabolic research or balance studies, nor are they accurate enough to plan diets for patients on very restricted diets. Food analysis of brand-name products or specific information from food manufacturers, however, could be used in research studies or for planning restricted diets.

We should use databases knowledgeably and not become unduly alarmed about uneven quality (for example, more detailed descriptions and more nutrient data for some foods than others) or inconsistencies. However, we should not accept unreasonable data and should try to determine the reasons for values that clearly appear to be out of line compared with values for similar foods. Several sources are available to address concerns or questions about the nutrient content of foods. The USDA and food trade associations are good sources of information regarding the composition of basic and traditional foods. The USDA should be contacted for concerns about data in the USDA Nutrient Database for Standard Reference (4). Food companies should be contacted regarding nutrient data for brand-name products. Food labels provide addresses and telephone numbers for food companies. The headquarter of fast-food chains or other restaurants should be contacted for information on the nutrient content of restaurant foods.

OUTLOOK FOR FOOD COMPOSITION DATABASES

Food composition databases have continued to improve with time and will continue to improve. Work will continue to improve analytic methods, quality assurance techniques, and statistical analysis of results. More food samples analyzed by better analytic techniques and monitored by better quality control procedures produce more and better results. Needs for current databases are to fill in the missing values for nutrients with analytic values and to analyze foods for which data are most needed (for example, prepared entrees and restaurant foods). As new data become available, they replace the older or missing values. Several publications (29,30) indicate that when databases are updated, changes in dietary intake of nutrients are observed (in other words, changes to the

database affect the results from food consumption surveys). Thus, maintaining and improving food composition data are important to obtain reliable information about dietary status and diet-health relationships.

Improvements in food composition data quality do not result in decreased data variability. However, improved data quality does allow variability to be more readily measured. As more data become available for the same food, outlying values are more clearly identified and can be omitted when averages are determined. For the future, better ways of determining and expressing nutrient variability and of validating nutrient data in compiled databases should be found so that nutrition professionals can more easily evaluate the results of their nutrition surveys and studies.

REFERENCES

1. Greenfield H, Southgate DAT. *Food Composition Data: Production, Management, and Use*. London, England: Elsevier Applied Science; 1992.
2. *Official Method of Analysis*. 17th ed. Gaithersburg Md: Association of Official Analytical Chemists; 1998.
3. Rand WM, Pennington JAT, Murphy SP, Klensin JC. *INFOODS Guidelines for Compiling Data for Food Composition Databases*. Tokyo, Japan: UNU Press; 1992.
4. USDA. *Nutrient Database for Standard Reference*. Available at: http://www.nal.usda.gov/fnic/foodcomp. Accessed January 7, 2003.
5. USDA. *Survey Nutrient Database* [survey on CD-ROM]. Springfield, Va: National Technical Information Service. Accession no. PB1998-500457.
6. Truswell AS, Bateson DJ, Madafiglio KC, Pennington JAT, Rand WM, Klensin JC. INFOODS guidelines for describing foods: a systematic approach to facilitate international exchange of food composition data. *J Food Comp Ann.*. 1991;4:18–38.
7. McCann A, Pennington JAT, EC Smith, JM Holden, D Soergel, RC Wiley. FDA's Factored Food Vocabulary for food product description. *J Am Diet Assoc.* 1988;88:336–342.
8. Pennington JAT, EC Smith, MR Chatfield, TC Hendricks. LANGUAL: a food description language. *Terminology.* 1995;1:277–289.
9. Pennington JAT. Issues of food description. *Food Chem.* 1996;57:145–148.
10. Pennington JAT. Cuisine: a descriptive factor for foods. *Terminology.* 1996;3:155–169.
11. Pennington JAT. *Bowes & Church's Food Values of Portions Commonly Used*. 17th ed. Philadelphia, Pa: JB Lippincott Co; 1998.

12. Murphy SP. Integrity checks for nutrient databases. In: Stumbo PJ, ed. *Proceedings of the Fourteenth National Nutrient Databank Conference.* Ithaca, NY: CBORO Group Inc; 1990:89–91.

13. Rittenbaugh C, Peng YM, Aickin M, Graver E, Branch M, Alberts DS. New carotenoid values for foods improve relationship of food frequency questionnaire intake estimates to plasma values. *Cancer Epidemiol Biomarkers Prev.* 1996;5:907–912.

14. Granado F, Olmeddilla B, Blanco I, Gil-Martinez E, Rojas-Hidalgo E. Variability in the intercomparison of food carotenoid content data: a user's point of view. *Crit Rev Food Sci Nutr.* 1997;37:621–633.

15. Goldbohm RA, Brants HA, Hulshof KF, van den Brandt PA. The contribution of various foods to intake of vitamin A and carotenoids in The Netherlands. *Int J Vitam Nutr Res.* 1998;68:378–383.

16. Nebeling LC, Forman MR, Graubard BI, Snyder RA. Changes in carotenoid intake in the United States: the 1987 and 1992 National Health Interview Surveys. *J Am Diet Assoc.* 1997;97:991–996.

17. Yong LC, Forman MR, Beecher GR, et al. Relationship between dietary intake and plasma concentrations of carotenoids in premenopausal women: application of the USDA-NCI carotenoid food-composition database. *Am J Clin Nutr.* 1994;60:223–230.

18. Forman MR, Lanza E, Yong LC, et al. The correlation between two dietary assessments of carotenoid intake and plasma carotenoid concentrations: application of a carotenoid food-composition database. *Am J Clin Nutr.* 1993;58:519–524.

19. Bravo L. Polyphenols: chemistry, dietary sources, metabolism, and nutritional significance. *Nutr Rev.* 1998;56:317–333.

20. Linseisen J, Radthk J, Wolfram G. Flavonoid intake of adults in a Bavarian subgroup of the national food consumption survey. *Z Ernahrungswiss.* 1997;36:403–412.

21. Peterson J, Dwyer J. Taxonomic classification helps identify flavonoid-containing foods on a semiquantitative food frequency questionnaire. *J Am Diet Assoc.* 1998;98:677–682.

22. Marlett JA, Cheung TF. Database and quick methods of assessing typical dietary fiber intakes using data for 228 commonly consumed foods. *J Am Diet Assoc.* 1997;97:1139–1148.

23. Shimbo S, Hayase A, Murakami M, et al. Use of a food composition database to estimate daily dietary intake of nutrient or trace elements in Japan, with reference to its limitation. *Food Addit Contam.* 1996;13:775–786.

24. MacIntosh DL, Williams PL, Hunter DK, et al. Evaluation of a food frequency questionnaire-food composition approach for estimating dietary intake of inorganic arsenic and methylmercury. *Cancer Epidemiol Biomarkers Prev.* 1997;6:1043–1050.

25. Ashton BA, Ambrosini GL, Marks GC, Harvey PW, Bain C. Development of a dietary supplement database. *Aust NZ J Public Health.* 1997;21:699–702.

26. Newman V, Rock CL, Faerber S, Flatt SW, Wright FA, Pierce JP. Dietary supplement use by women at risk for breast cancer recurrence. The Women's Healthy Eating and Living Study Group. *J Am Diet Assoc.* 1998;98:285–292.

27. Costello RB, Saldanha LG. *Annual Bibliography of Significant Advances in Dietary Supplement Research 1999.* Bethesda, Md: NIH Office of Dietary Supplements; 1999. Also available at: http://dietary-supplements.info.nih.gov/publications/publications.html.

28. Buzzard IM, Price KS, Warren RA. Considerations for selecting nutrient-calculation software: evaluation of the nutrient database. *Am J Clin Nutr.* 1991;54:7–9.

29. Guenther PM, Perloff BP, Vizioli TL Jr. Separating fact from artifact in changes in nutrient intake over time. *J Am Diet Assoc.* 1994;94:270–275.

30. Guilland JC, Aubert R, Lhuissier M, et al. Computerized analysis of food records: role of coding and food composition database. *Eur J Clin Nutr.* 1993;47:445–453.

Biomarkers in Nutrition Research

Cheryl L. Rock, Ph.D., R.D., F.A.D.A., and Johanna W. Lampe, Ph.D., R.D.

A *biomarker* is most simply defined as a biological marker or indicator. As used in nutrition research, this term encompasses diverse biological markers that differ in conceptual basis, interpretation, and use. For example, biomarkers of particular interest in nutrition research include biological markers or indicators of dietary intake, which are useful in the validation of dietary intake measures or as a way of quantifying exposure to various foods or dietary factors (1,2). Another type of biomarker reflects the biological or cellular activity of dietary constituents (or pharmacologic agents), although the activity may not be the primary mechanism by which the constituent or agent affects the disease process (3). Finally, biological markers that are useful in nutrition research as surrogate end point biomarkers are the molecular or cellular markers that reliably predict disease risk (4), typically reflecting a specific molecular mechanism that appears to play a role in the promotion or inhibition of the disease process. These biomarkers are cellular, biochemical, molecular, or genetic alterations by which a normal or abnormal biological process can be identified or monitored, and they are measurable in tissues, cells, or body fluids. As disease precursors, these alterations reflect inherited or acquired genetic susceptibility, metabolism of carcinogens, damage or repair of genetic material, abnormal cellular proliferation, or another aspect of the pathophysiological process of disease. In nutrition research on diseases that are preceded by a defined pathological lesion or morphological tissue changes, cytological or histological characteristics of tissues can also be used as biomarkers.

By definition, using biomarkers in nutrition research involves measuring biological materials, such as blood or urine samples, surgical specimens, or tissue biopsies. Blood collection enables the measurement of several different components or circulating pools, such as serum (the fluid portion remaining when blood has been allowed to clot and the clotted material discarded), plasma (the fluid portion remaining when clotting has been inhibited and the formed elements, red and white blood cells, removed), and red and white blood cell fractions. Although blood and the various components of blood are liquid at ambient temperature, blood should be considered (and described) as tissue, as one would consider and describe peripheral or solid tissue, such as cervix or skin. The collection of urine allows the measurement of excretory products and urinary metabolites that may reflect dietary intake or be responsive to interventions. Urine collections used in nutrition research are typically timed collections (for example, urine collected over a 24-hour period).

Biological samples are considered biohazardous materials, because exposure to microorganisms during the collection and processing of these samples presents a potential health risk. Health care facilities and research units or institutions at which biological materials are collected, handled, or measured must adhere to strict guidelines for the handling of the samples, and careful monitoring and documentation of these procedures is necessary. Universal precautions that must be employed to safely handle biological materials are described in detail elsewhere (5).

The factors being measured in biological samples are likely to be present in very small concentrations and are usually vulnerable to degradation once outside their normal environment, the biological system. Thus, scrupulous collection and handling procedures are necessary to obtain quality data on biomarkers. Collection and processing procedures are nearly always specific to the biomarker of interest, so one should determine the measurements desired prior to beginning the sample collection and processing so that appropriate procedures and supplies are used from the beginning of the study.

This chapter is not intended to be a comprehensive review, but instead it presents the basic concepts and key issues involved in the use of biomarkers in nutrition research. It focuses on the concepts and principles, and also some areas of current interest, with an emphasis on clinical and community-based research applications. Most of the examples presented relate to cancer research; however, the basic principles and key issues are uniformly applicable to any aspect of nutrition research in which biomarkers would enhance the ability to answer a research question.

BIOMARKERS: NUTRITION ASSESSMENT AND DIETARY INDICATORS

Biomarkers are used as in nutrition assessment for several reasons. One basic reason is to provide biochemical data on nutrition status by generating objective evidence that enables evaluation of dietary adequacy or ranking of individuals on exposure to particular nutrients or dietary constituents. Biochemical or biological measurements may also be collected to provide objective evidence of a dietary pattern, such as overall fruit and vegetable consumption, or to validate dietary assessment instruments or self-reported dietary data. Another possible purpose for obtaining these biological measures is to establish the biological link between the nutritional factor and a physiological or biochemical process, when the concentration of the micronutrient or dietary constituent in the target peripheral tissue is measured.

Biological Measures in Nutrition Assessment

Biochemical measures of nutrients or other dietary constituents can be a valuable component of nutrition assessment and monitoring. Overall, the usefulness of biochemical indicators of nutrition status or exposure is based on knowledge of the physiological and other determinants of the measure. For several micronutrients, the concentration of the nutrient in the circulating body pool (for example, serum) appears to be a reasonably accurate reflection of overall status for the nutrient. In contrast, the amount of some micronutrients in the circulating pool may be homeostatically regulated when the storage pool is adequate, or it may be unrelated to intake, and thus has little relationship to total body reserves or overall status. Figure 17.1 illustrates the relationships between various compartments or body pools that may be sampled in the measurement of biological indicators.

Knowledge of the influencing nondietary factors is particularly important for accurate interpretation of the nutrient concentration in tissues. For example, tocopherols and carotenoids are transported in the circulation nonspecifically by the cholesterol-rich lipoproteins (6,7), so higher concentrations of these lipoproteins are predictive of higher concentrations of the associated micronutrients in the circulation, independent of dietary intake or total body pool. Smoking and alcohol consumption need to be considered in the interpretation of serum and other tissue concentrations of several micronutrients, particularly compounds that may be subject to oxidation (for example, vitamin C, tocopherols, carotenoids, and folate). Knowledge of the relationship between the indicator and the risk of nutrient depletion, in addition to knowledge of the responsiveness of the indicator to interventions or change, is also necessary (8). For some nutrients, such as calcium and zinc, a specific sensitive biomarker of diet or biochemical status indicator has not yet been identified.

Practical considerations in the use of a biochemical measure of status include the ability to conveniently access the body compartment for measurement, the procedures necessary to collect and process the sample, subject burden, and the resources for laboratory analysis. For example, accurate quantification of vitamin C or folate in a circulating body pool requires processing steps that must be conducted immediately after blood collection to preserve the sample appropriately and prevent degradation that would otherwise make the resulting measurement inaccurate. These extra steps can add time and effort to the labor of blood processing, making these measurements more difficult to obtain in a large study in which resources are limited.

Technological challenges (and capabilities) are also often linked with the biochemical measurement capabilities. For example, the development of high-performance

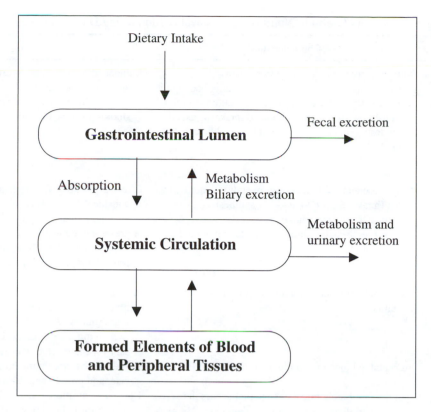

FIGURE 17.1 Relationships between compartments or body pools sampled in the measurement of biological indicators of nutrition status of exposure.

liquid chromatography (HPLC) in the 1970s and improved detection technologies that are currently emerging allow the separation and quantification of many micronutrients and other dietary constituents that are present in very low concentrations in biological samples. The development of specialized cell separation tubes for blood collection now permits easier separation of the leukocyte pool, allowing much easier measurement of micronutrients in this pool; vitamin C and zinc are notable examples.

Table 17.1 lists several examples of biochemical measures of micronutrients that may be useful in nutrition assessment or monitoring dietary intake. An important concept is that a static measurement (for example, a tissue concentration) is typically not as sensitive as a functional marker in the assessment of status. Also, functional measures, such as the in vitro activity of an erythrocyte-derived enzyme with and without the micronutrient cofactor, will more directly reflect the body function (9,10). However, a good functional measure is still lacking in many instances, or the extra labor involved in the procedures limits the ability to use the functional mea-

sures in large-scale studies. In-depth reviews of biological status indicators for the various micronutrients give more details (9–15).

Biomarkers as General Dietary Indicators

Monitoring overall dietary patterns or changes in patterns in response to dietary interventions presents additional challenges. The goal is to assess and monitor the intake of certain types of foods or food groups, rather than specific nutrients; therefore, these dietary indicators ideally should be distributed generally within certain types of foods. Table 17.2 provides examples of several biochemical indicators that are useful as biomarkers of plant-based diets, illustrating the use of biomarkers as objective evidence of an overall dietary pattern.

Plasma carotenoids provide a good example of the use of biomarkers as a dietary indicator when the goal is to assess and monitor dietary patterns. Vegetables and fruits contribute the vast majority of carotenoids in the diet, and plasma carotenoid concentrations have been

TABLE 17.1 Biological Indicators Useful in Nutrition Assessment or Monitoring Dietary Intakes[a]

Nutrient	Characteristics	Comments[b]
Tocopherols, plasma or serum	Vary directly with vitamin E (tocopherol) intake; slow tissue turnover and relatively large body pool	Influenced by cholesterol-carrying lipoprotein and smoking status
Carotenoids, plasma or serum (beta carotene, alpha carotene, lycopene, lutein, β-cryptoxanthin, zeaxanthin)	Vary directly with carotenoid intakes, although relationship with specific calculated intakes is usually modest; generally reflects total vegetable and fruit intake	Influenced by cholesterol-carrying lipoprotein levels, smoking status, body mass, and alcohol intake
25-Hydroxyvitamin D, plasma or serum	Good biochemical indicator of overall vitamin D status (intake plus endogenously synthesized in response to sun exposure)	Effect of skin pigmentation can be great and should be considered in interpretation of results; seasonal changes can also be notable
Vitamin C, plasma or serum	Varies directly with vitamin C intake only up to a threshold level	A preservative must be incorporated into the sample immediately after blood collection and separation, prior to preparing aliquots and freezing; influenced by smoking status
Folate, whole blood or erythrocyte	Acceptable biochemical indicator of long-term folate status	A preservative must be incorporated into the sample immediately after blood collection, prior to freezing; influenced by smoking status; hemoglobin (which must be conducted with fresh blood) necessary for interpretation of results
Pyridoxal-5-phosphate, plasma	Acceptable biochemical indicator of vitamin B-6 status	Influenced by circulating albumin concentration, exercise, and protein and carbohydrate intakes
Vitamin B-12, plasma or serum	Not the first biochemical change that occurs in response to dietary vitamin B-12 deficiency, but a definitive indicator of prolonged vitamin B-12 inadequacy	Low concentrations can result from several physiological abnormalities (e.g., pernicious anemia, atrophic gastritis, hypochlorhydria, and gastric surgery), in addition to dietary inadequacy
Ferritin, serum	Considered the most sensitive and specific indicator of overall iron status; increased concentration in response to excess iron uptake and body stores	Reference (normal) ranges vary depending on method used; increased in several physiological abnormalities in which normal uptake regulation is overridden (e.g., hereditary hemochromatosis), resulting in excessive accumulation of iron
Fatty acids, serum phospholipids or plasma	Modified in response to inadequate fat intake and also in response to substantial changes in n-6 and n-3 fatty acid ingestion	Used as a biomarker of compliance with supplementation in fish oil supplement studies

[a]Good or acceptable biochemical indicators of status have been established for several nutrients not on this list, but the effort involved in the analytic procedures precludes their usefulness in large clinical or community-based nutrition research studies. Also not listed are several nutrients (e.g., zinc, copper, and calcium) for which serum or plasma concentrations are easily measured and may contribute to the evaluation of status but the values produced need substantial additional information for accurate interpretation.

[b]Includes additional measures needed to be obtained concurrently for interpretation, as well as other factors crucial in the usefulness of values obtained. Notably, demographic characteristics (e.g., age, gender, and racial/ethnic group) are also useful in the interpretation for all of these measures.

Data are from Jacob 1990 (9), Food and Nutrition Board 1998 (12), Blanchard et al 1997 (15), Meydani et al 1991 (22).

shown to be useful biomarkers of vegetable and fruit intakes in cross-sectional descriptive studies, controlled feeding studies, and clinical trials (1,2,16–18). The consistency of this relationship across diverse groups and involving various concurrent diet manipulations (with differences in amounts of dietary factors that could alter carotenoid bioavailability) is notable, although considerable interindividual variation in the degree of response is typically observed. Also, nondietary factors that are among the determinants of plasma carotenoid concentrations (for example, body mass and plasma cholesterol concentration) will influence the absolute concentration that is observed in response to dietary intake.

Although vitamin C also is provided predominantly by fruits and vegetables in the diet, this measure is much less useful as a biomarker of this dietary pattern, because

TABLE 17.2 Biochemical Indicators Useful as Biomarkers of Plant-based Diets[a]

	Biochemical Indicators						
Measured in	β-cryptoxanthin (P)	α-carotene and β- (P)	Lycopene (P)	Lutein (P)	Isoflavones (P/U)	Lignans (P/U)	Dithiocarbamate (U)
Vegetables		X		X			
Soy					X		
Cruciferous vegetables							X
Tomatoes and tomato products			X				
Green-leafy vegetables				X			
Fruit	X	X				X	
Grains						X	

[a]P, plasma; U, urine.

the relationship between vitamin C intake and plasma concentration is linear only up to a certain threshold (15). The use of vitamin C supplements (which is common) often increases the intake level beyond the range in which linearity between intake and plasma concentration occurs, and it also obscures the relationship between food choices and tissue concentrations.

Lignans are a group of compounds that are present in high-fiber foods, particularly cereals and fruits (19). These compounds are not found in animal products and, like carotenoids, are useful markers of a plant-based diet (20). Lignans provide an example of how using dietary constituents as biomarkers requires an understanding of the metabolism of the compounds. Lignans in plant foods are altered by intestinal microflora, so the specific compounds monitored in plasma or urine are actually bacterial metabolites. Generally, enterolactone and enterodiol are measured. Because of this bacterial conversion, lignan concentrations in urine or plasma in response to a similar dietary dose will vary significantly among individuals. In addition, nondietary factors (for example, orally administered antibiotics) will reduce enterolactone and enterodiol production (21).

As another example, the fatty acid composition of membrane phospholipids is in part determined by the n-6 and n-3 fatty acid composition of the diet. Thus, the fatty acid pattern of serum phospholipids or plasma aliquots has been used as a biomarker of compliance with n-3 fatty acid supplementation in clinical trials (22,23). Although enzyme selectivities and other physiological factors are also important determinants of the fatty acid composition of phospholipids, a diet high in n-3 polyunsaturated fats will result in increased amounts of eicosapentaeneoic and docosahexaenoic acids in circulating tissue pools.

Specific fatty acids also can be associated with certain types of foods. Pentadecanoic acid (15:0) and heptadecanoic acid (17:0) are fatty acids produced by bacteria in the rumen of ruminants. These fatty acids, with uneven numbers of carbon atoms, are not synthesized by humans; therefore, their presence in human biological samples can be indicative of dietary exposure to milk fat. Proportions of 15:0 and 17:0 in adipose tissue and concentrations of 15:0 in serum have been found to correlate with milk-fat intake in men and women (24,25).

Biomarkers of Phytochemical Intakes

Although not recognized as essential for life, numerous dietary components—particularly of plant origin—have demonstrated biological activity and are thought to play an important role in the prevention of chronic disease (16–18). These phytochemicals are absorbed, often metabolized in the intestinal epithelium and liver, and excreted; thus, the metabolites can be monitored in urine, serum, or plasma.

Dietary exposure to flavonoids and other polyphenols can be monitored in urine or plasma (26). The isoflavones daidzein and genistein are highly concentrated in soybeans and soy products. Much remains to be learned about their metabolism in human beings (27,28). These compounds can be measured in urine and plasma by HPLC with diode array or coulometric array detection, gas chromatographymass spectrometry, or immunoassay. Urinary isoflavone excretion is associated strongly and directly with soy protein intake under controlled dietary conditions (29). In observational studies of populations that usually consume soy, soy food intake and urinary isoflavonoid excretion also are positively correlated (30–32). Because the plasma half-lives of the isoflavones genistein and daidzein are short (6 hours to 8 hours) (33), intermittent soy consumption may be severely underestimated or overestimated if isoflavone exposure is monitored in plasma or spot urine specimens. The metabolism of isoflavones is also inextricably linked to the health of colonic bacterial populations, and plasma and urinary levels may be influenced by the effects of diet and drugs on the colonic environment.

Other compounds that have been utilized as biomarkers of dietary intake, such as sulforaphane and other isothiocyanates in cruciferous vegetables, have been of interest because of putative chemopreventive effects. Dithiocarbamates (metabolites of isothiocyanates) can be quantified in urine, following extraction and measurement by HPLC, and provide a measure of cruciferous vegetable exposure (34).

Biomarkers of Energy Intake

To date, there are few biological measures that objectively monitor energy intake, and those measures that are available are cumbersome in free-living populations, expensive, or both. Under steady-state conditions, indirect calorimetry provides an estimate of energy expenditure and some insight about intake. Indirect calorimetry estimates the rate of oxidation or energy expenditure from the rate of oxygen consumption (VO_2) and the rate of carbon dioxide production (VCO_2). This technique is relatively inexpensive and portable, although some subject effort is required. These traits lend the technique to clinical applications (35).

The chief premise behind indirect calorimetry is that VO_2 and energy metabolism are proportional. All energy-dependent metabolic processes depend on energy liberated from adenosine triphosphate (ATP) hydrolysis. The ATP utilization rate dictates substrate oxidation (36). Total body oxygen storage is very small compared with oxygen consumption. Given the first law of thermodynamics, energy from oxidative metabolism is converted into heat and work. If the subject is resting in a thermoneutral environment, heat released by oxidation and measurable by indirect calorimetry is equal to heat lost to the environment measurable by direct calorimetry.

Indirect calorimetry produces two types of information: resting energy expenditure (REE) and the respiratory quotient (RQ). The REE estimates fasting energy expenditure in an awake, resting person and is approximately 10 percent greater than basal energy require-

ments. The REE correlates with lean body mass (37). The RQ is the ratio of carbon dioxide produced divided by oxygen consumed (VCO_2/VO_2), and the ratio indicates contributions from each substrate. An RQ of 1.0 suggests 100 percent glucose utilization, whereas an RQ of 0.7 corresponds to oxidation of 100 percent fat. Protein utilization results in an RQ near 0.8. However, urinary nitrogen excretion is used to determine what portion of the VCO_2 and VO_2 are contributed by protein utilization. Exclusion of the effects of protein produces the nonprotein respiratory quotient (NPRQ). Thus, for NPRQs between 0.7 and 1.0, proportions of fat and carbohydrate oxidation can be identified (38,39). It is important to note that the RQ represents substrate oxidation, which may or may not equal exogenous macronutrient intakes. In using the RQ to determine substrate oxidation, two assumptions are made: the subject is in a metabolically steady-state condition, and all expired carbon dioxide measured represents substrate oxidation (35).

Various types of equipment are used in indirect calorimetry, with both open- and closed-circuit systems available. The closed-circuit system allows the subject to breathe from a pure-oxygen reservoir and calculates oxygen consumption from disappearance data. The more sophisticated open-circuit system, in which subjects breathe room air and detectors calculate the difference in gases inhaled versus those exhaled, is more widely available in the United States. The apparatus used to collect respiratory gases may take the form of a tentlike canopy, a fitted face mask, or a mouthpiece with nose clips directing all inhalation and expiration through the mouth. The canopy system may be best suited to clinical and research applications, because it is comfortable and requires no fitting (40), whereas the face mask system has been tested in healthy adults restricted to bed (41). Despite validation in healthy subjects, indirect calorimetry is generally applied to critically ill individuals.

The limitations of indirect calorimetry in the community-based setting are significant. If the REE is measured, participants must provide accurate typical activity records for adjustment to total energy expenditure. Such records introduce reporting bias and general inaccuracy. Indirect calorimetry can be used to measure total energy expenditure, but long data collection periods are necessary to control error associated with extrapolation, and it is likely that usual activity would be hindered by even the most mobile system. Even measuring energy expenditure for a full day would leave day-to-day variability unacknowledged (42).

Energy expenditure can also be measured using a

doubly labeled water (DLW) technique (43). This method uses nonradioactive isotopes of hydrogen (^2H) and oxygen (^{18}O) to measure free-living total energy expenditure by monitoring urinary isotope excretion. Energy expenditures determined by room calorimetry, indirect calorimetry, and DLW are not significantly different within the calorimeter environment; however, in free-living subjects, DLW energy expenditures are found to be 13 percent to 15 percent higher than energy expenditures from other methods (42). The DLW method has the distinct advantage of allowing the subjects to go about their usual activities, with energy expenditure calculated after a study period of 7 days to 14 days. Unfortunately, the ^{18}O isotope required to conduct DLW studies is expensive and often in short supply. Although DLW studies are suited to nutrition research aimed at quantifying total energy expenditure for specific groups, the cost for large samples limits their broad use.

One of the most important and relevant uses of DLW methodology in community-based nutrition research has been to produce an estimate of energy requirements, which can then be compared to the reported energy intakes that are obtained from various dietary assessment methodologies (44). Underreporting is a recognized problem in dietary assessment, and DLW may be used to validate (or calibrate) assessment methods such as dietary recalls and food frequency questionnaires. Although the data produced are objective and the approach is less disruptive to normal life activities than indirect calorimetry, measurement error does occur and can be compounded by estimates of various physiological factors and assumptions that are used in the calculations. Furthermore, one of the most notable findings from the use of DLW methodology is that total daily energy expenditure varies dramatically among healthy, free-living human beings (45).

BIOMARKERS OF BIOCHEMICAL ACTIVITY AND SURROGATE END POINT BIOMARKERS

If a nutritional factor or dietary constituent has a known biochemical activity, measuring markers of that activity can be useful. One purpose is to identify the dosage or concentration necessary to achieve a clinically meaningful effect. Often, a biochemical activity may have been linked to the pathogenesis of disease, but the biomarker cannot be considered a surrogate end point biomarker unless its modulation has been shown to be indicative of

progression or reversal of the disease process. In an intervention trial, the use of surrogate end point biomarkers (rather than the diagnosis of disease) requires substantially less time and fewer resources in the evaluation of efforts aimed toward reducing risk for chronic diseases such as cancer, cardiovascular disease, and osteoporosis. To date, very few markers have been established as true surrogate end point biomarkers.

Biomarkers of Oxidative Stress

Biochemical indicators of oxidative stress illustrate a type of biomarker that reflects a biological activity. Oxidative stress has been suggested to play a role in the pathophysiological disease process in cancer, atherosclerotic cardiovascular disease, and many other acute and chronic conditions (46), although the specific relationship to the disease process remains to be established in most instances. Cellular damage caused by reactive oxygen species, which are generated from cellular respiration, co-oxidation during metabolism, and the activity of phagocytic cells of the immune system is controlled by antioxidant defense mechanisms that involve several micronutrients. Oxidative stress describes the condition of oxidative damage resulting when the balance between free-radical generation and antioxidant defenses is unfavorable. Direct measurement of active oxygen and related species in biological samples is very challenging, mainly because these compounds have very short half-lives. Thus, the oxidative stress biomarkers used in studies of human beings are typically adducts or end products that reflect reactions that have occurred between free radicals and compounds such as lipids, proteins, carbohydrates, DNA, and other molecules that are potential targets (47).

One frequently described assay used as an oxidative stress biomarker is the thiobarbituric acid reactive substances assay. This assay basically quantifies a product of malondialdehyde, which presumably reflects lipid hydroperoxides in the sample. However, this assay has some serious limitations in specificity, and the product measured cannot be interpreted as directly reflecting lipid peroxidation in vivo (47). Direct measurement of malondialdehyde in biological samples using HPLC has also been examined as an alterative approach, although the specificity of the more direct HPLC measurement has also not been established to the level desirable.

Measurement of breath pentane is another biomarker of oxidative stress that has been used in studies of human beings (48). The approach basically involves collecting exhaled air for the measurement of the products of peroxidation of unsaturated fatty acids, a portion of which are volatile and released in the breath, using GC methods. However, the specific measurement methodologies vary a great deal and are not always reliable; standardization of the procedure and knowledge of various influencing factors are needed to improve the usefulness of this approach (47).

Another biomarker of oxidative stress involves the measurement of urinary 8-hydroxydeoxyguanosine (8OHdG) using HPLC and electrochemical detection (49). The 8-hydroxylation of the guanine base is a frequent type of oxidative DNA damage, and 8OHdG is subsequently excreted without further metabolism in the urine after repair in vivo by exonucleases. In previous studies, certain demographic factors and physiological characteristics, such as gender and body mass (50), have been observed to influence urinary 8OHdG concentration, so these factors may need to be considered in interpretation. Urinary 8OHdG is increased in association with conditions known to be characterized by increased oxidative stress, such as smoking, whole body irradiation, and cytotoxic chemotherapy (49–51). Prostaglandin-like compounds produced by nonenzymatic free radical-catalyzed peroxidation of arachidonic acid, termed F_2-isoprostanes are currently of great interest as useful biomarkers of oxidative damage. Specific GC-mass spectrometry assays for the measurement of some of these compounds, such as $iPF_2\alpha$-III (also called 8-iso-$PGPF_2\alpha$) and $iPF_2\alpha$-VI, have been developed and used to quantify them in urine and blood samples. These markers have been shown to be less variable than 8OHdG (52), and elevated levels have been observed in plasma and urine samples from subjects under a wide variety of conditions of enhanced oxidative stress (53,54).

Another approach to measuring DNA oxidative damage that appears to be useful in human nutrition research is the measurement of 5-hydroxymethyluracil levels in DNA in blood. 5-Hydroxymethyluracil is produced when DNA is exposed to oxidants, is relatively stable when compared with other oxidation products, and can be quantified with GC-mass spectrometry (55,56). In a small cross-sectional study, 5-hydroxymethyluracil concentration was observed to be inversely associated with cooked vegetable intakes and directly related to beef and pork intakes in the diets of women enrolled in a low-fat diet intervention trial (57).

Oxidative damage to low-density lipoproteins (LDL) has been specifically linked to atherogenesis, and in an application of this biological activity, measurement of LDL oxidation ex vivo has been used in clinical stud-

ies as a biomarker of oxidative stress (58). Basically, this process involves isolating the LDL fraction from a blood sample, exposing this fraction to oxidants such as Cu^{2+}, and measuring the lag time before oxidation. Although this biomarker might appear to be specific to cardiovascular disease risk, results from this assay have not yet been specifically linked with risk for disease, so results should be interpreted as simply another approach to the assessment of oxidative stress (47). Also, a variety of specific methodologies are used across laboratories, and the lack of standardization in the approaches in use constrains the ability to make comparisons across studies.

Several other approaches to measuring biomarkers of oxidative stress have been proposed and are under study. Handelman et al provide a useful review of this topic (47).

Biomarkers of Metabolizing Enzyme Activity

Understanding how diet influences enzyme systems is important in developing strategies for disease prevention and treatment. For example, dietary modulation of enzymes involved in carcinogen metabolism may be important in reducing cancer risk. Dietary intervention that reduces the expression of rate-limiting enzymes in cholesterol synthesis may alter cardiovascular disease risk. Direct measurement of enzyme expression or activity in human studies is a challenge, however. Often the enzymes of interest are located primarily in tissues that are not readily accessible (for example, liver, intestine, or lung).

One approach to meeting this challenge is to measure the enzymes in more accessible tissue; for example, enzymes that are present in high levels in the liver can often be measured in plasma or serum as a result of normal hepatocyte turnover. Enzyme activity of glutathione—transferase (GST), a biotransformation enzyme important in carcinogen detoxification, can be measured spectrophotometrically in serum (59), or concentrations of the enzyme itself can be determined in serum by immunoassay (60). Serum concentration of the GST isoenzyme GST-α has been shown to increase when cruciferous vegetables are added to the diet (60). A limitation of using serum measures of a hepatic enzyme is that the assumption is made that liver function is normal. Thus, including other measures of liver function in the data collection is important to verify that there is no underlying hepatic disease that may result in spurious GST values. Additionally, some enzymes are present in isoforms in various tissues. GST-μ, another GST isoenzyme, is present in lymphocytes as well as in liver; therefore, for this isoenzyme, GST activity or protein concentration can be measured in cells extracted from blood samples.

Another approach is to use a drug probe to measure enzyme activity. Many of the same xenobiotic metabolizing enzymes that metabolize carcinogens also are induced by, and metabolize, commonly used drugs. The metabolites of these drugs can be monitored in serum, plasma, or urine and used to determine enzyme activities. Caffeine metabolites measured in urine samples collected 4 hours after consumption of 500 mg caffeine allows determination of cytochrome P-450 1A2, *N*-acetyltransferase, and xanthine oxidase activities (61). Similarly, acetaminophen (paracetamol) is used to measure UDP-glucuronosyltransferase and sulfotransferase activities (62). Drugs can be administered as probes following a nutrition intervention to determine the degree of change in enzyme activity in response to diet (63,64).

Biomarkers Reflecting Other Biochemical Activities

The specificity of the biochemical activities of the dietary constituent of interest means that a wide variety of biomarkers that are indicators of biological activity may be useful in nutrition research. For example, folate is an essential micronutrient in DNA methylation. The degree of methylation in DNA extracted from tissue samples has been used in human studies as a biomarker of folate function (65). A possible link to disease process is that DNA hypomethylation is known to be an early step in colon carcinogenesis (66). However, it is possible that the effect of dietary folate is modified by other influencing factors, such as dietary methyl donors and certain genetic polymorphisms (67), and specific areas of hypermethylation of genes have also been identified in colon carcinogenesis (66). Thus, measuring the degree of DNA methylation has been examined as a possible biomarker of folate biochemical activity, although a direct link between dietary folate, methylation abnormalities, and human colon carcinogenesis has not yet been established.

Measurement of arachidonic acid metabolism—which involves measuring the concentration of prostaglandins, leukotrienes (metabolic products), or enzymes in the eicosanoid metabolic pathway (cyclooxygenase)—provides another example. Altered arachidonic acid metabolism is among the biochemical activities of nonsteroidal anti-inflammatory agents and may also be influenced by antioxidant micronutrients, such as vitamin E (68), and quantitative changes in these products or enzymes in tissues serve as biomarkers of this activity (69). Similar to the link between disease process and DNA hypomethylation, a reasonable amount of biological evidence suggests some role for this enzymatic pathway in colon carcinogenesis (70); however, the overall relationship with disease process is still under investigation.

Cellular Biomarkers

Cellular markers of proliferation, differentiation, and apoptosis (programmed cell death) can be useful as biomarkers in research focused on nutrition factors and cancer, although the measured effect is more of a general indicator of an altered cell growth regulation effect than a measure of specific biochemical activity.

As a general rule, increased proliferation of undifferentiated cells is one aspect or characteristic of carcinogenesis, and in colon cancer this relationship has been well established. For example, cell proliferation occurs at the base of the colonic crypts, and as cells migrate from the crypts to the luminal surface, they become increasingly differentiated and mature and lose their proliferative capabilities (71). The shift in which the proliferative zone extends to the surface, so that cells on the luminal surface retain proliferative capabilities and are immature and underdifferentiated, may be considered a field defect that sets the stage for current and future neoplastic changes (72–74).

Early work in this area relied on the incorporation of tritiated thymidine or bromodeoxyuridine into the DNA of dividing cells during incubation of a biopsy specimen. These methods required that the tissue be freshly obtained so that cells were viable and replicating. Often, label incorporation was incomplete. With increased sensitivity in immunohistochemical techniques, proteins present in proliferating cells (for example, proliferating cell nuclear antigen [PCNA] and Ki67) now are used more widely to quantify proliferative activity in tissue specimens. Labeling indexes involving tritiated thymidine and PCNA have been used to quantify the proliferative activity in colonic mucosal samples from human subjects (73) and have been used successfully as end points in several nutrition intervention studies to prevent colon cancer (74,75). These indexes are being further refined by staining for proteins present during apoptosis (for example, Bax, Bcl-2) and in differentiated cells, in order to provide a more complete picture of cell dynamics.

In cases where specific genetic mutations may be indicative of disease risk or progression or may be modified by nutritional factors, genetic markers can also be useful biomarkers. Various molecular techniques have been developed to help characterize genetic abnormalities or differences. Genetic factors are important to consider in nutrition research for several reasons. One reason is that it is increasingly evident that genetic polymorphisms (that is, variations in DNA coding sequences of genes) may contribute substantially to differences in the response to environmental and dietary exposures (76) and analysis by subgroup according to differences in genetic susceptibility permits a more refined evaluation and interpretation of the observed effect of nutrition interventions and associations. For example, genetic variations in the expression of the xenobiotic metabolizing enzymes may mediate the potentially carcinogenic effect of heterocyclic amines (obtained from meat cooked at high temperatures) (77,78). Also, results from laboratory animal studies suggest that dietary modifications can promote alterations in genetic factors (79), so measuring genetic abnormalities may be considered an approach to demonstrating a biological link between dietary factors and disease risk. These approaches are increasingly possible and useful in clinical and community-based nutrition research because of improved molecular methodologies, and they are feasible if appropriate tissue samples and technologies are available. With microdissection and immunohistochemical analysis using small tissue specimens, molecular markers can thus be used to monitor the effects of dietary modifications on the altered physiological processes that may be present even prior to the diagnosis of clinical disease.

In colon cancer, several genetic alterations in the course of disease progression have been well defined and so can serve as biomarkers of carcinogenesis (70). In contrast, none of the currently available molecular biomarkers suggested for breast cancer has been accepted as a surrogate end point biomarker, although a number of cellular growth factors, markers of disordered cell signaling, markers of oncogene overexpression, and cell cycle markers are currently under study in clinical trials (3). Figure 17.2 lists examples of several types of biomarkers of biochemical activity or genetic alterations that are currently considered promising or are in use in cancer prevention studies.

Biomarkers Involving Physiological Characteristics and Pathological Lesions

In some instances, physiological characteristics have been used as biomarkers of disease and thus may be useful in measuring the effect of nutrition interventions. Al-

though not a biological measurement, increased breast density, which can be measured noninvasively through imaging techniques, has been used as a type of biological marker in nutrition research. Increased breast density is associated with increased breast cancer risk (80), and some studies have suggested that it may be reversible and responsive to changes in the hormonal milieu. In one clinical trial, reduced breast density was observed in association with a low-fat diet intervention (81).

Precursor lesions are known to occur in carcinogenesis, and when the lesions may be reversible, cytological and histological examination of tissues provides a useful approach to using biomarkers as a measure of efficacy of nutrition intervention. One of the best examples occurs in cervical carcinogenesis, which is characterized as a progression from cervical dysplasia to carcinoma in situ and, finally, invasive cancer (82). In several clinical trials, the effect of nutrient supplements or dietary modification on cervical cancer risk has been monitored by serial examination of cervical tissue lesions in human subjects (83), with reversal of the lesion being the positive outcome desired. Another example of this type of approach is found in research studies on colon cancer prevention. The earliest lesion of colonic neoplasia is the polyp, and it is generally accepted that most cancers of the colon are preceded by an adenomatous polyp (71). The occurrence of polyps basically indicates an early abnormal tissue characteristic that occurs in the continuum of colon carcinogenesis. The major outcome under study in numerous colon cancer prevention trials using various nutrition interventions has been recurrence of polyps in subjects who have had them removed (84–87). A reduced rate of recurrence of these adenomatous polyps, indicating that the tissue abnormality is being corrected, would theoretically provide biological evidence suggesting a reduction in risk for colon cancer.

BIOMARKERS IN NUTRITION RESEARCH: PRACTICAL CONSIDERATIONS

Practical considerations in the use of biomarkers in nutrition research involve all the details and issues that are necessary for the appropriate collection, handling, processing, and storage of biological samples. Prior to selecting the biomarkers to examine, the nutrition researcher must know what is reflected in the pool or compartment to be measured and the various factors that might influence the interpretation of results.

Proliferation indexes and markers:
  Ki67
  Proliferating cell nuclear antigen
  Tritiated thymidine incorporation
  Mitotic frequency (MPM-2)
  Bromodeoxyuridine incorporation
Markers of oncogene overexpression (Her-2/neu [breast])
Growth factors and related markers:
  Epidermal growth factor receptor (EGFR)
  Insulin-like growth factor receptor (IGFR)
  Serum insulin-like growth factor (IGF-1)
  Serum IGF-1 binding protein (IGFBP-3)
Apoptosis markers:
  Bcl-2:Bax ratio
  TdT-mediated dUTP nick end labeling (TUNEL) assay
Tumor suppressors (p53, Rb)
Alteration of differentiation signals (C-myc)
Differentiation markers:
  Transforming growth factor β (TGFβ, TGF-β2)
  Retinoic acid receptors
  Lectin labeling
  Fibrillar proteins (keratins) (cervix)
Cell cycle markers (cyclin D1)
DNA abnormalities:
  DNA methylation abnormalities
  Loss of heterozygosity
Genetic instability markers (chromosome polysomy, aneuploidy)
Genetic markers (colon: K-*ras,* adenomatous polyposis coli gene/product)
Estrogen receptor overexpression (breast)
Human papillomavirus (HPV) oncogene expression (cervix):
  Presence of viral DNA
  Expression of E2, E6, and E7 proteins
Polyamine metabolism markers
  Ornithine decarboxylase
  Spermidine
Arachidonic acid metabolism markers:
  Prostaglandins, leukotrienes
  Cyclooxygenase and lipoxygenase enzymes
Detoxifying enzyme markers:
  Cytochrome P450 genes (e.g., *CYP1A1*)
  Glutathione-*S*-transferase gene (GSTM1)

FIGURE 17.2 Examples of biomarkers of biochemical activity or genetic alterations. Data from Fabian et al (3); Vargas and Alberts (75); Ruffin et al (82).

Collection of Blood and Other Tissues

Although the risk involved in blood collection may be minimal, it is an invasive procedure, and subjects must be informed of all inherent risks. Trained and certified personnel must be responsible for the procedure. There are some variations in the requirements for training and certification across institutions, but a key factor to consider for subject comfort is the experience of the individual responsible for the phlebotomy and how frequently the individual performs the procedure. Experienced phlebotomists should have the knowledge and skills to cope with the challenges that can arise. For example, collecting blood from even a healthy adult can be very difficult if the subject is somewhat dehydrated. Most research studies specify a protocol (for example, how many attempts are to be made before allowing another phlebotomist to try or before a subject may be dismissed to return for another attempt at later time). When blood collections are very frequent over a very short period (say, 12 hours), an indwelling catheter enabling access without repeated venipuncture may be necessary.

The selection of the collection tube for blood collection is determined by the compartment to be measured (for example, serum, plasma, erythrocytes, or leukocytes). The selection of tubes for plasma collection contain various anticlotting chemicals. These chemicals may have either positive or negative effects on the constituents being measured, so the specific tube choice will be driven by the effect on the measurement. If white blood cells are needed to extract cellular constituents such as DNA, the heterogeneous "buffy coat" mixture of blood cells (the whitish layer of cells between the red blood cells and the plasma following centrifugation) is an appropriate fraction to remove and collect. If the leukocyte compartment is specifically desired, specialized cell separation tubes must be used. For many constituents of interest, especially constituents subject to oxidation by light exposure, the tube with collected blood may need to be protected from light immediately, using an amber sample bag or aluminum foil, during the processing steps when the tube is not in the centrifuge. If the erythrocyte pool is to be measured, the red blood cells remaining after the plasma has been removed typically need to be "washed"; this washing involves twice adding an equal volume of normal saline, centrifuging, and discarding the supernatant so that the plasma material adhering to the red blood cells is rinsed away.

The processing of the blood samples is often quite specific to the constituent to be measured. For example, extra processing steps to better preserve the constituent may need to be performed immediately after the blood has been collected and before the sample is placed in cryovials for storage or analysis. Additional considerations relevant to blood sample collection involve nonfasting versus fasting samples (and how many hours postprandial are considered acceptable) and timing of the sample collection (which would be important if diurnal variations were known to occur). In planning the study design and protocol, seasonal effects on the biochemical measurement may need to be considered.

When solid tissue samples are examined or measured, the exact tissue type needs to be considered prior to collection and processing, even if normal tissue is the target. For example, a surgical biopsy sample of normal tissue from either breast or fat depots will often typically include connective tissue, adipose tissue, and glandular tissue (if the sample is from the breast). Different distributions of micronutrients or other dietary constituents are usually present in these tissue types, so dissection and examination is necessary prior to static measures of the sample. Before storage, solid tissue samples must be rinsed of blood with normal saline, and depending on the measurement to be made, a chemical preservative may need to be added before storage. If the biopsy sample is a surgical sample of a possible or known lesion, the first priority is for sufficient tissue for histopathological examination for diagnosis and medical care; tissue for research purposes is considered a lower priority.

Urine Collection

Urine is an easily accessible pool for measurement of numerous biomarkers; however, urinary markers of diet generally reflect recent intake. Timing and length of collection, as well as handling and processing methods, are determined by the biomarkers being measured. Collections may vary from a "spot urine" (a convenience sample, usually less than 100 mL, collected during a clinic visit) to days of complete urine collection (24- or 72-hour urine collections). Additional collection strategies include overnight collection (approximately a 10-hour collection) or first-voided fasting morning collection (collected upon waking in the morning). A first-voided morning specimen is usually the most concentrated sample of the day and is affected least by recent dietary intake.

It is difficult to collect 24- and 72-hour urine samples in free-living individuals. The collection procedure involves significant participant burden and can impair participant recruitment, retention, and compliance. Nonetheless, these total urine collections are often necessary to provide a useful measure of dietary exposure. Participants must be provided an adequate supply of easy-to-use, leak-proof collection containers; clear instructions for collection, labeling, and handling; and if necessary, commode specimen systems and transport coolers. Sometimes urine collection containers need to be pretreated with additives. For example, some biomarkers that undergo oxidation require the use of collection containers that have ascorbic acid (1 g per 1-L bottle) added to them prior to collection. To monitor the completeness of a 24-hour collection, *para*-aminobenzoic acid (PABA) can be used. This compound is ingested with meals (80 mg, three times per day) and is rapidly and completely excreted in the urine (88). A urine collection containing less than 85 percent of the administered dose of PABA is considered incomplete.

For population studies, spot, overnight, and first-voided urine collections are more feasible than 24-hour collections. These collections are especially useful when a ratio of markers is determined (for example, drug metabolites to parent drug or one hormone metabolite to another). Urinary excretion of a marker also can be normalized to the creatinine content of the sample (milligrams of the marker per milligram of creatinine) to correct for diurnal variation and urine volume.

Fecal Collection

Fecal collection is less frequently used than urine and blood collection in nutrition research, in part because of the logistics of, and aversion to, collection. However, absorption studies, as well as and dietary interventions with outcomes related to gut function, bile acid metabolism, and colonic microfloral changes, rely on fecal samples for biomarkers. As with urine collections, minimizing participant burden is an important consideration for fecal collections. This includes devising the least offensive method of sample collection that still meets the study's needs, identifying the shortest time over which samples need to be collected, and carefully arranging sample storage and transport.

Sample handling is specific to the measurements planned. Various additives may need to be provided to participants to add directly to the specimen at the time of collection. Often, samples must be frozen immediately to prevent continued microbial degradation of dietary fiber.

Samples used for microbiological cultures may need to be collected with minimal exposure to air and processed immediately to minimize alterations in microfloral populations. A careful understanding of the biology involved and testing of the collection protocol by the researchers is necessary to ensure that the samples are collected appropriately for the biomarker under investigation.

General Considerations

Unless the biological measurement is conducted immediately after sample collection, storage issues must be considered. Thawing and refreezing may promote degradation of the constituents, so it is usually best to divide the sample into several aliquots for storage so that only portions of the material collected are removed for analysis at any one time. Regular laboratory refrigeration (for example, a refrigerated centrifuge) is typically at a temperature of 4 degrees Celsius, and biological samples nearly always must be stored at −20 degrees Celsius, or preferably at −70 degrees Celsius to −80 degrees Celsius, for best preservation. The ultralow freezers necessary for the lower temperature range and better preservation have an additional compressor unit, so they are considerably more expensive. Additionally, storage of the samples in liquid nitrogen is necessary for some types of cellular measurements. Stability of the biological markers to be measured should be verified in the process of planning the time span between collection and analysis.

Needless to say, freezers used to store biological samples for biomarker measurements should have an emergency backup power source and an alarm for notification when power is lost or the temperature rises above a preset level. Freezer space needs can be substantial in a study in which numerous aliquots are produced, and early planning can prevent later problems.

Quality Assurance

All compounds measured in biological samples have a certain amount of biological variability, reflecting the inherent fluctuation that is normal in the biological system because the constituents are not static but are continuously influenced by rates of metabolism and flux across body pools. For that reason, biochemical measurements may need to be replicated (if possible) or even measured in duplicate or triplicate (if the cost and effort of the measurement permit) to accurately characterize the situation.

More important, knowledge of biological variability is simply an important consideration in the interpretation of actual values obtained from the measurements; the researcher must recognize that quantified values are not absolutes but estimates, even when the best procedures and methods are in place.

Although biological variability is to be expected, other sources of variation are ideally anticipated and minimized in the measurement methodologies used (89). Biochemical methods used in the measurements of biological samples should always be tested for reliability prior to use in a research study. This aspect of quality assurance (QA) typically involves repeated measurements at several levels of set concentrations using various matrixes so that procedural sources of variation can be identified. The concentrations used to test the accuracy of the method should be in the range of the concentrations expected in the biological samples. As an example, coefficients of variation obtained from these QA procedures for HPLC methods produce figures for both run-to-run and day-to-day variability. External assistance with QA may be possible through the National Institute of Standards and Technology, from which samples with known concentrations of micronutrients and some other dietary constituents may be purchased for comparative testing of validity of the methods in use in the researcher's laboratory. For micronutrients, the institute conducts a round robin QA program in which samples with unknown concentrations are sent to participating laboratories for measurement as a type of blinded evaluation of laboratory performance (90).

Several other strategies can be used to improve the quality of biochemical measurement data produced, as well as the interpretation and conclusions based on these data. For example, conducting the analysis of samples from a given subject collected at baseline and after intervention in the same batch may help minimize the potential effect of some sources of methodological variation. However, with large numbers of samples from intervention studies that are conducted over years, it may be impossible to measure baseline and endpoint samples within the time span of the research project. In this case, measurements from a pooled "generic" sample (for example, aliquots of pooled plasma samples from several subjects that have been combined and stored) are obtained with each batch of samples that are measured. This allows examination of the values produced for possible shifts or errors over time so that the methods and instrumentation can be adjusted accordingly. If the nutrition researcher is considering sending samples to a service or clinical laboratory for biochemical measurements, information about these types of QA procedures should be requested for evaluation prior to making a commitment to use the service or laboratory.

REFERENCES

1. Martini MC, Campbell DR, Gross MD, Grandis GA, Potter JD, Slavin JL. Plasma carotenoids as biomarkers of vegetables intake: the University of Minnesota Cancer Prevention Research Unit feeding studies. *Cancer Epidemiol Biomarkers Prev.* 1995;4:491–496.
2. Polsinelli ML, Rock CL, Henderson SA, Drewnowski A. Plasma carotenoids as biomarkers of fruit and vegetable servings in women. *J Am Diet Assoc.* 1998;98:194–196.
3. Fabian CJ, Kimler BF, Elledge RM, Grizzle WE, Beenken SW, Ward JH. Models for early chemoprevention trials in breast cancer. *Hem Oncol Clin N Am.* 1998;12:993–1017.
4. Meyskens FL. Principles of human chemoprevention. *Hem Oncol Clin N Am.* 1998;12:935–941.
5. *Biosafety in Microbial and Biomedical Laboratories.* Washington, DC: US Dept of Health and Human Services, Centers for Disease Control, and National Institutes of Health; 1993. HHS publication no. (CDC) 93-8395.
6. Clevidence BA, Bieri JG. Association of carotenoids with human plasma lipoproteins. *Methods Enzymol.* 1993;214:33–46.
7. Romanchik JE, Morel DW, Harrison EH. Distribution of carotenoids and α-tocopherol among lipoproteins do not change when human plasma is incubated in vitro. *J Nutr.* 1995;125:2610–2617.
8. Habicht JP, Pelletier DL. The importance of context in choosing nutritional indicators. 1990;120(suppl):1519–1524.
9. Jacob RA. Assessment of human vitamin C status. *J Nutr.* 1990;120(suppl):1480–1485.
10. Shils ME, Olson JA, Shike M, Ross AC, eds. *Modern Nutrition in Health and Disease.* 9th ed. Philadelphia, Pa: Williams & Wilkins; 1999.
11. Ziegler EE, Filer LJ, eds. *Present Knowledge in Nutrition.* 7th ed. Washington, DC: ILSI Press; 1996.
12. Food and Nutrition Board, Institute of Medicine. *Dietary Reference Intakes for Calcium, Phosphorus, Magnesium, Vitamin D, and Fluoride.* Washington, DC: National Academy Press; 1997.
13. Food and Nutrition Board. *Dietary Reference Intakes for Thiamin, Riboflavin, Niacin, Vitamin B6, Folate, Vitamin B12, Pantothenic Acid, Biotin, and Choline.* Washington, DC: National Academy Press; 1998.
14. Food and Nutrition Board. *Dietary Reference Intakes for Vitamin C, Vitamin E, Selenium, and Carotenoids.* Washington, DC: National Academy Press; 2000.

15. Blanchard J, Toxer TN, Rowland M. Pharmacokinetic perspectives on megadoses of ascorbic acid. *Am J Clin Nutr.* 1997;66:1165–1171.

16. Campbell DR, Gross MD, Martini MC, Grandits GA, Slavin JL, Potter JD. Plasma carotenoids as biomarkers of vegetable and fruit intake. *Cancer Epidemiol Biomarkers Prev.* 1994;3:493–500.

17. Rock CL, Flatt SW, Wright FA, et al. Responsiveness of carotenoids to a high vegetable diet intervention designed to prevent breast cancer recurrence. *Cancer Epidemiol Biomarkers Prev.* 1997;6:617–623.

18. Le Marchand L, Hankin JH, Carter FS, et al. A pilot study on the use of plasma carotenoids and ascorbic acid as markers of compliance to a high fruit and vegetable diet intervention. *Cancer Epidemiol Biomarkers Prev.* 1994;3:245–251.

19. Mazur W, Fotsis T, Wähälä K, Ojala S, Salakka A, Adlercreutz H. Isotope dilution gas chromatographic-mass spectrophotometric method for the determination of isoflavonoids, coumestrol, and lignans in food samples. *Analytical Biochem.* 1996;233:169–180.

20. Lampe JW, Campbell DR, Hutchins AM, et al. Urinary isoflavonoid and lignan excretion on a Western diet: relation to soy, vegetable, and fruit intake. *Cancer Epidemiol Biomarkers Prev.* 1999;8:699–707.

21. Borriello SP, Setchell KDR, Axelson M, Lawson AM. Production and metabolism of lignans by the human faecal flora. *J Appl Bacteriol.* 1985;58:37–43.

22. Meydani SN, Endres S, Woods MM, et al. Oral (n-3) fatty acid supplementation suppresses cytokine production and lymphocyte proliferation: comparison between young and older women. *J Nutr.* 1991;121:547–555.

23. Soyland E, Funk J, Rajka G, et al. Effect of dietary supplementation with very-long-chain n-3 fatty acids in patients with psoriasis. *N Eng J Med.* 1993;328:1812–1816.

24. Wolk A, Vessby B, Ljung H, Barrefors P. Evaluation of a biologic marker for dairy fat intake. *Am J Clin Nutr.* 1998;68:291–295.

25. Smedman AEM, Gustafsson I-B, Berglund LGT, Vessby BOH. Pentadecanoic acid in serum as a marker for intake of milk fat: relations between intake of milk fat and metabolic risk factors. *Am J Clin Nutr.* 1999;69:22–29.

26. Gross MD, Pfeiffer M, Martini M, Campbell D, Slavin J, Potter J. The quantitation of metabolites of quercetin flavonols in human urine. *Cancer Epidemiol Biomarkers Prev.* 1996;5:711–720.

27. Coward L, Barnes NC, Setchell KDR, Barnes S. Genistein, daidzein and their β-glycoside conjugates: antitumor isoflavones in soybean foods from American and Asian diets. *J Agric Food Chem.* 1993;41:1961–1967.

28. Franke AA, Custer LJ, Cerna CM, Narala K. Quantitation of phytoestrogens in legumes by HPLC. *J Agric Food Chem.* 1994;42:1905–1913.

29. Karr SC, Lampe JW, Hutchins AM, Slavin JL. Urinary isoflavonoid excretion in humans is dose-dependent at low to moderate levels of soy protein consumption. *Am J Clin Nutr.* 1997;66:46–51.

30. Adlercreutz H, Honjo H, Higashi A, et al. Urinary excretion of lignans and isoflavonoid phytoestrogens in Japanese men and women consuming a traditional Japanese diet. *Am J Clin Nutr.* 1991;54:1093–1100.

31. Franke AA, Custer LJ. High-performance liquid chromatography assay of isoflavonoids and coumestrol from human urine. *J Chromatogr B Biomed Appl.* 1994;662:47–60.

32. Maskarinec G, Singh S, Meng L, Franke AA. Dietary soy intake and urinary isoflavonoid excretion among women from a multiethnic population. *Cancer Epidemiol Biomarkers Prev.* 1998;7:613–619.

33. Watanabe S, Yamaguchi M, Sobue T, et al. Pharmacokinetics of soybean isoflavones in plasma, urine, and feces of men after ingestion of 60 g baked soybean powder (kinako). *J Nutr.* 1998;128:1710–1715.

34. Shapiro TA, Fahey JW, Wade KL, Stephenson KK, Talalay P. Human metabolism and excretion of cancer chemoprotective glucosinolates and isothiocyanates of cruciferous vegetables. *Cancer Epidemiol Biomarkers Prev.* 1998;7:1091–1100.

35. McClave SA, Snider HL. Use of indirect calorimetry in clinical nutrition. *Nutr Clin Prac.* 1992;7:207–221.

36. Jequier E, Felber JP. Indirect calorimetry. *Baillieres Clin Endocrinol Metab.* 1987;1:911–935.

37. Owen OE. Resting metabolic requirements of men and women. *Mayo Clin Proc.* 1988;63:503–510.

38. Lusk G. Animal calorimetry: analysis of the oxidation of mixtures of carbohydrate and fat [a correction]. *J Biol Chem.* 1994;59:41–42.

39. Peronnet F, Massicotte D. Table of nonprotein respiratory quotient: an update. *Can J Sport Sci.* 1991:16:23–29.

40. Isbell TR, Klesges RC, Meyers AW, Klesges LM. Measurement reliability and reactivity using repeated measurements of resting energy expenditure with a face mask, mouthpiece, and ventilated canopy. *JPEN J Parenter Enteral Nutr.* 1991;15:165–168.

41. Leff ML, Hill JO, Yates AA, Cotsonis GA, Heymsfield SB. Resting metabolic rate: measurement reliability. *JPEN J Parenter Enteral Nutr.* 1987;11:354–359.

42. Seale J. Energy expenditure measurements in relation to energy requirements. *Am J Clin Nutr.* 1995; 62(suppl):1042–1046.

43. Speakman JR. The history and theory of the doubly labeled water technique. *Am J Clin Nutr.* 1998; 68(suppl):932–938.

44. Sawaya AL, Tucker K, Tsay R, et al. Evaluation of four methods for determining energy intake in young and older women: comparison with doubly labeled water measurements of total energy expenditure. *Am J Clin Nutr.* 1996;63:491–499.

45. Schultz LA, Schoeller DA. A compilation of total daily energy expenditures and body weights in healthy adults. *Am J Clin Nutr.* 1994;60:676–681.

46. Rock CL, Jacob RA, Bowen PA. Update on the biological characteristics of the antioxidant micronutrients: vitamin C, vitamin E, and the carotenoids. *J Am Diet Assoc.* 1996;96:693–702.

47. Handelman GJ, Pryor WA. Evaluation of antioxidant status in humans. In: Papas AM, ed. *Antioxidant Status, Diet, Nutrition, and Health.* New York, NY: CRC Press; 1999:37–62.

48. Lemoyne M, Gossum AV, Kurian R, Ostro M, Azler J, Jeejeebhoy KN. Breath pentane analysis as an index of lipid peroxidation: a functional test of vitamin E status. *Am J Clin Nutr.* 1987;46:267–272.

49. Kasai H, Crain PF, Kuchino Y, Nishimura S, Oostsuyama A, Tanooka H. Formation of 8-hydroxyguanine moiety in cellular DNA by agents producing oxygen radicals and evidence for its repair. *Carcinog.* 1986;7:1849–1851.

50. Loft S, Vistisen K, Ewertz M, Tjonneland A, Overvad K, Poulsen HE. Oxidative DNA damage estimated by 8-hydroxydeoxyguanosine excretion in humans: influence of smoking, gender, and body mass index. *Carcinog.* 1992;13:2241–2247.

51. Tagesson C, Kallberg M, Klintenberg C, Starkhammar. Determination of urinary 8-hydroxydeoxyguanosine by automated coupled-column high performance liquid chromatography: a powerful technique for assaying oxidative DNA damage in cancer patients. *Eur J Cancer.* 1995;31A:934–940.

52. Morrow JD, Harris TM, Roberts LJ. Noncyclooxygenase oxidative formation of a series of novel prostaglandins: analytical ramifications for measurement of eicosanoids. *Ann Biochem.* 1990;184:1–10.

53. Morrow JD, Roberts LJ. The isoprostanes: unique bioactive products of lipid peroxidation. *Prog Lipid Res.* 1997;36:1–21.

54. Patrono C, FitzGerald GA. Isoprostanes: potential markers of oxidant stress in atherothrombotic disease. *Arterioscler Thromb Vasc Biol.* 1997;17:2309–2315.

55. Djuric Z, Lu MH, Lewis SM, et al. Oxidative DNA damage levels in rats fed low-fat, high-fat, or calorie-restricted diets. *Toxicol Appl Pharmacol.* 1992;115:156–160.

56. Djuric Z, Heilbrun LK, Reading BA, Boomer A, Valeriote FA, Martino S. Effects of a low-fat diet on levels of oxidative damage to DNA in human peripheral nucleated blood cells. *J Natl Cancer Inst.* 1991;83:766–769.

57. Djuric Z, Depper JB, Uhley V, et al. Oxidative DNA damage levels in blood from women at high risk for breast cancer are associated with dietary intakes of meats, vegetables, and fruits. *J Am Diet Assoc.* 1998;98:524–528.

58. Mosca L, Rubenfire M, Mandel C, et al. Antioxidant nutrient supplementation reduces the susceptibility of low density lipoprotein to oxidation in patients with coronary artery disease. *J Am Coll Cardiol.* 1997;30:392–399.

59. Habig WH, Pabst MJ, Jakoby WB. Glutathione S-transferases: the first enzymatic step in mercapturic acid formation. *J Biol Chem.* 1974;249:7130–7139.

60. Bogaards JJP, Verhagen H, Willems MI, van Poppel G, van Bladeren PJ. Consumption of brussels sprouts results in elevated alpha-class glutathione S-transferase levels in human blood plasma. *Carcinog.* 1994;15:1073–1075.

61. Kashuba ADM, Bertino JS, Kearns GL, et al. Quantitation of three-month intraindividual variability and influence of sex and menstrual cycle phase on CYP1A2, -acetyltransferase-2, and xanthine oxidase activity determined with caffeine phenotyping. *Clin Pharmacol Ther.* 1998;63:540–551.

62. Pantuck EJ, Pantuck CB, Anderson KE, Wattenberg LW, Conney AH, Kappas A. Effect of brussels sprouts and cabbage on drug conjugation. *Clin Pharmacol Ther.* 1984;35:161–169.

63. Sinha R, Rothman N, Brown ED, et al. Pan-fried meat containing high levels of heterocyclic aromatic amines but low levels of polycyclic aromatic hydrocarbons induces cytochrome P4501A2 activity in humans. *Cancer Res.* 1994;54:6154–6159.

64. Kall MA, Vang O, Clausen J. Effects of dietary broccoli on human drug metabolising activity. *Cancer Lett.* 1997;114:169–170.

65. Fowler BM, Giuliano AR, Piyathilake C, Nour M, Hatch K. Hypomethylation in cervical tissue: is there a correlation with folate status? *Cancer Epidemiol Biomarkers Prev.* 1998;7:901–906.

66. Hamilton SR. Molecular genetics of colorectal carcinoma. *Cancer.* 1992;70:1216–1221.

67. Chen J, Giovannucci EL, Hunter DJ. MTHFR polymorphism, methyl-replete diets and the risk of colorectal carcinoma and adenoma among US men and women: an example of gene-environment interactions in colorectal tumorigenesis. *J Nutr.* 1999;129(suppl):560–564.

68. Lauritsen K, Laursen LS, Bukhave K, Rask-Madsen J. Does vitamin E supplementation modulate in vivo arachidonate metabolism in human inflammation? *Pharmacol Toxicol.* 1987;61:246–249.

69. Ruffin MT, Krishnan K, Rock CL, et al. Suppression of human colorectal mucosal prostaglandins: determining the lowest effective aspirin dose. *J Natl Cancer Inst.* 1997;89:1152–1160.

70. Krishnan K, Ruffin MT, Brenner DE. Clinical models of chemoprevention for colon cancer. *Hematol Oncol Clin North Amer.* 1998;12:1079–1113.

71. Boland CR. The biology of colorectal cancer. *Cancer.* 1993:71(suppl):4181–4186.

72. Einspahr JG, Alberts DS, Gapstur SM, Bostick RM, Emerson SS, Gerner EW. Surrogate end-point biomarkers

as measures of colon cancer risk and their use in cancer chemoprevention trials. *Cancer Epidemiol Biomarkers Prev.* 1997;6:37–48.

73. Lipkin MH. Effect of added dietary calcium on colonic epithelial-cells proliferation in subjects at high risk for familial colonic cancer. *N Eng J Med.* 1985;313:1381–1384.

74. Bostick RM, Fosdick L, Lillemoe TJ, et al. Methodological findings and considerations in measuring colorectal epithelial cell proliferation in humans. *Cancer Epidemiol Biomarkers Prev.* 1997;6:931–942.

75. Vargas PA, Alberts DS. Primary prevention of colorectal cancer through dietary modification. *Cancer.* 1992;70:1229–1235.

76. Lai C, Shields PG. The role of interindividual variation in human carcinogenesis. *J Nutr.* 1999;129(suppl):552–555.

77. Rock CL, Lampe JW, Patterson RE. Nutrition, genetics, and risks of cancer. *Ann Rev Pub Health.* 2000;21:47–64.

78. Sinha R, Caporaso N. Diet, genetic susceptibility, and human cancer etiology. *J Nutr.* 1999;129(suppl):556–559.

79. Kim YI, Pogribney IP, Basnakian AG, et al. Folate deficiency in rats induces DNA strand breaks and hypomethylation within the p53 tumor suppressor gene. *Am J Clin Nutr.* 1997;65:46–52.

80. Byrne C. Studying mammographic density: implications for understanding breast cancer. *J Natl Cancer Inst.* 1997;89:531–533.

81. Knight JA, Martin LJ, Greenberg CV, et al. Macronutrient intake and change in mammographic density at menopause: results from a randomized trial. *Cancer Epidemiol Biomarkers Prev.* 1999;8:123–128.

82. Ruffin MT, Ogaily MS, Johnston CM, Gregoire L, Lancaster WD, Brenner DE. Surrogate endpoint biomarkers for cervical cancer chemoprevention trials. *J Cell Biochem Suppl.* 1995;23:113–124.

83. Rock CL, Michael CW, Reynolds RK, Ruffin MT. Prevention of cervix cancer. *Crit Rev Oncol Hematol.* 2000;33:169–185.

84. MacLennan R, Macrae F, Bain C, et al. Randomized trial of intake of fat, fiber, and beta carotene to prevent colorectal adenomas. The Australian Polyp Prevention Project. *J Natl Cancer Inst.* 1995;87:1760–1766.

85. Greenwald P. Colon cancer overview. *Cancer.* 1992;70(suppl):1206–1215.

86. Byers T. Diet, colorectal adenomas, and colorectal cancer. *N Eng J Med.* 2000;342:1206–1207.

87. Schatzkin A, Lanza E, Corle D, et al. Lack of effect of a low-fat diet on the recurrence of colorectal adenomas. *N Eng J Med.* 2000;342:1149–1155.

88. Bingham S, Cummings JH. The use of 4-aminobenzoic acid as a marker to validate the completeness of 24 hr urine collections in man. *Clin Sci.* 1983;64:629–635.

89. Guilliano AR, Matzner MB, Canfield LM. Assessing variability in quantitation of carotenoids in human plasma: variance component model. *Methods Enzymol.* 1993;214:94–101.

90. Duewer DL, Thomas JB, Kline MC, MacCrehan WA, Schaffer R, Sharpless KE. NIST/NCI Micronutrients Quality Assurance Program: measurement repeatabili-ties and reproducibilities for fat-soluble vitamin-related compounds in human sera. *Ann Chem.* 1997;69:1406–1413.

Further Reading

Armstrong BK, White E, Saracci R. Monographs in Epidemiology and Biostatistics. Vol 21. New York, NY: Oxford University Press; 1994.

Hulka BS, Wilcosky TC, Griffish JD, eds. New York, NY: Oxford University Press; 1990.

18

Research Methods for Human Sensory System Analysis and Food Evaluation

Richard D. Mattes, M.P.H., Ph.D., R.D.

"Sensory appeal" is arguably the principal determinant of food selection and ingestion. In surveys, more than 90 percent of consumers rank taste as more influential on their food selection and ingestion choices than other factors, such as nutrition, price, or safety (1,2). Professionals in academia, industry, medicine, and government also indicate that taste takes precedence over nutrient content, price, convenience, and health concerns (3). Furthermore, concern over sacrificing the sensory pleasure of eating is a primary explanation for failure to adopt a more healthful diet. Consequently, it is vital for health care providers, and especially dietitians, to understand how the sensory properties of foods and the sensory abilities of humans interact to influence food choice in health and disease.

TERMINOLOGY

Taste is used colloquially to refer to the sensory properties of foods. However, to a sensory scientist, the term *taste* is restricted to those sensations arising from chemical stimulation of taste receptor cells. These cells are located on the tongue, soft palate, pharynx, epiglottis, larynx, and upper esophagus. The repertoire of sensations is limited to sweetness, sourness, saltiness, bitterness, and probably umami (the sensation elicited by monosodium glutamate). Detection systems for dietary starch and fat have recently been proposed, but the evidence is very preliminary.

In contrast, the array of food odors is vast, and most believe there is no limited set of primary qualities. Food odors are detected by specialized receptor cells in the olfactory epithelium, located at the apex of the superior turbinate. Odor molecules may reach the olfactory epithelium via the orthonasal route and the retronasal route. The former pathway involves the passage of odor molecules through the nares (for example, when sniffing food), whereas the latter entails access of volatile compounds derived from food in the mouth through the back of the throat. Retronasal stimulation accounts for much of the flavor of foods.

The chemically mediated irritancy (for example, the burning of pepper or the coolness of menthol) and mouth feel (for example, astringency of foods and beverages) is referred to as *chemesthesis*. This input is conveyed by trigeminal innervation, which is widely dispersed throughout the nasopharyngeal region. Foods also provide an array of nonchemically mediated sensations (for example, visual, auditory, and thermal sensations).

The combination of all of this input is referred to as *flavor*. Any alteration of a component part will result in a different flavor, much as the omission of selected pieces can alter the overall appearance of a puzzle. Because each of us differs in our innate and acquired sensitivities and affective responses to the plethora of chemicals in foods and beverages, the perception of flavor is idiosyncratic.

STUDY OF FLAVOR PERCEPTION

The study of flavor perception can be broadly divided into two tracks. One track concerns the sensory properties of foods and is largely in the domain of food scientists. The focus is on gaining a better understanding of the physiochemical properties of foods and beverages that determine a their sensory characteristics. The most widely used definition of such sensory evaluation is that it is a scientific method used to evoke, measure, analyze, and interpret responses to products perceived through the senses of sight, smell, touch, taste, and hearing (4). Generally, the approach is to identify and train a panel of judges who will be able to provide reliable and detailed information about the sensory attributes of complex stimuli (real foods). It is important to recognize that sensory evaluation is a science based on the principles of the scientific method, including hypothesis testing through objective and reproducible measurements. The skills necessary to conduct this work are varied, but they are largely drawn from statistics, psychology, and food science. The information generated by sensory professionals in the food industry has multiple uses (Figure 18.1). These are described more fully, along with the suitable testing methodologies, in several references (5–7).

The second track in the study of flavor perception, referred to as *psychophysics,* is primarily concerned with the psychological perception of physical stimuli. The aim is a better understanding of the factors that influence the sensory capabilities of judges (consumers). Thus, the approach is to measure individual variability in responses to standardized, typically simple stimuli (for example, a single compound in water). Such work has been dominated by psychologists, physiologists, and neuroscientists. The goals are to understand the basic mechanisms of sensory systems, as well as their contribution to, and complications from, pathological processes. Hence, psychophysical testing is useful in the clinical setting.

The array of chemosensory disorders is listed in Table 18.1. In general, olfactory disorders are more prevalent than gustatory disorders (8,9). Anosmia is the most common diagnosis among patients evaluated at taste and smell centers, followed by hyposmia and dysosmia and then phantosmia. The majority of problems stem from upper respiratory tract infections, head trauma, and nasal and paranasal sinus disease. Ageusia is extremely rare. Diminutions of sensation and distortions are more prevalent. Taste disorders most commonly follow upper respiratory tract infections, middle ear surgery and disease, and head trauma. A number of references describe the etiology, diagnosis, incidence, and management of these abnormalities (8–20).

The outcome variables for these two branches of sensory science are quite similar, but the experimental approaches often differ. Common questions in both approaches concern (1) the minimal level of stimulus intensity that can be detected or characterized, (2) the relationship between growth of sensation and physical concentration, (3) spatial-temporal influences on responsiveness, and (4) hedonic judgments. Combined, these measures characterize an individual's sensory capabilities and experiences fairly well. Individually, each measure provides information about a segment of the sensory spectrum, but because they are poorly correlated, knowledge

---

Dietary Implications of Sensory Function
>   Quality of life
>   Food safety
>   Food selection
>   Digestion and nutrient metabolism

Applications of Sensory Evaluation in the Food Industry
>   New product development
>   Product reformulation
>   Cost reduction
>   Quality control
>   Quality assurance
>   Monitoring the competition
>   Shelf-life studies
>   Assessment of raw materials
>   Support of advertising claims

FIGURE 18.1 Functions of sensory systems and sensory evaluation in dietetics and food science.

TABLE 18.1   Chemosensory Disorders

Taste	Smell	Description
Ageusia	Anosmia	Loss of sensation
Hypogeusia	Hyposmia	Diminished sensation
Hypergeusia	Hyperosmia	Enhanced sensation
Dysgeusia	Dysosmia	Distorted sensation
Phantogeusia	Phantosmia	Sensation without known stimulation

of one segment does not provide a basis for assumptions about another segment. For example, during recovery following radiation therapy administered to the head and neck, the ability to detect low concentrations of stimuli may return well before the ability to assign increasing intensity ratings to graded concentrations of stronger stimuli (21). Neither threshold sensitivity nor responsiveness to suprathreshold stimuli holds predictive power for hedonic judgments, because hedonic judgments are strongly influenced by culture and dietary experiences.

There are multiple methods for assessment of the different facets of chemosensory function. Several of the more common methods are described in this chapter. The interested researcher is encouraged to consult one or more of the references for a more comprehensive description of test procedures and the issues that warrant control when using them. In addition, a number of short courses are offered for intensive training in various aspects of sensory science. Additional information may be obtained from the following Web sites: http://www.sensoryspec trum.com, http://www.ifpress.com, http://www.infosense. com/courses, and http://www.tragon.com.

THRESHOLD MEASUREMENT

A *threshold* is a measure of the lowest limits of sensitivity of a sensory system. If the task is to determine simply whether a stimulus is present or if one sample contains a stimulus while a comparison sample does not, the threshold is called a *detection threshold*. It is not necessary to be able to characterize the stimulus; a determination of its presence alone is sufficient. If the task is to determine the lowest concentration at which the quality of the stimulus can be identified, the threshold is termed a *recognition threshold*. *Discrimination thresholds* represent the increment in stimulus intensity required to detect a difference between paired samples. In actuality, detection thresholds are just one level of a discrimination threshold where the comparison stimulus level is zero.

It is often incorrectly assumed that thresholds reflect an inherent characteristic of an individual. Rather, they are probabilistic measures that may be defined as the lowest concentration of a stimulus that can be detected (or recognized, or discriminated) at greater than some set level of probability under a given set of conditions. Generally, as one is exposed to increasing concentrations of a stimulus, the likelihood of detecting its presence rises as a sigmoidal function. The probability level is customarily set at the level of chance performance for the task. Thus, if two sam-

ples are rated, the probability of guessing correctly is 50 percent. If three samples are being compared, the probability of correct guessing is 33 percent. However, the criterion is arbitrary, and if the experimenter wants to decrease the risk of a false-positive identification (type I error), this probability level may be raised to a higher level. The medium in which the stimulus is to be identified is also critical. A stimulus in a simple medium, such as water, is more easily detected than the same stimulus incorporated in a complex food system. Thus, thresholds are generally lower in model solutions.

There are three common methods for measuring thresholds in sensory evaluation, although a number of variations on them are used. They may be the method of choice when attempting to determine subtle differences in products possibly due to reformulation or processing changes, monitoring quality control, or performing shelf life studies.

Paired Comparison Test

The paired comparison test may be directional or nondirectional. In the former case, the nature of the stimulus is known, and the judge is required to indicate which of the two samples presented contains the target sensory attribute. In this two-alternative forced choice test, the judge must make a choice even if unsure of the correct answer. If the nature of the stimulus is not known, the judge is asked to indicate if the two samples are alike or different in the simple difference or same-different test. In both cases, pairs of samples are presented in random order. Typically, sufficient time or a means to clear the first stimulus prior to administration of the second (for example, rinsing with water or breathing air without a stimulus) is used. For both tests the probability of correct guessing is 50 percent. Because the experimenter knows the correct response, a one-tailed test is used to establish statistical significance, which is determined by comparing the proportion of correct responses to the binomial distribution. Strengths of the paired comparison test are that it is conceptually simple and, as a result, quite sensitive and resistant to confusion errors. Because few samples need to be tested, fatigue is minimized.

Duo-Trio Test

The duo-trio test involves presenting judges with three samples. One sample is labeled as a reference, and two samples are unknowns; the task is to determine which of the unknowns is similar to the reference. The reference is sampled first, followed by the two unknowns, which are presented in counterbalanced orders in duplicate trials. This test is nondirectional, because the basis for making a match decision need not be specified, and it will not be known. The probability of correct guessing is 50 percent. Analysis is based on comparison with the binomial distribution in a one-tailed test.

The advantage of this procedure is that it can be used to assess sensitivity to changes of a product without knowing what attribute of the product has actually changed. This characteristic is also a drawback, because the test may not provide insights on the component responsible for the difference between samples. Furthermore, it requires more sampling than the paired comparison test, is slightly less powerful, and is more susceptible to reversal errors (i.e., judge reports which are the "odd sample," rather than the match).

Triangle Test

The triangle test entails the simultaneous presentation of three samples; two are alike and one is different. The samples are rated in random order, and the task is to identify the odd sample. This test is nondirectional, because the basis for selecting the odd sample need not be specified, and it will not be known. The probability of guessing is 33 percent. Analysis is based on comparison with the binomial distribution in a one-tailed test.

The advantage of the triangle test is that the probability of correct guessing is lower, so fewer subjects may be required to determine whether differences exist. This characteristic may reduce time and sample costs. The fact that it is nondirectional can be a strength (if the nature of the target sensation is not known) or a weakness (the basis for a judgment is not known), depending on the desired outcome of testing. Because the triangle test requires exposure to more samples than does the paired comparison test, there is increased risk of fatigue and loss of sensitivity, especially for samples that are difficult to clear from the mouth or nose.

Staircase Procedure

The staircase procedure is widely used in psychophysical studies (22), although the previously discussed methods may also be appropriate under certain conditions. In the staircase procedure, the judge may be offered two samples and asked to indicate which contains a particular stimulus. Alternatively, the judge may be offered a single sample and asked whether a stimulus is present or not. If

the response is incorrect, a higher concentration is then presented, along with a sample of the vehicle or medium without the stimulus (in the paired comparison situation). Another incorrect response is followed with a still higher concentration. This activity continues until a correct response is obtained. Because there is a 50 percent probability of guessing, it is common practice to present an identical concentration a second time after a correct response to confirm that the stimulus was indeed detected. Following repeated correct responses, an incrementally lower concentration is presented. If the response to this pair is again correct, the concentration declines again on the next trial. This procedure continues until a single incorrect response is obtained.

The concentrations where ascending and descending trials originate are termed *reversal points*. The first reversal point is typically discarded as unreliable because of orienting effects. The subsequent reversal concentrations are averaged to derive an estimated threshold. An equal number, commonly two to three of the ascending-to-descending trials and two to three of the descending-to-ascending trials, are included. This rigorous method can provide a reasonable estimate of an individual's limit of sensitivity, but it is extremely time-consuming to administer.

General Concerns About Threshold Tests

Researchers using threshold tests should keep potential problems in mind. First, all threshold procedures are in fact estimating the ability to discriminate differences between a signal and a background level of stimulation (because of other food constituents, water, air, or whatever the vehicle may be that carries the stimulus). When there is a higher level of background stimulation, it is more difficult to detect a small increment in stimulus intensity than when there is little background noise. For example, detecting the change in illumination of a dark room when one lightbulb is on is easier than detecting the contribution of one lightbulb when added in a room containing 100 other lighted bulbs. Thus, the absolute value of a threshold estimate is highly dependent on the test conditions. Indeed, a reported value cannot be interpreted without knowledge of the mode of sensory stimulation.

Another problem with threshold tests involves learning. Familiarity with the testing procedure leads to improved performance. Thus, it is important to have a run-in period so that judge performance is stable before actual testing.

Fatigue is another problem. Prolonged testing can

lead to reduced attention and adaptation of sensory receptors to the stimuli under study. These effects will raise threshold levels. If feasible, it may be preferable to test individuals on two occasions so fewer stimuli will be sampled in a single session. Habituation may hamper interpretation of threshold tests. In the single-sample staircase procedure, judges may simply continue to respond positively or negatively, overshooting concentrations where reversals should occur. Care should be taken to avoid providing the judge with clues about the testing paradigm. Selecting stimulus concentration steps that are small enough to be difficult to discriminate will reduce learning. At the same time, if the steps are so small that discrimination is extremely difficult, the test may take an inordinate amount of time to administer. Half-log steps or serial half-dilutions often work well.

Another problem, anticipation, is the opposite of habituation. Judges may attempt to anticipate a concentration reversal and prematurely switch their response. Again, taking steps to reduce the judges' knowledge of the testing sequence should reduce this problem.

When two stimuli are presented, the second stimulus sampled is often rated as stronger because of memory decay. This problem can be avoided by counterbalancing sample presentation.

Another issue with threshold testing involves position bias. Judges tend to favor one position (for example, they might select the sample on the right), so samples should be presented in different positions.

As has been noted, absolute threshold values reflect testing conditions. Variability of motivation can alter threshold estimates. If a reward (for example, a monetary bonus) is provided for performance leading to a low threshold without penalty for guessing, judges may adopt a different response strategy than they would if there were a penalty (for example, reduction of monetary remuneration) for incorrect responses.

Extraneous cues may confound test results. Subtle differences in attributes not intentionally manipulated (for example, temperature, color, or viscosity), rather than the target stimulus, may be the basis of judgments. A wide array of subject attributes, including mood, alertness, hunger level, health status, and oral hygiene, may alter performance in unpredictable ways. Thus, test-retest reliability can be low. Attempts to recruit a homogenous sample of judges or to control various relevant behaviors (for example, forbidding eating, smoking, and drinking for some period prior to testing) should reduce variability and permit identification of subtle changes that occur over time, which is often the primary dependent variable in clinical assessments.

Another concern is that sensory evaluation studies often are conducted with the hope of finding no significant difference between samples. To ensure that reasonable conclusions are drawn, it is especially critical in this case to design the test to have sufficient statistical power. This goal may be achieved by using trained judges, by lowering the critical value for significance, or by increasing the sample size.

Finally, it cannot be assumed that threshold sensitivity correlates with other measures of sensory function or food selection. As noted previously (21), threshold sensitivity can change independently of other indexes of sensory function—for example, because of the administration of therapeutic modalities (for example, medications or radiotherapy) or the progression of disease.

SCALING PROCEDURES

Scaling procedures are used to evaluate the association between sensation and suprathreshold (above-threshold) concentrations of stimuli. In contrast to threshold assessment, scaling procedures can provide insights on the perceived intensity of stimuli over a wide range of concentrations. Some stimuli (for example, sucrose and sodium chloride) lead to disproportionately large increments in sensation relative to gradations in physical concentration, a phenomenon termed *expansion*. The perceived intensity of some stimuli grows in proportion to steps of physical concentration, whereas the perceived intensity of other stimuli (for example, fat) leads to lesser increments in sensation than predicted by changes in physical concentration. The latter phenomenon is referred to as *compression*. Knowledge of these relationships is vital in the food industry for product development and reformulation. The rate of growth of sensation with increasing stimulus concentration is also an index of the function of the sensory system being stimulated. There are several response formats (e.g., ranking, category and visual analog scales, magnitude estimation) for scaling stimuli, each with advantages and disadvantages. Different formats generate different levels of data.

Ordinal Data

Ranking is perhaps the simplest form of scaling. It generates data at the ordinal level. The judge is asked to sample a set of stimuli and order them along a stipulated dimension (for example, odor intensity). This procedure does not require the assignment of numerical intensity ratings to the stimuli, which is an advantage when working with very young children or people unfamiliar or uncomfortable with number use. The drawback is that no information is obtained regarding the perceived magnitude of difference between successive stimuli. It is also necessary to make multiple comparisons to assign ranks, which may lead to fatigue. Thus, the number of stimuli that can be evaluated is limited. Ranked data do not meet the assumptions underlying parametric statistics, so nonparametric tests must be used to assess test results.

Interval Data

Category scales permit the assignment of numerical responses to stimuli that reflect the magnitude of differences between them. However, because they have no true zero, they yield interval-level data. Figure 18.2 shows some of the many variations of category scales. Judges are presented with a set of stimuli and asked to rate each stimulus on a given scale. The samples are presented in random order, preferably in duplicate or triplicate, with adequate time or procedures to reduce carryover effects from the previous sample. Samples are coded with 3-digit random numbers to avoid biasing responses. As a general rule, judges are comfortable with 7 category options. Given that judges may avoid the extreme response options (end effect) (23,24), the effective scale is often 2 categories fewer than presented. Thus, 3- and 5-point scales provide a very limited array of response options. Scales with more than 9 options appear to provide greater flexibility to judges, but it must be determined whether the judges are really able to make the fine discriminations that these scales imply. Given end effects, a 9-point scale (the most commonly used) yields an adequate (7-point) response format.

By having an odd number of categories, it is possible to have a bipolar scale with a neutral point in the center. This type of scale is used more frequently for hedonic rating, but it can be used for intensity judgments as well if ratings are being made relative to a reference sample. In this case, the center rating would indicate no difference. The choice of descriptors attached to scales is critical. They must be unambiguous to all judges, isolate a single sensory attribute (intensity and hedonic terms should not be mixed, for example), and cover the range of sensations judges will experience.

The strength of category scales is that they permit rapid acquisition of intensity judgments over a wide segment of an individual's sensory range. Furthermore, they are simple, familiar response scales that can be adapted to almost any audience. Because all judges are responding on a fixed scale, the calibration of responses is straightforward.

A drawback is that it is not known if the sensation difference between ratings of 2 and 3 is really equal to the difference between ratings of 7 and 8. Indeed, the differences probably are not equal. Sensation maps better on a roughly logarithmic scale, with better discrimination for small differences between weak stimuli than strong ones. The labeled magnitude scale (25,26) captures this characteristic and has found wide application in psychophysical studies (see Figure 18.2). This scale also helps address the issue of whether comparable ratings reflect equal sensation of different judges. The use of verbal descriptors helps to anchor responses, but it does not ensure that ratings reflect a common experience.

Another threat to the validity of category scales is termed the *range-frequency effect* (23,27). Judges tend to use the allotted range of response options regardless of the range of sensations experienced. In addition, they are uncomfortable assigning too many samples to a single category and thus tend to distribute responses to adjacent, lesser used categories. This problem requires that all between-study comparisons using category scale response formats be based on similar sample sets and response options. Furthermore, less distortion in responses is likely if an equal number of stimuli of each intensity level are presented. Differences in reported intensity between moderately to widely discrepant concentrations of stimuli are exaggerated when the judge has received repeated exposure to a set of samples clustered around a particular concentration (28–31).

Visual Analog Scales

Visual analog scales provide a response format that yields interval-level data without the need for number assignment. Judges are asked to place a mark along a line anchored with semantic labels that reflect their impression of the intensity of the attribute being rated (see Figure 18.2). Ratings are interpreted by measuring the distance from a set point (typically one anchor) to the judge's mark. Analysis is time-consuming and prone to error if done by manual measurement with a ruler. Several computer-based data collection programs now offer this response format and compute the distances automatically.

Scales that generate interval level data do not meet the assumptions underlying parametric statistical tests. Consequently, data derived from them are most appropriately analyzed by nonparametric tests. However, the

Category Scales

Example 1

1	2	3	4	5	6	7	8	9
No sweetness								Extremely sweet

Example 2

|----------------|----------------|----------------|----------------|----------------|----------------|----------------|----------------|

Weak burn   Strong burn

Example 3

□   □   □   □   □   □   □   □   □

Not at all fishy   Extremely fishy

Example 4

Extremely oily
Very oily
Moderately oily
Slightly oily
Not oily

Example 5

|----------------|----------------|----------------|----------------|----------------|----------------|----------------|----------------|

Weaker than   Same as the   Stronger than
the reference   reference   the reference

Labeled Magnitude Scale

— Strongest imaginable

— Very strong

— Strong

— Moderate

— Weak
— Barely detectable

Visual Analog Scale

No sensation   Strongest imaginable sensation

Pictorial Scale

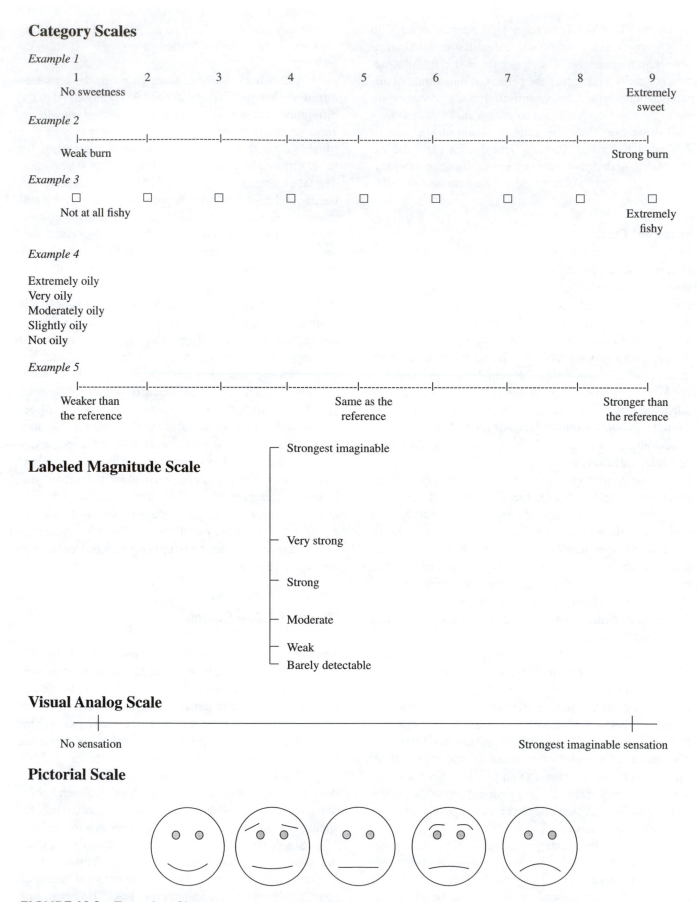

FIGURE 18.2 Examples of interval-level scales of intensity.

more powerful and familiar parametric tests generally lead to comparable results and are widely applied. If a parametric test (*t* test or F test) is used, the outcome should be interpreted as approximate and verified by the comparable nonparametric procedure.

Ratio Scales

Ratio scales permit judges to assign numbers to stimuli that reflect their intensity, with the only restriction being that the ratings reflect the proportional sensation differences between stimuli. For example, with the magnitude estimation procedure, judges are instructed to sample and assign an intensity rating—whatever number seems appropriate—to one stimulus. Subsequent samples are then rated relative to this initial assessment. If a subsequent sample is half as intense, the sample is assigned a rating half as large as the former; if it is four times stronger, it is assigned a rating four times greater.

Because of individual differences in number use that may not reflect true differences in perceived intensity, it is necessary to normalize all responses to a common scale. A variety of techniques have been proposed for this purpose. One approach is to determine the arithmetic mean of all sensory responses and to divide this value into 10 (an arbitrary number). The result is a factor by which each individual response is then multiplied to normalize the data. Another solution involves providing judges a reference sample with an assigned intensity score. All ratings are then made relative to the reference, so they are already normalized. The disadvantage of this approach is that judges may not be comfortable with the number assigned by the researcher, which could bias their subsequent ratings. Another method to adjust for discrepancies in number use is to have judges concurrently rate stimuli in another modality (for example, taste and loudness of tones). In the clinical setting, a modality presumed to be unaffected by a patient's condition is selected (for example, estimation of the loudness of tones or brightness of lights when assessing salt taste in patients with hypertension). This method is termed *cross-modality matching* (32). The responses to the second modality are then used to normalize responses to the target stimuli.

Once the data are normalized, the least squares regression line for the plot of stimulus concentration versus intensity ratings is determined. The slope of the line is the metric used to evaluate the growth of sensation with physical concentration. The y-axis intercept also provides information about the absolute strength of sensation. Often log-log plots are used to linearize the data (a permissible transformation only with ratio-level data), but this technique should be used only after determining the function that best describes the data. If a log transformation is used, responses of zero intensity become problematic. Suggested treatments for this problem include omitting zero ratings; however, there is little justification to ignore valid responses, and if the number of such ratings is large, analyses could be distorted. Replacement of zeros with a small number has been used but accomplishes little, because the log of a very small number is extremely small and can distort the data. Another method is to use the median response of all judges at each concentration, but this method can result in the loss of important information. Finally, the geometric mean of responses can by "be" computed.

As a general rule, a minimum of 5 stimulus levels are used in the sample set, and there should be at least 20 observations per stimulus level. Ideally, these observations would be independent, but replicates from a smaller panel of judges can be used. The number of samples that may be rated in a session will be determined by the nature of the stimuli. Fewer presentations will be possible for stimuli that are difficult to clear (for example, peanut butter). Overall, sessions should not last longer than approximately 45 minutes, after which the attention and motivation of judges may wane. Further discussion of ratio scaling is available in a number of sources (6,24,33–37).

The strength of ratio scales lies in the level of data generated. Ratio-level data are amenable to potentially useful transformations and the full array of parametric statistical procedures. The primary concern lies in the level of sophistication required of judges. They must be comfortable assigning numbers on an open scale that reflect proportional relationships between stimuli. For example, such a scale would not be appropriate with small children.

With appropriate training of judges and control over potential biases, the different scaling methods overall have comparable sensitivity and yield similar results (6). A decision about which method to use in a study should be guided by the study objectives, the nature of the study population, and the resources available for data analyses (38–42).

TIME-INTENSITY PROCEDURES

The procedures described thus far require judges to integrate or summate sensations derived from a stimulus and report the experience with a single number. Consequently, all information about the time course of sensation is lost. Time-intensity procedures involve evaluation of the intensity of stimulus characteristics at specified time points (43).

Following exposure to a stimulus, there is usually a delay or lag time before it is detected. The sensation then grows in intensity to a peak and begins to decline. However, the time course of these phases differs for each stimulus component because of their varying physical-chemical properties. This idea is easily illustrated for a food placed in the oral cavity. If it is a solid item, it is masticated, resulting in mechanical degradation. Volatiles are also released by this process and, in the case of cold items, by warming in the oral cavity. The speed with which the released taste and odor compounds are transported to their receptive site is determined by the degree to which they stimulate salivary flow and water-lipid-air partitioning coefficients. Chemical interactions may modify all of these steps.

To capture time-intensity information, sensory ratings may be obtained using a wide variety of response formats (for example, category scales, visual analog scales, or magnitude estimation). Tracings of the growth and decline of sensation may also be made with the zero control of a strip-chart recorder or the joystick or sliding bar potentiometer on a computer (43). The timing of ratings will be determined by the product under consideration. Rapid ratings would be required to assess the carbonation level of a beverage consumed under natural conditions. Less frequent responses would be needed to trace the perceived burn of a spicy sauce, and still longer interrating intervals might be suitable for evaluating the sweetness of chewing gum. Because the task requires a high degree of attention to the sensory attribute under study, it is not advisable to rate more than one attribute at a time.

Analyses of time-intensity data generally focus on four dimensions: (1) time-related events, such as the lag time from stimulus delivery to onset of sensation or to peak intensity; (2) rate-related parameters, such as the rate of growth or decline of sensation; (3) intensity-related attributes, including peak sensation; and (4) events-related indexes, such as breathing or swallowing. Recommendations for analyses of these parameters have been published (44–46).

Time-intensity ratings are highly susceptible to error due to fatigue; reduced motivation; and depending on the nature of the attribute being rated (for example, odor),

poor control over stimulus onset and elimination. These ratings are best obtained using trained judges. The potential biases that judges bring to the task remain largely uncharacterized (47). Thus, the data must be interpreted cautiously.

SPATIAL TESTING

Experimental exploitation of regional differences in sensation have provided new insights of clinical importance. Although the notion that there is a regional tongue map has been largely discredited (48), there are differences in neural innervation patterns in the oral cavity. By stimulating localized sites, it is possible to gain insights on the fundamental mechanisms of taste reception and to diagnose selective neural damage that may account for taste disorders (49,50). This stimulation is accomplished by swabbing stimuli on selected sites with a cotton applicator (51).

Another use of spatial testing is to permit differentiation of the contributions of olfactory and chemesthetic stimulation from volatile compounds. This problem arises because nearly all odorants also have a pungent quality that is mediated by the trigeminal nerve. As a consequence, the diagnosis of anosmia may be complicated. By testing a patient's ability to localize inhaled stimuli, it may be possible to identify a potential contribution of the trigeminal sense to test performance. A blank sample is presented to one nostril, and a true stimulus is simultaneously presented to the other nostril; the patient is asked to indicate which nostril has the stimulus.

Finally, by manipulating the route of olfactory stimulation, it has been possible to better determine the nature of olfactory complaints in a range of patient populations, notably the elderly. Odors may reach the olfactory epithelium orthonasally or retronasally. Sensory disturbances attributable to stimulant access to receptors can thus be identified by testing performance to both routes of stimulus delivery. This testing involves having individuals rate stimuli after sniffing or holding them in the oral cavity with the nose both open and pinched. Such studies have demonstrated that the elderly experience a greater decline in retronasal than orthonasal olfaction, and the former is the larger contributor to the flavor of food (52–54). The full potential for various forms of spatial testing to reveal insights on sensory mechanisms, flavor perception, and clinical disorders has yet to be realized.

IDENTIFICATION TESTS

As has been described, the ability of individuals to identify stimuli alone or in mixtures at threshold levels is an index of sensory sensitivity called a *recognition threshold*. Such a task is also used with suprathreshold stimulus concentrations in both the food industry and clinical settings. Because of the limited number of taste sensations, identification tests generally are conducted with odors alone or flavors during food ingestion. Odor profiling, identification of the component parts of a complex odor, may be used in the food industry for a variety of purposes, such as evaluation of a competitor's product, formulation of new products, quality control, and checking product stability. However, human beings have a limited ability to identify single odor compounds in mixtures (55,56), so odor profiling requires considerable training and may lend itself to instrumental methods.

Odor identification has gained wide acceptance as a means to diagnose olfactory disorders. Patients are presented an array of common odors matched on intensity and are required to identify the quality. One limitation of the test is that it depends heavily on memory to generate the correct labels. To minimize this potential confounding factor, a multiple-choice answer format is often used.

Descriptions of several tests have been published (8,57–61). They vary in the source (blended foods versus pure chemicals) and array of odors used, as well as the format of odor delivery (for example, sniffing the head space over the stimulus in a solid container or squeeze bottle or the use of scratch-and-sniff microencapsulated odors).

Odor identification test results correlate well with results of threshold tests, but they may have better reliability and require much less time to administer (14,62). The primary concerns with odor identification tests are control over stimulus delivery (if stimuli are of different intensity, it may alter performance) and memory demands.

DESCRIPTIVE ANALYSIS

Because of the diversity of products that many companies market, the increasing sophistication of food science, and the huge economic consequences of decisions based on sensory data, reliance on the expert opinions of single individuals to guide sensory evaluation in the food industry

has diminished. It has been replaced by a wide array of sophisticated approaches, termed *descriptive analysis,* that involve the discrimination and description of the qualitative and quantitative attributes of products. Descriptive testing attempts to produce a total product profile. It is used to guide research, support or interpret instrumental or other sensory analysis methods, and provide quality control information.

Broadly, descriptive analysis involves assembling a group of individuals who, through the development of a common lexicon, identify and rate the proportional contributions of salient attributes of products. Depending on the approach, the lexicon may be developed through panel consensus or more formal training with preestablished standards. The attributes rated may be determined by allowing the panel to identify the salient characteristics of the product or by externally imposed criteria. Ratings may be made by a variety of techniques, including category or visual analog scales or magnitude estimation.

Some approaches train panelists to rate a limited set of products, and others train judges to be generalists able to evaluate a broad range of products. In either case, considerable time and effort are typically invested to train and maintain the skills of judges. Consequently, it is essential to select panelists carefully. Criteria used include normal sensory ability judged by threshold and scaling tests, availability for training and service, and motivation. Personality is also important, because panelists must work as a team. Domineering or passive individuals may hurt (change to "impede") productivity.

Some approaches culminate in the development of a consensus report, whereas other approaches are amenable to statistical analysis. A more detailed discussion of descriptive analysis techniques may be found in the literature (63–72), and a number of professionals offer short, intensive training courses. Advertisements for these courses are published in *Food Technology* and the newsletter of the Sensory Division of the Society for Food Science and Technology.

AFFECTIVE TESTS (TESTS OF HEDONICS)

Hedonics refers to the pleasantness or appeal of stimuli (foods and beverages, in this case). The sensations measured by the previously outlined techniques provide the substrate upon which hedonic judgments are made. Some sensations appear to be inherently pleasing (for example, sweetness and saltiness) or inherently unpleasant (for example, bitterness), but in light of evidence that maternal diet during pregnancy or lactation may influence the neonate's responsiveness to flavors (73,74), delineation of the role of genetics and learning is problematic.

Perhaps the most important point from a dietetics perspective is that the affective interpretation of different forms and intensities of sensory stimulation is not immutable. It can change with varying physiological status, including hunger (75,76), pathological conditions (8–20), and dietary experience (77). Dietary experience, in particular, provides an avenue for dietary interventions. One of the most powerful, but complex, influences on palatability is frequency of exposure. Familiarity enhances acceptability (78). A second strong influence is culture. Foods seasoned according to the flavor principles of an individual's culture are generally well accepted, whereas other foods are less well liked despite there being no clear biological basis for the superiority of any particular cuisine.

Purposeful manipulation of exposure frequency can support therapeutic diets. By restricting sensory exposure to salt, fat, or sugar, the preferred level of these flavor modifiers declines (79–81). Conversely, increased exposure will lead to a preference for higher levels of the constituents (82,83). However, exposure at too high a level can result in monotony and a decline in acceptability (84). This principle also has been used therapeutically to promote reduced energy intake (for example, diets relying on free consumption of single foods). However, the success of such diets has been poor because of the overpowering desire for sensory variety and resultant diet rejection.

Another method of modifying the valence of sensory stimuli is through learned associations. If ingestion of an item is followed by malaise, its future acceptability may be diminished. Taste, odor, and texture are the attributes of food that provide the basis for this shift (85). At the same time, repeated pairing of items with positive experiences, both biological and cultural, may enhance the appeal of foods. This mechanism may be the basis for desiring certain items, such as the craving for chocolate when one is under stress or depressed (86).

Hedonics is a multidimensional attribute that is not adequately captured by a single test. Knowledge of the optimal level of a sensory characteristic in a food (one hedonic index) does not provide insights on the desired frequency of consumption of the item (a second index). Furthermore, knowledge of the optimal frequency of consumption of an item characterized by some sensory property does not necessarily provide insights on liking for a range of items with that particular prominent sensory attribute (a third index). Thus, an attempt to capture more fully the appeal of the target product should include either carefully selected tests addressing the measure of interest or a battery of tests.

To measure the optimal concentration of an ingredient in a product, samples with graded levels of the key constituent can be presented in random order and rated for palatability. Multiple response formats may be used to capture the information. These formats include measurement of autonomic nervous system responses (for example, respiratory or heart rate) or videotaped mimetic responses to stimulus presentation in subjects unable to respond by more conventional scales (for example, infants or illiterate subjects). Pictorial scales (for example, faces) may also be used when numerical responses are not viable. Category and visual analog scales are used most commonly. Depending on the product, optimization procedures are also possible (87,88). These procedures permit the panelists to actually adjust the level of the target constituent in a food to an optimal point or to indicate how each sample of an array can be manipulated to yield a more palatable product. One potential problem is deciding which food or beverage to use as a model system, because responses to one food may not be predictive of impressions for another food. One solution is to conduct dietary surveys of the target population in order to use the products that are regularly consumed and are important components of the diet. When measuring the optimal concentration, it is important to recognize that rarely is there a single optimal level of a constituent. More commonly, there is a range of equally palatable, but sensorially distinguishable, formulations (39).

The optimal frequency of exposure to, or consumption of, a stimulus can be measured by scales with appropriate descriptors, questionnaires, food records, monitored plate waste, or garbage analysis. Such information is critical for menu planning in institutional settings.

Liking for items with a given set of sensory characteristics can be ascertained by questionnaires, analyses of diet records that include information about the predominant sensory characteristics of the foods consumed, information on intent to purchase items, or sensory testing with a broad range of products. It is important to understand that liking and preference are distinct measures. One product may be preferred over another, but both may be acceptable or unacceptable. Preference implies a comparison between two or more stimuli, whereas liking is relative only to an internal standard. Paired-preference testing requires judges to indicate which stimulus from a pair is most appealing. The task is conceptually very simple and may be done by children, people who are illiterate, and people who do not understand the language of the test. The primary limitation of preference testing is that the results provide no insights on the absolute acceptability of the sample.

Frequently, researchers ask study participants to rate concurrently the intensity and palatability of stimuli. Some researchers believe the former task confounds the latter because it creates an orientation that is more analytical than is the case under normal dietary conditions. Other researchers feel that the threat is minimal and that it is efficient to obtain both forms of information concurrently (89). Analyses of preference testing may be based on the binomial distribution, chi-square statistic, or z test on proportions.

In preference testing, judges may have the option of indicating no preference. The advantages are that consumers with no real preference have a logical response option, and the researcher gains insight into the proportion of judges falling into this category. However, this option complicates data analysis and interpretation. The tests previously described assume that a choice between samples was required, so "no preference" ratings must be omitted or recoded according to some arbitrary rule (for example, distributing the "no preference" scores to each product on 50:50 basis or in proportion to the true preference choices). When judges are not required to make a decision, each judge is free to adopt his or her own criteria as to how strong a feeling he or she must hold to be willing to choose one sample over the other. This characteristic introduces an uncontrolled level of variability into the data.

If preferences among a set of more than two samples are to be determined, judges may be allowed to rank the samples. The disadvantage is that the magnitude of differences is not known, and if real foods are used, the attributes upon which decisions are made are not known and may vary across samples. A strength of the approach is that its simplicity makes it suitable for use with almost any type of sample population. Nonparametric procedures (for example, the Friedman test) are used for analysis.

The interpretation of hedonic data requires several fundamental considerations. Whereas threshold, scaling, time-intensity, and descriptive tests conducted in an industrial setting may be optimized by using trained panelists, this is not the case for hedonic testing. Here, the key outcome is to capture the impressions of potential consumers, whose responses may be based on an entirely different set of influences (for example, convenience, cost, or availability). Another consideration is the fact that hedonic data may be especially susceptible to modification by cognitive factors. For example, providing brand-name information along with test samples can markedly skew responses (90). This brand name may be important information to collect, but it is more a tool of marketing than of sensory evaluation. Health beliefs are another cognitive factor that can modify responses differentially on various scales. For example, ice cream may be regarded as more pleasant than cottage cheese, but the latter may be preferred for health reasons. Finally, hedonic judgments are strongly influenced by temporal cues. Foods customarily consumed in the morning may be less acceptable in the evening and vice versa (91). Threshold sensitivity and intensity judgments are less affected by time factors.

PARTICIPANT RECRUITMENT CONSIDERATIONS

Participant selection is critical in the successful outcome of psychophysical studies and sensory evaluation. In the latter case, the expectation for all kinds of evaluation except affective testing is that judges will function as objective, sensitive, and reliable assays. Although people have a range of innate abilities, screening to identify individuals with exceptional sensitivity is not a common practice. Training and standardization of individuals with average abilities can raise performance substantially, and such individuals are more commonly encountered and may have other characteristics (for example, motivation, availability, or team spirit) that make them better suited for sensory studies.

Nevertheless, some individual characteristics may be important to consider during recruitment. These traits may include, but are by no means restricted to, the characteristics listed in Table 18.2. Other issues that vary on a daily basis should be considered, such as the judges' state of hunger, recent diet, and current health status. A judge who has eaten a large meal prior to testing may give lower hedonic ratings to foods and be less motivated to identify subtle differences between stimuli. Olfactory testing on days when an individual is experiencing nasal congestion due to allergies clearly would be inadvisable. In addition to subject characteristics, a host of issues pertaining to the testing protocol must be addressed prior to test initiation. Table 18.3 lists a few selected issues, but the relevant factors will vary according to the nature of the study.

TABLE 18.2　Selected Potentially Important Individual Characteristics in Subject Recruitment for Sensory Evaluation Studies

Characteristic	Examples of Rationale
Age	May be performance limitations at age extremes.
Gender	Sensitivity is generally slightly higher in females; different expectations.
Smoking status	Smokers have a slight decline in sensitivity, especially olfactory sensitivity.
Genetic traits	Taste blindness and specific anosmia (insensitivity to selected taste and odor stimuli, respectively) are common and may relate to the proposed test stimuli.
Ethnic origin	Varying experience with potential stimuli or innate responsivity to them may bias reporting
Health status	Acute and chronic health conditions may alter (generally decrease) sensory function. Changes may be in quality (e.g., sweet vs. bitter) or modality (taste vs. smell) and may be specific or generalized.
Medication use	May alter (generally decrease) sensory function.
Prior experience with stimuli	May influence test performance (e.g., ratings for the burn of certain spices may be skewed by individuals who never use them or regularly consume them; affective ratings for unfamiliar foods may be low because of neophobia).
Acute food constituent interactions	Recent oral exposure to spices (e.g., capsaicin) may decrease the perceived intensity of other irritants.
Health beliefs	May bias judgment (e.g., concern about fat, sugar, or salt may result in biased responses for stimuli containing these substances).
Dietary patterns	May influence orientation to stimuli (e.g., ratings for breakfast foods may be negatively biased if this meal is not regularly consumed).

Because the aim of psychophysical studies often is to learn about the mechanisms of sensory function and the basis for individual differences, recruitment strategies may entail the purposeful selection of individuals with contrasting characteristics and capabilities. The same considerations of subject and testing issues must be made before undertaking these types of studies, although the decisions may vary from those made for sensory evaluation studies to reflect the different aims of such work. The fundamental point is that for either type of study, the researcher should attempt to establish the optimal conditions for examining the issue under consideration, and reaching this goal requires thoughtful planning. Subtle, uncontrolled influences may invalidate entire studies.

TESTING ENVIRONMENT

A typical sensory testing facility in the food industry includes a waiting area for panelists, a food preparation area, a series of individual booths for product sampling, a group meeting area for descriptive analysis work, an office for the sensory professionals, and a sufficient amount of cold and dry storage capacity. Specifications for each of these components and other functional features have been published (6,7). The need for strict adherence to the various specifications is not clear. Indeed, facilities vary widely across industries, while each serves its intended purpose.

The most critical features are perhaps the most intuitive. The environment should be free of distractions, such as noise, worker traffic, and odors. Red lighting, which masks visual cues from products, may enable some questions to be addressed. However, these questions are not likely to be important to consumers who do not view or consume food under such conditions. There is increased reliance on computerized data acquisition software, which may expedite data collection while reducing coding errors and analysis time. Some programs generate forms that may be optically scanned and thus may be used at sites distant from the home facility. Others require direct entry of responses into a computer. However, paper-and-pencil formats are still functional. A suitable system for presenting and removing samples, as well as dealing with expectorated waste, is also important, as accumulations may distract or confuse judges.

Assessments of patient sensory function may be conducted in clinical settings. The same principles about the environment hold. Subjects should not view needles, blood, or instruments that might distract them from their task or potentially bias their responses. Extraneous odors should also be eliminated.

INSTRUMENTAL ANALYSES

Interest in instrumental methods for analysis of foods and beverages, including artificial noses and tongues, is growing rapidly. Analytic methods offer a number of unique advantages. They are better able to analyze foods for nutrient composition, as well as for certain ingredi-

TABLE 18.3 Selected Potentially Important Testing Issues in Sensory Evaluation Studies

Testing Issue	Examples of Rationale
Time of day	Cultural norms determine appropriateness of certain stimuli (e.g., alcohol or ice cream) at different times of day, and there is slight diurnal variation in sensory system sensitivity.
Nature of stimulus exposure	Stimulus consumption is more "natural" than chewing and expectorating but likely to elicit metabolic feedback that may alter responsivity over time.
Sample size	Must be determined prior to study initiation to establish feasibility. Power must be balanced with allocation of resources, time, and money.
Time trends	If testing is to be conducted over time, trends in dietary experiences and health beliefs may alter test performance.
Fatigue	The number and nature of stimuli to be presented and the pace will influence sensitivity and motivation (e.g., rapid presentation of numerous, strong stimuli that are difficult to clear will reduce sensitivity).
Blinding	Unless cognitive influences are being studied, stimuli identifiers or labels that may be perceived to offer clues about their content (e.g., plus and minus symbols, sequential numbers) may bias responses.
Randomization	Failure to randomize the presentation order of stimuli may lead to systematic rating biases (e.g., if weak stimuli always follow strong ones, intensity rating for the former may be disproportionately low, or repeated presentation of a particular class of stimuli in one position may lead to uncritical reporting based only on expectations).
Sample presentation	To enhance the ecological validity of testing results, samples should be presented in a format that most closely resembles their intended use. There are no immutable rules for sample size, temperature, and other characteristics except that all nonexperimental attributes should be alike so that subjects rate them on the property under study. The timing of sample presentation will be dictated by stimulus characteristics; odors and beverages may permit more rapid presentation rates than tastes of lipophilic compounds. It is generally preferable to randomize the order of sample presentations, but when one sample will alter perception of another, it may be best to present it at the end of a session.
Data handling	Sensory studies often yield large amounts of data and, especially in the food industry, may need to be analyzed quickly. Plans for data coding, storage, and analyses should be made prior to study initiation to avoid loss or corruption.
Subject Appreciation	Adequate provisions must be made for subjects to access the test center, wait comfortably and for a reasonable amount of time prior to and between testing sessions, and receive adequate compensation for their time and effort; otherwise, attrition may threaten data integrity.

ents and contaminants that are not strong sensory stimuli. In addition, they can often yield data more rapidly, at lower cost, and with higher precision. They are also ideal for situations where continuous data are needed (e.g., on a processing line that runs 24 hours a day) and where information is needed on products that may contain unpleasant or dangerous constituents. The principal disadvantage is that such data cannot reflect the affective dimension of sensory evaluation. Predictive models may be developed, but their functionality will always be tied to human sensory studies. The two approaches are complementary.

STATISTICAL ANALYSES

The outcomes of sensory studies may be the basis of multimillion-dollar decisions about product formulation or the diagnosis and management of health disorders. Con-

sequently, conclusions drawn for sensory tests must be based on sound statistical analyses. Excellent, easily readable discussions of basic statistical treatment of commonly used sensory tests are available (6,92). It is recommended that researchers consult such references or a statistician prior to study initiation if they are not confident in their statistical skills. There is no point in conducting a study that is destined to fail because of poor design.

CONDUCTING A SENSORY TEST

The following is a general outline of the steps involved in planning and conducting a sensory test:

1. Clearly define the study objective in measurable terms.
2. Determine the appropriate testing methodology, including the types and concentrations of stimuli

to be used and the number of replications. If possible, it is valuable to have participants rate a stimulus unrelated to the one of interest or, in the case of clinical studies, a stimulus unaffected by the patient's condition. This procedure serves as a control for test performance alone and aids in determination of the specificity of responses. For example, if it is hypothesized that diabetes leads to a reduced ability to perceive the sweetness of monosaccharides and disaccharides, testing should include another quality, such as saltiness or sourness, to determine whether noted changes are due to a general decrement in sensory function or a decrement that is sweet specific.

3. Determine the risks of type I (false-positive) and type II (false-negative) errors, expected measurement error, within-subject variability, critical effect size, and the required sample size.

4. Estimate the costs of conducting the study.

5. Determine the availability of required resources, including space, facilities, and support staff.

6. Determine the eligibility and exclusionary criteria for subjects and the availability of individuals meeting the stipulated criteria.

7. Obtain approval to use human subjects from a local institutional review board.

8. If practical, purchase all supplies needed to complete the study. This step is especially critical if commercial products will be used, because their availability and formulation may change midway through the study. Plan for waste.

9. Prepare all instructional materials, response forms, and consent forms, and assemble a full set of forms for each prospective participant. Set up files in a data acquisition computer, if needed. All forms should have space for subject identification number, date, time, and testing order information.

10. Create randomization orders for subjects if different treatments will be administered and for test stimuli presentation.

11. Create a master sheet of sample presentation orders, and label sample presentation containers with blinding codes. Use codes that cannot be perceived to convey information about the sample.

12. Practice all test procedures, and have all response forms checked by an independent party.

13. Recruit study participants. Based on prior experi-

ence, estimate attrition rates; oversample to account for this so the final sample will meet the projected power requirements.

14. Train participants until performance is optimal and stable. Training is not appropriate for affective testing and may not be feasible for clinical patients.

15. Prior to arrival at the test site, prepare test stimuli, and portion them out to appropriately labeled containers. All stimuli should be prepared and handled similarly, because subtle differences in temperature, appearance, and other attributes not intended to vary may serve as the basis for responses.

16. Conduct the test.

17. Compile, check, and analyze data.

REFERENCES

1. Giese J. Modern alchemy: use of flavors in food. *Food Technol.* 1994;48:106–116.

2. Glanz K, Basil M, Maibach E, Goldberg J, Snyder D. Why Americans eat what they do: taste, nutrition, cost, convenience, and weight control concerns as influences on food consumption. *J Am Diet Assoc.* 1998;98:1118–1126.

3. National Dairy Council. Dietary Guidelines and Children's Nutrition: A Survey of Health Care Professionals. Rosemont, Ill: National Dairy Council; 1995.

4. Stone H, Sidel JL. Sensory Evaluation Practices, 2nd ed. San Diego, Calif: Academic; 1993.

5. Dethmers AE, Civille GV, Eggert JM, et al. Sensory evaluation guide for testing food and beverage products. *Inst Food Technol.* 1981;11:50–59.

6. Lawless HT, Heymann H. *Sensory Evaluation of Food: Principles and Practices.* New York, NY: Chapman and Hall; 1998.

7. Meilgaard M, Civille GV, Carr BT. *Sensory Evaluation Techniques.* 2nd ed. Boca Raton, Fla: CRC Press; 1991.

8. Doty RL, Bartoshuk LM, Snow JB. Cause of Olfactory and Gustatory Disorders. In: Getchell TV, Doty RL, Bartoshuk LM, Snow JB. *Smell and Taste in Health and Disease.* New York, NY: Raven Press; 1991.

9. Mott AE, Leopold DA. Disorders in taste and smell. *Med Clin North Am.* 1991;75:1321–1353.

10. Davidson TM, Jalowayski A, Murphy C, Jacobs RD. Evaluation and treatment of smell dysfunction. *West J Med.* 1987;146:434–438.

11. Gent JF, Goodspeed RB, Zagraniski RT, Catalanotto FA.

Taste and smell problems: validation of questions for the clinical history. *Yale J Biol Med.* 1987;60:27–35.

12. Goodspeed RB, Gent JF, Catalanotto FA. Chemosensory dysfunction: clinical evaluation results from a taste and smell clinic. *Postgrad Med.* 1987;81:251–257, 260.

13. Cain WS, Gent JF, Goodspeed RB, Leonard G. Evaluation of olfactory dysfunction in the Connecticut Chemosensory Clinical Research Center. *Laryngoscope.* 1988;98:83–88.

14. Smith DV. Assessment of patients with taste and smell disorders. *Acta Otolaryngol Suppl.* 1988;458:129–133.

15. Cain WS. Testing olfaction in a clinical setting. *Ear Nose Throat J.* 1989;68:316, 322–328.

16. Snow JB, Doty RL, Bartoshuk LM. Clinical Evaluation of Olfactory and Gustory Disorders. In: Getchell TV, Doty RL, Bartoshuk LM, Snow JB. *Smell and Taste in Health and Disease.* New York, NY: Raven Press; 1991.

17. Mattes RD, Cowart BJ. Dietary assessment of patients with chemosensory disorders. *J Am Diet Assoc.* 1994;94:50–56.

18. Rankin KM, Mattes RD, Massaro EJ, eds. *Handbook of Human Toxicology.* New York, NY: CRC Press; 1997:347–368.

19. Mattes RD. In: Shils ME, Olson JA, Shike M, Ross AC, eds. *Modern Nutrition in Health and Disease.* 9th ed. Baltimore, Md: Williams & Wilkins; 1999:667–677.

20. Cullen MM, Leopold DA. Disorders of smell and taste. *Med Clin North Am.* 1999;83:57–74.

21. Bartoshuk LM. The psychophysics of taste. *Am J Clin Nutr.* 1978;31:1068–1077.

22. Cornsweet TN. The staircase-method in psychophysics. *Am J Psychol.* 1962;75:485–491.

23. Riskey DR. Use and abuses of category scales in sensory measurement. *J Sens Stud.* 1986;1:217.

24. Moskowitz HR. *Product Testing and Sensory Evaluation of Foods: Marketing and R&D Approaches.* Westport, Conn: Food and Nutrition Press; 1983.

25. Green BG, Shaffer GS, Gilmore MM. Derivation and evaluation of a semantic scale of oral sensation magnitude with apparent ratio properties. *Chem Senses.* 1993;18:683–702.

26. Green BG, Dalton P, Cowart B, Shaffer G, Rankin K, Higgins J. Evaluating the "Labeled Magnitude Scale" for measuring sensations of taste and smell. *Chem Senses.* 1996;21:323–334.

27. McBride RL. Stimulus range influences intensity and hedonic ratings of flavour. *Appetite.* 1985;6:125–131.

28. Lawless H. Contextual effects in category ratings. *J Testing Eval.* 1983;11:346–349.

29. Rankin KM, Marks LE. Differential context effects in taste perception. *Chem Senses.* 1991;16:617–629.

30. Schifferstein HNJ. Contextual effects in difference judgments. *Perception Psychophys.* 1995;57:56–70.

31. Hulshoff Pol HE, Hijman R, Baare WFC, van Ree JM. Effects of context on judgments of odor intensities in humans. *Chem Senses.* 1998;23:131–135.

32. Stevens JC, Marks LE. Cross-modality matching functions generated by magnitude estimation. *Perception Psychophys.* 1980;27:379–389.

33. Stevens SS. The surprising simplicity of sensory metrics. *Am Psychol.* 1962;17:29.

34. Doehlert DN. Methods for measuring degree of subjective response. In: *Basic Principles of Sensory Evaluation.* Philadelphia, Pa: American Society for Testing and Materials; 1968:58. ASTM special technical publication 433.

35. Poulton EC. The new psychophysics: six models for magnitude estimation. *Psychol Bull.* 1968;69:1.

36. Moskowitz HR. Magnitude estimation: notes on what, how, when, and why to use it. *J Food Qual.* 1977;1:195–227.

37. American Society for Testing and Materials. *Manual on Sensory Testing Methods.* Philadelphia, Pa: American Society for Testing and Materials; 1968. ASTM special technical publication 434.

38. Giovanni MA, Pangborn RM. Measurement of taste intensity and degree of liking of beverages by graphic scales and magnitude estimation. *J Food Sci.* 1983;48:1175.

39. Mattes RD, Lawless HT. An adjustment error in optimization of taste intensity. *Appetite.* 1985;6:103–114.

40. Lawless HT, Malone GJ. A comparison of rating scales: sensitivity, replicates and relative measurement. *J Sens Stud.* 1986;1:155.

41. Lawless HT. Logarithmic transformation of magnitude estimation data comparison of scaling methods. *J Sens Stud.* 1989;4:75.

42. Jaeschke R, Singer J, Guyatt GH. A comparison of seven-point and visual analogue scales. Data from a randomized trial. *Control Clin Trials.* 1990;11:43–51.

43. Lee WE, Pangborn RM. Time-intensity: the temporal aspects of sensory perception. *Food Technol.* 1986;40:71.

44. Liu Y-H, MacFie HJH. Methods for averaging time-intensity curves. *Chem Senses.* 1990;15:471.

45. van Buuren S. Analyzing time-intensity responses in sensory evaluation. *Food Technol.* 1992;2:101–104.

46. MacFie HJH, Liu YH. Developments in the analysis of time-intensity curves. *Food Technol.* 1992;11:92–97.

47. Lawless HT, Clark CC. Psychological biases in time-intensity scaling. *Food Technol.* 1992;11:81–90.

48. Bartoshuk LM, Beauchamp GK. Chemical Senses. *Annu Rev Psychol.* 1994;45:419–449.

49. Lehman CD, Bartoshuk LM, Catalanotto FA, Kveton JF, Lowlicht RA. Effect of anesthesia of the chorda tympani nerve on taste perception in humans. *Physiol Behav.* 1995;57:943–951.

50. Yanagisawa K, Bartoshuk LM, Catalanotto FA, Karrer

TA, Kveton JF. Anesthesia of the chorda tympani nerve and taste phantoms. *Physiol Behav.* 1998;63:329–335.

51. Bartoshuk LM, Desnoyers S, O'Brien M, Gent JF, Catalanotto FA. Taste stimulation of localized tongue areas: the Q-tip test. *Chem Senses.* 1985;10:453.

52. Stevens JC, Cain WS. Smelling via the mouth: effect of aging. *Perception Psychophys.* 1986;40:142–146.

53. Cain WS, Reid F, Stevens JC. Missing ingredients: aging and the discrimination of flavor. *J Nutr Elder.* 1990;9:3–15.

54. Duffy VB, Cain WS, Ferris AM. Measurement of sensitivity to olfactory flavor: application in a study of aging and dentures. *Chem Senses.* 1999;24:671–677.

55. Laing DG, Livermore BA, Francis GW. The human sense of smell has a limited capacity for identifying odors in mixtures. *Chem Senses.* 1991;16:392.

56. Laska M, Hudson R. A comparison of the detection thresholds of odour mixtures and their components. *Chem Senses.* 1991;16:651–662.

57. Schiffman S. Food recognition by the elderly. *J Gerontol.* 1977;32:586–692.

58. Cain WS, Krause RJ. Olfactory testing: rules for odor identification. *Neurol Res.* 1979;1: 1–9.

59. Wright HN. Characterization of olfactory dysfunction. *Arch Otolaryngol Head Neck Surg.* 1987;113:163–168.

60. Hummel T, Sekinger B, Wolf SR, Pauli E, Kobal G. "Sniffin' Sticks": olfactory performance assessed by the combined testing of odor identification, odor discrimination, and olfactory threshold. *Chem Senses.* 1997;22:39–52.

61. Doty RL, Marcus A, Lee WW. Development of the 12-item cross-cultural smell identification test (CC-SIT). *Laryngoscope.* 1996;106:353–356.

62. Cain WS, Rabin MD. Comparability of two tests of olfactory functioning. *Chem Senses.* 1989;14:479.

63. Stone H, Sidel J, Oliver S, Woolsey A, Singleton RC. Sensory evaluation by qualitative descriptive analysis. *Food Technol.* 1974;11:24–34.

64. Schiffman SS, Reynolds ML, Young FW. Theory, Methods, and Applications. In: Schiffman SS, Reynolds ML, Young FW. *Introduction to Multidimensional Scaling.* New York, NY: Academic Press; 1981.

65. Giovanni M. Response surface methodology and product optimization. *Food Technol.* 1983;11:41–45.

66. Drewnowski A. New techniques: multidimensional analyses of taste responsiveness. *Int J Obes.* 1984;8:599–607.

67. Drewnowski A, Moskowitz HR. Sensory characteristics of foods: new evaluation techniques. *Am J Clin Nutr.* 1985;42:924–931.

68. Rutledge KP. Accelerated training of sensory descriptive flavor analysis panelists. *Food Technol.* 1992;11:114–118.

69. MacFie HJH. Assessment of the sensory properties of food. *Nutr Rev.* 1990;48:87–93.

70. Stone H, Sidel JL. Quantitative descriptive analysis: developments, applications, and the future. *Food Technol.* 1998;8:48–52.

71. Szczesniak AS. Sensory texture profiling—historical and scientific perspectives. *Food Technol.* 1998;8:54–57.

72. Schutz HT. Evolution of the sensory science discipline. *Food Technol.* 1998;8:42–46.

73. Schaal B, Marlier L, Soussigan R. Human foetuses learn odours from their pregnant mother's diet. *Chem Senses.* 2000;25:729–737.

74. Mennella JA. Infants' suckling response to the flavor of alcohol in mother's milk. *Alcohol Clin Exp Res.* 1997;21:581–585.

75. Pangborn RM. Influence of hunger on sweetness preferences and taste thresholds. *Am J Clin Nutr.* 1959;7:280–287.

76. Moskowitz HR, Sharma KKN, Jacobs HL, Sharma SD. Effects of hunger, satiety, and glucose load upon taste intensity and taste hedonics. *Physiol Behav.* 1976;16:471–475.

77. Mattes RD. Innate and acquired taste preferences for the macronutrients and salt. In Guy-Grand B, Ailhaud G, eds. *Progress in Obesity Research.* London, England: John Libbey & Co.; 1999:173–185.

78. Birch LL, Marlin DW. I don't like it; I never tried it: effects of exposure on two-year-old children's food preferences. *Appetite.* 1982;3:353–360.

79. Bertino M, Beauchamp GK, Riskey DR, Engelman K. Taste perception in three individuals on a low-sodium diet. *Appetite.* 1981;2:67–73.

80. Bertino M, Beauchamp GK, Engelman K. Long-term reduction in dietary sodium alters the taste of salt. *Am J Clin Nutr.* 1982;36:1134–1144.

81. Mattes RD. Discretionary salt and compliance with reduced sodium diet. *Nutr Res.* 1990;10:1337–1352.

82. Bertino M, Beauchamp GK. Increasing dietary salt alters taste preference. *Physiol Behav.* 1986;38:203–213.

83. Tepper BJ, Harfiel LM, Schneider SH. Sweet taste and diet type II diabetes. *Physiol Behav.* 1996;60:13–18.

84. Schutz HG, Pilgrim FJ. A field study of food monotony. *Psychol Rep.* 1958;4:559–565.

85. Blank DM, Mattes RD. Exploration of the sensory characteristics of craved and aversive foods. *J Sens Stud.* 1990;5:193–202.

86. Weingarten HP, Elston D. The phenomenology of food changes. *Appetite.* 1990;15:231–246.

87. Moskowitz HR. Subjective ideals and sensory optimization in evaluating perceptual dimensions in food. *J Appl Psychol.* 1972;56:60–66.

88. Sidel JL, Stone H. An introduction to optimization research. *Food Technol.* 1983;11:36–38.

89. Mela DJ. A comparison of single and concurrent evalua-

tions of sensory and hedonic attributes. *J Food Sci.* 1989;54:1098–1100.

90. Moskowitz HR. Mind, body and pleasure: an analysis of factors which influence sensory hedonics. In: Kroeze JHA, ed. *Preference Behavior and Chemoreception.* London, England: Info Retrieval Ltd; 1979.

91. Birch LL, Billman J, Richards SS. Time of day influences food acceptability. *Appetite.* 1984;5:109–116.

92. O'Mahony M. *Sensory Evaluation of Food: Statistical Methods and Procedures.* New York, NY: Marcel Dekker; 1985.

Part 7

—ɯɯ—

Key Aspects of Research in Food, Nutrition, and Dietetics

Opportunities for research continue to expand as our knowledge base sharpens and broadens in such diverse areas as human genetics, changes in behavior, complementary medicine, foodservice, marketing, and economic analyses of outcomes and effectiveness of care. All these areas are vital in dietetics education and its research component.

Economic analysis (Chapter 19) relies on several analytic methods—namely, cost minimization, cost-effectiveness, cost benefit, cost utility, and clinical decision analysis. Chapter 19 presents examples related to the economics of practice. Costs and benefits can be classified as being direct to the patient (for example, costs of special food products), direct to the health care sector (for example, expenditures avoided because of nutrition intervention), indirect to the patient (for example, improved functional ability of the patient), or intangible (for example, positive or negative changes in the quality of life). Through careful analysis of the data generated, including a consideration of ethical issues, recommendations for action may be formulated.

As we learn more about human genetics and diet through research on diet-gene interactions and genetic predisposition, we will be able to provide more effective nutrition counseling and improved patient care. Chapter 20 presents valuable information regarding genes and disease risk, the role of genetic markers, collecting and archiving DNA, and the impact of poly-

morphism. Observational and ethical clinical studies, primarily using cohort and case-control designs, will extend our capabilities.

Behavior theory–based research (Chapter 21) is shedding new light on attitudes and beliefs as they relate to an individual's diet and health behavior. The six theories in behavioral research are the theory of reasoned action, the theory of planned behavior, the transtheoretical model (stages of change), the health belief model, social cognitive theory, and reciprocal determinism. The constructs of each of these theories are laid out in Chapter 21, and the researcher should tailor and validate interventions accordingly prior to initiating a research study.

Chapter 22 points out the need for evaluating the effectiveness of protocols in complementary and alternative medicine and reminds researchers to apply the rigorous research designs presented in other chapters of this text. Such research is essential before adopting alternative or complementary medicine in therapeutic regimens. Research in foodservice management also relies on observational studies, as well as controlled designs (Chapter 23). A wide matrix may be addressed where human resources (for example, staffing and performance), products (for example, menus, production, and food safety), and customers interact.

Various designs for marketing research are presented in Chapter 24. Price, product, place, and promotion are key extensions of marketing strategies to assess and ensure customer satisfaction. A detailed table of external data services is provided. It is appropriate that the last chapter in Part 7 focuses on descriptive and analytic research approaches to dietetics (Chapter 25). Re-searchers are alerted to the value of thoughtful research design and observer training in minimizing the negative impact of both halo and Hawthorne effects.

ERM, Editor

19

Outcomes Research and Economic Analysis

Patricia L. Splett, Ph.D., R.D., F.A.D.A.

Across the health care system, organizations are examining the structure and processes of care, its outcomes, and its cost; they are then using these data to improve the consistency, effectiveness, and efficiency of care. These activities have taken many forms over the years, including peer review, quality assurance, total quality management, continuous quality improvement, and more recently, outcomes measurement and performance improvement. Most organizations have mechanisms to monitor selected indicators of performance. Some use standard measures, such as the measures developed for the Health Plan Employers Data and Information Set, and many participate in quality certification programs, such as the National Committee for Quality Assurance. Some health care organizations have outcomes management units and systems and care improvement departments that are responsible for monitoring quality indicators and conducting special outcomes studies. In addition, individuals and teams initiate special studies within their units or work collaboratively to study outcomes across departments or across institutions. At the department and organizational levels, outcomes studies provide information to guide adjustments in operations and clinical practices so that clinical effectiveness, patient satisfaction, and cost management are achieved. Outcomes research and economic analysis are important research approaches to apply in these challenging situations. Dietitians are encouraged to make outcomes research a standard part of their practice (1).

On another level, outcomes research is used to evaluate the impact of health care, including discrete interventions as well as broader programmatic or system interventions, on the health outcomes of patients and populations (2). The goal is to shape policy; affect clinical practice, such as through clinical practice guidelines; define programs; and ultimately, improve health outcomes across the country. At this level, greater weight is given to the external validity and generalizability of findings so that they can be applicable across settings and population groups. When planned at this level, outcomes research is also referred to as *medical effectiveness research,* and its results become the evidence, or part of the evidence, behind evidence-based practice.

OUTCOMES RESEARCH

Outcomes and Effectiveness Research

Attention to outcomes (that is, the results of a procedure, treatment, or program) has greatly increased since the beginning of the outcomes movement in the late 1980s (3,4), and the movement continues to attract the attention of health care systems, decision makers, and practitioners (5–7). Outcomes research/medical effectiveness research (now also called *outcomes and effectiveness research*) is used to evaluate the effectiveness of preventive, diagnostic, and therapeutic procedures, treatments, and programs. It answers the following questions: Does it work?

What is the magnitude of effect? Is the effect large enough to be clinically meaningful? Outcomes research investigates the results of interventions as they are used in typical practice settings (measures effectiveness), as opposed to the strictly controlled conditions of randomized clinical trials (which are used to determine efficacy). (The concepts of efficacy and effectiveness are discussed in Box 19.1.) A range of outcomes of concern to patients, practitioners, health care administrators, payers/buyers, and policy makers are considered in outcomes and effectiveness research. Carefully selected evaluation and research methods are used to determine whether the procedure or care process does lead to the desired results (7). An aim of outcomes and effectiveness research is to determine what approaches work best for most patients or clients in routine settings and at what cost.

There is some debate over the types of studies used to determine effectiveness. How the conclusion is to be applied determines the rigor of the study required. When evidence of effectiveness is used to develop broadly disseminated guidelines, such as the National Institute of Health's Obesity Guidelines, studies at the top of the hierarchy are desired (see Chapter 12, on evidence-based medicine, for a hierarchy of study types). The Cochrane Database of Abstracts of Reviews of Effectiveness, an international collection of structured literature abstracts, limits its collection to randomized controlled trials that have been critically appraised using explicit quality criteria to minimize bias and maximize internal and external validity. This chapter takes a more liberal view of outcomes and effectiveness studies; it considers situations in which dietitians conduct outcomes studies to assess the effects of nutrition interventions in a more localized environment.

Costs can also be investigated in outcomes studies. Costs include both the cost of delivering specific interventions and the costs associated with the resulting consequences, such as health care resources saved by positive health outcomes (8). This cost concern closely links outcomes and effectiveness research to cost-effectiveness analysis. Methods of economic analysis (discussed later in this chapter) examine effectiveness and costs to determine the cost-effectiveness of competing interventions.

The findings from outcomes research inform decisions about implementing, expanding, or changing care processes. The findings are also used, along with findings from other research approaches, to develop protocols, clinical practice guidelines, and clinical pathway or care maps that foster the use of the most effective and cost-effective practices across the system (9,10). Outcomes research also aids planning and decision making by providing data on which to base prediction of future clinical, cost, and patient outcomes if specific interventions, procedures, or treatments are adopted.

Types of Outcomes

Three outcome categories are generally assessed: clinical outcomes, patient outcomes, and cost outcomes. Numerous outcomes could be measured in each of these areas. When the outcomes study is planned, the analyst defines the outcomes most relevant to the study question and purpose.

Clinical Outcomes

Clinical outcomes are the health status-related outcomes and can include mortality, risk factors, changes in the development or progression of signs or symptoms of disease and its sequelae, and complications resulting from the disease or condition or its treatment. The clinical outcomes selected for evaluation are relevant and important indicators of health or disease progress in the specific life cycle stage, condition, or disease state. What is relevant does change depending on the time horizon of the study. In some situations, biochemical or clinical signs in the

---

Efficacy refers to the scientific bases for determining that a causal relationship exists between a specific intervention and a significant clinical result. It determines the level of effect possible when the intervention is applied by experts under ideal circumstances. *Randomized clinical trials* are used to measure efficacy.

Effectiveness is the level of outcome achieved when the intervention is delivered under ordinary circumstances by usual practitioners for typical patients. *Outcomes and effectiveness research* determines the magnitude of effect in real-world settings using naturalistic, quasi-experimental, and other studies, in addition to controlled trials.

Efficacy proves that something "can work." Effectiveness verifies that it "does work" when applied in routine practice.

BOX 19.1   Efficacy Versus Effectiveness

next few days are of interest; in other situations, the outcome of interest is disease occurrence several years out. The exact outcome indicators that will be measured and the specification of clinically meaningful changes in the indicators are based on scientific studies, expert judgment, or established norms (11).

Patient Outcomes

Patient outcomes emphasize attention to the consequences of intervention that are of concern to patients and their families. These consequences include survival, symptom relief, adverse effects of the condition or its treatment, functional status, quality of life, and satisfaction with care (12). Nutrition status has been shown to be related to patients' functional status, including psychological and cognitive performance, psychosocial status, and activities of daily living (13). Patient-related outcomes extend from the individual to community systems (14).

Assessment of patients' perceptions of nutrition care services and the effect of nutrition on quality of life are relatively new areas in nutrition research and outcomes assessment. An early study identified a range of health and nonhealth benefits that patients gained from nutrition counseling, including reassurance, sense of control, and relief of symptoms (15). Other studies have shown a link between nutrition-related biochemical parameters and patients' quality of life (16).

Outcomes as perceived by the patient and family are also related to the willingness of individuals and society in general to pay for health and nutrition care. If it is perceived that improved health outcomes result from nutrition intervention, then individuals and society demand, and are willing to pay for, these interventions. Demand and willingness to pay diminish however, if care is perceived to be of poor quality, have little effect, and be of high cost (17).

Cost Outcomes

All the financial implications of a specific intervention or procedure are considered to be cost outcomes. Thus, cost outcomes includes the input cost to plan and deliver the intervention or procedure, as well as the cost consequences of the outcomes produced—which may be positive or negative (18). Cost outcomes are of major importance to health care administrators and policy makers. The topic of costs is discussed in more detail later in the chapter.

Methods Used in Outcomes Research

The challenge of outcomes research is to determine the magnitude of effect attributable to the intervention (19). Many designs have been used, including observational, quasi-experimental, and randomized controlled trials. All can provide information to quantify the effect, but well-designed quasi-experimental and experimental designs are needed to confirm the causal relationships linking the intervention to the outcomes.

There is debate about which methods are suitable (2,20–22). The essence of the debate is the relative merits of observational versus randomized studies. Although observational studies have the advantage of most closely approximating usual care, they cannot provide definitive answers to many questions about comparative clinical effectiveness. Trotter emphasizes that prospective studies that are naturalistic in design produce results with greater validity to actual practice than do tightly controlled trials with rigid eligibility criteria and tightly defined protocols (23). Others recommend more traditional randomized controlled designs because they overcome the potential bias of observational and quasi-experimental studies (24). However, randomized clinical trials lack generalizability across the range of settings and patients encountered in usual practice. An answer to this dilemma may be prospective effectiveness trials that afford randomization of similar patients to intervention alternatives, but that are conducted in routine practice settings. Another factor influencing the selection of study design selection is the type and amount of existing research in the practice area. Often observational studies precede randomized trials.

Observational and quasi-experimental studies have several advantages over randomized controlled trials, including lower costs, greater timeliness, and inclusion of a greater range of patients. These designs are used when there are practical or ethical barriers to conducting randomized trials. Before and after studies without a comparison group are weak designs subject to many threats to validity and generally are not recommended. If this study design is used, findings must be interpreted with great caution. Controlled before and after studies (in which a population with similar characteristics serves as the comparison, and data are collected in both populations at the same time using the same methods) can give an estimate of effect. However, this study design requires a well-matched comparison group and appropriate statistical analysis. Other quasi-experimental designs, their strengths and weaknesses, and recommended statistical analysis approaches have been described (20).

Two questions can be used when considering a study design: How likely is it that bias could affect the findings? and How certain of the results is it necessary to be in order to change policy or practice? (2). In outcomes and effectiveness research, as in any research effort, the design and methods selected must match the research question, the planned application of the findings, and the resources available to conduct the study while minimizing threats to validity (20). These issues are addressed throughout this book. In spite of the controversy, a common process, outlined in Figure 19.1, is used to plan and conduct outcomes and effectiveness studies.

Results of Outcomes Research

The final result of an outcomes study should be a quantitative estimate of (1) the magnitude of effect in outcome

---

Define the research purpose and question or questions:

- Describe the intervention, procedure, or program to be evaluated.
- Identify and describe its alternatives.

Determine the key outcome or outcomes:

- Specify indicators of the key outcome and the appropriate time period for their measurement.
- Identify other important positive and negative outcomes to be tracked.

Design the study, and specify procedures for data collection:

- Define the relevant population.
- Determine the sample size and the method of sampling.
- Establish points to measure outcome and other indicators, considering the period of time necessary for the effect to occur.
- Define all data elements to be included (with the aim of "controlling" relevant elements either through design or by statistical analytic techniques), considering intervention details, patient or client characteristics, key outcomes and other outcomes, and intervening and confounding factors.
- Develop and pilot test forms and procedures for data collection.
- Determine data analysis methods.

Collect data according to procedures:

- Train data collectors.
- Monitor quality and completeness of data.

Analyze the data:

- Code and enter the data.
- Assess the clinical importance of the data.
- Assess the data's statistical significance.

Interpret and report the results.

Act on the findings.

FIGURE 19.1   Outcomes and effectiveness research: planning and conducting a study.

associated with, or attributed to, the studied interventions or interventions; and (2) the proportion of patients, clients, or the population that benefits from access to, and participation in, the intervention. Other results that can be presented in quantitative or qualitative terms are variation in provision of the intervention, costs, client characteristics associated with positive or negative outcomes, other important outcomes, and intervening or confounding factors.

Challenges of Outcomes Research

Outcomes research can be conducted prospectively or retrospectively. Prospective studies are carried out from the present to the future. The advantages are the ability to control for confounding factors and potential bias; as a result, a prospective study is a more powerful design for establishing cause and effect. A challenge is allocating sufficient staff and necessary resources to implement the study and oversee its management over a period of time. Standardized measurements and consistent documentation should be used throughout the study. A disadvantage is the potential for investigator or provider bias when either is aware of the alternatives being studied.

Retrospective studies, which are conducted in the present and look into the past, can be divided into three general approaches: retrieval of data from source documents such as medical records; retrieval from existing databases; and meta-analyses, or systematic reviews of previously conducted and reported studies. The retrospective approach requires complete and consistent documentation at the time the record was created. A limitation is that important confounding variables frequently have not been consistently assessed and documented and therefore cannot be controlled. It also can take considerable resources and skill to access and use archival data. Adding to the challenge of undertaking valid and reliable retrospective studies is the fact that procedures for measurement and recording can change over time, and terminology is often used inconsistently. The expansion of computerized charting and electronic databases offers promise for improving retrospective studies (25). Well-designed observational studies, including controlled cohort studies and case-controlled studies, can provide useful data on the effectiveness of interventions. (See Chapters 2 and 6 for information on these types of studies.)

Outcomes studies often involve practitioners in providing and documenting the care under study. Data collection can be done by an outside investigator, be performed by the dietitian, or be delegated to other nutrition staff, medical records personnel, students, or volunteers. The individuals involved must be trained in the study protocol and committed to not introducing bias arising from their knowledge and experience and their desire for a positive result of the study. The study must be designed and conducted to prevent bias and ensure validity.

Evaluating the effectiveness of nutrition therapy, programs, and services is challenging. There are many confounding factors in nutrition care research. A study must be designed carefully and the appropriate methodologies used. The better the study, the more valuable the results will be to the profession and to individual decision makers (26). However, no study is perfect; each has limitations. Dietitians need to tackle these challenges and go forward with outcomes research and economic analysis (27,28). Suggestions for making them a regular part of dietetics practice include planning studies to address problems encountered regularly in your patient population; selecting areas where you have control and will be able to implement changes shown to be effective; beginning with a small study that can be finished in a few months and building on experience to plan larger studies; collaborating with others (team members, colleagues at other facilities, and faculty at nearby colleges or universities) who have interest, experience, and expertise in research design; constructing databases; and performing statistical analysis and outcomes evaluation (27).

ECONOMIC ANALYSIS

Economic analysis examines outcomes in relation to costs; it determines efficiency. The methods of economic analysis are used to identify the most efficient intervention, that is, the one that achieves more of the desired outcomes for the lowest or most reasonable investment of resources. Economic analysis requires a systematic process of defining, measuring, and valuing the costs and outcomes of two or more competing alternatives for accomplishing something (18). Six steps of economic analysis, discussed later in the chapter, are based on a synthesis of the principles and current recommendations for economic analysis (28).

Opportunity cost is a concept integral to economic analysis. As nutrition interventions or programs are implemented and produce outcomes, they consume resources. The consumed resources are then unavailable for another purpose. Opportunity cost is the value that would have been gained if the resource had been used for the next best alternative. This competition for scarce resources is the foundation of economic analysis.

Economic Analysis in Nutrition

Before 1979, economic evaluation was rare in the nutrition literature. At that time, the American Dietetic Association (ADA) proposed a model for estimating the economic benefits of nutrition (29). The model, which provides a firm foundation for considering logical and scientifically based linkages of nutrition services and interventions to outcomes, is shown in Figure 19.2.

In 1989 Disbrow summarized data on costs, health status (outcomes) and economic benefits, and results of economic analysis (30). In 1991, following a critical analysis of existing studies in four areas of practice, the ADA published summary documents that justify nutrition care in terms of its effectiveness, intermediate-term cost savings, and economic gains (31). In that publication, research designs were proposed for assessing the effectiveness and cost-effectiveness of nutrition care defined by practice guidelines. In 1995 the ADA published a position paper summarizing the body of literature supporting the cost-effectiveness of medical nutrition therapy (32). A critique of nutrition effectiveness and cost studies was

also published by the Agency for Health Care Policy and Research (33).

During this same time, economic evaluation was increasingly used throughout health care and public health to evaluate new and old medical procedures and technology, as well as public health interventions. The methods of economic analysis as applied to health also have been evolving. In the early 1990s an expert panel was convened by the U.S. Public Health Service to review the theory and practice of cost-effectiveness analysis (CEA) and make recommendations for standardizing cost-effectiveness analysis methodology in health and medicine (18). Staff of the Centers for Disease Control and Prevention also reviewed methods and described methodology for cost-effectiveness analysis as it applies to public health intervention and prevention (34). Current recommended methods merge the theoretical base of economic analysis with its practical application for decision making in the health care sector.

Analytic Methods Used in Economic Analysis

Several analytic methods are used in economic analysis, including cost minimization analysis, cost-effectiveness analysis (CEA), cost-benefit analysis (CBA), cost-utility

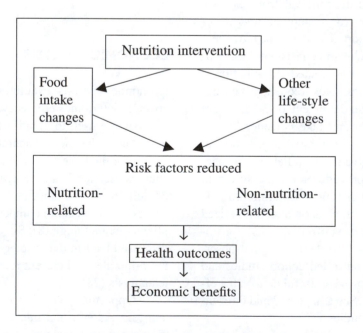

FIGURE 19.2   Expanded model for measuring the benefits of nutritional care. Adapted from Olendsky MC, Tolpin HG, Buckley EL. Evaluating nutrition intervention in atherosclerosis: some theoretical and practical considerations. *J Am Diet Assoc.* 1981;79:9–16. Copyright 1981, used with permission from Elsevier Science.

TABLE 19.1   Analytic Methods Used in Economic Analysis[a]

Method	Focus	Application Example	Outcomes	Costs	Ways to Report
Cost minimization analysis	Identifies the lowest-cost way to do something.	Should an R.D., R.D.T., or R.N. do nutrition assessment at hospital admission?	No data; assumes outcomes are equal	Cost analysis and comparison using cost of inputs	Costs of inputs for each alternative ($ per activity, day, patient, or course of treatment)
Cost-effectiveness analysis	Compares the efficiency of two or more alternatives for a specified outcome.	Should a special oral supplement be recommended for HIV/AIDS patients?	Biochemical, clinical, or quality-of-life measures for each alternative	Cost of each alternative or net cost (cost of inputs + cost of consequences)	Amount of successful outcome per $ investment, net cost per unit of outcome, or $ per unit of improvement
Cost-benefit analysis	Assigns dollar value to resource inputs and health outcomes; may compare alternatives with different goals.	Is it cost-beneficial to initiate nutrition intervention to prevent pressure ulcers?	Dollar value assigned to outcomes	Cost of inputs over complete course of intervention	Net consumption of resources, the ratio of $ of outcomes to $ of inputs (benefit-cost analysis), or $ of input to $ of outcome (cost-benefit analysis)
Cost-utility analysis	Relates cost to quality-of-life differences. Other preference or satisfaction measures can also be used.	Is nutrition support via enteral feeding or total parenteral nutrition worth QALY for terminally ill patients?	Weeks or months of life extended and patients' perceptions of quality of life with or without intervention	Net cost for each alternative (input cost + cost of complications, cost of medical care for extended life, and any medical cost savings)	Net cost per QALY; $ per QALY
Clinical decision analysis	Uses estimates from published studies or expert opinion to construct probability of events (diagnosis, treatment response, complication rate, survival)	What outcomes can be expected if elemental vs. nonelemental enteral formula is used for surgical patients with hypoalbuminemia?	Intermediate and clinical outcomes	Probability estimates used to develop predictions of input costs and medical cost savings and cost of complications for each decision alternative	Decision tree with outcome probabilities and net cost estimates

[a]QALY indicates quality-adjusted life years.

analysis, and clinical decision analysis. The objectives of the investigation determine which analytic method is appropriate. Table 19.1 compares the methods and gives examples of their application in clinical dietetics.

Cost minimization analysis and CEA are used to determine the lower-cost way to achieve a specified outcome. In cost minimization analysis, the outcomes of nutrition alternatives are assumed to be equal, and only costs are measured. In CEA, the magnitude of outcome produced by each alternative is measured, along with the cost to produce the outcome. A ratio of cost per unit of effect (outcome) is calculated for each alternative and compared to determine which alternative is more cost-effective.

CBA considers the monetary (dollar) value of both inputs and outcomes. In a cost-benefit ratio, the dollar value of input costs is related to the dollar value of outcomes (positive and negative) produced. Cost-utility analysis relates costs to the patient's quality of life. Quality-adjusted life years (QALY) is the common unit of measure used in cost-utility analysis (see Box 19.2) (18,34). Results are expressed as cost per QALY. Because of the standardized units, CBA and cost-utility analysis can be used to compare the efficiency of activities in different areas. Thus, they can be used to inform policy and resource allocation decisions across different areas of health care or different sectors of the economy (for example, health care versus education and training). Clinical decision analysis uses estimates of outcome probabilities and net cost to evaluate intervention alternatives (34,35,36).

Steps of Economic Analysis

As shown in Figure 19.3, the process of planning, conducting, and reporting in economic analysis can be divided into six steps (28).

Step 1: State the Objective

The first step is to determine the objective of the economic analysis. In general terms, the objective is to arrive at an unbiased determination of how to use scarce resources most efficiently for a specific purpose. The type of intervention or program, its intended purpose (nutrition or health aims), competing alternatives, and the context for application are included in the objective. How the information will be used and the primary and other expected users of the information are also stated in the purpose.

Step 2: Define the Framework for Analysis

The framework for the analysis involves decisions about three things: perspective, alternatives, and time horizon.

Perspective. The study perspective identifies whose resources are at stake. It is the basis for choosing the type of economic analysis to undertake, including the type of cost to include in the analysis. As shown in Table 19.2, different groups of people are interested in different types of information. The perspective must be specified at the planning stage, because it influences which costs and outcomes are most relevant to measure for the analysis. The perspectives of the intervention provider (the program or organization) or the payer are commonly selected when comparing medical or nutrition therapies. The perspectives of the health care sector and society are frequently used in policy analysis, health care reform, and planning (18,34,37).

Alternatives. To evaluate a nutrition intervention for efficiency and effectiveness, it must be compared with one or more alternatives. All reasonable alternatives should be evaluated, but at least two are necessary. The alternatives to be included are described in detail. The selected alternatives should meet the following criteria:

Quality-adjusted life years is a universal measure of health status that is expressed as the length of healthy life. It assumes that the goal is to extend the state of good health as long as possible and minimize periods of ill health or disability.

QALY takes two things into account:

- Length of life.
- Quality or state of health (well-being) during various periods of time.

Length of life comes from a life table of the population. Life tables specify the proportion of the population of people living and dying at each age interval.

Measures of well-being include mental, physical, and social functioning, as well as pain and suffering. For example, social functioning includes an individual's limitations in performing usual social roles of work, school, homemaking, and the like; physical functioning can be measured in terms of being confined to a bed, chair, or home because of health reasons.

Various tools have been developed to assign a quality-of-life or well-being score (a number ranging from 0.0 [death] to 1.0 [optimal health]) to an individual's functioning (12,34).

QALY is calculated by multiplying years times quality of life during those years.

BOX 19.2   Quality-Adjusted Life Years (QALY)

```
┌─────────────────────────────────────────────────────────────────────────┐
│                    ┌───────────────────────────────┐                      │
│                    │   Step 1. State OBJECTIVE.     │                      │
│                    └───────────────────────────────┘                      │
│                    ┌───────────────────────────────┐                      │
│                    │   Step 2. Define FRAMEWORK:    │                      │
│                    │                                │                      │
│                    │      • Perspective             │                      │
│                    │      • Alternatives            │                      │
│                    │      • Time horizon            │                      │
│                    └───────────────────────────────┘                      │
│  ┌────────────────────────────────┐ ┌────────────────────────────────┐    │
│  │ Step 3. Determine COSTS:       │ │ Step 4. Determine OUTCOMES:     │    │
│  │                                │ │                                 │    │
│  │ Microcosting:                  │ │    • Define key outcomes        │    │
│  │    • List all activities.      │ │    • Select design              │    │
│  │    • Identify principal.       │ │    • Measure for each alternative│   │
│  │    • Measure consumption.      │ │    • Analyze and compare        │    │
│  │    • Assign monetary value.    │ │                                 │    │
│  │                                │ │ Discount if necessary.          │    │
│  │ Gross costing:                 │ │                                 │    │
│  │    • Identify economic events. │ │                                 │    │
│  │    • Measure or estimate number.│ │                                │    │
│  │    • Assign monetary value.    │ │                                 │    │
│  │                                │ │                                 │    │
│  │ Discount if necessary.         │ │                                 │    │
│  └────────────────────────────────┘ └────────────────────────────────┘    │
│                    ┌───────────────────────────────┐                      │
│                    │ Step 5. RELATE cost to outcomes:│                     │
│                    │                                │                      │
│                    │      • Ratio                   │                      │
│                    │      • Array table             │                      │
│                    │      • Net benefit (net cost)  │                      │
│                    │                                │                      │
│                    │ Conduct sensitivity analysis.  │                      │
│                    │ Consider ethical issues.       │                      │
│                    └───────────────────────────────┘                      │
│                    ┌───────────────────────────────┐                      │
│                    │ Step 6. Summarize, INTERPRET, USE│                    │
│                    │ and REPORT the findings.       │                      │
│                    └───────────────────────────────┘                      │
└─────────────────────────────────────────────────────────────────────────┘
```

FIGURE 19.3   Six steps of economic analysis. Adapted from Splett 1996 (28).

- address the same preventive or therapeutic aim;
- represent current practice and new innovations;
- consider available scientific evidence;
- include alternatives that have political and professional support.

Sometimes the option of no intervention is included as a studied alternative.

Time horizon.   Many economic analyses track patients through a relatively short course of therapy to clinical end points. Nutrition intervention can impact longer-term outcomes, such as the patient's functional capacity at home, relapse rate, future need for health care services, or even incidence of disease or complications many years in the future.

When discussing the time horizon, economists use

TABLE 19.2   Perspectives for Economic Analysis

Perspective	Information Interest
Clinician	• Cost of preventive, diagnostic, therapeutic, and rehabilitative alternatives • Clinical outcomes and their associated costs
Provider organization	• Cost to the organization • Resources required to deliver the intervention, such as personnel, supplies, and equipment • Cost consequences associated with the clinical outcomes (such as extended length of stay and complications) • Impact on budget
Payer	• Volume and intensity of service provided • Claims to be paid (charges for pharmacy, ambulatory care, inpatient stays, and emergency room visits) • Expenditures that could be avoided
Managed care organization	• Costs to provide preventive, diagnostic, therapeutic, rehabilitative, and palliative care, as well as costs associated with the outcomes, such as illness or hospitalization prevented
Patient	• Out-of-pocket costs for diagnosis and treatment regimens • Convenience/inconvenience, satisfaction with care • Pain and suffering • Functional ability and quality of life
Health care sector of economy	• Resource demands across the health care system • Hospital, community, long-term care, and outpatient services are viewed as a whole • Considers input costs and the cost consequences of outcomes
Society	• Most complex and comprehensive perspective • Includes total economic impact of health care, disease, and disability, regardless of who bears the cost • Can include indirect costs such as education potential and lost worker productivity due to disability or early death

the terms *cost stream* and *benefit stream*. The cost stream is the period of time over which intervention resources must be invested. The benefit stream is the period of time over which outcomes and associated costs of consequences are accumulated. The time horizon of a study, then, refers to the defined time periods for tracking cost and benefit streams for the economic analysis. In cardiovascular disease, for example, the objective of the study could be the outcomes of care during the hospital stay for coronary artery bypass grafting, through a period of cardiac rehabilitation, or several years in the future to track cardiac events.

After the framework for analysis has been specified, the next two steps are to determine costs and to determine outcomes of the compared alternatives. These procedures are undertaken for both costs and outcomes by identifying (listing and defining), measuring (quantifying the amount used and/or produced), and valuing (assigning units to be reported—natural units, dollars, or QALY). These steps are listed in this discussion as Step 3 and Step 4, but they can be conducted simultaneously.

Step 3: Determine Costs

The process of quantifying costs is called *cost analysis* or *cost identification*. It provides a systematic and defensible estimation of resources consumed, which is necessary for all types of economic analysis. Costing often focuses on the input cost of the intervention, but it is also used to determine the monetary value of outcomes for net cost-effectiveness and for CBA. The process is not complicated, but it must be approached in a systematic and careful manner (8,18,34).

Types of costs. Economists traditionally categorize costs into direct, indirect, and intangible costs, as illustrated in Table 19.3. The analyst decides which costs to include and how to measure them based on the objectives of the analysis and the information needs of the decision makers who will use the results.

Direct costs receive attention in most economic analyses of nutrition care and programs. Direct costs include resources consumed in the prevention, diagnosis,

TABLE 19.3 Types of Costs Used in Economic Analysis

Cost	Definition	Examples
Direct health care (or other sector) cost	Costs associated directly with the nutrition intervention and related health care	Nutrition education and counseling; enteral or parenteral nutrition support
	Health care or other costs resulting from the intervention	Medication use, related medical visits, hospitalization
Direct patient costs	Costs borne by patients or their families	Transportation to clinic; out-of-pocket costs for the intervention and special food products
Indirect costs	Cost of reduced productivity as a result of the condition/illness and/or the nutrition intervention	Time lost (from work, school, or normal activities) because of the condition; preparation of special feedings; time needed to participate in the intervention/program
Intangible costs	Costs difficult to quantify in monetary terms, such as the cost of pain and suffering and quality-of-life changes	Impaired mental functioning; social limitation due to dietary restriction; lost sense of control

treatment, and rehabilitation of a disease. In nutrition, direct costs are defined as those resources used by the provider in the delivery of nutrition and related care to achieve the health goals or outcome objectives of the intervention or program. They are estimated from principal resource components incurred by the provider organization. Other perspectives for analysis would require the inclusion of other kinds of costs.

Cost analysis. Cost analysis can be done in two ways, using either a microcosting approach, which accounts for all costs in detail, or a gross costing approach, which considers only significant economic events (18). Cost analysis must be carried out with equal precision for all alternatives being compared.

In the microcosting/accounting approach, principal resource components are identified, tracked, and assigned a dollar value based on prevailing market prices. Principal resource components commonly included are personnel, fringe benefits, food and nutrition products and supplies, office supplies, education materials, equipment, laboratory tests, other diagnostic and monitoring procedures, other ancillary services, continuing education and training of staff, facility/space, and administrative overhead (8,18,34).

In microcosting, the analyst systematically goes through the following steps:

- List all activities.
- Identify principal resource components for activities (as previously described).
- Estimate resource consumption for each principal resource component by tracking/measuring actual utilization or using secondary data.
- Assign a monetary value to each component and activity using market prices.
- List all assumptions made for possible sensitivity analysis.
- Calculate total, average, incremental, marginal, and/or net cost.
- Perform discounting, if necessary.

Personnel costs are a large part of the costs for nutrition interventions. Time studies may be necessary to determine accurately the quantity of personnel time required for an intervention (28). Time and activity records or data from productivity studies carried out in the organization could also be used to estimate time for specific activities.

The steps of gross costing are as follows:

- Identify significant economic events relevant to the intervention (inputs) and/or outcomes. These might include outpatient care; hospitalization; nursing home placement; home health services; services of a registered dietitian, physician, or other professional; medication; and durable medical equipment.
- Measure or estimate the quantity of significant events used or produced.
- Assign value to significant events using fees schedules, actual charges, or payments.
- List all assumptions made for possible sensitivity analysis.
- Calculate total, average, incremental, marginal, and/or net cost.
- Perform discounting, if necessary.

Assigning monetary value. The value assigned to the component or significant economic event is either the actual market price paid by the buyer or an assigned value. When the buyer is the provider/health care organization, the value can be based on the price paid for resources consumed, the amount billed (charges), or the amount received as payments or reimbursements. When the buyer is the third-party payer (for example, Medicare, an insurance carrier, or a health plan), the value assigned is usually based on records of claims paid or estimates using organization, industry, state, or national reports of health care utilization and cost under various circumstances. Sources of such data are described by Gold et al (18). See Appendix 19B of this chapter for an example illustrating gross costing using administrative data from the Special Supplemental Nutrition Program for Women, Infants, and Children (WIC), as well as Medicaid files.

Market price and charges often exceed the actual resource cost. To adjust for this fact, a cost-to-charge ratio is used (18,34). Payments made by third parties are often less than charges because the amount paid includes discounts and denied claims. Thus, determining the bases for valuing health care resources requires thought.

The value of patients' or clients' time associated with receiving the service or experiencing its consequences is an additional important cost. Time costs, including time waiting for a service to begin, travel costs, time lost from work, and child-care costs, are all potential indirect costs to patients and are very important to the people receiving the service. These costs are very influential in patients' decisions to keep appointments and adhere to the treatment regimen. Economists translate these indirect costs into time lost from work and lost productivity (18,34). Wages are frequently used to value indirect costs, and in spite of the potential inequities for women, minorities, and youth, wages are considered by economists to be the best measure of value. Wages must be used with caution and with the acknowledgment that indirect costs may be underestimated for some groups and overestimated for others. The perspective of the study determines whether or not indirect costs are included in the analysis.

The fear, grief, worry, and pain experienced by patients, clients, and family members are intangible costs. These costs are difficult to measure and even more difficult to value in dollars terms, but they are very real to patients, clients, and families. All illnesses and treatments have intangible costs. They are less commonly addressed, although they may be very influential pieces of information for decision makers.

Each alternative included in the analysis requires a cost analysis. The same types of costs and assumptions should be used in the cost analysis for each alternative, if not, any differences must be described. The approaches to cost analysis and means of valuing costs produce different results; therefore, methods and sources used must be fully disclosed in the report. In addition, when calculating costs, assumptions are frequently used to identify relevant resource costs, estimate the amount of resources consumed, and/or assign a value for each resource component or significant economic event. All assumptions should be documented and subjected to sensitivity analysis (described later in the chapter).

Summarizing and reporting costs. The findings of the cost analysis can be summarized and reported in a number of ways, including full (total) cost, average cost, marginal cost, and net cost. Full (or total) cost is the cost of the intervention over a period of time (usually 1 year or the usual course of treatment). Total costs estimates are made up of fixed costs (stable costs not related to the volume of service) and variable costs (resource utilization that varies with the volume [number served] or intensity [frequency and type of contact] of service). Average cost is the cost per unit of output/outcome, determined by dividing total costs involved by the number of units of service (for example, cost per nutrition assessment or cost per low-birth-weight infant prevented). Incremental cost is the cost difference between one alternative and another (such as the extra cost of managing hypercholesterolemia with pharmaceutical intervention compared with dietary intervention).

When the cost of providing a little more or a little less of the intervention is calculated, it is a marginal cost calculation (for example, the added cost of a second nutrition follow-up visit for people completing a weight-loss program).

EXAMPLE. A substantial amount of resources are consumed to develop a program and system to deliver nutrition messages through local grocery stores. Once the program is developed, adding another store greatly expands the number of families reached, but the marginal costs are considerably less than the original cost of introducing the program in the first store.

Net cost (or net benefit, when positive) refers to the balance when the cost of doing the intervention (inputs) is added to the monetary value of positive consequences or outcomes (resources saved) and negative consequences or outcomes (additional resource consumption) (18,34).

> **EXAMPLE.** Montgomery and Splett found a net benefit to society when WIC infants were exclusively breast-fed for 3 months. The net benefit was calculated from WIC food cost (input) and resulting Medicaid expenditures during the first 6 months of life (outcome) (38).

Incremental or marginal costs are more relevant to economic analysis than are total or average costs, because incremental or marginal costs relate to the extra resource requirements to produce each added effect (and the opportunity costs of removing those resources from other purposes). Total and unit costs are especially useful for budgeting, establishing fees, and negotiating reimbursement rates.

Special considerations in costing. In an economic analysis covering multiple years or using cost data gathered at different times in the past, dollar values for all alternatives must be expressed as a standard base year. This calculation is called *adjusting to present value,* and it uses the Consumer Price Index to adjust for inflation over time. This adjustment is done before costs are related to outcomes and before discounting is done. (See Box 19.3 for more information about the Consumer Price Index. Also, Sikand and colleagues [39] offer an example of this calculation in a cost-benefit study.)

Discounting is a mathematical procedure used to convert future costs and future outcomes to present value. Two factors make discounting necessary in long-term analyses: (1) inflation reduces the value of money over time, and (2) there is a tendency to prefer both dollars and benefits now, rather than in the future. Discounting can be done using computer accounting or statistical analysis software. The discount rate used can range between 2 percent and 10 percent per year, with 5 percent as the most common rate (18). Discounting is discussed in greater detail after Step 4, because it is applied to both costs and outcomes.

Applying cost analysis. The following example illustrates how a nutritionist might determine the cost of nutrition services in prenatal care from the perspective of the public health center, using data from the current program year:

The Consumer Price Index reflects the average change in prices of defined goods and services over specified periods. The U.S. Department of Labor collects prices of selected items each month at multiple sites across the country, summarizes them, and compares them to past prices. These indexes are reported monthly by the Bureau of Labor Statistics in the *Consumer Price Index Detailed Report* and summarized annually in *Statistical Abstracts of the United States*. Separate indexes specific to food and beverages and medical care are most relevant when evaluating nutrition programs and medical nutrition therapy. In an economic analysis covering multiple years or when using cost data from different years, the Consumer Price Index is used to bring dollar values to a standard base year.

BOX 19.3   Consumer Price Index

1. Prepare a flow chart of all activities involved in providing nutrition services to pregnant clients, including activities such as client recruitment and outreach, nutrition assessment and counseling of clients, record keeping and scheduling, client follow-up and monitoring, and program administration and evaluation.

2. Identify the principal resource components necessary for each activity. This might include nutrition and clerical personnel, fringe benefits, nutrition education materials and equipment, laboratory tests to monitor anemia, office and clinic space, nutrition reference materials, office supplies, and administrative overhead.

3. Specify ways costs will be measured. Use work schedules and existing reports such as service statistics or accounting records (after verifying their completeness and accuracy), conduct time studies or productivity studies, or use other methods to accurately estimate the quantity of principal resource components necessary to carry out each activity.

4. Work with the accounting staff to assign a monetary value based on the actual cost to the organization for each cost component. Keep track of all assumptions made along the way.

5. Calculate the total cost for prenatal nutrition services; then divide by the number of women served

to get an average or unit cost. If the cost analysis looked only at nutrition costs as a component of an existing prenatal care program, the cost could be considered incremental cost (the amount added to prenatal care costs for nutrition services).

Similar steps with similar assumptions should be carried out for each alternative to be compared. For example, freestanding nutrition services delivered at a different location requiring separate staffing and facilities would likely have significantly different, and probably higher, costs.

Step 4: Determine Outcomes

Once the objectives of the service are defined and the type of analysis has been determined, the effect or benefit anticipated from the dietetics services can be identified, measured, and valued. The magnitude of the outcome (effect or benefit) associated with or attributed to the nutrition intervention is determined in Step 4. The analyst must have a defensible estimate of the effect of each alternative to include in the economic analysis. These estimates are made through an outcomes study, as described earlier in this chapter, or through other research methods described throughout this book. In some situations the analyst uses effectiveness results reported by others. Meta-analysis is recommended as a method for critically appraising and integrating the results of past studies into an estimate of effect (35).

Regardless of the source of outcomes data, they must be logically and scientifically linked to the interventions being studied. Furthermore, data must be appropriate, given the framework of the economic analysis (alternatives, perspective, and time horizon). The end point for the analysis can be short-term or longer-term results. Short- to intermediate-term outcomes might be a change in nutrition-related behaviors with an improvement in a biochemical or physiological measure, a change in the signs or symptoms of the disease, a change in the complication rate, or a change in days of hospital stay. In longer-term studies, these measures or their associated state of health, functional ability, quality of life, and health care utilization could be measured.

In dietetics practice, it is assumed that people who receive nutrition services and programs improve their nutrient intake or nutrition practices, that this produces improved health status, and that improved health status results in reduced consumption of other medical services and therefore saves resources. This chain of assumptions,

and particularly the key outcome of interest, must be verified through scientifically sound studies—either previously reported or conducted specifically for the economic analysis. Information on the magnitude of change is required.

For CEA, a key outcome (effect) is measured and reported in natural units (for example, pounds of weight loss, percentage reduction in cholesterol, or proportion of persons with diabetes who improve their blood glucose levels). For CBA, important outcomes (benefits) are measured in or converted to monetary units (dollars). The magnitude of outcomes is related to cost data from Step 3 for the actual economic analysis. Relating outcomes to benefits is explained in Step 5.

Types of benefits. Like costs, economists classify benefits as direct, indirect, and intangible. Direct benefits of nutrition care are in the expenditures that would otherwise have been spent on health care had the intervention not been effective. Direct benefits represent all types of health resources that are not consumed as a result of the intervention; in other words, they represent resources saved or expenditures avoided because of the nutrition intervention. Direct benefits also accrue to individuals. For example, people with improved nutrition status and health outcomes may save out-of-pocket expenses when medications can be reduced.

Indirect benefits of nutrition care are improvements in functional ability and capacity to carry out the daily tasks of living and resume normal social roles (for example, worker, homemaker, or student). In some studies, improvements in work attendance and performance are used as proxies for improved health status. Estimates based on measures used in the National Health Interview Survey, the National Health and Nutrition Examination Survey, and the National Medical Expenditure Survey, among others, are useful when determining the indirect benefits of health care to consumers and to society and translating those benefits into economic consequences (18,34). The dollar savings that are due to indirect benefits are estimated as part of the burden of illness (40).

Improvements in the quality of life also represent important benefits that are difficult to measure. Intangible benefits express subjective judgments of well-being, improved independence and mobility, and the avoidance of pain and suffering. These intangible benefits are very real to the people who experience them and therefore should contribute to the decision-making process. The development of quality-of-life assessments has enabled measurement of the patients' perception of the impact of disease and disability and of the course of treatment selected on their lives and functioning (12,18,34).

All payers are interested in direct benefits, because they want to reduce their expenditures. Insurance companies pay for certain services and procedures when evidence shows that savings accrue in other areas, such as reduced hospital costs. In contrast, payers and organization administrators are less concerned about indirect benefits and intangibles, because they do not produce specific dollar savings for the organization. All three categories of benefits can and do occur in the same situation; for economic analysis, however, the perspective determines which categories are measured and included in the analysis.

Study design. After consideration of the above points, the research design and methods to measure outcomes (effects or benefits) of the compared alternatives can be determined. A strong research design is the controlled experiment, which usually randomizes clients into at least two groups: one that receives the dietetics service under study and another that receives an alternative course of care (see Chapter 7). When randomized clinical trials are not feasible, a carefully constructed quasi-experimental design may be used successfully (7,22). The inclusion of a comparison is a required aspect of these designs. Furthermore, economic efficiency is always based on a comparison with the next available alternative. The stronger the design, the greater the validity of results and the greater the usefulness of the economic analysis.

Data need to be collected on factors that could potentially confound the interpretation of the results of the effectiveness study. For example, age, race/ethnicity, socioeconomic status, smoking and other lifestyle factors, and concurrent medical care can have an effect on the measured outcome. Other factors, such as seasonal variation of illness and deaths, must also be considered (41). The study design should control these factors to ensure valid results.

Summarizing and reporting outcomes. After the data are collected, they are analyzed to determine the magnitude of effect achieved by each alternative. This analysis involves aggregating the raw data into summary statistics that include a measure of variation (for example, mean with standard deviation or confidence interval), determining the statistical and clinical significance of outcomes, and making comparisons between alternatives. Appropriate statistical tests, which are determined by the design of the study and the type of variables measured,

must be used. For each alternative the following should be reported:

- Descriptive data about the sample studied and the population it represents.
- Magnitude of outcome associated with, or attributed to, the intervention.
- Assessment of the clinical importance of the outcome achieved.
- Comparison of results between alternatives to determine if they are significantly different and/or to determine the incremental effectiveness.
- Descriptive data about any intervening or confounding factors.
- Statistical adjustments of the magnitude of the outcome for preexisting group differences and for intervening factors.
- Quantitative or qualitative summary of other outcomes.
- Relationship of the degree of outcome to the amount of exposure to the nutrition intervention.

Application examples. In CEA, two or more alternatives for achieving the same outcome objective are compared, and the units of measure are the same. In the CEA case study in Appendix 19A, the effectiveness of a work site program for hyperlipidemia was compared with the effectiveness of lipid screening without education. The outcome measure was the percentage decrease in total serum cholesterol level. Cost-effectiveness was reported as participant program cost per percent reduction. Compared with CBA, CEA is easier to carry out, because it uses natural units that are commonly measured and documented in health care. However, CEA can require considerable time and expense to access records and abstract data.

Economic analysis can use data that are actually measured for the study, as well as values that are estimated from other data sources. The clinical effect of medical nutrition therapy, for example, could be measured, but the value of the effect to an organization, third-party payers, or society might be estimated by using data from other sources. A frequently used application of CBA is to compare the length of stay of a group of patients receiving a new or added procedure or treatment, such as medical nutrition therapy, with the length of stay reported for patients with the same diagnosis in a national study or existing database. The benefit then can be calculated from the cost differences if a shorter length of stay is found in the group receiving the nutrition therapy. In the Lewin study, future health care utilization and resulting costs were compared between adults who had or did not have nutrition counseling (42).

For a societal perspective in CBA, information collected by the government through state, regional, and national studies is often used. The National Center for Health Statistics conducts the National Health Survey and publishes the results on a regular basis through the *Vital and Health Statistics* series. In CBA, the benefits are expressed in dollar terms (for example, cost per day of hospital stay), so they can be directly compared with the input costs. The CBA case study of breast-feeding in Appendix 19B provides an example of the use of existing data from state WIC and Medicaid files.

As mentioned earlier, intangible benefits may be identified, but not measured. These benefits are important to consumers and, depending on the perspective, may be of interest to the decision maker. A legislator considering a Medicare or Medicaid reimbursement policy, for instance, would be interested to know that the constituents' quality of life has improved through a reduction in pain or an increased ability to ambulate and care for themselves. The Medicare administrator, however, would not find this information as useful, because it has no impact on the direct cost of the Medicare program. When significant intangible benefits are produced by an intervention, it is useful to describe them in the report. They represent added value beyond the value reflected in the cost-benefit ratio.

Discounting costs and benefits. Whenever the time horizon of an analysis extends beyond a year or when data for input costs or outcome estimates for compared alternatives come from different years, the issues of present value and discounting must be addressed. Discounting adjusts for the preference people have for immediate consumption over future consumption (18): a bird in the hand is worth two in the bush. If money is invested in a service now, people prefer to have the benefits immediately rather than in 5 or 40 years in the future. Thus, immediate benefits have higher value, and future benefits are discounted, or reduced in value.

Discounting is important when the costs and benefits are expressed in different periods. For example, if a heart-healthy program is begun this year for 10-year-old schoolchildren with the expectation of reducing the morbidity and mortality from heart disease when they are 50-year-olds, the money spent now is of higher preference to society than the savings in 40 years, even if the estimated future cost savings would be very large relative to the cost of the program now. However, that advantage might be significantly reduced when the future costs are discounted.

The discounting procedure adjusts estimates of cost and/or outcomes that will be experienced in a future time period. The interest rate is commonly used for discounting. Economists recommend making and reporting a range of calculations to include conservative and more optimistic projections, including rates of 2, 3, 5, and 10 percent (18). If a low discount rate is used, the value of long-term costs and benefits is increased; in contrast, a higher discount rate increases the value of short-term costs and benefits. According to a rule of thumb, an analyst should apply discounting to any study when the time difference between investment and benefit is greater than 1 year. When necessary, cost, outcomes, or both are discounted before Step 5. Present value tables in economics and accounting reference books and on computer spreadsheet software programs simplify the process of discounting.

The formula for discounting follows (34):

$$PV_{C/B} = C/B_{(0)} + \frac{C/B_{(1)}}{(1 + r)} + \frac{C/B_{(2)}}{(1 + r)^2} + \ldots + \frac{C/B_n}{(1 + r)^n}$$

where $PV_{C/B}$ = Present value of costs or benefits.
$C/B_{(0)}$ = Dollar value of costs or benefits during the immediate period.
$C/B_{(1)}$ = Dollar value of costs or benefits during the first year.
$C/B_{(2)}$ = Dollar value of costs or benefits during the second year.
$C/B_{(n)}$ = Dollar value of costs or benefits during each subsequent year until the end of the expenditures or the last year in which benefits are expected to accrue.
r = The discount rate.

Step 5: Relate Costs to Outcomes

After accurate and defensible estimates of costs and outcomes have been gathered (in Steps 3 and 4), they are related to each other so that judgments about the relative economic efficiency of the compared alternatives can be made. This economic analysis can be done and presented in several ways—ratios, net benefit or net cost-effectiveness, or an array table. The method is determined by the objectives of the study, the type of economic analysis, and the nature of the data, as well as by considerations about what form will be most understandable and helpful to potential users of the results.

Ratio. The ratio communicates the cost for a unit of outcome and allows direct comparison between the efficiency of one alternative and the efficiency of another alternative. The use of a cost-effectiveness ratio is illustrated in Appendix 19A, where the chosen outcome variable was lowered blood cholesterol level as an intermediary for preventing coronary artery disease. The cost-effectiveness results for Alternative I (screening and the intervention) was $6.75 for each percentage point decrease in the serum cholesterol level. For Alternative II (screening and referral to customary medical care), it was $25.56 for no reduction in serum cholesterol level.

Ratios provide a succinct, and often memorable, way of communicating results. The results of the 1990 WIC cost-benefit study (43) are commonly stated as, "Every $1 invested in WIC saves $3." However, the ratio does not tell the whole story in this case. A more accurate summary of the WIC study would be, "On the average, each $1 invested in WIC for pregnant women results in $3 savings in Medicaid cost for newborns and their mothers during the first 60 days after birth. The benefit-cost ratio varied considerably among the five states studied. The benefit-cost ratios for the three study states were Florida, 1.77; North Carolina, 3.13; Minnesota, 1.83; South Carolina, 2.44; and Texas, 2.44" (43).

Ratios have other drawbacks. When a ratio is used, it is difficult to visualize the total costs of implementing the intervention. Furthermore, the actual magnitude of change is not evident, so clinicians cannot determine whether the amount of change is clinically meaningful. Decision makers will need additional descriptive or graphic information to consider the budgetary ramifications and numbers of persons who are likely to have access to the defined nutrition intervention and to benefit from it. Additionally, various audiences may be interested in other outcomes beyond the key outcomes identified for the cost-effectiveness or cost-benefit ratio.

Array table. Many of the drawbacks of ratio use are overcome by presenting results in an array. Showing actual costs and outcomes in an array table allows audiences to consider simultaneously more than one outcome measure in relation to the resource requirements to produce the outcomes. Table 19.4 shows an array presentation of the findings from a study of nutrition practice guidelines for non-insulin-dependent diabetes mellitus. The results of the same study are summarized in Table 19.5 using cost-effectiveness ratios (44).

From ratio to net benefit. A ratio is traditionally used to express the results of CBA research. It may be a cost-benefit ratio, in which the numerator is the cost of inputs and the denominator is the monetary value of benefits (outcomes), or it may be a benefit-cost ratio, in which the numerator is the benefits and the denominator is the costs:

$$\text{Cost-benefit ratio} = \frac{\text{Cost of inputs in dollars}}{\text{Benefit (outcomes) in dollars}} = 1{:}3$$

$$\text{Benefit-cost ratio} = \frac{\text{Benefit (outcomes) in dollars}}{\text{Cost of inputs in dollars}} = 3{:}1$$

TABLE 19.4 Nutrition Visits, Costs, Outcomes, and Cost Savings for Two Levels of Medical Nutrition Therapy for Non-Insulin-Dependent Diabetes Mellitus[a]

Level of nutrition care	No. of visits	Mean contact time (h)	Total costs[b]	Per-patient cost[b]	Mean change in fasting plasma glucose level (mmol/L)[c]	Mean change in HbA$_{1c}$ assay (% point)	No. of changes in therapy	Mean cost savings due to changes in therapy
BC group ($n = 85$)	1	1	$3,565.55	$41.95	-0.41 ± 2.74	-0.69 ± 1.67	9	$3.13
PGC group ($n = 94$)	3	2.5	$10,534.33	$112.07	-1.07 ± 2.77	-0.93 ± 1.63	17	$31.49

[a]BC indicates basic nutrition care and PGC, practice guidelines nutrition care.

[b]Incremental costs for medical nutrition therapy as a component of diabetes care, expressed in 1993 dollars.

[c]To convert mmol/L glucose to mg/dL, multiply mmol/L by 18.0. To convert mg/dL glucose to mmol/L, multiply mg/dL by 0.0555. For example, a glucose level of 6.0 mmol/L = 108 mg/dL.

Adapted with permission from Franz MJ, Splett PL, Monk A, et al. Cost-effectiveness of medical nutrition therapy provided by dietitians for persons with non-insulin-dependent diabetes mellitus. *J Am Diet Assoc.* 1995;95:1018–1026.

TABLE 19.5 Cost-Effectiveness Ratios for Medical Nutrition Therapy for Non-Insulin-Dependent Diabetes Mellitus Under Differing Salary, Laboratory, and Outcome Assumptions[a]

Variable	Fasting plasma glucose (mmol/L)		
	Low	Mean	High
	←	$[b]	→
High salary ($19.20/h)			
BC	X[c]	6.58	2.70
PGC, extra laboratory test	14.42	6.86	4.50
PGC, no laboratory test	12.56	5.97	3.92
Low salary ($13.94/h)			
BC	X[c]	4.71	1.93
PGC, extra laboratory test	10.21	4.85	3.18
PGC, no laboratory test	8.35	3.97	2.60

[a]BC = basic nutrition care; PGC = practice guidelines nutrition care.
[b]Cost per unit of change.
[c]The cost-effectiveness ratio cannot be calculated.

Reprinted with permission. Franz MJ, Splett PL, Monk A, et al. Cost-effectiveness of medical nutrition therapy provided by dietitians for persons with non-insulin-dependent diabetes mellitus. *J Am Diet Assoc.* 1995;95:1018–1026.

Net benefit (or net cost) is the dollars gained (or lost) when the monetary value of all resources consumed is subtracted from the total estimate of cost savings or averted expenditures when the alternative is implemented. It uses the same values that are used in the numerator and denominator of the cost-benefit ratio. Compared with the ratio, the net benefit calculation does a better job of communicating the magnitude of resources at stake and can be applied more directly to budgetary planning.

Presenting only the ratio conceals the magnitude of the resources at stake. For example, benefits of $3 million dollars gained from an expenditure of $1 million results in a 1:3 cost-benefit ratio. A benefit of $3,000 from an investment of $1,000 is also a 1:3 cost-benefit ratio. However, the net benefits would be reported as $2 million and $2,000, respectively, which certainly tells a different story.

Some experts advocate presenting the results of a CEA as net cost-effectiveness. In this method, the monetary value of cost savings generated by the improved health or averted deterioration is calculated (usually using gross costing to assign value to economically significant events). From this value, the input (intervention) costs are subtracted. The resulting figure is related to a key outcome presented in natural units (18,34,35).

Sensitivity analysis and ethical issues in economic analysis. Before the final conclusions can be drawn, the analyst should consider discounting (discussed earlier), sensitivity analysis, and ethical issues. Once the analysis has been done, sensitivity analysis is used to check the robustness of the conclusions. Sensitivity analysis involves the reanalysis of data using different estimates for assumptions or uncertainties. It informs the analyst and decision maker of the degree to which specific assumptions affect the results. For example, in a study of medical nutrition therapy in non-insulin-dependent diabetes mellitus, the impact of different assumptions about dietitians' salaries, variations in the use of laboratory tests, and the magnitude of glucose control outcome were assessed (44).

In sensitivity analysis, what-if scenarios are used to determine the impact of substitute assumptions (or other uncertainties) on the conclusions. Several rounds of reanalysis are done using more-conservative and more-liberal estimates. Reanalysis is not difficult. Using computer spreadsheets or statistical software programs, revised estimates can be substituted for a value used in the original analysis, and the computer quickly recalculates the results.

Reports of CEA and CBA should describe the assumptions made and how sensitivity analysis was used to explore the impact of the assumptions on the analysis and its conclusions. If a conclusion holds up under varying assumptions, it is said to be *robust*. If changing some of the assumptions used to assign value to resources significantly changes the conclusion, greater efforts should be directed toward determining the true value for the cost component or the outcome estimate. When this effort is not possible, the analyst must state explicitly that the results are "sensitive to" the value assigned to that component. In the report of a non-insulin-dependent diabetes mellitus study, the authors stated, "The results indicate that cost-effectiveness conclusions were sensitive to the outcome indicator selected." They went on to report the impact of dietitians' salaries, laboratory tests, and outcome variations on conclusions (44).

In reports of studies about the cost-effectiveness of nutrition services, questions can arise about assumptions used in the estimates of costs or outcomes. Dietitians and others conducting these studies must identify the potential areas for questioning. They must use sensitivity analysis to understand the strengths and limitations of the analysis and openly report them along with conclusions and recommendations.

The results of economic analysis indicate the preferred alternative based on the criterion of economic efficiency—that is, the alternative that produces the greater amount of outcomes for the lower cost. However, additional criteria come into play when setting policies, making administrative decisions, or recommending clinical practices. The findings of CBA or CEA could favor targeting medical nutrition therapy or a nutrition program to younger, more compliant patients with less severe disease. But is it ethical to withhold therapy from older or more acutely ill persons? And although delivering a nutrition program via the Internet may be very efficient, is it ethical to exclude persons who cannot afford a computer or Internet access? Ethical issues like these must be considered when conducting economic analyses.

When an ethical issue, such as access to nutrition care for people without insurance, is incorporated into the objectives of the CEA or CBA, the study can be designed to measure and value the issue. Ethical issues can also come to light during the study and interpretation of results. Relevant ethical issues should be explored, identified, and discussed, even if it is not possible to measure or place a dollar value on them (28). Many people—especially advocates, legislators, planners, and policy analysts—who use reports about the economic implications of nutrition services and programs have no nutrition training. Ethical issues related to food and nutrition may not be evident and thus must be brought to their attention. Whenever ethical issues are identified, their implications should be explored and presented as a part of the findings. Roth-Yousey presents additional discussion of ethical issues in nutrition and their analysis (45).

Step 6: Interpret and Use the Results

When the analysis is complete, the last step is to interpret the findings and make recommendations for action. The results should increase knowledge of the cost, effectiveness, and efficiency of nutrition programs and services. The study and its findings must be presented to decision makers who can use the information. Clinical nutrition managers benefit from a CEA that identifies areas in which expected outcomes are not being reached or patients' health outcomes could be achieved with fewer inputs. The results can support changes in practice necessary to make dietetics services more effective and efficient. Providing results of CBA to health plans and insurance companies can support coverage of medical nutrition therapy (46), and CBA results are strong factors in policy decisions at state and federal levels.

Every study has limitations that must be acknowledged. Nutritionists in Washington State, for example, collected case studies of the impact of nutrition services for children with special health care conditions and used them to estimate health care averted and associated eco-

nomic benefits. The report described limitations of the study and offered appropriate application of the findings and the need for further study (47).

The report of an economic analysis must include enough information for users to be able to understand the conclusion, judge its accuracy, and determine the context in which it can be applied. The following is a checklist of items needed in preparing reports or reviewing reports of economic analysis prepared by others:

- Statement of the purpose and objectives of the analysis.
- Description of compared alternatives and why they were selected, the perspective for analysis, the time frame for inputs and outcomes, and the key outcome or outcomes.
- Procedures for determining costs, cost components included, sources of data, assumptions made, costing approach, the base year for standardizing costs, the computed monetary value of inputs (and outcomes, if monetized), and discounting, if done.
- Procedures for determining effectiveness/outcome, including study design, sources of data, assumptions made, methods of statistical analysis, proportion of the target population that benefited and their characteristics, the magnitude of effect for each alternative and its variation, discounting if done, any problems or limitations encountered, and significant intervening or confounding factors affecting the interpretation of results.
- The relative efficiency of each alternative-relating costs to outcomes in a ratio, array, and/or net cost (benefit) equation, as well as sensitivity analysis to explore the robustness of conclusions under more conservative or liberal assumptions.
- Ethical issues and their role in interpreting findings.
- Conclusions and recommendations for action, when appropriate.

APPLICATIONS IN DIETETICS PRACTICE

Economic Analysis in Clinical Nutrition

The following examples illustrate the range of opportunities for incorporating economic analysis in nutrition research and outcomes studies. Gallagher-Allred et al reviewed studies that demonstrated how appropriate nutrition support is associated with reduced morbidity and mortality and lower costs among hospital patients (48). Together the studies build a case for early and appropriate medical nutrition therapy (MNT). Specific studies, such as work by Hedberg et al (49), help quantify the resource requirements for appropriate and effective nutrition care.

Brannon et al examined the cost-effectiveness of two methods of nutrition education delivered through physicians' offices for children with hypercholesterolemia (50). They calculated CEA ratios two ways, one relating program costs to changes in calories consumed from fat, and another relating program costs to reduction of low-density lipoprotein cholesterol at 3 and 12 months. They noted that the findings were sensitive to the time horizon for measurement, assumptions about children's contact with primary care, and availability of someone to administer the intervention (parent or dietitian). They also noted that third-party payment favored one method over another.

Sikand et al conducted a cost-benefit study of MNT versus lipid drug therapy for a sample of adults with hypercholesterolemia (39). Their comprehensive report included MNT and lipid costs; change in lipids, body mass index, and drug eligibility as outcomes; and reported CBA results as annualized net benefits;, cost-effectiveness ratios for different intensities of nutrition care;, and a cost-benefit ratio of MNT to drug therapy. The Massachusetts Dietetic Association used the results of a cost-benefit study to influence payment/reimbursement policies for MNT (46).

Using a large longitudinal database from a health maintenance organization, Sheils et al measured the relationship between MNT and health care spending for diabetes, cardiovascular disease, and renal disease (42). They used multiple regression to separate the effect of other factors that could impact health care utilization in addition to MNT. The outcome indicator was differences in health care utilization measured as change in physician visits per quarter. The cost of MNT provided by dietitians was estimated using the average Medicare reimbursement rate for physicians, and Medicare claims data were used to estimate the health care utilization and its costs. The investigators found significant reductions in utilization for persons with diabetes and cardiovascular disease but not renal disease, and they projected net savings of $369.7 million beginning after 3 years of the program. This study demonstrates the use of administrative databases as the data source for economic analysis of nutrition intervention.

Following work with a CEA study, Naglak et al offered advice about what to include and what to avoid in future CEA (51). They discuss issues of sample size, compliance with MNT and alternate therapies, following patients long enough to assess the effects of recidivism, and selection of the outcomes measure for the efficiency calculation. They also recommend consulting with a statistician early in the process.

Economic Analysis in Public Health

The Basic Assessment Scheme for Intervention Costs and Consequences (BASICC) has been recommended as a methodology for determining the cost and consequences of prevention programs (52). The BASICC approach provides a minimum standard for analyzing the cost-effectiveness of new and existing prevention programs. It is used to inform public health decisions and to set priorities for prevention strategies. The six data elements necessary for completing the BASICC and calculating net cost are as follows:

- A complete description of the program, the units in which services are provided, and the time frame of the program.
- Health outcomes averted by the prevention program and the estimated time between its implementation and when the negative health outcome is averted.
- Rates and the societal burden of the health outcome.
- The preventable fraction for the health outcome; that is, the proportion of the health outcome averted when the program is in place.
- Intervention costs per unit of intervention, including the costs of any intervention adverse effects.
- Direct medical treatment cost of the health outcome prevented.

Prevention programs should have a specific objective related to the public health goals of improving the quality of life, reducing the incidence or severity of disease or injury, and reducing premature death through early detection or interventions to reduce risk or exposures associated with the incidence of disease or injury. Determining the incidence and prevalence of the specific health outcome is the target of the analysis, and the magnitude of the effect is expressed as the preventable fraction. Data about the effect of the program are related to the usual rate of the health outcome in the population and geographic area of interest. The formula for calculation of the preventable fraction follows (52):

$$\text{Preventable fraction} = \frac{R_{(I)} - R_{(O)}}{R_{(O)}} \times p_r \times p_c$$

where R refers to the rate of the health outcomes with the intervention program *(I)* and without *(O)* the program; p_r is the proportion of the population reached; and p_c is the proportion of the population who comply. The preventable fraction is related to the resources required to conduct the program during a specified time period to produce the measure of efficiency (the cost-effectiveness).

The microcosting, resource-based approach to costing is used to determine program costs, and actual or reported estimates of averted medical care costs are used. Although a societal perspective is recommended, in practice only direct costs to the program and direct costs associated with the outcome (such as medical treatment costs and nonmedical household assistance or hospice costs) are computed. The economic analysis is expressed as a net cost, which is the cost of the intervention and its adverse effects for 10^n persons, minus the direct cost associated with the expected number of cases averted in the same 10^n persons. Table 19.6 illustrates the information used to calculate the cost-effectiveness (expressed as a net cost of intervention costs minus discounted medical costs) of a hypothetical smoking cessation program.

Under the leadership of the Centers for Disease Control and Prevention, extensive work has been done to link the principles and analytic techniques of economic analysis and epidemiology to improve the quality of CEA studies of prevention (34,52). *Prevention Effectiveness: A Guide to Decision Analysis and Economic Evaluation* presents extensive coverage of the topic (34).

DIETETICS RESEARCH

Dietetics practitioners in all practice settings can contribute to knowledge about the effectiveness and efficiency of nutrition care. Using data collected for quality assurance purposes and outcomes measurement can ease the burden of conducting a CEA. Dietitians with management responsibilities can allocate time for staff to spend on planning, conducting, and reporting outcome studies and economic analyses.

Studies may be small and carried out in one facility, or several locations may collaborate. They can be planned and implemented prospectively or conducted retrospectively using medical records and existing databases. All will add to the information needed to refine, im-

TABLE 19.6 Net Cost Calculation for a Prevention Program

Information Necessary for Net Cost Calculation	Hypothetical Data
Cost of intervention per participant	$86.13
Medical care cost per case of smoking-related disease	$55,000
Rate of smoking-related disease among smokers who are not participants	10 cases per 1,000 smokers
Rate of disease among program participants	2 cases per 1,000 nonsmokers
Net Cost Calculation for 1,000 Persons	Calculation
Intervention costs	$1,000 \times \$86.13 = \$83,130$
Cases of smoking-related disease averted	$10 - 2 = 8$
Medical costs of disease averted	$8 \times \$55,000 = \$440,000$
Medical costs equally spaced and discounted, 3%/yr, over 24 yr	$0.7056 \times \$440,000 = \$310,470$

prove, and promote nutrition care. The results need to be shared through professional and scientific meetings and publications. It is up to dietitians, along with other researchers and economists, to conduct the research and make the results available to the administrators, planners, regulators, legislators, and third-party payers who need this information to make informed decisions about the allocation of resources to nutrition care. By working with these policy makers, dietitians will learn about their different information needs and therefore be better able to plan, conduct, and report studies that can influence clinical administrative and policy decisions.

CEA and CBA are not a panacea for the dietetics profession. They are tools to provide more information about nutrition care and its cost and effectiveness. If used wisely, these tools will enable dietitians to continue to improve their services, increase their visibility with payers and other decision makers, and provide nutrition services that will have greater impact on the health of the public.

REFERENCES

1. Eck LH, Slawson DL, Williams R, Smith K, Harmon-Clayton K, Oliver D. A model for making outcomes

research standard practice in clinical dietetics. *J Am Diet Assoc.* 1998;98:451–457.

2. Agency for Health Care Policy and Research. *The Outcome of Outcomes Research at AHCPR.* Silver Springs, Md: Agency for Health Care Policy and Research; 1999. AHCPR publication 99-RO44.

3. Ellwood PM. Shattuck lecture—outcomes management: a technology of patient experience. *N Engl J Med.* 1988;318(23):1549–1556.

4. Epstein AM. The outcomes movement—will it get us where we want to go? *N Engl J Med.* 1990;323(4)266–270.

5. Porter C, Matel JL. Are we making decisions based on evidence? *J Am Diet Assoc.* 1998;98:404–407.

6. Dobzykowshi EA. The methodology of outcomes measurement. *J Rehabil Outcomes Meas.* 1997;1(1):8–17.

7. Kane RL. *Understanding Health Care Outcomes Research.* Gaithersburg, Md: Aspen Publishers Inc; 1997.

8. Splett PL. *Cost Outcomes of Nutrition Intervention, Part 3: Economic and Cost Analysis of Nutrition Interventions.* Evansville, Ind: Mead Johnson and Co Inc; 1996.

9. Splett PL. *Developing and Validating Evidence-Based Guides for Practice: A Tool Kit for Dietetics Professionals.* Chicago, Ill: The American Dietetic Association; 2000.

10. Hayward RSA, Wilson MC, Tunis SR, Bass EB, Guyatt G. Users' guides to the medical literature, VIII: How to use clinical practice guidelines. A. Are the recommendations valid? *JAMA.* 1995;274:570–574.

11. Kushner RF, Ayello EA, Beyer PL, et al. National Coordinating Committee clinical indicators of nutrition care. *J Am Diet Assoc.* 1994;94:1169–1177.

12. Spilker B, ed. *Quality of Life and Pharmacoeconomics.* 2nd ed. Philadelphia, Pa: Lippincott-Raven; 1996.

13. Gallagher-Allred CR, Voss AC, Finn SC, McCamish MA. Malnutrition and clinical outcomes: the case for medical nutrition therapy. *J Am Diet Assoc.* 1996;96:361–396.

14. Splett PL, Weddle DO. *A White Paper on Measuring Outcomes. Prepared for the Administration on Aging.* Washington, DC: Dept of Health and Human Services; 1999.

15. Hauchecorne CM, Barr SI, Sork TJ. Evaluation of nutrition counseling in clinical settings: do we make a difference? *J Am Diet Assoc.* 1994;94:437–440.

16. Kulkarni K, Gregory R, Holmes A, et al. Nutrition Practice Guidelines for Type I Diabetes Mellitus positively affect dietitian practices and patient outcomes. *J Am Diet Assoc.* 1998;98:62–70.

17. Splett PL. *Cost Outcomes of Nutrition Intervention, Part 1: Outcomes Research.* Evansville, Ind: Mead Johnson and Co Inc; 1996.

18. Gold MR, Siegel JE, Russell LB, Weinstein MC. *Cost-Effectiveness in Health and Medicine.* New York, NY: Oxford University Press; 1996.

19. Splett PL. *Cost Outcomes of Nutrition Intervention, Part 2: Measuring Effectiveness of Nutrition Interventions.* Evansville, Ind: Mead Johnson and Co Inc; 1996.

20. Cook TD, Campbell DT. *Quasi-experimentation: Design and Analysis Issues for Field Settings.* Boston, Mass: Houghton Mifflin Company; 1979.

21. Heithoff K. *Effectiveness and Outcomes in Health Care.* Washington, DC: National Academy Press; 1990.

22. Hornberger J, Wrone E. When to base clinical policies on observational versus randomized trial data. *Ann Intern Med.* 1997;127:697–703.

23. Trotter JP. *The Quest for Cost-Effectiveness in Health Care.* Chicago, Ill: American Hospital Publishers; 1995.

24. August D. In: Ireton-Jones CS, Gottschlich MM, Bell SJ. *Practice-Oriented Nutrition Research: An Outcomes Measurement Approach.* Gaithersburg, Md: Aspen; 1998.

25. Zeilstorff RD. Capturing and using clinical outcome data: implications for information design systems. *J Am Med Infromatics Assoc.* 1995;2:191–199.

26. Eddy DM, Billings J. The quality of medical evidence: implications for quality of care. *Health Aff (Millwood).* 1998;7(1):19–32.

27. Schiller MR, Moore C. Practical approaches to outcomes evaluation. *Top Clin Nutr.* 1999;14(2)1–12.

28. Splett PL. *A Practitioner's Guide to Cost-Effectiveness Analysis of Nutrition Interventions.* Arlington, Va: National Center for Education in Maternal and Child Health; 1996.

29. Mason M, ed. *Cost and Benefits of Nutrition Care: Phase 1.* Chicago, Ill: The American Dietetic Association; 1979.

30. Disbrow DD. The cost and benefits of nutrition services: a literature review. *J Am Diet Assoc.* 1989;89(suppl 4):3–66.

31. Splett PL. Effectiveness and cost effectiveness of nutrition care: a critical appraisal with recommendations, Phase III: research designs for future studies. *J Am Diet Assoc.* 1991;91(suppl):9–35.

32. American Dietetic Association. Cost-effectiveness of medical nutrition therapy. Position paper of The American Dietetic Association. *J Am Diet Assoc.* 1995;95:88–91.

33. Barr JT. *Clinical Effectiveness in Allied Health Practices.* Silver Springs, Md: US Dept of Health and Human Services, Agency for Health Care Policy and Research; 1993.

34. Haddix AC, Teutsch SM, Shaffer PA, Dunet DO. *Prevention Effectiveness: A Guide to Decision Analysis and Economic Evaluation.* New York, NY: Oxford University Press; 1996.

35. Petti DB. *Meta-Analysis, Decision Analysis, and Cost-Effectiveness Analysis: Methods for Quantitative Synthesis in Medicine.* 2nd ed. New York, NY: Oxford University Press; 2000.

36. Gill TM, Feinstein AR. A critical appraisal of the quality of quality-of-life measurements. *JAMA.* 1994;272:619–626.

37. Russell LB, Fryback DG, Sonnenberg FA. Is the societal perspective in cost-effectiveness analysis useful for decision makers? *Jt Comm J Qual Improv.* 1999;25:447–454.

38. Montgomery DL, Splett PL. The economic benefits of breastfeeding infants enrolled in the WIC Program. *J Am Diet Assoc.* 1997;97:379–385.

39. Sikand G, Kashyap ML, Yang I. Medical nutrition therapy lowers serum cholesterol and saves medication costs. *J Am Diet Assoc.* 1998;98:889–894.

40. Rice DP. *Estimating the Cost of Illness.* Washington, DC: US Dept of Health Education and Welfare; 1966. Health Economic Series 6, Public Health Service.

41. Veney JE, Kaluzny AD. *Evaluation and Decision Making for Health Services Programs.* Englewood Cliffs, NJ: Prentice-Hall Inc; 1984.

42. Sheils JF, Rubin R, Stapleton DC. The estimated costs and savings of medical nutrition therapy: the Medicare population. *J Am Diet Assoc.* 1999;99:428–435.

43. Devaney B, Bilheimer L, Schore J. *The Savings in Medicaid Costs for Newborns and Their Mothers from Prenatal Participation in the WIC Program.* Washington, DC: US Dept of Agriculture, Food, and Nutrition Service, Office of Analysis and Evaluation; 1990.

44. Franz MJ, Splett PL, Monk A, et al. Cost-effectiveness of medical nutrition therapy provided by dietitians for persons with non-insulin-dependent diabetes mellitus. *J Am Diet Assoc.* 1995;95:1018–1026.

45. Roth-Yousey L. Ethics in Community Nutrition. In: Owen AL, Splett PL, Owen GM. *Nutrition in the Community: The Art and Science of Delivering Services.* 4th ed. Boston, Mass: WBC McGraw-Hill; 1999.

46. McGehee MM, Hohnson EQ, Rasmussen HM, Sahyoun N, Lynch MM, Carey M. Benefits and costs of medical nutrition therapy by registered dietitians for patients with hypercholesterolemia. *J Am Diet Assoc.* 1995;95:1041–1043.

47. Lucas B, Nardella M. *Cost Considerations: The Benefits of Nutrition Services for a Case Series of Children with Special Health Care Needs in Washington State, Seattle.* Olympia, Wash: Washington State Department of Health; 1998.

48. Gallagher-Allred GR, Voss AC, Finn SC, McCamish MA. Malnutrition and clinical outcomes: the case for medical nutrition therapy. *J Am Diet Assoc.* 1996;96:366–369.

49. Hedberg AM, Lairson DR, Aday LA, et al. Economic implications of an early postoperative enteral feeding protocol. *J Am Diet Assoc.* 1999;99:802–807.

50. Brannon SD, Tershakovec AM, Shannon BM. The cost-effectiveness of alternative methods of nutrition education for hypercholesterolemic children. *Am J Public Health.* 1997;87:1967–1970.

51. Naglak M, Mitchell DC, Kris-Etherton P, Harkness W, Pearson TA. What to consider when conducting cost-effectiveness analysis in a clinical setting. *J Am Diet Assoc.* 1998;98:1149–1154.

52. Centers for Disease Control and Prevention. Assessing the effectiveness of disease and injury prevention programs: cost and consequences. *MMWR Morb Mortal Wkly Rep.* 1995;44(No. RR-10):1–10.

—⁓—

Appendix 19A
Cost-Effectiveness Analysis Case Study[a]

OBJECTIVE AND FRAMEWORK OF THE ECONOMIC ANALYSIS

A prospective, two-group comparison study was conducted to evaluate the effectiveness of a worksite nutrition intervention program designed to lower total serum cholesterol levels. The target population was a group of 450 professional firefighters, all of whom participated in the worksite program. Of the 450 firefighters, 52 men with elevated cholesterol levels volunteered to be in the study. A comparison group was made up of 44 male volunteers from adjacent fire department districts. The perspective was the fire department's worksite wellness program, and the time horizon was 6 months. Costs are based on 1983 dollars, as documented at the time of the study, and are calculated using a micro-costing approach.

INTERVENTION PROTOCOL

A three-phase intervention program was delivered to 450 firefighters. Phase I included a lipid screening and height and weight measurements. A questionnaire was also administered to collect information on diagnoses, medication use, family history of coronary heart disease (CHD), dietary practices, and so forth.

In phase II, the treatment phase, dietitians interpret-

---

[a]Adapted from Disbrow DD and Dowling RA. Cost-effectiveness and cost-benefit analysis: research to support practice. In: Monsen ER, ed. *Research: Successful Approaches.* Chicago, Ill: American Dietetic Association; 1992:285–288.

ed laboratory results for each participant and provided an individualized behavior change plan based on those results. Phase II also included educational sessions, cooking demonstrations, and exercise prescriptions. Classes were $2^{1}/_{2}$ hours long, and each had 20 to 25 participants.

Phase III was the evaluation phase. A 6-month follow-up lipid panel analysis was completed. The laboratory results were reviewed, and individual progress toward meeting specific goals was discussed. Motivational materials were provided to encourage continued compliance after completion of the program.

The comparison group had the lipid panel analysis at the beginning and end of the project. They did not participate in the intervention program but were referred for standard medical care if elevated lipid levels were identified.

DETERMINATION OF OUTCOMES

Treatment Group (Alternative I)

At the 6-month follow-up, the mean percentage change in total serum cholesterol level for the 52 men in the group was a 10.4 percent decrease. Forty-five of the 52 men in this group (86.5 percent) had decreased their total serum cholesterol level. The mean decrease for the 45 men was 32 mg/dL, with a range of 3 mg/dL to 79 mg/dL.

Comparison Group (Alternative II)

Six of the 44 volunteers in the comparison group were lost to follow-up; repeat lipid panel analyses were completed for 38 men. Although the serum cholesterol level had decreased for 14 men (36.8 percent), the mean percentage change in total serum cholesterol for the comparison group during the follow-up period was a 4.9 percent increase.

DETERMINATION OF COSTS

The following costs determination uses the micro-costing approach. Costs to deliver the program are based on documented resource utilization for principal cost components. Total program cost can be reported and the cost per participant can be calculated.

Principal Resource Component, Amount Used, Bases for Calculating Monetary Value	Subtotal	Total
Alternative I: Screening plus intervention ($n = 52$)		
A. Personnel costs (personnel time × personnel cost/hour)		
1. Registered dietitian (R.D.)—Program development, admin-strative activities:		
3.6 hours × R.D. cost/hour ($21.60 [$18.00/hour + 20% fringe benefits])	$77.76	
2. R.D.—Teaching, development of classes, and individualized treatment plans:		
38.5 hours × R.D. cost/hour	$831.60	
3. Nutrition assistant—Teaching, counseling, blood draws:		
38.5 hours × nutrition assistant cost/hour ($13.20 [$11.00/hour + 20% fringe benefits])	$508.20	
4. Clerical—Typing, filing:		
16.64 hours × clerical cost/hour ($6.60 [$5.50/hour + 20% fringe benefits])	$108.90	
B. Total personnel costs		$1526.46
C. Material and supply costs		
1. Blood lipid tests:		
2 per participant × $11.00 = $22.00/participant	$1144.00	
2. Assessment forms (documented expense)	$14.04	
3. Education materials (documented expense)	$86.84	
4. Supplies (documented expense)	$14.82	
5. Computer time and software 16 hours × $11.18/hour	$178.88	
D. Total material and supply costs		$1438.58
E. Administrative overhead costs		
1. Travel:		
75 miles × $0.23 per mile	$17.25	
2. Advertising (pro-rated at $12.39)	$12.39	

3. Office space and equipment allocated to program based on square feet of space $657.28

F. Total administrative costs $686.92

G. Total program costs (personnel costs + material/supply costs + administrative costs) $3651.96

H. Total cost per participant (total program costs ÷ number of participants [52]) $70.23

Alternative II: Screening with referral to standard medical care (*n* = 38); because this group did not receive any intervention, the only costs are for the lipid analyses completed at the beginning and end of the project.

A. Personnel costs (personnel time × personnel cost/hour)
   1. Nutrition assistant—blood draws:
      10.26 hours × nutrition assistant cost/hour ($13.20 [$11.00/hour + 20% fringe benefits]) $135.43

B. Total personnel cost $135.43

C. Material and supply costs
   1. Blood analyses:
      2 per participant × $11.00 = $22.00/participant $836.00

D. Total material and supply costs $836.00

E. Administrative overhead costs $0

G. Total costs for Alternative II $971.43

H. Total cost per comparison group participant (total program costs ÷ number of participants [38]) $25.56

RELATING COSTS TO OUTCOMES

Results

Alternative I. Screening plus intervention (*n* = 52)

A. Magnitude of outcome: 10.4 percent mean decrease in total cholesterol

B. Value of inputs (program costs): $70.23 per participant

C. Express as ratio of cost per effect (outcome): It cost $70.23 per participant to achieve a 10.4 percent mean decrease in total cholesterol, or $6.75 per each 1 percent decrease. $70.23 per 10.4 percent decrease

Alternative II. Screening with referral to standard medical care (*n* = 38)

A. Magnitude of outcome: No benefit; participants had a mean increase in total serum cholesterol of 4.9 percent

B. Value of inputs (screening costs): $25.56 per participant

C. Express as ratio of cost per effect (outcome): It cost $25.56 per participant, yet no decrease in serum cholesterol level was achieved. $25.56 per no decrease

The 10.4 percent reduction in serum cholesterol was clinically meaningful. The worksite intervention program was judged effective in achieving the goal of reduction in serum cholesterol and, theoretically, reducing the risk of the participants for coronary heart disease. The results support the use of worksite screening plus cholesterol education interventions by an R.D. when compared with cholesterol screening with no worksite education.

DISCUSSION OF THE CASE STUDY

The members of the treatment group and the comparison group, all with elevated cholesterol levels, were self-selected volunteers, not randomly selected to participate. Therefore, they were not necessarily representative of all the firefighters. Further, because there was no random assignment to groups, confounding factors that could impact the outcomes cannot be ruled out.

Keeping in mind these limitations, the results of the screening-plus-intervention study can be used to promote the continuation and expansion of this worksite program. Other fire districts, as well as other public employee groups such as police and bus drivers, would be other prospective clients for the wellness program. Data like these would be of interest to health maintenance organizations and other health plans that are structured to control health care costs by risk reduction and prevention of disease. With additional information, the study results could provide a basis for a cost-benefit study. Estimating future health care costs related to coronary heart disease for treatment and comparison group participants over time could reveal differences between the groups that would further support nutrition intervention provided by an R.D. at the worksite.

— ⁓ —

Appendix 19B
Cost-Benefit Analysis
Case Study[a]

Is it "worth it" to promote exclusive breast-feeding by participants in the Special Supplemental Nutrition Program for Women, Infants, and Children (WIC)? To answer this question in Colorado, WIC cost and Medicaid expenditures were tracked to determine the economic benefit of 3 months of exclusive breast-feeding of WIC infants.

A two-group cohort design was used to measure outcomes, and the gross costing approach was used to determine input and outcome costs for a cost-benefit analysis. The source of the data was existing computerized databases.

OBJECTIVE AND FRAMEWORK OF THE ECONOMIC ANALYSIS

The objective of the analysis was to determine whether the method of feeding low-income infants enrolled in WIC affected their health outcomes during the first 6 months of life and the degree to which feeding method affected WIC costs and Medicaid expenditures. Medical costs resulting from infants' health outcomes were determined from Medicaid expenditures and related to WIC program costs for the infants and their mothers. This was a benefit-cost study planned from the perspective of the government programs and the taxpayers supporting those programs. The time horizon was 6 months. Costs are based on 1993–1994 dollars documented at the time of the study.

---

[a]Adapted from Montgomery DL, Splett PL. The economic benefits of breastfeeding infants enrolled in the WIC program. *J Am Diet Assoc.* 1997;97:379–385.

BACKGROUND AND STUDY PROCEDURES

WIC provides monthly vouchers for a package of supplemental food that is tailored to the nutrition needs of participants (for example, lactating women get more than women who are formula feeding their infants). Nationally, WIC strongly encourages breast-feeding; however the level of breast-feeding education and support varies from state to state and from site to site within each state. WIC participants have varying levels of breast-feeding initiation and breast-feed exclusively for varying lengths of time. The results of this study document the economic value of breast-feeding and help clarify whether it is worth it to promote exclusive breast-feeding (that is, no feeding of supplemental formula for a significant number of months).

The population studied was made up of WIC infants who were born healthy and had their healthcare paid for by Medicaid on a fee-for-service basis. Using 1993 WIC records, infants who were enrolled in WIC within 1 month of birth and who were either exclusively breast-fed or exclusively formula fed during the first 3 months of life were identified. Those records were linked with birth certificates and Medicaid files to determine study eligibility. Multiple births and infants with low birth weight, congenital anomalies, or other abnormal conditions were excluded. The final sample included 406 breast-fed infants and 470 formula-fed infants and their mothers.

Defining the sample and getting the data for analysis involved many people. Following administrative approval by the state WIC and Medicaid administrations, information specialists and computer programmers/analysts within WIC and Medicaid retrieved the archived 1993 files and wrote programs to abstract the defined sample and specific data requested by the study investigators. Another statistician hired for the study merged the data files to conduct the outcomes and cost analyses.

DETERMINATION OF OUTCOMES

Medicaid enrollment and claims files were used as the data source for health outcomes and associated costs of medical care for illnesses and injuries for each infant. Health problems were summarized for descriptive purposes, but the key outcome was Medicare expenditures (claims paid) for each infant during the first 6 months of life. Mean Medicaid expenditures for each group of infants were calculated (Table 19B.1). An adjusted analysis, using multiple linear regression, was used to adjust for the

TABLE 19B.1 Mean 6-Month Medicaid Expenditures for a WIC Infant

Feeding Method	6-month Medicaid Expenditures
Breast-feeding	$484.80
Formula feeding	$586.67
Group differences	$102.00

Cost savings to Medicaid for breast-feeding compared with formula-feeding equal $101.87 (or $111.63 after statistical adjustment for relevant factors).

TABLE 19B.2 Mean 6-Month WIC Costs for Infant-Mother WIC Pairs

Significant Cost Components	Monetary Value
Breast-fed infants	
• Infant formula and food	$33.08
• Food package for lactating mothers	$236.48
Total cost for mother-infant pair	$269.56
Formula rebate adjustment	−$29.60
Addition for administration	$70.08
WIC cost for breast-fed group	$310.04
Formula-fed infants	
• Infant formula and food	$381.10
• Food package for postpartum mothers	$187.00
Total cost for mother-infant pair	$568.10
Formula rebate adjustment	−$346.77
Addition for administration	$147.71
WIC cost for formula-fed group	$369.04

Cost savings to WIC for breast-feeding compared with formula feeding equal $59.00 over 6 months for each infant-mother pair.

effect of factors found to be different between groups (for example, mother's age, employment during pregnancy, and smoking) and other variables found to affect health outcomes, including infant sex and, birthweight.

DETERMINATION OF COSTS

The inputs were WIC cost. This cost included the cost of redeemed vouchers for infant formula and the mothers' food packages, as well as a calculated allowance for WIC administrative costs (operating costs, client certification, voucher issuance, and nutrition education). Administrative cost was calculated at the Colorado rate of 26 percent of the WIC food costs. An additional factor in the cost calculation was an adjustment for a formula rebate returned to the Colorado WIC by the formula manufacturer for each can of formula purchased. The value of the rebate was calculated by multiplying the contracted rebate amount by the number of cans of formula purchased with WIC vouchers during the 6-month period. Total WIC costs were food cost plus administrative overhead minus formula rebate. Table 19B.2 shows costs reported in 1993–1994 dollars as documented at the time of the study.

RELATING COSTS TO OUTCOMES

Benefit-Cost Ratio

A benefit-cost ratio for each group was calculated to express the relationship of outcome (Medicaid dollars) per unit of input (WIC costs). The relative efficiency was found to be about the same. The benefit-cost ratios were:

- Breast-fed group: $484.80 ÷ $310.04 = 1.56
- Formula-fed group: $586.67 ÷ $369.04 = 1.59

Net Benefit

The net benefit calculation reflects the savings (or excess cost) of one alternative compared with the other. This calculation is much more useful for policy and budget purposes. The following net benefit formula was used:

$$\text{Net benefit} = \left(\begin{array}{c} \text{Medicare \$ for breast-fed infants} \\ - \text{Medicare \$ for formula-fed infants} \end{array} \right)$$

$$+ \left(\begin{array}{c} \text{WIC \$ for breast-fed infants} \\ - \text{WIC \$ for formula-fed infants} \end{array} \right)$$

$$\text{Net benefit} = (\$484.80 - \$586.67)$$

$$+ (\$310.04 - \$369.04) = \$160.87$$

Thus, each WIC infant who is exclusively breast-fed for at least 3 months saves $160.87 over the first 6 months of life. In other words, the economic advantage of exclusive breast-feeding over formula feeding is $160.87.

SENSITIVITY ANALYSIS

To see how robust the results were, other assumptions were tested. This testing included recalculations using the national WIC administrative cost rate of 20 percent and examination of the costs and benefits for subgroups based on the number of months of exclusive breast-feeding

TABLE 19B.3   Net Benefits by Duration of Exclusive Breast-feeding

Duration of Breastfeeding (months)	Net Benefit for First 6 Months of Life
3	$118.68
4	$194.83
5	$292.21
6	$157.07

(3, 4, 5, and 6 months). Net benefits increased with exclusive breast-feeding of 4 or 5 months (Table 19B.3).

REPORTING AND USING RESULTS OF THE STUDY

WIC and Medicaid programs both benefit when WIC mothers are encouraged to exclusively breast-feed their infants. During the first 6 months of life, WIC saves about $60, and Medicaid gains more than $100, for each WIC infant exclusively breast-fed at least 3 months compared with the infant's formula-fed counterpart. The findings become even more compelling when applied to the number of infants participating in WIC in Colorado and across the country. Using breast-feeding rates from an-

other Colorado report, it was estimated that $25,803 is saved monthly by the 17.5 percent of Colorado WIC infants who are breast-fed for 6 months.

DISCUSSION OF THE CASE STUDY

The cohort design with WIC infants sorted by exposure to breast milk (exclusive formula feeding and exclusive breast-feeding) provides a fairly strong basis for attributing outcome differences to method of feeding. Statistical adjustment to remove possible confounding factors further strengthens the analysis, and sensitivity analysis verifies the robustness of the findings. Accessing and using existing databases for economic analysis has its challenges, but it affords a much larger sample size and access to cost data in a consistent, standardized form that can be tracked over time.

The results of this study demonstrate an economic benefit of exclusive breast-feeding at least 3 months compared with formula feeding. These benefits accrue to federal and state budgets and, ultimately, to taxpayers. In addition, WIC families experience the intangible benefits of healthier infants and avoid the stress of caring for sick infants. These additional benefits cannot be quantified in monetary terms, but contribute to the quality of life of families.

20

Research in Diet and Human Genetics

Ruth E. Patterson, Ph.D., R.D., Johanna W. Lampe, Ph.D., R.D., and
Cheryl L. Rock, Ph.D., R.D., F.A.D.A.

Considerable research has focused on identifying exposures (for example, dietary intake) that increase the risk of disease, but it is evident that not all individuals exposed to the same risk factors will develop the associated disease (1). For example, although it is well accepted that smoking causes lung cancer, only 10 percent to 15 percent of smokers will be diagnosed with the disease in their lifetime (2). We are beginning to understand the impact of differential genetic susceptibility in the etiology and pathogenesis of common diseases such as coronary heart disease and cancer. This new biology offers promise of an individualized approach to preventive medicine through risk profiling and the provision of information on how to modify the potential results of genetic predisposition via dietary modification or other environmental changes (3).

The objective of this chapter is to review the basic genetic mechanisms, describe the concepts underlying research in diet and human genetics, review important study designs for conducting research in this area, present tools and techniques for the collection and archiving of DNA, discuss informed consent for studies involving genetic markers, and comment upon the future of research in diet-gene interactions.

BASIC GENETIC MECHANISMS

To understand the new advances in human genetics, it is useful to review the fundamentals of molecular genetics.

This review is brief and therefore necessarily simplistic; we refer the interested reader to texts by Mueller and Young (4) and Alberts et al (5), from which the following overview is largely synthesized.

The genetic material within our cells contains the complete set of instructions for making an organism, called its *genome*. The human genome is organized into 46 chromosomes. Of these chromosomes, 44 are in 22 pairs (autosomes) in which 1 chromosome is inherited from the mother and 1 chromosome from the father. In addition, females inherit an X chromosome from each parent, whereas males inherit an X chromosome from the mother and a Y chromosome from the father.

Each chromosome contains many genes. A gene is a segment of a chromosome that encodes instructions that allow a cell to produce a specific protein, such as an enzyme, receptor, or carrier protein. The human genome is estimated to contain about 35,000 genes (6). Each gene is composed of long stretches of DNA that can be divided into three separate classes (Figure 20.1). The parts of a gene that actually provide the specific "instructions" (the coding region) for making a protein are called *exons*. In most genes, multiple exons are present, but they are separated by noncoding stretches of DNA called introns. In addition to exons and introns, each gene also contains a noncoding region at its beginning (the 5′ end) that serves to regulate when, and to what extent, the gene is expressed. This is referred to as the regulatory region of the gene, and it can be envisioned as a series of on/off switches that respond to signals (for example, proteins and

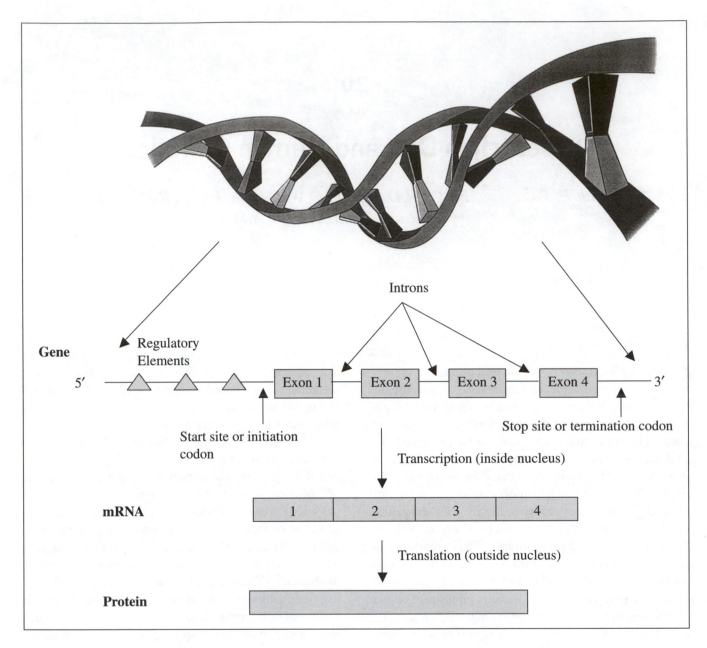

FIGURE 20.1   DNA and a diagram of a typical human structural gene. Reprinted with permission from Patterson RE, Eaton EL, Potter JP. The genetic revolution: change and challenge for the profession of dietetics. *J Am Diet Assoc.* 1999;99:1412–1420.

hormones) from within the cell, from neighboring cells, and from more distant parts of the organism.

Genes are composed of DNA, which exists as two paired or complementary strands forming a double helix (see Figure 20.1). Each strand is composed of millions of chemical building blocks, called *bases*. There are four different chemical bases in DNA: adenine, thymine, cytosine, and guanine. The four bases are strung along a repetitive sugar (deoxyribose) phosphate backbone. The two strands of DNA are held together by pairing of the chemical bases. Adenine forms hydrogen bonds with thymine, and cytosine forms hydrogen bonds with guanine.

Every three bases (called a *triplet*) along a strand of DNA specifies an amino acid to be incorporated into a protein, in what is called the *genetic code*. For example, a triplet composed of the bases guanine, cytosine, and adenine, in that order, is the genetic triplet code for the amino acid alanine. Certain combinations of bases (for example, thymine adenine adenine [TAA]), called *termination* or *stop codons,* will terminate the gene product. Mathematically, 4 bases could form up to 64 unique triplet codes; however, there are only 20 amino acids. This redundancy in the genetic code is called *degeneracy.*

When a cell is "switched" on to make a protein, the information from a gene is copied, base by base, from DNA into a single new strand of complementary RNA. RNA differs from DNA in three ways: (1) RNA is single stranded, whereas DNA is double stranded; (2) the sugar-phosphate backbone of RNA is composed of ribose, whereas in DNA it is composed of deoxyribose; and (3) RNA contains the base uracil, whereas DNA contains the base thymine. This primary RNA molecule is spliced to remove intron sequences so that only the coding sequence from the exons are used to produce messenger RNA (mRNA). The mRNA travels out of the nucleus into the cytoplasm, where it directs the complex set of reactions that occur on a ribosome and results in the assembly of amino acids that fold into completed protein molecules. Two other types of RNA, transfer RNA (tRNA) and ribosomal RNA (rRNA) are used in the cell to facilitate the synthesis of proteins from the mRNA template. In addition, some RNA molecules in cells have been found to function as enzymelike catalysts rather than serving as a template for protein synthesis.

Genes, through the proteins they encode, control all aspects of our cell function, including how efficiently we process foods, how effectively we metabolize compounds such as endogenous hormones and exogenous toxins, and how vigorously we respond to infections.

Human Genetic Variation, Mutations, and Polymorphism

Although thousands of random changes occur every day in the DNA of a cell as a result of heat energy and metabolic accidents, only a few stable changes accumulate in the DNA sequence of an average cell in a year. The rest of the changes are eliminated with remarkable efficiency by a variety of DNA repair mechanisms. Nearly all these repair mechanisms depend on the existence of two copies, or alleles, of the genetic material. If one DNA strand is accidentally changed, information is not lost irretrievably because an unaltered (complementary) copy of the altered strand remains and can act as a template to repair the damaged strand. DNA mutations that occur in germ cells (sperm or ova) are called *germ-line mutations.* These inheritable DNA mutations determine the charac-

teristics of offspring, including their susceptibility to disease. It is important to recognize that DNA mutations can occur in other body cells (that is, somatic cells). Somatic mutations are acquired from the environment (for example, from tobacco) and can result in the transformation of a normal cell to a malignant cell, which can then give rise to a tumor by clonal expansion. However, this overview of diet-gene interactions focuses entirely on germ-line mutations.

The effect of a change or alteration in DNA depends on a large variety of factors. If it occurs in an intron, there may be no effect on the functioning of an organism. When a gene is altered, the protein encoded by that gene may or may not be modified. For example, the most common type of mutation involves a single changed base in the DNA, called a *single-nucleotide polymorphism (SNP).* However, because the triplet genetic code is degenerate, an SNP may still code for the same amino acid (called a *silent mutation*). Even if a DNA sequence alteration produces a change in an amino acid, it may not significantly affect the protein, because the amino acid may not be at a site that is crucial to the protein's function. In contrast, other DNA alterations result in protein changes that can be disabling. For example, some alterations include the loss (or gain) of a base, resulting in a frame-shift mutation such that all the codons downstream are now out of their usual sequence of triplets. Other alterations can convert a coding triplet into a stop codon, which tells the cell to end the protein prematurely. DNA alterations can also include multiplication or disappearance of long segments of DNA, which can severely impair (or rarely, augment) protein function.

A genetic polymorphism is a variation in DNA that is inherited in the population at levels high enough that it could not be maintained by random DNA changes alone (conventionally defined as more than 1 percent of the population). Studies of enzyme and protein variability have indicated that in human beings, at least 30 percent of gene loci are polymorphic. Polymorphisms occur with great frequency outside coding regions, where the alterations have little consequence on gene expression.

Genes and Disease Risk

The relative influences of environmental and genetic factors in disease causation is variable and results in a spectrum with diseases that are largely environmentally determined (for example, highly infectious diseases) at one end and genetically determined (for example, severe inherited metabolic disorders) at the other (7). Probably the best known genetic factors that increase risk of disease are the highly penetrant, dominant mutations associated with high disease risks. An example of this type of mutation is breast cancer gene 1 (*BRCA1*) and breast cancer gene 2 (*BRCA2*). Although this type of genetic variation can appreciably increase the individual risk of disease, the public health significance is less clear, because the majority of women who develop breast cancer do not have this mutation or other highly penetrant mutations that have been identified. For example, *BRCA1* and *BRCA2* mutations appear to account for 5.3 percent of breast cancer cases in women younger than 40 years, 2.2 percent of cases in women aged 40 to 49 years, and only 1.1 percent of cases in women aged 50 to 70 years (8). In addition, recent studies in low-risk populations suggest that many women with *BRCA1* or *BRCA2* do not develop breast cancer (8,9).

Compared with highly penetrant, dominant mutations, genetic variants that affect susceptibility to common diseases can have a much greater effect on a population level, even though they may pose relatively low individual risk (10). Although these genes determine susceptibility to diseases such as coronary heart disease, hypertension, diabetes, and some types of cancer, environmental factors (for example, dietary intake) determine who among the susceptible subgroup will develop the associated disease. Table 20.1 gives several examples of known or hypothesized diet-gene interactions.

One intense area of research concerns polymorphisms in genes that code for xenobiotic metabolizing enzymes (for example, cytochromes P450 and glutathione-*S*-transferases), which play an important role in activating and/or detoxifying foreign compounds, such as carcinogens (Figure 20.2). Dietary constituents (including micronutrients and nonnutrient compounds) act as inducing agents through several molecular mechanisms and are well-known substrates of some of these enzymes. Interactions between these enzymes and dietary intake likely play a large role in cancer etiology (11,12). Another area of interest in susceptibility genes includes polymorphisms in apolipoproteins, which influence serum lipid responsiveness to dietary intake and thereby modify the development of cardiovascular disease (12).

Polymorphisms that alter enzyme activities often have high prevalence in the population, so even modestly increased absolute risk can lead to a rather high popula-

TABLE 20.1 Examples of Known and Hypothesized Diet-Gene Interactions

Polymorphism (Gene or *Gene Product*)	Gene Product Function	Environmental Exposure(s) (risk factor)	Associated Condition or Disease (phenotype)
Known Diet-Gene Interactions			
Glucose-6-phosphate dehydrogenase (G6PD)	Metabolism	Fava bean consumption	Hemolytic anemia
Phenylketonuria (PKU) gene	Metabolism of phenylalanine	Dietary phenylalanine	Phenylketonuria
Hemochromatosis (HFE) gene	Iron absorption	Dietary iron	Hemochromatosis
Hypothesized Diet-Gene Interactions			
Glutathione-S-transferase M1 (GSTM1)	Detoxification	Smoking combined with diet low in antioxidants	Lung cancer
Epoxide hydrolase (EH), glutathione-S-transferase M1 (GSTM1)	Detoxification	Consumption of aflatoxin (fungal contaminant, especially of peanuts)	Liver cancer
Apolipoprotein E (Apo E), apolipoprotein B	Lipoprotein metabolism	Dietary cholesterol and fat	Increased responsiveness to dietary cholesterol and fat intake
Methylenetetrahydrofolate reductase (MTHFR)	Metabolism of folate, affecting plasma homocysteine levels	Low folate status, multivitamin nonuse	Coronary heart disease, stroke, colon cancer, and neural tube defects
Leptin (ob) gene	Regulatory hormone	High-fat diet	Obesity

Reprinted with permission from Patterson RE, Eaton EL, Potter JP. The genetic revolution: change and challenge for the profession of dietetics. *J Am Diet Assoc.* 1999;99:1412–1420.

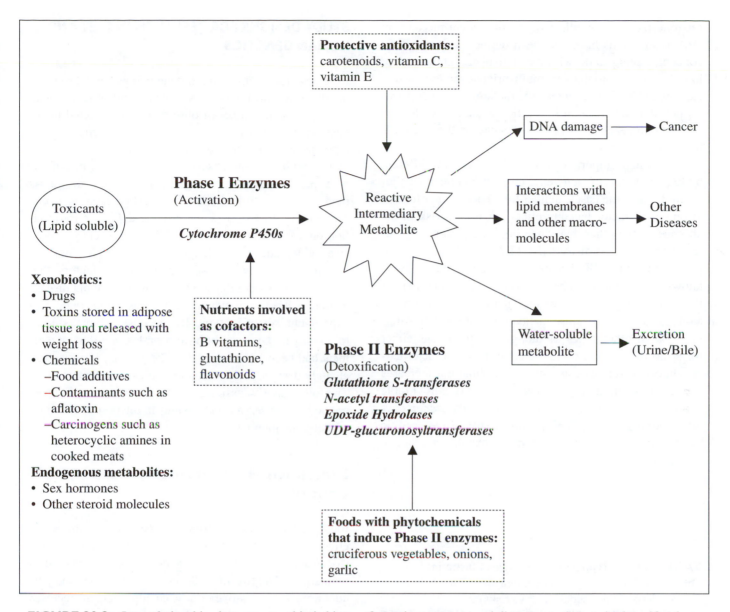

FIGURE 20.2 Interrelationships between xenobiotic biotransformation enzymes and dietary constituents in detoxification pathways. Reprinted with permission from Patterson RE, Eaton EL, Potter JP. The genetic revolution: change and challenge for the profession of dietetics. *J Am Diet Assoc.* 1999;99:1412–1420.

tion-level risk when there is appropriate exposure (3). For example, McWilliams et al conducted a meta-analysis in which they concluded that deficiency of a certain enzyme (glutathione-*S*-transferase M1) results in approximately a 40 percent increased risk of lung cancer among smokers (13). Although the increased risk to an individual is fairly small, both cigarette smoking and the enzyme deficiency are so prevalent that this polymorphism may result in approximately 29,000 new cases of lung cancer each year in the United States.

Diet-Gene Interactions

Several definitions for diet-gene interactions have been proposed. From a biological perspective, interaction between two factors (for example, genotype and dietary intake) has been defined as their co-participation in the same causal mechanism of disease development (14,15). Alternatively, interaction is often thought of as a situation in which joint exposure to two or more factors results in a greater number of cases of diseases than the sum of the separate factors, regardless of the biological mechanism (16). Interactions have also been defined as a statistical concept, having to do with the statistical significance of joint-predictor variables in multivariable models of disease risk (15). This chapter uses the simplest and broadest possible definition of interaction as being two factors that act upon each other (17), in this case in the modification of disease risk.

It is also important to note that there are different biological types of gene-environment interactions. For example, in some cases, neither the genotype nor the environmental factor has any effect on disease risk in the absence of the other, but when both are present, the interaction increases disease risk (Table 20.2a). An example of this kind of diet-gene interaction that is well known to dietitians is phenylketonuria, in which neither the abnormal genotype nor the environmental exposure alone is sufficient to cause mental retardation (18). Alternatively, in other types of diet-gene interactions either (or both) the genotype and the environmental factor carry some risk for disease, but the combination increases disease risk additively or even synergistically (Table 20.2b). The critical point is that the term *interaction* covers a variety of biological phenomena, and the specific form of the interaction is as important as the fact that an interaction exists.

TABLE 20.2   Hypothetical Examples Illustrating Two Difference Types of Diet-Gene Interactions That Increase Disease Risk (expressed as relative risks)

a. Neither dietary intake nor the genotype are independent risk factors, but interaction results in disease risk.

Nutrient Intake	Genotype	
	Wild Type ("normal")	Variant
Low	1.00	1.00
High	1.00	2.00

b. Both dietary intake and the genotype are independent risk factors, and the interaction increases disease risk synergistically.

Nutrient Intake	Genotype	
	Wild Type ("normal")	Variant
Low	1.00	2.00
High	2.00	10.00

STUDY DESIGNS FOR RESEARCH IN DIET AND HUMAN GENETICS

Research studies involving human beings can be roughly divided into two types: experimental and observational. An experiment is a set of observations conducted under controlled circumstances, in which the investigator manipulates the conditions to ascertain what effect such manipulation has on the observations (19). In studies of human beings, the main experimental study design is randomized controlled trials, also called *clinical trials*. These controlled studies can provide definitive information on a research question, but they are usually expensive and logistically challenging. In addition, it is not ethical to knowingly expose individuals to factors that increase their risk of disease simply to learn about disease causation. Therefore, when it is not feasible to conduct an experiment, scientists typically use observational studies to investigate what might have been learned if an experiment had been conducted (19). The primary observational study designs include cohort and case-control studies. The following discussion provides an overview of experimental and observational designs in relation to the study of diet-gene interactions.

Experimental Design: Randomized Controlled Trials

Randomized controlled trials prospectively examine the effect of an exposure (for example, diet) on an outcome (for example, a disease, a risk factor for a disease, or a biomarker). The two main designs are crossover and parallel arm. In a crossover study, each participant receives all test diets in a randomized order. Important considerations regarding crossover designs are the potential for carryover effects and the time between experimental conditions that is necessary to achieve baseline conditions (that is, the washout period). In a parallel-arm design, each participant is assigned at random to only one test diet. and therefore different groups of participants receive different test diets. Each design has advantages and disadvantages related to sample size, duration of the study, and design considerations (20). Both study designs lend themselves to studying diet-gene interactions, so the design should be selected on the basis of the hypothesis being tested.

Another important consideration in the design of an experimental study is the degree of dietary control required. The stringency of dietary control (for example, a controlled diet provided by the investigators versus supplementation of a usual diet versus dietary counseling) is determined in part by the expected size of the response variable of interest and the length of the treatment period required. For instance, if the interindividual variation in the response variable is high (possibly as a result of normal dietary differences), standardizing the diet (for example, by using a controlled feeding study) may improve the capacity to detect an effect of a particular nutrient or dietary constituent. However, if the required dietary treatment period exceeds several months, a controlled feeding study is usually not logistically or financially viable.

Two different approaches to testing gene-diet interactions in randomized controlled trials are used. One approach is to select participants a priori on the basis of genotype. This requires that the investigator identify a candidate genetic polymorphism and have some knowledge or hypothesis regarding the genotype response. In studies of this type, individuals are recruited, genotyped for the polymorphism of interest, and then block randomized to treatment or treatment order by genotype. This design ensures that there is adequate, balanced representation of each genotype, which is especially valuable if the frequency of the polymorphism is low.

Another approach is to select participants for a study, conduct the intervention or feeding study, genotype individuals, and test for diet-gene interactions in the statistical analysis. This approach is feasible in studies with large sample sizes and for polymorphisms that are highly prevalent. For example, if the frequency of a particular genetic variant is 50 percent and the variant (1) does not phenotypically influence eligibility for the study and (2) does not bias willingness to participate in the study, one would expect relatively equal representation of the wild type (that is, the "normal" genotype) and the variant. In contrast, if the variant frequency is low (for example, 10 percent), the distribution may be unbalanced, and it is unlikely that there will be enough individuals with the variant genotype to make it possible to test for the diet-gene interaction.

Clinical trials provide a useful platform for testing effects of genetic polymorphisms in response to particular dietary treatments, and this approach to researching diet-gene interactions is gaining popularity. A clinical trial is a rigorous study design, because participants with factors that might influence the disease or other end point being studied (for example, diet quality, physical activity, or cancer screening behavior) are equally likely to be randomized into the intervention or the control group. However, as is the case with traditional feeding studies, these projects tend to be expensive and labor intensive and therefore may not be feasible.

Observational Design: Epidemiologic Studies

Ideally, the quality of evidence from an observational (nonexperimental) study would be as high as that from a well-designed experiment. However, in an experiment the investigator has the power to assign exposures, whereas in an observational design the investigator cannot control the exposure (19). For example, in a clinical trial the researcher can randomly assign an exposure (for example, vitamin E supplements) versus placebos to participants and thereby feel confident that any observed change in disease risk in the intervention group is solely the result of the supplement. In an observational study the investigator can collect data on self-reported use of vitamin E supplements and then assess whether there appears to be an association of supplement use with disease risk. However, if individuals who use dietary supplements also eat a healthier diet and exercise, any observed association between supplement use and disease risk might also be the result of factors correlated with supplement use (for example, diet and exercise).

A major limitation of all epidemiologic observational studies is the possibility of confounding, in which the exposure of interest is merely a surrogate for a different active agent. Although statistical models that control for confounding factors attempt to address this problem, an absence of confounding cannot be ensured, particularly if important confounding factors are unknown or not measured.

There are two primary types of observational study designs in epidemiology: the cohort study and the case-control study. The basics of these study designs and their application in research on diet-gene interactions will be reviewed.

Cohort Studies

The classic cohort study is a design in which one or more groups of people who are free of disease and who vary in exposure to a potential risk factor (for example, dietary intake) are followed over time and examined with respect to the development of disease. The major advantage of cohort studies is that exposure to potential risk factors is assessed before the development of disease. Therefore, risk factors, such as serum micronutrient concentrations, cannot be influenced by the disease process. In addition, these types of studies can examine many different exposures in relation to many different disease outcomes.

A cohort study is generally a large enterprise, because most diseases affect only a small proportion of a population, even if the population is followed for many years. These studies typically have sample sizes exceeding 50,000, can have a total cost in excess of $100 million, and require that the cohort be followed for at least 10 years (15).

Because of the large size of these studies, the analysis of biological markers (for example, serum micronutrient concentrations or genotype) of all participants is prohibitively expensive. Therefore, these studies typically rely on specimen repositories or frozen banks of substances such as serum, white blood cells, and DNA to conduct future nested case-control studies. In a nested case-control study, a sample of cohort participants who develop a disease, such as breast cancer (cases), are matched to other individuals in the cohort who do not develop the disease (controls). Biological samples from cases and controls are then pulled from the freezer and analyzed for genetic polymorphisms. Statistical analyses are performed to determine whether there are differences in prevalence of the polymorphism and other exposures (such as dietary intake) between the cases and the controls. This design can be efficient and powerful, and it avoids many of the pitfalls of retrospective case-control studies (see the next section).

Case-Control Studies

In a case-control study, individuals are identified and studied according to a single disease outcome. In the classic case-control study, individuals who have recently been diagnosed with a disease (say, colon cancer) are queried about their past exposure to diet and other risk factors, and they often provide a blood sample. A matched set of control individuals, usually drawn from the same population, are also enrolled in the study. The major advantage of this design is that an entire study can be completed in 4 years, typically with as few as 400 cases and 400 controls. However, this design can answer only questions about a single disease outcome. In addition, these studies can introduce biases that are absent in cohort or nested case-control studies.

Two major concerns with case-control studies are recall bias and selection bias. In studies of chronic disease, investigators typically ask participants to recall behaviors and other exposures (for example, dietary intake) from 5 years to 10 years in the past. Bias can occur when individuals in the case group recall exposure to potential risk factors differently than do individuals in the control group. Selection bias can occur when response rates for controls are low, and those controls who agree to participate join the study because of an interest in health and therefore are more likely to practice other healthy behavior (for example, to eat a healthy diet). When this type of selection bias occurs, the higher prevalence of healthy behavior in the controls appears to be associated with reduced risk of disease, when actually it is associated with willingness to participate in a research study on health.

Another problem with case-control studies is that many biomarkers (for example, serum micronutrient concentrations) are affected by the disease process and therefore may not be reliable measures of predisease status (risk) in cases. However genetic polymorphisms are not altered by disease and therefore remain valid markers of individual susceptibility to disease, even in this study design where the cases have already developed the disease of interest.

Sample Size Considerations in Studies of Diet-Gene Interactions

A major concern in all studies of diet-gene interactions is adequate sample size. Interaction effects can be thought of as the identification of subgroups of the population for whom the exposure of interest imparts a particularly high risk. The sample size required to study interactions is dependent upon the percentage of the sample exposed to both the main effects (for example, fat intake and a particular polymorphism), the degree of increased risk conferred by each of the main effects separately, and the increased risk conferred by the interaction (21).

For example, a sample size of approximately 750 cases and 750 controls is required to detect, with reasonable statistical confidence ($\alpha = 0.05$ [one sided], $1 - \beta = 0.95$), a two-fold increased risk among individuals with a variant genotype who are also exposed to a specific diet, assuming no increased risk among those exposed to diet or the genotype alone (see Table 20.2a)—*if* 50 percent of the population is exposed to the genotype (21). If only 10 percent of the population is exposed to the genotype, the minimal study size to detect the interaction effect is approximately 1,800 cases and 1,800 controls.

In general, to detect an interaction effect of the same magnitude as a postulated main effect always requires an increase in the size of a study by a factor of approximately four, and in some circumstances considerably more (21). Therefore, unless a study is designed to test for diet-gene interactions, it is unlikely to have enough power to detect such an interaction; indeed, much of the published literature on diet-gene interactions has that limitation.

TOOLS AND TECHNIQUES: COLLECTING AND ARCHIVING DNA

Several factors related to study logistics and planned use of DNA specimens should be considered when choosing a method of DNA collection and storage. For example, What is the study sample size? Do you need blood for measuring other biomarkers? Where will the DNA specimens be collected? How many assays are you planning to run on the sample? Are you collecting the samples for long-term storage? How are you going to retrieve the samples from storage? Many of these considerations are generic issues that relate to collection and storage of all types of biological specimens for biomarker measurement (see Chapter 17 for a general discussion); however, other issues are DNA specific. Note that information on methods for analyzing polymorphisms are beyond the scope of this chapter; interested readers should refer to recent papers and texts on the topic (22).

Traditionally, DNA for genetic analyses has been extracted from white blood cells (leukocytes) collected from whole blood. This approach yields substantial amounts of DNA (approximately 100 (g DNA from 10 mL whole blood). However, to participants, venipuncture is probably the least attractive method of providing genomic DNA. It is invasive and uncomfortable, is unacceptable to some for cultural or religious reasons, and usually requires that participants come to a central location to have blood drawn. These undesirable aspects of venipuncture mean that participant refusal rates for blood collection can be high (20 percent to 40 percent) (23). In addition, for molecular epidemiologic studies, blood specimen collection is expensive and can be a logistical challenge when sample sizes are large and people are scattered geographically.

For studies where only DNA is needed (in other words, blood samples are not also being collected for plasma), there are other approaches to collecting genom-

ic DNA. Improved sensitivity in molecular biological techniques means that very small quantities of DNA are often sufficient for many assays. Thus, biological samples obtained by less invasive methods, but providing lower yields of DNA, can be sources of DNA for genotyping (Table 20.3). DNA for genetic analysis can be extracted from urine, hair roots, finger-stick blood, saliva, and buccal cells obtained by cheek scraping, brushing, or oral rinsing. Some of these methods are moderately invasive or unpleasant (finger stick, cheek scraping or brushing, and urine collection) or provide lower yields (urine, hair roots, and saliva) or lower-quality DNA (that is, short fragments) (23,24,25).

Tissues obtained at surgery that are fixed and embedded in paraffin provide another source of DNA. The ability to isolate DNA from paraffin-embedded tissues, as well as from serum and plasma, facilitates genetic analysis of archived samples from prospective cohort studies (26); however, the ethical and legal issues of analyzing archived tissues must be addressed, and appropriate institutional review board approval must be obtained. (This topic will be covered in more detail later in the chapter.)

Guidelines for collecting, processing, and banking DNA have been published (26–28). Although the extraction of DNA from fresh samples is optimal, storage of whole blood for up to 3 days at room temperature does not appear to adversely affect DNA recovery (27). This fact provides researchers with some leeway when samples are collected at remote sites and then shipped to a central laboratory for processing.

Currently, DNA is purified from biological samples by one of three major methods that are fast and yield good-quality DNA. These methods include salt precipita-

TABLE 20.3 DNA Yields From Human Tissues and Body Fluids

Biological Specimen	DNA Yield (μg, mean [range])
Whole blood, 10 mL	~100
Serum, 250 μL	0.16–1.06
Plasma, 250 μL	0.16–0.37
Paraffin-embedded tissue, 5- to 20-μm sections	1–11.7
Buccal cells, mouthwash method	49.7 (0.2–134.0)
Buccal cells, 1 swab	1.3
Buccal cells, 10 swabs	32 (3.2–110.8)

Data are from references 23 (whole blood; buccal cells, mouthwash method), 24 (buccal cells, 10 swabs), 25 (buccal cells, 1 swab), and 26 (serum, plasma, paraffin-embedded tissue).

tion (29), phenol/chloroform extraction (30), and solid-phase extraction (31,32). Differences in DNA extraction procedures do not appear to affect DNA yields, which are more influenced by how the blood or tissue is collected and stored (26). Carefully handled lymphocytes obtained from whole blood can be frozen in liquid nitrogen for 20 years or more without losing their viability. Thus, they can be stored and processed at a later date, or they can be immortalized to provide a stable, indefinite source of DNA (33).

Storing or banking DNA offers researchers the option of testing new hypotheses about gene-diet interactions in relation to disease risk many years after the blood or tissue specimen has been collected. The use of DNA banks requires appropriate long-term storage conditions and meticulous record keeping (28).

INFORMED CONSENT ISSUES

Increasing knowledge regarding disease etiology and treatment is generally good for both society and the individuals whose care is improved by more complete understanding of disease (34). Despite the desirability of increased knowledge, however, research can risk harming the individuals who are being studied. Therefore, the legal and ethical precept is that people participate in research only after they have given their informed consent. From the perspective of individuals, consent provides information about the nature of the project and the risks and benefits that accompany participation so that they can decide whether to participate. For the investigator, obtaining informed consent reduces the risk that participants will pursue legal actions when their expectations about the study are not met (34).

Although not unique to genetic research, the issues related to potential discrimination based on genetic profiling, the retrospective use of archived tissue samples, and the adequacy of protections for privacy and confidentiality have triggered public concerns about the pace and scale of technological change (35). Two characteristics of genetic testing make it especially controversial. First, the implications of genetic information are both individual and familial; second, genetic testing often identifies disorders for which there are no effective treatments or preventive measures (36). Obtaining informed consent for genetic testing is particularly challenging in view of the complexity of the genetic information, the controversial nature of clinical options such as abortion or prophylactic

surgery of unknown efficacy, and the social and psychological implications of testing (37).

Informed Consent for Genetic Testing

For conditions in which a polymorphism confers a fairly high risk of developing the associated disease, the consequences of knowledge of genotype are complex. On the basis of family history alone, individuals at risk of relatively uncommon and highly penetrant conditions (for example, Huntington disease) have found it difficult to obtain health insurance and have faced employment discrimination. The ethical response to these concerns has been to mandate detailed informed consent with pretest, and sometimes posttest, counseling of participants (38). However, the paradigm for consent in genetic research may not be appropriate for all applications. For research on common low-risk genotypes, it is not clear that the risks to participants warrant counseling, particularly if little is known about the risk of the genotype. Hunter and Caporasa have suggested that, as in most other aspects of research, the level of consent should be proportional to the degree of risk involved, and thus less stringent consent procedures may be appropriate for low-risk genotypes than for high-risk genotypes (38).

Informed Consent for Genetic Research on Stored Tissue Samples

It is widely accepted that individuals must provide informed consent for projects that involve their direct involvement. However, the role of informed consent is much less clear for research that does not require such personal involvement, but rather can be performed using stored tissue samples.

From a historical perspective, the use of banked serum samples in the study of both chronic and infectious disease has a long and distinguished history in public health and medicine (39). Many important studies in these areas came about only after stored samples provided the material to test hypotheses that could not have been formulated at the time of specimen collection. Similarly, genetic research is evolving rapidly, and most hypotheses will emerge because of future research. Suggestions have been made that specific informed consent be required for all genetic testing (34). If it were necessary to recontact participants, however, most studies could not be performed. Recontacting participants would be prohibitively expensive and time-consuming, and it would be impossible to reach many participants because they had moved or died. In addition, this process has the potential to introduce bias, making the research findings less valid. One approach to this dilemma is asking participants to approve genetic testing of their biological samples on the condition that all identifying information be removed. The results of these tests could not be matched to the individual participant in the study, at any time or by any investigator. However, even this procedure is controversial (34).

Summary: Informed Consent and Genetic Testing

The current regulations regarding genetic testing are unclear, and expert groups offer conflicting advice. A survey of informed consent forms from seven different testing facilities found that the forms demonstrated substantial variation in content and organization (40), indicating that the institutional approaches to these questions can vary substantially. It is critical that the debate on measures to prevent the misuse of genetic information in research be conducted by scientists and professional societies. Otherwise, well-intentioned, but ill-informed, efforts to protect the rights of individuals and groups could hurt everyone by blocking the progress of research.

RESEARCH OUTLOOK

Research on diet-gene interactions can greatly improve our understanding of the influence of nutrition factors on risks for common diseases. If only a subgroup of individuals is sensitive to dietary factors, the effect on disease risk may be diluted, or even undetectable, when the entire population is the focus of study. Continued research in this area will also clarify the underlying mechanisms of many nutrition factors by delineating their biological roles in relation to variations in enzyme activity. Eventually, increased knowledge will allow us to target disease-preventing diet interventions to individuals most likely to benefit by diet modification, based on their genetic susceptibility.

In spite of the substantial potential benefits in this area of study, there are also notable constraints:

- There are substantial challenges involved in accurately identifying and characterizing exposures to nutrition factors in epidemiologic studies, and even the best methods for nutrition and dietary assessment used in population-based research have well-known limitations and weaknesses (41).
- Given the potential importance of recently recognized phytochemicals (for example, isoflavones) in diet-gene interactions, considerable research is needed to improve our understanding of the bioavailability and other pharmacokinetic properties of these compounds; exacerbating the problem is the fact that in most cases, a food content database that would allow quantification of intake of these compounds is not available.
- Biomarkers and biological assays that are used to characterize the susceptibility of individuals based on genetic variation must be readily available, at low cost, with demonstrated and understood validity in the targeted populations.
- Studies must be carefully designed so that sample sizes are large enough to detect diet-gene interaction effects.

Even at this early stage of research, evidence suggests that diet-gene interactions are likely to contribute considerably to the observed individual variation in disease risk in response to nutrition factors (11). In the future, we will be able to define more precisely the molecular mechanisms underlying human health and disease; subdivide clinically indistinguishable diseases and conditions (for example, obesity) into more distinct entities, thereby improving our ability to choose rational preventive and treatment measures; identify genotypic markers that predict metabolic responses to dietary interventions; stratify the population into groups at higher or lower risk of chronic diseases such as cancer, allowing dietary intervention to be appropriately targeted; and develop dietary recommendations that take into account genetically determined taste preferences (12). Diet-gene interactions represents an exciting and important new interdisciplinary research area for dietitians in collaboration with epidemiologists and molecular scientists.

REFERENCES

1. Khoury MJ. Genetic epidemiology. In: Rothman K, Greenland S, eds. *Modern Epidemiology*. 2nd ed. Boston, Mass: Little, Brown, and Company; 1998.
2. American Cancer Society. *Cancer Facts and Figures 1995*. Atlanta, Ga: ACS; 1995.

3. Eaton DL, Farina F, Omiecinski CJ, Omenn GS. Genetic susceptibility. In: Rom William N, ed. *Environmental and Occupational Medicine*. 3rd ed. Philadelphia, Pa: Lippincott-Raven; 1998:209–221.

4. Mueller RF, Young ID. *Emery's Elements of Medical Genetics*. 9th ed. New York, NY: Churchill Livingstone; 1995.

5. Alberts B, Bray D, Lewis J, Raff M, Roberts K, Watson JD. *Molecular Biology of The Cell*. 3rd ed. New York, NY: Garland Publishing Inc; 1994.

6. Ewing B, Green B. Analysis of expressed sequence tags indicated 35,000 human genes. *Nat Genet*. 2000;25:232–234.

7. Garte S, Zocchetti C, Taioli E. Gene-environmental interactions in the application of biomarkers of cancer susceptibility in epidemiology. In: Toniolo P, Boffetta P, Shuker DEG, Rothman N, Hulka B, Pearce N, eds. *Applications of Biomarkers in Cancer Epidemiology*. Lyon, France: IARC Scientific Publications; 1997. Publication 142.

8. Sellers TA. Genetic factors in the pathogenesis of breast cancer: their role and relative importance. *J Nutr*. 1997;127(suppl 5):929–932.

9. Malone KE, Daling JR, Thompson JD, O'Brien CA, Francisco LV, Ostrander EA. BRCA1 mutations and breast cancer in the general population: analyses in women before age 35 years and in women before age 45 years with first-degree family history. *JAMA*. 1998;279:922–929.

10. Perera FP. Environment and cancer: who are susceptible? *Science*. 1997;278:1068–1073.

11. Rock C, Lampe J, Patterson RE. Nutrition, genetics, and risks of cancer. *Annu Rev Public Health*. 2000;21:47–64.

12. Patterson RE, Eaton DL, Potter JP. The Genetic Revolution: change and challenge for the profession of dietetics. *J Am Diet Assoc*. 1999;99:1412–1420.

13. McWilliams JE, Sanderson BJS, Harris EL, Richert-Boe KE, Henner WD. Glutathione *S*-transferase M1 (GSTM1) deficiency and lung cancer risk. *Cancer Epidemiol Biomarkers Prev*. 1995;4:589–594.

14. Yang Q, Khoury MJ. Evolving methods in genetic epidemiology. III. Gene-environment interaction in epidemiologic research. *Epidemiol Rev*. 1997;19:33–43.

15. Rothman KJ. Types of epidemiologic studies. In: Rothman KJ. *Modern Epidemiology*. Boston, Mass: Little, Brown, and Company; 1986.

16. Blot WJ, Day NE. Synergism and interaction: are they equivalent. *Am J Epidemiol*. 1979;110:99–100.

17. Flexner SB, Hauck LC, eds. *The Random House Dictionary of the English Language*. 2nd ed. New York, NY: Random House; 1987.

18. Elsas LJ, Acosta PB. Nutrition support of inherited metabolic disease. In: Shils ME, Olson JA, Shike M, eds. *Modern Nutrition in Health and Disease*. 8th ed. Philadelphia, Pa: Lea & Febiger; 1994.

19. Rothman KJ, Greenland S. Types of epidemiologic studies. In: Rothman K, Greenland S, eds. *Modern Epidemiology*. 2nd ed. Boston, Mass: Little, Brown, and Company; 1998.

20. Derr JA. Statistical aspects of controlled diet studies. In: Dennis BH, Ershow AG, Obarzanek E, Clevidence BA, eds. *Well-Controlled Diet Studies in Humans: A Practical Guide to Design and Management*. Chicago, Ill: The American Dietetic Association; 1997.

21. Smith PG, Day NE. The design of case-control studies: the influence of confounding and interaction effect. *Int J Epidemiol*. 1984;13:356–365.

22. Burczak JD, Mardis E, eds. *Polymorphism Detection and Analysis*. Natick, Mass: BioTechniques Books Publication, Eaton Publishing Company; 2000.

23. Lum A, Le Marchand L. A simple mouthwash method for obtaining genomic DNA in molecular epidemiological studies. *Cancer Epidemiol Biomarkers Prev*. 1998;7:719–724.

24. Meulenbelt I, Droog S, Trommelen GJM, Boomsma D I, Slagboom P E. High-yield noninvasive human genomic DNA isolation method for genetic studies in geographically dispersed families and populations. *Am J Hum Genet*. 1995;57:1252–1254.

25. Freeman B, Powell J, Ball D, Hill L, Craig I, Plomin R. DNA by mail: an inexpensive and noninvasive method for collecting DNA samples from widely dispersed populations. *Behav Genet*. 1997;27:251–257.

26. Blomeke B, Bennett WP, Harris CC, Shields PG. Serum, plasma, and paraffin-embedded tissues as sources of DNA for studying cancer susceptibility genes. *Carcinogenesis*. 1997;18:1271–1275.

27. Austin MA, Ordovas JM, Eckfeldt JH, et al. Guidelines of the National Heart, Lung, and Blood Institute Working Group on blood drawing, processing, and storage for genetic studies. *Am J Epidemiol*. 1996;5:437–441.

28. Yates JR, Malcolm S, Read AP. Guidelines for DNA banking. Report of the Clinical Genetics Society working party on DNA banking. *J Med Genet*. 1989;26:245–50.

29. Miller SA, Dykes DD, Polesky HF. A simple salting out procedure for extracting DNA from human nucleated cells. *Nucleic Acids Res*. 1988;16:1215.

30. Strauss WM. Preparation of genomic DNA from mammalian tissue. In: Ausubel FM, Brent R, Kingston RE, et al, eds. *Current Protocols in Molecular Biology, Vol. 1. Molecular Biology—Technique*. New York, NY: John Wiley & Sons Inc; 1998.

31. Hawkins TL, O'Connor-Morin T, Roy A, Santillan C. DNA purification and isolation using a solid-phase. *Nucleic Acids Res*. 1994;22:4543–4544.

32. McCormick RM. A solid-phase extraction procedure for DNA purification. *Anal Biochem*. 1989;181:66–74.

33. Louie LG, King MC. A novel approach to establishing permanent lymphoblastoid cell lines: Epstein-Barr virus

transformation of cryopreserved lymphocytes. *Am J Hum Genet.* 1991;69:383–387.

34. Clayton EW, Steinberg KK, Khoury MJ, et al. Informed consent for genetic research on stored tissue samples [Consensus Statement]. *JAMA.* 1995;274:1786–1792.

35. Fears R, Poste G. Building population genetics resources using the UK NHS. *Science.* 1999;284:267–268.

36. Burgess MM. Beyond consent: ethical and social issues in genetic testing. *Nat Rev Genet.* 2001;2:147–151.

37. Burgess MM, Laberge C, Knoppers BM. Bioethics for clinicians: 14. Ethics and genetics in medicine. *Can Med Assoc J.* 1998;158:1309–1313.

38. Hunter D, Caporaso N. Informed consent in epidemiologic studies involving genetic markers. *Epidemiol.* 1997;8:596–599.

39. Kelsey KT. Informed consent for genetic research [letter]. *JAMA.* 1996;275:1085.

40. Durfy SJ, Buchanan TE, Burke W. Testing for inherited susceptibility to breast cancer: a survey of informed consent forms for BRCA1 and BRCA2 mutation testing. *Am J Med Genet.* 1998;75:82–87.

41. Willett W. *Nutritional Epidemiology.* 2nd ed. Oxford, England: Oxford University Press; 1998.

21

Behavioral Theory–Based Research

Geoffrey W. Greene, Ph.D., R.D., L.D.N., and Alma J. Blake, Ph.D., R.D.

This chapter discusses the importance of behavioral theory–based research, provides guidelines on using theories in nutrition research, and describes the practical aspects of conducting research based on commonly used behavioral theories. The material is only an introduction to the behavioral theories and is not intended as a comprehensive review (1). The more established theories, such as the health belief model, social cognitive theory, and reciprocal determinism, are discussed only briefly, because they are extensively reviewed in the literature. In contrast, the newer theories—the theory of reasoned action, the theory of planned behavior, and the transtheoretical (stages-of-change) model—are discussed in greater depth to provide researchers with a better understanding of how to apply them.

IMPORTANCE OF BEHAVIORAL THEORY–BASED RESEARCH

Theory describes the mechanisms of how attitudes and beliefs related to diet and health influence behavior. Theories consist of a set of variables in a specified relationship (2). Research based on a theory involves measuring variables and, depending on the study design, using interventions designed to affect those variables (3). Describing these mechanisms and relationships is critical for behavioral science to be seen as scientifically rigorous. Behavioral theory–based research guides an orderly investigation of these mechanisms and relationships, which results in a better understanding of how people change from high-risk to health-promoting dietary behavior.

By increasing understanding of the basic mechanisms, behavioral theory–based research has the potential for increasing the efficiency and efficacy of interventions for both individuals and populations. This potential also exists in qualitative research, where theory provides a starting place and a framework for qualitative designs (which may generate new or revised theories) (4), and in quantitative research, where theory provides validated instruments measuring key variables associated with behavior change (2). Thus, researchers can avoid "reinventing the wheel." If properly conducted, theory–based research will produce meaningful results, both positive and negative, as well as study findings that are more easily interpretable. Theory-based research facilitates funding or approval of a thesis, as well as publishing research results.

Most theories used in nutrition have been applied to behavior change for health promotion. However, these theories may be applied to behavior change in clinical and management situations as well. The health belief model has defined *perceived severity* as a key variable predicting change. For example, if a patient does not believe that his "touch of diabetes" is likely to affect his health, he won't be motivated to change his diet. Increasing this patient's awareness of his risk for diabetic complications may increase his motivation to change.

Similarly, the stages-of-change model has been applied to organizational change (5). Key variables in this model are *stage of change* and *decisional balance*. If a worksite is in the "contemplation stage" and employees perceive the disadvantages to change as being greater than the benefits, they are likely to resist change. The model suggests that management prepare for change by explaining to employees how the change will benefit them and providing mechanisms for employee input in solving or reducing problems.

GUIDELINES FOR APPLICATION OF THEORIES IN RESEARCH

Theories lay out the big picture and are defined in terms of constructs. For example, the health belief model postulates that people change those behaviors that are threatening if the perceived benefits are greater than the perceived barriers or costs of change. Perceived benefits and barriers are key constructs in this model, as well as other models (see Table 21.1). Similarly, social cognitive theory suggests that a person's belief that he or she can change a behavior (the construct of self-efficacy) is critically important in the decision to change.

Constructs are abstract concepts that cannot be measured directly. They need to be made concrete (operationalized) by variables that can be measured. In general, variables are measured by a set of questions on a questionnaire (instrument). Individual questions are called *items*. At least three to five items that are highly correlated (that is, that have a Chronbach $\alpha > .7$) will provide a relatively stable measurement of a construct, provided that expert opinion has determined that the set of items is a valid representation of the construct (6,7). Constructs

should be measured using only validated instruments, and the instruments must be selected or developed and tested with the target population prior to the study. Although each theory develops its own constructs, several constructs are analogous across different theories (see Table 21.1).

The researcher should start by selecting the theory best suited for his or her goals and study it thoroughly. The second step is to define the research question in terms of the theory (for example, the intervention will test the efficacy of a theory–based intervention, the survey will assess key constructs of a theory, or the study will develop/validate instruments measuring constructs). The third step is to clearly define dependent variables (for example, the percentage of energy from fat or servings of fruits and vegetables in a day). Key dependent variables may be called *primary outcomes*. In addition to primary outcome variables, the researcher can use constructs as intermediate outcome variables. Thus, even if the primary outcome goal of dietary change is not attained, the researcher can identify change in intermediate outcomes (for example, an increase in motivational readiness to change). A fourth step is to define the independent variables (for example, the intervention group). The final step for experimental studies is to determine the expected effect size (the amount of change in the dependent variable due to the independent variable) in order to conduct statistical power calculations for the estimation of sample size (8). In general, previous studies based on the theory can provide an estimate of the effect size.

In addition to outcome analyses, researchers can conduct correlational analyses looking at the relationships between constructs. They also can conduct process-to-outcome analyses looking at the proportion of the variance in the dependent variable that can be explained by a

TABLE 21.1   Similarities in Key Constructs by Behavioral Theory[a]

Construct	Theory			
	Health Belief Model	Social Cognitive Theory	Theory of Reasoned Action	Transtheoretical (Stages-of-Change) Model
Self-efficacy	*	Self-efficacy	*	Confidence/temptation
Benefits	Perceived benefits	Positive outcome expectancies	Positive attitudes toward behavior	Pros
Barriers	Perceived barriers	Negative outcome expectancies	Positive attitudes toward behavior	Cons

[a]The health belief model postulates (in part) that people change behavior if the perceived benefits are greater than the perceived costs. Perceived benefits and costs are constructs. Similarly, social cognitive theory suggests that a person's belief that he or she can change a behavior (the construct of self-efficacy) is critically important in the decision to change. This table lists what analogous constructs are called in the four theories.

*Although not part of the original theory, this construct has been added by some researchers (1).

construct [r^2]. Cohen (8) defined a large effect in the behavioral sciences as an effect that explains at least 14 percent of the variance in outcome. However, the lack of precision in the assessment of dietary intake usually attenuates the effect size (9). Nevertheless, from a public health perspective, even a relatively small change in diet can have enormous economic and social significance. Ostler and Thompson (10), for example, estimated that decreasing saturated fat intake by 1 percent of energy would reduce the incidence of cardiac events by 32,000 per year for a savings of $4.1 billion.

USING MAJOR BEHAVIORAL THEORIES

Health Belief Model

The first theory in health behavior was the health belief model (11), which was developed more than 4 decades ago (12–14). The health belief model hypothesizes that individuals are more likely to change behavior if they perceive that (1) they are threatened by an adverse health condition and (2) the change will provide greater benefits than costs. The health belief model is defined by the constructs of perceived susceptibility, perceived severity, perceived benefits, and perceived barriers. Perceived susceptibility measures a person's belief in his or her vulnerability to the adverse health condition (How likely is it that you will get it?). Perceived severity measures a person's belief in the severity of the adverse health condition if he or she does get it. The construct of perceived benefits measures a person's belief in the efficacy of the behavior change both to reduce the threats and to provide other benefits. The construct of perceived barriers measures a person's evaluation of the cost or problems associated with behavior change.

One of the difficulties in using this theory is the necessity of developing instruments measuring the constructs for the specific health problem in the target population. Other difficulties arise when there is little variance in the constructs (for example, cancer is considered by most people to have extremely severe health consequences). The strength of the model is in identifying and measuring perceived threat as an important mediating variable in predicting how people respond to perceived benefits and barriers. This model was one of the first to define benefits and barriers and how these constructs may affect change. These constructs are generally believed to be associated with behavior, as demonstrated in Table 21.1. In the past, the health belief model has not been credited with success

in explaining dietary behavior change (13). However, recent data suggest that the magnitude of the correlation between its constructs and dietary variables is similar to that of other theories (15,16).

Social Cognitive Theory and Reciprocal Determinism

Bandura initiated development of the social cognitive theory in 1962, defined principles of behavior modification (an application of the theory) in 1969, added the construct of self-efficacy in 1977, and broadened the scope for population-based interventions in 1978 with reciprocal determinism (17–22). Social cognitive theory postulates that behavior is not random but is a predictable result of antecedents and consequences that either increase or decrease the likelihood that the behavior will be repeated. However, the constructs of self-efficacy (the confidence one has to perform a particular behavior) and outcome expectancies (the anticipated positive and negative consequences) modulate this effect. New behaviors can be learned and old ones extinguished. The overall goal of an intervention is to increase the likelihood of performance of the health-promoting behavior and minimize the likelihood of the risky health behavior. Interventions focus on skills training designed to break down complex behaviors into small steps to maximize the chance of success and to provide practice in learning new behaviors. Practice and success will increase self-efficacy and create positive outcome expectancies.

Using social cognitive theory for individual change, a process referred to as *cognitive behavior modification,* involves behavioral analysis and the design of a specific, individualized intervention (18). Social cognitive theory has been successfully used in group treatment for weight control following a one-size-fits-all type of approach (23). However, this approach has been less successful with minority groups and groups with literacy deficits (23).

Reciprocal determinism broadens the application from group to community (21). A strength of reciprocal determinism is that it focuses on the reciprocal relationship between person, environment, and behavior. A person influences the environment and in turn is influenced by the environment. Environmental interventions can increase positive outcome expectancies, as well as increase "positive" antecedents (16,21,22,24). Social cognitive theory and reciprocal determinism have been used in a variety of community-based interventions with mixed results. Despite early promise, community-based interventions involving over 600,000 participants found no consistent results (25), and there was no effect found for a 15–year, school-based smoking cessation intervention in 40 school districts (26). In contrast, involving parents in school-based interventions has been successful in promoting dietary change in children (27) and increasing the availability of fruits and vegetables, which is critical in increasing children's intake (28). Although the translation of social cognitive theory and reciprocal determinism from the individual and group to the community has been disappointing, many of the constructs in these theories have proved important predictors of behavior; for example, self-efficacy has consistently been identified as a key moderating or intermediate outcome variable (16,29–32).

Theory of Reasoned Action and Theory of Planned Behavior

The theory of reasoned action, developed in 1967 by Fishbein and Ajzen (33,34) and modified in 1980 (35), proposes that behavior change is ultimately the result of changes in beliefs. Therefore, to influence behavior, people need to be exposed to information, which will change their beliefs (36). A strength of the theory of reasoned action is that it facilitates deciphering actions by identifying, measuring, and combining beliefs that are relevant to individuals or groups in making decisions about health. Behavioral beliefs and normative beliefs are linked to behavioral intention and behavior by attitude and subjective norm (Figure 21.1), resulting in the following equation (34,35):

Behavior = Behavioral intention

= Attitude + Subjective norm

The theory of reasoned action is unique in its potential for extension with the addition of sensory factors, such as taste and texture, to the link between attitude, subjective norm, and behavior, making the theory particularly attractive to food scientists (37–42).

The theory of reasoned action assumes that (1) human beings are usually quite rational and consider the implications of their actions and (2) most actions of social relevance are under volitional control, and therefore a person's intention is the immediate determinant of the action (34,35). However, many researchers have added the use of measured behavior in the model to confirm intention (37–40).

A study by Brewer and coworkers (39), investigating the ability to predict consumption of four milk types (whole, reduced fat, low fat, and nonfat) by adult females, provides an example of the extended theory of reasoned action. The researchers added components measuring milk consumption and sensory attributes leading to a modified equation:

Behavior = Behavioral intention

= Attitude + Sensory score + Subjective norm

Constructs were represented with three to six items, which were assessed on a 7-point Likert scale.

The *attitude (A)* is the learned predisposition to respond in a consistently favorable or unfavorable manner toward an object or an act and is the sum of the *salient*

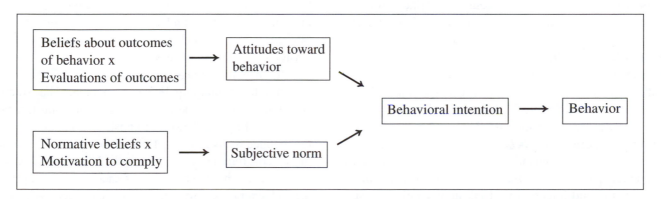

FIGURE 21.1 Model of the theory of reasoned action. Reprinted with permission from Brewer J, Blake AJ, Rankin SA, Douglass LW. The Theory of Reasoned Action predicts milk consumption in females. *J Am Diet Assoc.* 1999;99:30–44.

beliefs (b$_i$) about the outcomes, which is multiplied by the *evaluations (e$_i$)* of whether these outcomes are important to the individual:

$$A = \Sigma b_i e_i$$

Health-related belief item scores for nonfat and low-fat milk were significantly higher than scores for reduced-fat and whole milk, but the opposite was found for taste-related scales. That is, milk drinkers preferred the taste of higher fat milks. Nevertheless, evaluation scores (importance to the individual) were highest for health-related belief items. Therefore, overall attitude scores were higher for nonfat and low-fat milk than for reduced-fat or whole milk.

The *subjective norm (SN)* is the individual's perception of social pressure to perform a particular behavior. It is the product of the *normative beliefs (NB$_j$)*, which is what specific people or groups of people think the individual should do multiplied by the individual's *motivation to comply (MC$_j$)*, or how much the individual wishes to comply with his or her normative influences:

$$SN = \Sigma NB_j MC_j$$

The theory of reasoned action assumes a multiplicative relationship. That is, the likelihood and desirability of each outcome should be multiplied and their products added, reflecting the assumption that threats will be ignored if either severity or their likelihood and desirability is zero (40). Because *SN* did not have a significant effect in this study, it was omitted in the overall predictive equation.

The hedonic testing protocol produced a *sensory score* evaluating the taste of four milks under blinded taste testing according to the attributes of overall appeal/liking using a 9-point Likert scale (1 = Like extremely to 9 = Dislike extremely). Whole milk was liked by subjects significantly more than nonfat and low-fat milk. However, sensory scores contributed minimally to the final equation (Figure 21.2).

Behavioral intention (BI) is the likelihood that a person will perform the *behavior (B)*, which was defined as milk intake or avoidance measured by a dairy product frequency questionnaire. Intention was a strong predictor of behavior, and intention to drink nonfat milk was significantly higher than intention to drink the other milks. Therefore, it appears that health concerns prevailed over

beliefs about taste and sensory scores in determining milk choice by milk drinkers.

The final equation in the study was as follows:

Behavior = Behavioral intention

= Attitude + Sensory score

Figure 21.2 shows that the regression model with behavior of "milk as a beverage" as the dependent variable explained 67 percent of the variability for nonfat milk use, 45 percent for low-fat milk use, 60 percent for reduced-fat milk use, and 67 percent for whole milk use. Correlational analyses between variables showed that attitudes for all milks correlated significantly with behavioral intention; however, the standardized regression coefficients were higher for nonfat and low-fat milk (Figure 21.2). Key findings in this study were that (1) the model was the strongest in predicting whether an individual would use whole or nonfat milk, (2) intention was a strong indicator of actual milk intake behavior as reported in the dairy frequency questionnaire, and (3) attitudes and beliefs about health outweighed the sensory response in milk drinkers.

The model seems best suited for studying specific behavior, such as drinking low-fat milk or eating low-nutrient snacks (38–40), as well as single food/nutrient consumption behavior, such as consumption of high-fat food, sugar, or milk (16,41–45). The theory of reasoned action does not specify particular beliefs about a behavior. Therefore, it is necessary to generate items for the model based on formative research (elicitation interviews) unless items have previously been validated for the target population and behavior (34,35,39).

The theory of reasoned action does not deal with behavior that is not under volitional control. In an effort to account for factors outside the individual's control that may affect intention and behavior, Ajzen and Madden (46) developed the theory of planned behavior as an extension of the theory of reasoned action. The theory is insightful in that it covers more diverse motivational factors (beliefs) for explaining decision making. The authors added the concept of perceived behavioral control, which is measured by the following constructs: (1) *control belief*, defined as likelihood of occurrence of each facilitating or constraining condition, and (2) *perceived power*, defined as the perceived effect of each condition in making behavioral performance difficult or easy. Although these additions reflect important concepts, they have not been fully validated (16,36,47,48)

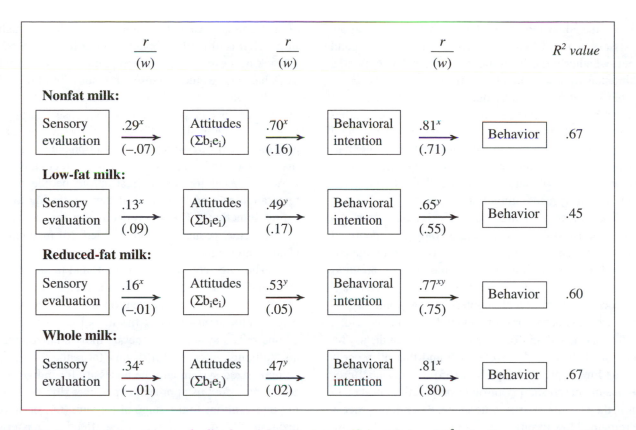

FIGURE 21.2 Correlations (r), standardized partial regression coefficients (w), and R^2 value for components of the Ajzen and Fishbein model (35). Correlation coefficients above 0.47 are significant at $P < .0001$, and correlation coefficients above 0.29 are significant at $P < .001$. Values in a column with the same superscript do not differ significantly. Reprinted with permission from Brewer J, Blake AJ, Rankin SA, Douglass LW. The Theory of Reasoned Action predicts milk consumption in females. *J Am Diet Assoc.* 1999;99:39–44.

Transtheoretical (Stages-of-Change) Model

During the last 2 decades, the transtheoretical model, also known as the stages-of-change model, has become one of the most influential theoretical models for health-related behavior change. The model consists of four dimensions: the central organizing construct, stage of change (the temporal dimension), and the three additional dimensions of decisional balance, self-efficacy (or temptation), and process of change (49,50). Of these four dimensions, stages of change is the most widely researched dimension; during the last decade, decisional balance and self-efficacy also have received considerable attention. The least-investigated dimension is process of change.

Stage of change is the temporal dimension of motivational readiness to change a health behavior. The stages are as follows: precontemplation (no intention of changing in the foreseeable future), contemplation (intending to change, but not soon), preparation (intending to change within the next few weeks), action (recent change), and maintenance (maintaining change). Stage defines when change occurs and can be used in interventions to show individuals where they are in the change process. Like all dimensions of the model, stage is a dynamic variable, and people are expected to move from one stage to another. Although stage change is sometimes conceptualized as linear, a spiral appears to best express stage movement because of the dynamic nature of change. For example, regressing from preparation or action to an earlier stage is just as likely as progressing to the next stage (50,51). In the area of smoking cessation, self-changers averaged three serious quit attempts (action stage) over 7 years before succeeding (50).

Developing a good staging algorithm is critical to all applications of the model. However, to measure stage, it is necessary to define the target behavior and the criterion for effective action (52). Once the criterion is defined, the algorithm should be constructed to allow self-assessment of whether the criterion has been met and if met, whether it has been met for longer than 6 months (maintenance) or less than 6 months (action). If the criterion has not been met, individuals should have an idea of the amount of change necessary to meet the criterion (behavioral distance) in order to assess whether they intend to change in the next month (preparation), they intend to change in the next 6 months (contemplation), or they have no intention of changing to meet the criterion in the next 6 months (precontemplation) (53,54).

The stages-of-change model originated from an analysis of 18 systems of psychotherapy that identified common processes of change (49). Processes are the covert and overt activities that people use to progress through the stages; they are *how* people change. Experiential processes focus on thoughts, feelings, and experiences, whereas behavioral processes focus on behaviors, social support, and reinforcement. In a study of dietary fat reduction, Greene and coworkers found that all process use was low in precontemplation (55). Experiential process use increased sharply through preparation, peaked in action, then decreased in maintenance. Behavioral process use remained low through contemplation, and it then rose sharply and linearly through action before decreasing in maintenance.

Decisional balance measures the balance or relative importance to the individual of the pros (advantages or benefits) and cons (disadvantages, barriers, or costs) of change. Prochaska and colleagues (56) found that for 12 health behaviors, including dietary fat reduction, pros had to outweigh cons for all behaviors before action. Progress from precontemplation to action required an increase in the pros of approximately 1 standard deviation (57). This progress was associated with a decrease in the cons of approximately half a standard deviation. Shifting decisional balance so that pros outweigh cons appears to be important in explaining why people make a commitment to change behavior in the near future.

The self-efficacy construct represents situation-specific confidence people have that they can engage in the desired behavior change; it is usually operationalized in interventions as confidence (58). This construct was adapted from Bandura's self-efficacy theory (20). The converse of confidence is situation-specific temptation (for example, how tempted a person feels to eat high-fat foods across different situations). Both confidence and temptation have the same measurement structure, with three distinct factors: positive social occasions, negative

affective situations, and challenging situations (situations in which it is difficult to obtain low-fat foods) (58,59). In a smoking cessation study, temptation predicted which self-changers would relapse and start smoking again (58). For dietary fat reduction, Greene found that temptation was low in precontemplation, rose sharply to a peak in contemplation, dipped slightly in preparation, and then declined somewhat in action and sharply in maintenance (55). The low values in precontemplation may be typical for dietary restriction; people perceive temptation as a problem only if they are trying to avoid eating something. The sharp decline in maintenance illustrates the reduced effort needed to maintain the change after 6 months.

The stage construct has been found to be an important predictor of change in several intervention studies (31,60–65). Tailoring intervention materials to stage as well as other constructs of the model is possible using computerized systems to generate individualized materials. Although effective for dietary fat reduction (63), the computerized system and the necessity for individual assessment make this approach expensive. However, tailoring interventions to the stage of a group (64) or an organization (5) has been found to be effective. It is critical for all applications of the model that a good staging algorithm be used. The algorithm should include a behavioral criterion for action or maintenance; a method of self-assessment, so individuals can identify intention to change in the future; and ideally, a method for self-assessment of the behavioral distance required to meet the criterion.

REFERENCES

1. Glanz K, Lewis FM, Rimer B, eds. *Health Behavior and Health Education: Theory, Research, Practice.* 2nd ed. San Francisco, Calif: Jossey Bass Publishers; 1997.
2. Glanz K, Lewis FM, Rimer B. Linking Theory, Research, and Practice. In: Glanz K, Lewis FM, Rimer B, eds. *Health Behavior and Health Education: Theory, Research, Practice.* 2nd ed. San Francisco, Calif: Jossey Bass Publishers; 1997: 19-35.
3. Guthrie JF. Quantitative nutrition education research: approaches, findings, outlook. *J Nutr.* 1994; 124(suppl):1814–1819.
4. Kirby S, Baranowski T, Reynolds K, Taylor G, Binkley D. Children's fruit and vegetable intake: socioeconomic, adult child, regional, and urban-rural influences. *J Nutr Educ.* 1995;27:261–271.

5. Prochaska JM. A transtheoretical model approach to organizational change: family service agencies' movement to time-limited therapy. *Fam Soc.* 2000;81:76–84.

6. DeVellis RF. *Scale Development: Theory and Applications.* Newbury Park, Calif: Sage Publications; 1991.

7. Spector PE. *Summated Rating Scale Construction: An Introduction.* Newbury Park, Calif Sage; 1992.

8. Cohen J. *Statistical Power Analysis for the Behavioral Sciences.* Rev ed. New York, NY: Academic Press; 1977.

9. Gibson R. *Principles of Nutrition Assessment.* New York, NY: Oxford University Press; 1990.

10. Ostler G, Thompson D. Estimated effects of reducing dietary saturated fat on the incidence and costs of coronary heart disease in the United States. *J Am Diet Assoc.* 1996;96:127-131.

11. Becker MH, ed. *The Health Belief Model and Personal Behavior.* Thorofore, NJ: C. B. Flack; 1974.

12. Rosenstock IM. Historical origins of the health belief model. *Health Educ Monogr.* 1974;12:328–335.

13. Strecher VJ, Rosenstock IM. The Health Belief Model. In: Glanz K, Lewis FM, Rimer B, eds. *Health Behavior and Health Education: Theory, Research, Practice.* 2nd ed. San Francisco, Calif: Jossey Bass Publishers; 1997: 41–59.

14. Janz NK, Becker MH. The health belief model. A decade later. *Health Educ Q.* 1984;11:1–47.

15. Kloeblen AS. Folate knowledge, intake from fortified grain products, and periconceptional supplementation patterns of a sample of low-income pregnant women according to the Health Belief Model. *J Am Diet Assoc.* 1999;99:33–38.

16. Baranowski T, Cullen K, Baranowski J. Psychosocial correlates of dietary intake: advancing dietary intervention. *Ann Rev Nutr.* 1999;19:17–40.

17. Bandura A. Social Learning Through Imitation. In: Jones MR, ed. *Nebraska Symposium on Motivation.* Vol 10. Lincoln, Neb: University of Nebraska Press; 1962.

18. Bandura A. *Principles of Behavior Modification.* Austin, Tex: Holt, Rinehart, and Winston; 1969.

19. Bandura A. *Social Learning Theory.* Englewood Cliffs, NJ: Prentice Hall; 1977.

20. Bandura A. Self efficacy. Toward a unifying theory of behavior change. *Psychol Rev.* 1977;84:191–215.

21. Bandura A. The self system in reciprocal determinism. *Am Psychol.* 1982;37:122–147.

22. Baranowski T, Perry CL, Parcel GS. Social Cognitive Theory. In: Glanz K, Lewis FM, Rimer B, eds. *Health Behavior and Health Education: Theory, Research, Practice.* 2nd ed. San Francisco, Calif: Jossey Bass Publishers; 1997:153–178.

23. Expert Panel on the Identification, Evaluation, and Treatment of Overweight in Adults. Clinical guidelines on the identification, evaluation, and treatment of overweight and obesity in adults: executive summary. *Am J Clin Nutr.* 1998;68:899–917.

24. Cusatis DC, Shannon BM. Influences on adolescent eating behavior. *J Adolesc Health.* 1996;18:27–34.

25. Luepker RV, Murray DM, Jacobs DR, et al. Community education for cardiovascular disease prevention: risk factor changes in the Minnesota Heart Health Program. *Am J Public Health.* 1994;84:1383–1393.

26. Peterson AV, Kealey KA, Mann SL, Marcek PM, Sarason IG. Hutchinson Smoking Prevention Project: Long-term randomized trial in school-based tobacco use prevention. Results on smoking. *J Natl Cancer Inst.* 2000;92:1979–1991.

27. Luepker RV. Outcomes of a trial to improve children's dietary patterns and physical activity: The child and adolescent trial for cardiovascular health. *JAMA.* 1996;275:768–776.

28. Hearn MD, Baranowski T, Baranowski J, Doyle C, Smith M. Environmental influences on dietary behavior among children: availability and accessibility of fruits and vegetables enables consumption. *J Health Educ.* 1998;29:26–32.

29. AbuSabha R, Acterberg C. Review of self efficacy and locus of control for nutrition-health related behavior. *J Am Diet Assoc.* 1997;97:1122–1132.

30. Nestle M, Wing R, Birch L, et al. Behavioral and social influences on food choice. *Nutr Rev.* 1998;55(suppl):50–74.

31. Campbell MK, Symons M, Demark-Wahnfried W, Polhamus B, Bernhardt JM. Stages of change and psychosocial correlates of fruit and vegetable consumption among rural African-American church members. *Am J Health Prom.* 1998;12:185–191.

32. Havas S, Treiman K, Langenberg P, et al. Factors associated with fruit and vegetable consumption among women participating in WIC. *J Am Diet Assoc.* 1998;98:1141–1148.

33. Fishbein MH, ed. *Readings in Attitude Theory and Measurement.* New York, NY: Wiley; 1967.

34. Fishbein M, Ajzen I. *Belief, Attitude, Intention, and Behavior: An Introduction to Theory and Research.* Reading, Mass: Addison-Wesley; 1975.

35. Ajzen I, Fishbein M. *Understanding Attitudes and Predicting Social Behavior.* Englewood Cliffs, NJ: Prentice Hall; 1980.

36. Montano DE, Kasprzyk D, Taplin SH. The theory of reasoned action and the theory of planned behavior. In: Glanz K, Lewis FM, Rimer B, eds. *Health Behavior and Health Education: Theory, Research, Practice.* 2nd ed. San Francisco, Calif: Jossey Bass Publishers; 1997:85–112.

37. Shepherd R, Sparks P, Belliers S, Raats M. Attitudes and choice of flavored milks: extension of Fishbein and Ajzen's theory of reasoned action. *Food Q Preference.* 1991;3:157–164.

38. Arvola A, Lahteenmaki L, Tuorila H. Predicting the intent

to purchase unfamiliar and familiar cheeses, the effects of attitudes, expected liking and food neophobia. *Appetite.* 1999;32:113–126.

39. Brewer J, Blake AJ, Rankin SA, Douglass LW. The Theory of Reasoned Action predicts milk consumption in females. *J Am Diet Assoc.* 1999;99:39–44.

40. Weinstein ND. Testing four competing theories of health protective behavior. *Health Psychol.* 1993;4(12):324–333.

41. Freeman R, Sheiham A. Understanding decision-making processes for sugar consumption in adolescence. *Dent Oral Epidemiol.* 1997;25:228–232.

42. Mester I, Oostveen T. Why do adolescents eat low nutrient snacks between meals? An analysis of behavioral determinants with Fishbein and Ajzen models. *Nutr Health.* 1994;10(1):33–47.

43. Raats MM, Shephard R, Sparks P. Attitudes, obligations, and perceived control. Predicting milk selection. *Appetite.* 1993;20:239–241.

44. Stafleu A, de Graff C, van Staveren WA, de Jong MA. Attitudes toward high-fat foods and their low fat alternatives: reliability and relationship with fat intake. *Appetite.* 1994;22:183–196.

45. Saunders RP, Rahilly SA. Influences on intention to reduce dietary intake of fat and sugar. *J Nutr Educ.* 1990;22:169–176.

46. Ajzen I, Madden TJ. Prediction of goal-directed behavior: attitudes, intentions, and perceived behavioral control. *J Exp Soc Psychol.* 1986;22:453–474.

47. Raats MM, Shephard R, Sparks P. Attitudes, obligations, and perceived control. Predicting milk selection. *Appetite.* 1993;20: 239–241.

48. Park K, Ureda JR. Specific motivations of milk consumption among pregnant women enrolled in or eligible for WIC. *J Nutr Educ.* 1999;31:76–85.

49. Prochaska JO, DiClemente CC. *The Transtheoretical Approach: Crossing the Traditional Boundaries of Therapy.* Homewood, Ill: Irwin; 1984.

50. Prochaska JO, DiClemente CC, Norcross JC. In search of how people change: applications to addictive behaviors. *Am Psychol.* 1992;47:1102–1114.

51. Greene GW, Rossi SR. Stages of change for dietary fat reduction over 18 months. *J Am Diet Assoc.* 1998; 98:529–534.

52. Reed GR, Velicer WF, Prochaska JO, Rossi JS, Marcus BH. What makes a good staging algorithm: examples from regular exercise. *Am J Health Prom.* 1997;12:57–66.

53. Greene GW, Rossi SR, Reed GR, Willey C, Prochaska JO.

Stages of change for reducing dietary fat to 30% of total energy or less. *J Am Diet Assoc.* 1994;94:1105–1110.

54. Hargreaves M, Schlundt D, Buchowski M, Hardy RE, Rossi S, Rossi J. Stages of change and the intake of fat in African American women: improving stage assignment using the eating styles questionnaire. *J Am Diet Assoc.* 1999;99:1392–1399.

55. Greene GW, Rossi SR, Rossi JS, Velicer WF, Fava JS, Prochaska JO. Dietary applications of the Stages of Change Model. *J Am Diet Assoc.* 1999;99:673–678.

56. Prochaska JO, Velicer WF, Rossi JS, et al. Stages of change and decisional balance for twelve problem behaviors. *Health Psychol.* 1994;13:39–46.

57. Prochaska JO. Strong and weak principles for progressing from precontemplation to action on the basis of twelve problem behaviors. *Health Psychol.* 1994;13:47–51.

58. Velicer WF, DiClemente CC, Rossi JS, Prochaska JO. Relapse situations and self-efficacy: an integrative model. *Addict Behav.* 1990;15:271–283.

59. Rossi SR, Greene GW, Rossi JS, et al. Validation of decisional balance and temptations measures for dietary fat reduction in a large school-based population of adolescents. *Eating Behav.* 2001;2:1–18.

60. Campbell MC, DeVellis BM, Strecher VJ, Ammerman AS, DeVellis RF, Sandler RS. The impact of message tailoring on dietary behavior change for disease prevention in primary care settings. *Am J Public Health.* 1994;84:739–787.

61. Brug J, Steenhuis I, van Assema P, de Vries H. The impact of a computer-tailored nutrition intervention. *Prev Med.* 1996;25:236–242.

62. Brug J, Glanz K, van Assema P, Kok G, van Breukelen GJ. The impact of computer-tailored feedback and iterative feedback on fat, fruit, and vegetable intake. *Health Educ Behav.* 1998;25:517–531.

63. Greene GW, Rossi SR, Rossi JS, Fava JL, Prochaska JO, Velicer WF. An expert system intervention for dietary fat reduction [abstract]. *Ann Behav Med.* 1998;20(suppl):197.

64. Marcus BH, Emmons KM, Simkin-Silverman L, et al. Evaluation of tailored versus standard self-help physical activity interventions at the workplace. *Am J Health Prom.* 1997;12:246–253.

65. Steptoe A, Kerry S, Rink E, Hilton S. The impact of behavioral counseling on stage of change in fat intake, physical activity, and cigarette smoking in adults at increased risk of coronary heart disease. *Am J Public Health.* 2001;91:265–269.

22

Research Methods in Complementary and Alternative Medicine

Mark Kestin, Ph.D., M.P.H.

Awareness and use of complementary and alternative medicine (CAM) has increased significantly in recent years. In a landmark 1990 survey, Eisenberg et al found that 34 percent of the U.S. population reported using at least one alternative therapy in the previous year (1). When the survey was repeated in 1997, reported CAM use had increased to 42 percent of the population (2), with an estimated 629 million visits to alternative care practitioners and a cost of $21.2 billion dollars. In the same period, this population made only 386 million visits to primary care physicians.

Because of the frequent use of CAM services by people in the United States and the magnitude of their economic impact, it is important to understand what CAM is, how it relates to dietetics and nutrition, and what is involved in conducting dietetics and nutrition-oriented CAM research.

CAM: A DEFINITION

Complementary alternative medicine is a term that encompasses a variety of medical practices. *Complementary* refers to treatments provided alongside conventional medicine, and *alternative* implies treatments used instead of conventional medical treatments. The term *integrative medicine* is sometimes used to describe treatment that purposefully uses aspects of both alternative and conventional medicine.

CAM was functionally defined in 1993 as a group of medical practices not taught widely in medical schools, not generally available in U.S. hospitals, and not routinely reimbursed by third-party payers (1). A problem with this definition is that is says what CAM is not rather than what it is. Also, by 1998, most U.S. medical schools were offering elective courses in CAM (3).

The definition of CAM will probably remain fluid as some of its interventions become incorporated into conventional medical practice and are no longer considered alternative. An example is the 1997 National Institutes for Health (NIH) consensus statement that acupuncture should be incorporated into usual practice because there is good research evidence showing it to be effective in treating adult postoperative and chemotherapy nausea and vomiting, as well as in reducing postoperative dental pain (4). As these conditions are treated more commonly by acupuncture in the health delivery system and the services are reimbursed by third-party payers, at some point acupuncture may not meet the definition of CAM and would be considered conventional. However, when acupuncture is used to treat other medical conditions it may still be considered alternative until there is sufficient evidence of its effectiveness.

OVERVIEW OF CAM PRACTICES

CAM practices have been conceptually organized in many ways. Common elements in CAM practices include an emphasis on prevention and a holistic approach (an approach that considers all aspects of an individual, including physical, emotional, mental, social, and spiritual dimensions). The NIH National Center for Complementary and Alternative Medicine (NCCAM) groups CAM practices in to five major domains (5): manipulative and body-based methods, energy therapies, mind-body interventions, biologically based therapies, and alternative medical systems. Biologically based therapies and alternative medical systems are particularly relevant to nutrition and dietetics.

Biologically Based Therapies

Biologically based CAM therapies overlap both conventional medicine and nutrition. Nutrition-related practices include diet therapy, megadoses of nutrients, and supplementation with compounds not commonly defined as essential nutrients. An area that is both historic and burgeoning today is botanical medicine (also called *herbal therapy* or *phytotherapy*), which uses plants, parts of plants, and plant extracts as therapeutic agents (6). Some of the active ingredients of herbal medicines have been characterized, although many herbal medicine practitioners believe that an herb as a whole is more therapeutically effective than its parts and that the living properties of an herb are an important part of its action (6). Other biologically based CAM therapies include hormones (for example, melatonin) and supplements such as bee pollen and laetrile (5).

Alternative Medical Systems

Alternative medical systems are complete theoretical and practical systems independent of the conventional biomedical approach (5). They may have a long history of traditional practice or be of modern origin. The most developed traditional alternative medical systems are traditional Chinese medicine (TCM)—sometimes called *oriental medicine*—and Ayruveda, originating in India. Other traditional alternative medical systems have developed in Native American, Australian Aboriginal, African, Middle Eastern, Tibetan, Central American, and South American cultures (5).

Most traditional medical systems, and particularly TCM (7) and Ayruveda (8,9), use food as part of both diagnosis and therapy. TCM has significant influence in Korea and Japan. A modern offshoot of TCM is the macrobiotic diet, which is based on TCM principles (10).

Both TCM and Ayruveda have developed over thousands of years. More recently developed alternative medical systems founded in Western countries include homeopathy and naturopathy. Naturopathic medicine is an integrated medical system with a philosophical basis that emphasizes the body's abilities to heal itself. It has a vitalistic approach in that it claims that the body has an innate intelligence that strives for health and life and is "more than the sum of biochemical processes" (11). Naturopathic medicine uses nutrition as a major means of treatment, including diet therapy, fasting, and nutrition supplements (12). It also considers food intolerance to be a major cause of illness (12).

EVIDENCE-BASED MEDICINE, NUTRITION, AND CAM

Diet and nutrition therapies are commonly used in CAM practice. In the 1997 Eisenberg survey, 5.5 percent of the U.S. population reported having used "megavitamins" in the previous year, and 4.0 percent reported using "lifestyle diet" as part of CAM therapies (2). For convenience, nutrition therapies used in CAM can be divided into therapies aimed at changing dietary intake patterns and therapies using dietary supplements.

It is important to remember, however, that there is no clear distinction between an alternative diet therapy or dietary supplement use and a conventional one. Any nutrition therapy use in dietetics practice, whether alternative or conventional, should be based on evidence.

Evidence-Based Medicine

An evidence-based approach is currently preferred in scientific medicine—that is, any recommended therapy or preventive regimen should be based on the current best evidence from systematic research and clinical experience (13). Although multiple, large, randomized controlled trials often provide strong evidence about treatment efficacy, this study design is not always desirable or possible. Evidence can come from a variety of sources (14). Scientific evidence from any source should be critically reviewed, and schemas have been developed for evaluating a variety of studies to guide treatment decisions (15).

A 1998 editorial in the *Journal of the American Medical Association* (16) proposed that "there is no alternative medicine. There is only scientifically proven, evidence-based medicine supported by solid data or un-proven medicine, for which scientific evidence is lacking." This approach is a reasonable one to apply to diet and supplement use in dietetics practice.

Alternative Diet Therapies

Many dietary regimens have been advocated for disease prevention and treatment over the past hundred years. Such regimens have arisen from sources such as physicians, nutritionists and dietitians, CAM practitioners, and popular authors. Most of these diets have been at least loosely based on biomedical science, but for many the evidence is weak.

Over time there have been many profound changes in recommended dietary therapies, partly because they were not originally based on strong evidence. Examples include changing opinions on carbohydrate intake recommendations for non-insulin-dependent diabetes mellitus (17,18); attitudinal changes about the importance of dietary animal protein (19); and the abandonment of some dietary therapies, such as the Sippy diet for peptic ulcers (20).

An alternative diet may become conventional as evidence accumulates for its effectiveness and it becomes incorporated into conventional practice. For example, 19th-century advocates of whole grains and bulk (that is, dietary fiber), such as Sylvester Graham and Dr. John Harvey Kellog, were considered cranks until the 1970s (21). In contrast, current epidemiologic evidence emphasizes the use of whole grain consumption in the prevention of cardiovascular disease and cancer (22).

Many other diets that may be considered alternative are advocated for disease prevention and therapy. They vary from diets supported by evidence to diets based on little or no scientific data. Whether they are considered alternative or conventional is based on how accepted their use is in current conventional practice—opinions that are likely to change over time. However, the NCCAM generally classifies diet therapy and diet supplementation as alternative therapies (5). Examples of dietary practices that many consider alternative and that are based on scientific evidence include the following: vegan and vegetarian diets (19), whole food diets (that is, diets based on unrefined and minimally processed foods) (22), low-fat diets (23), Mediterranean diets (24), and elimination/exclusion diets (that is, the use of oligoantigenic diets to identify food intolerances) (25).

Evidence for using these diets is stronger for treating some disease states than others. For example, there is strong evidence that vegan and vegetarian diets reduce coronary heart disease risk factors (26) and that vegetarians, as a whole, have a lower incidence of coronary heart disease than nonvegetarians (19). In contrast, there is only slight evidence that a vegan diet alleviates rheumatoid arthritis (27). Even if there is evidence that a diet is effective in preventing a disease, the diet is not necessarily a useful treatment for that disease. For example, there is good epidemiologic evidence that a low-fat, high-fruit, and high-vegetable diet is associated with a lower incidence of cancer of some sites (28), but such a diet is not necessarily a good treatment for the same cancers.

There are a number of other alternative dietary practices without significant clinical or epidemiologic evidence of effectiveness (Table 22.1). This does not necessarily mean they are not efficacious, but rather that there is little current scientific evidence about their efficacy. Apart from the diet therapies outlined in Table 22.1, there are a number of other dietary regimens proposed for treating cancer that have little supporting evidence of efficacy, including the Kelly regimen, macrobiotic diets, the Harold Manner diet, the Hoxsley regimen, the Livingston Wheeler regimen, and the Wigmore treatment (29–31).

TABLE 22.1 Examples of Alternative Dietary Therapies With Little Evidence of Efficacy

Condition	Dietary Therapy	Description
General health	The Zone	Low in carbohydrate, high in protein
General health	Blood type diet	Type of diet should depend on ABO blood type
Obesity	The Zone, Protein Power	High to very high in protein
Obesity	Atkins Diet	Very low in carbohydrate
Obesity	Fit for Life	Proper food combinations important for digestion
Cancer	Gerson	Raw fruit, raw vegetables, and coffee enemas

Data are from references 29–31.

Dietary Supplements

The line between alternative and conventional practices in the use of dietary supplements is not always clear. The 1998 edition of Dietary Reference Intakes by the Food and Nutrition Board (FNB) of the Institute of Medicine shows a change in approach toward foods versus supplements as sources of nutrients since the 1989 publication of Recommended Dietary Allowances (RDAs). The FNB now recommends that women of childbearing age have 400 (g/day of folate from supplements or fortified foods (32). This recommendation, aimed at preventing neural tube defects, is based on the lower absorption rate of food-derived folate in comparison with supplemental folate (32). It represents a significant philosophical change for the FNB to conclude that sufficient folate for preventing neural tube defects cannot be practically obtained from unfortified food. Similarly, the FNB recommends that people older than 50 meet the RDA for vitamin B-12 primarily from supplements or fortified foods (32).

Ingesting nutrients in amounts much greater than the RDA to prevent or treat disease is controversial. The 1996 position statement of the American Dietetic Association on vitamin and mineral supplementation recommends taking nutrition supplements at "low levels of nutrients that do not exceed the RDA" (33).

In 1968 Linus Pauling introduced the term *orthomolecular* (or "right molecules") *medicine*. Practitioners of orthomolecular medicine believe that increasing or decreasing concentrations of molecules in the body is important in preventing and treating disease (34). The validity is obvious in treating scurvy with vitamin C, for example, but prescribing large doses of niacin to treat schizophrenia is more controversial (34). Many CAM practitioners—both those considering themselves orthomolecular medicine practitioners and those who do not—often recommend nutrition supplements in doses not obtainable from most diets. This practice can be termed *orthomolecular* or *meganutrient therapy*.

Various supplements are recommended by CAM practitioners, including dietary compounds not commonly considered conventional nutrients, such as inositol, taurine, coenzyme Q-10, and carnitine (35,36). As in diet therapy, the amount and quality of evidence for the prevention and treatment of disease varies for each nutrition supplement (36).

For some therapeutic uses of meganutrients, there is consistent evidence of effectiveness based on multiple randomized clinical trials (Table 22.2). In addition to the meganutrients shown in Table 22.2, many other meganutrients have been advocated for the prevention and treatment of many diseases (35). Again, the extent to which each use is considered alternative or conventional depends on how well they have been tested and whether or not they are incorporated into conventional practice.

In summary, CAM practitioners advocate many food-based and supplement therapies. Some of these therapies are not very different from the recommendations of all dietitians (for example, plant-based diets), but many are quite different. Whether a given diet or supplement therapy is recommended should be based on evidence of its effectiveness. Many CAM therapies, including the nutrition-based therapies, have not been evaluated using current standards of clinical research.

TABLE 22.2   Examples of Meganutrient Therapy with Good Evidence for Efficacy

Nutrient	Condition	Reference
Vitamin C	Common cold	Douglas RM et al. Vitamin C for preventing and treating the common cold (37)
Vitamin B6	Premenstrual syndrome	Wyatt KM et al. Efficacy of vitamin B-6 in the treatment of premenstrual syndrome (38)
Coenzyme Q10	Congestive heart failure	Mortensen SA. Perspectives on therapy of cardiovascular diseases with coenzyme Q10 (ubiquinone) (39)
Calcium	Osteoporosis	Food and Nutrition Board, Institute of Medicine. *Dietary Reference Intakes for Calcium, Phosphorus, Magnesium, Vitamin D, and Fluoride* (40)
Chromium	Type 2 diabetes	Anderson RA. Chromium in the prevention and control of diabetes (41)
Zinc	Common cold	Marshall S. Zinc gluconate and the common cold (42)
Fish oil	Hypertriglyceridemia	Harris WS. n-3 fatty acids and lipoproteins (43)
Fish oil	Rheumatoid arthritis	Fortin PR et al. Validation of a meta-analysis (44)

OVERVIEW OF RESEARCH IN CAM

To date, there has been much less research literature concerning CAM therapies than conventional medical therapies (45). The many reasons include the relative paucity of funding for CAM research (until recently), limited research training and interest in performing research by most CAM practitioners (46), and methodological research problems that may be inherent in the nature of some CAM therapies (29). However, the amount and quality of published CAM research has increased over the past decade. U.S. government funding of CAM research has also increased significantly. The NIH Office of Alternative Medicine (OAM) was founded in 1991 and had a budget of $2 million in 1993 (47). In 1999, the OAM was upgraded to a center, the National Center for Complementary and Alternative Medicine (NCCAM), administering a budget of $61.7 million for the year 2000 (47).

Some of the methodological problems in CAM research are similar to problems found in conventional medical and nutrition research; other problems pertain particularly to CAM research (29). This chapter focuses on clinical research, but the complete range of research techniques can be used in CAM research, including basic laboratory, qualitative, and descriptive techniques (for example, surveys).

METHODOLOGICAL ISSUES IN CAM RESEARCH

CAM therapies cover many modalities, so challenges in performing CAM research vary. For interventions in which a single agent (for example, a vitamin or herb) is being tested, the research issues are similar to issues in other areas of medical research. One exception is that the active ingredient in herbs can vary by such factors as season, storage, and growing conditions. Often the active ingredient or ingredients are unknown (6). Unknown ingredients are involved in some food-based nutrition research as well; for example, there is evidence that cranberry juice may reduce the frequency of urinary tract infections, although no one has determined the active agent (48).

The following are important methodological issues specific to clinical CAM research:

- Each treatment may be individualized, and patients are seen as unique.
- Treatments can be complex and multifactorial.
- Difficulties involve control groups, randomization, placebos, and blinding.
- The mechanisms of action of some CAM therapies seem implausible in Western scientific terms.

Individualized Treatments and Patients

In many CAM therapies, the treatment of individual patients may differ even when they have identical presenting symptoms. For example, there are various styles of acupuncture, and individual acupuncturists may insert needles at different sites (49). Part of the holistic aspect of CAM treatment is that the patient-practitioner relationship is an important part of the healing process, and many CAM practitioners believe that the same treatment would work differently with different practitioners and different patients. This issue can make a standard protocol in a trial situation difficult, because CAM practitioners may not be willing the use the same treatment for every patient and do not believe that other practitioners using the same protocol would necessarily have the same results. These views could be a barrier to standardized research.

However, the extent to which individualized treatment by CAM practitioners is a hindrance to conducting research depends on the research question being asked. If the purpose of the research is to test the efficacy of a given treatment modality rather than the mechanism of the process, rigorous and valid research can be undertaken, provided the end points of interest are carefully considered. If the outcomes are valid, quantifiable, reproducible, and objective, the issues of treatment variability can be obviated (50). For example, the NCCAM has funded a study comparing naturopathic medicine, TCM, and the usual conventional care for women experiencing temporomandibular disorder (51). The treatment each patient receives may vary within and between practitioners. Naturopaths may use none, some, or all of diet, supplements, herbs, physical medicine, and homeopathy to treat most disorders (11), so the treatment for temporomandibular disorder is likely to vary across patients. However, the study end points are validated measures of temporomandibular disorder, enabling valid comparison between treatments. However, even if the study found, for example, that naturopathic treatment was superior to conventional care, it would not be possible to isolate which aspects of the treatment were most effective.

Outcomes research may be particularly useful for

CAM investigations (14). In this kind of research, preexisting databases available to health insurers and health maintenance organizations are used in an observational manner to compare the effectiveness of various medical treatments (52). These types of studies lend themselves to the assessment of the effectiveness of a practitioner's treatment because they examine the treatment process as a whole rather than focusing on individual aspects of treatments.

Nonhomogeneity of Patients

Many CAM practitioners object to current clinical research methods in which patients with a given condition are seen as the same for randomization and evaluation purposes (46). Because CAM practitioners consider each patient as a unique individual, even biochemically (11), they want to be free to vary treatments across individuals, even people who have the same presenting symptoms.

The nonhomogeneity of patients is an issue for nutrition research as well. For example, the therapeutic response to protein and energy supplementation in patients with protein-energy malnutrition would differ from the response in normally nourished patients. Also, even though it is well known that nutrient requirements vary across individuals, the genetic basis for this is variation just emerging. An excellent example is polymorphism for the gene that encodes for the methyltetrahydrofolate reductase enzyme, used in folate metabolism. A subset of the population (perhaps 10 percent to 15 percent) is homozygous for a thermolabile variant of this enzyme that derives from one base substitution in the based sequence encoding the enzyme, and members of this subset may require a greater dietary folate intake than individuals with the more common variant for good folate status (53). Nonhomogeneity of patients can be addressed in clinical research by careful selection of study participants according to characteristics of interest. For example, participants may be stratified in, or excluded from, a folate supplementation study based on their genotype for the methyltetrahydrofolate reductase enzyme.

Complex and Multifactorial Treatments

Along with varying treatments by individuals, many CAM practitioners use complex and multifactorial treatments, making it difficult to pinpoint the effectiveness of any particular part of the treatment. For example, the work of Ornish and associates presents good evidence that a combination of a very low fat vegetarian diet, aerobic exercise regimen, stress reduction education, group support, and smoking cessation education can reverse coronary atherosclerosis, as measured angiographically (54). The relative effectiveness of diet, exercise, smoking cessation, group support, and stress reduction in reversing atherosclerosis cannot be individually assessed from the study design. This intervention follows a holistic approach, in which the body, mind, and spirit are all addressed. The work of Ornish et al is a good example of focusing on end points. The study was carefully designed and the results interesting and valid, even though the most effective aspect of the intervention cannot be isolated. In cases like this one, the whole is indeed greater than the sum of the parts.

This idea is further illustrated in diet therapy for hypertension. Studies in the early 1980s documented that lacto-ovo-vegetarians had lower blood pressure than nonvegetarians even controlling for body mass index and sodium intake, and nonvegetarians could lower their blood pressure by eating a vegetarian diet (55). Since then, attempts to isolate vegetarian diet characteristics that are responsible for lowered blood pressure have been unenlightening. A number of controlled studies on dietary fiber, type of fatty acids, animal and vegetable protein, magnesium, calcium, and potassium have been done without clear success (55).

A combination of nutritional characteristics of vegetarian diets were combined in the large Dietary Alternatives to Stop Hypertension (DASH) study that conclusively demonstrated that a "prudent" omnivorous diet—low in saturated fat and high in fruits, vegetables, and low-fat dairy products—effectively lowers blood pressure in participants with and without mild hypertension (56). The hypotensive effect of a prudent diet may be due to the additive or synergistic effect of many dietary factors. Thus, a reductionist approach (trying to find the single nutrient responsible for the hypotensive effect of vegetarian diets) was less successful than a more holistic study.

Placebos, Control Groups, Randomization, and Blinding

Placebos and Control Groups

The use of placebos is another of the CAM research design and performance issues that is paralleled by similar issues in conventional clinical nutrition research. A major issue is placebo definition and use. Traditionally, the placebo effect was seen as a nuisance getting in the way of testing a particular therapy (29). The placebo effect relies on the relationship between practitioner and patient and the expectations of both (29). The effect can be so strong that it can affect physiological processes such as postoperative swelling and gastric motility, as well as psychological processes (46). There is some disagreement, however, about the importance of the placebo response (57). Nocebo responses, or toxic placebo effects, have been documented; for example, in one study 30 percent of patients receiving a placebo in a chemotherapy trial lost their hair (58). The mechanisms involved in these effects are becoming more delineated, and the relatively new area of psychoimmunology is of particular interest (59).

Many CAM practitioners see the placebo effect, particularly the therapeutic effect of their personal relationship with patient, as a critical part of the healing process. This view makes finding a placebo or a suitable control difficult in some CAM research and makes some CAM practitioners skeptical of participating in randomized controlled trials. The choice of placebo or control groups is particularly difficult in physical CAM therapies such as acupuncture. Should no acupuncture, acupuncture at different sites, or acupuncture with needle insertion to a lesser depth be used as a control? Or should the control be something else altogether? (49)

Randomization and Blinding

Randomization can be a problem in research patients with a strong preference for a specific treatment, as they will often refuse to be randomized (51). Separating treatment and control groups can be difficult in some CAM trials because dietary supplements and other alternative therapies are available, thus potentially contaminating the control group if their use of treatments is unknown to the researchers (51).

Many CAM therapies have problems with blinding. Blinding of both participant and researcher can be difficult for physical therapies such as chiropractic, acupuncture, and massage. One solution being employed in a randomized trial of acupuncture in depression is to have different practitioners diagnose, treat, and evaluate the patient (51). Blinding is easier, but not always straightforward, for biotherapy treatments such as herbal or nutrition supplements. Because these agents are often available in encapsulated form, it is not difficult to make similar capsules as a blinded control treatment.

Dietary Intervention Studies

Placebos, control groups, and blinding are major issues for any dietary intervention studies using food (for example, community-based dietary interventions or controlled feeding studies). In most cases, it is difficult to have blinding of participant or researcher with a food-based diet. The choice of control diet can also be a problem when there is any manipulation of energy-providing nutrients; an increase in any given nutrient needs to be balanced with a decrease in another nutrient if weight gain is to be avoided.

Researchers of dietary intervention rely on having unbiased outcomes to compensate for the potentially negative effects of not being able to blind the participants about the nature of the intervention. It is usually possible to blind the researcher doing the outcome assessment (for example, the laboratory technician), even if the participant and the main researcher are not blinded.

One ingenious approach to this problem was used by Panush and co-workers in testing the effectiveness of the Dong diet (a popular diet proposing that a Chinese peasant diet would effectively treat rheumatoid arthritis) (60). Because many of the outcome measures in this study relied on participant self-assessment (for example, self-reported pain and stiffness), there was concern that the placebo effect arising from paying attention to diet might have an effect. The researchers thus invented an entirely arbitrary placebo diet that randomly allowed some foods and forbade others (for example, chicken was allowed, but turkey was not). This technique allowed control for any placebo effect of being on a restricted diet, such as gaining social support by participating in a study.

Implausible Mechanisms

Some CAM therapies propose mechanisms that cannot be easily explained in Western scientific terms and are based on paradigms that are hard to explain or measure in scientific terms; one example is *qi,* or a life force that flows through vital energy systems in the body (61). Homeopathy, for example, uses solutions of substances that are so dilute that there may not be one molecule of the substance of interest in the vial (62). Similarly, it is difficult to explain, in terms of current physics, how distant healing therapies (for example, distant prayer) would work when a practitioner is geographically distant from a patient). Practitioners of such therapies have tried to explain the mechanisms in terms of energy fields surrounding the body (63); however, these energy fields have not been directly observed or measured, and *energy* in this sense does not refer to the same energy forms familiar to physics (62).

For some scientists, the lack of a paradigm explainable in Western scientific terms invalidates research (64). However, it is important to differentiate research on the effectiveness of a treatment from research examining the underlying paradigm. There is evidence of effectiveness for both homeopathy (62) and distant prayer (63) from well-designed, double-blind, placebo-controlled, randomized clinical trials. A good example from the diet therapy literature is the demonstrated effectiveness of ketogenic diets in treating children with refractive epilepsy, despite there being no accepted mechanism for the action of these diets (65).

RECOMMENDATIONS FOR RESEARCH IN CAM

As part of a 1995 NIH Conference on Complementary and Alternative Research Methodology, the Quantitative Methods Working Group proposed a methodological manifesto for performing quantitative CAM research (14), providing a framework for planning CAM research. The main themes are (1) that CAM can be tested using current techniques and (2) that research should focus on well-accepted outcomes (end points). The group's suggestions may be summarized as follows (14):

- Different study questions require different methodologies.
- Researchers should use the strongest possible design and the most appropriate statistical procedures for a given study question.
- Clinical trials are "not the only game in town" (i.e., alternative methodologies should be considered).
- The results of observational studies can inform the design of intervention trials.
- Alternative therapies are acceptable, whereas alternative outcomes are not.
- Existing quantitative procedures are generally applicable in researching alternative therapies and complementary medical systems.
- Complex complementary medical systems can be studied as gestalts, or whole systems.

These suggestions can be applied to dietetics and nutrition research. For example, the diet for lowering blood pressure that was previously discussed is a good example of testing a gestalt. Focusing on outcomes allows for choice in testing therapies, including the possibility of preserving their holistic and individualistic nature. Although randomized controlled trials are often considered the gold standard in establishing causation, in many instances they cannot or should not be used (14,50).

However, because practical randomized controlled trial methodology can be powerful in testing medical treatments (50), an effort is under way to perform and publish systematic reviews of randomized controlled trials of CAM therapies through the Cochrane Collaboration, an international organization that produces, maintains, and disseminates systemic reviews in health care (66).

RESEARCH OUTLOOK

Dietitians are seeing an increasing number of clients who are using CAM therapies, including meganutrient supplements and therapeutic herbs, and the attitudes of dietitians toward CAM may be changing. In a recent Oregon survey of licensed dietitians (L.D.s), a large majority believed in the effectiveness and safety of functional foods and nutrient supplements for preventing and treating chronic and acute disease (67). About half of the L.D.s thought that herbs were effective for these uses, although only about a third had recommended herbs during the preceding year. Other indications of the increasing importance of CAM to dietitians is the inclusion of a chapter on CAM in the newest edition of the standard diet therapy text, *Krause's Food, Nutrition, and Diet Therapy* (68); the publication of a monograph on dietary supplements by the American Dietetic Association (36); and the establishment by the American Dietetic Association of a Nutrition and Complementary Care dietetic practice group.

The definition of CAM is fluid, and many of the diet and nutrient supplement therapies now considered alternative may be incorporated in future conventional dietetics practice if there is good evidence for their effectiveness. From a research perspective, all the research methods described in other chapters in this book should, in principle, be applied to CAM research. Issues in CAM research parallel many of the issues that complicate study design and performance in nutrition research. Dietetics researchers should use opportunities to learn about CAM and to initiate and collaborate in CAM research.

REFERENCES

1. Eisenberg DM, Kessler RC, Foster C, Norlock FE, Calkins DR, Delbanco TL. Unconventional medicine in the United States. *N Engl J Med.* 1993;428:246–252.

2. Eisenberg DM, Davis RB, Ettner SL, et al. Trends in the alternative medicine use in the United States, 1990–1997. *JAMA.* 1998;280:1569–1575

3. Wetzel MS, Eisenberg DM, Kaptchuk TJ. Courses involving complementary and alternative medicine at US medical schools. *JAMA.* 1998;280:784–787.

4. National Institutes for Health. Acupuncture. *NIH Consensus Statement.* 1997;15(5):1–34.

5. National Center for Complementary and Alternative Medicine. Major domains of complementary and alternative medicine. August 2000. Available at: http://nccam.nih.gov/nccam/fcp/classify/index.html. Accessed June 8, 2001.

6. Low Dog T. Phytomedicine. In: Jonas WB, Levin JS, eds. *Essentials of Complementary and Alternative Medicine.* Philadelphia, Pa: Lippincott Williams and Wilkins; 1999:355–368.

7. Lao L. Traditional Chinese medicine. In: Jonas WB, Levin JS, eds. *Essentials of Complementary and Alternative Medicine.* Philadelphia, Pa: Lippincott Williams and Wilkins; 1999:216–232.

8. Zysk KG. Traditional Ayruveda. In: Micozzi MS, ed. *Fundamentals of Complementary and Alternative Medicine.* New York, NY: Churchill Livingstone; 1996:233–242.

9. Lad DV. Ayruvedic medicine. In: Jonas WB, Levin JS, eds. *Essentials of Complementary and Alternative Medicine.* Philadelphia, Pa: Lippincott Williams and Wilkins; 1999:200–215.

10. Kushi M. *The Macrobiotic Way.* Wayne, NJ: Avery; 1985.

11. Pizzorno JE Jr. Naturopathic medicine. In: Micozzi MS, ed. *Fundamentals of Complementary and Alternative Medicine.* New York, NY: Churchill Livingstone; 1996:163–182.

12. Murray MT, Pizzorno JE Jr. Nutritional medicine. In: Jonas WB, Levin JS, eds. *Essentials of Complementary and Alternative Medicine.* Philadelphia, Pa: Lippincott Williams and Wilkins; 1999:369–380.

13. Sackett DL, Rosenberg WMC, Gray JAM, Haynes RB, Richardson WS. Evidence based medicine: what it is and what it isn't. *BMJ.* 1996;312:71–72.

14. Levin JS, Glass TA, Kushi LH, Schuck JR, Sreele L,

15. Schenbaum SC, ed. *Using Clinical Practice Guidelines to Evaluate Quality of Care.* Washington, DC: US Dept of Health and Human Services; 1995. AHCPR publication 95-0045.

16. Fontanarosa PB, Lundeberg GD. Alternative medicine meets science. *JAMA.* 1998;280:1618–1619.

17. Hockaday TD. High-carbohydrate and fibre diets in the treatment of diabetes. *Scand J Gastroenterol.* 1987;129(suppl):124–131.

18. Vessby B. Dietary carbohydrates in diabetes. *Am J Clin Nutr.* 1994;59(suppl):742–746.

19. Willett WC. Convergence of philosophy and science: the third international congress on vegetarian nutrition. *Am J Clin Nutr.* 1999;70(suppl 3):434–438.

20. Warner CW, McIsaac RL. The evolution of peptic ulcer therapy. A role for temporal control of drug delivery. *Ann NY Acad Sci.* 1991;618:504–516.

21. Deutsch RM. The new nuts among the berries. Palo Alto, Calif: Bull; 1977.

22. Marquart L, Jacobs DR Jr, Slavin JL. Whole grains and health: an overview. *J Am Coll Nutr.* 2000;19(suppl 3):289–290.

23. Lichtenstein AH, Kennedy E, Barrier P, et al. Dietary fat consumption and health. *Nutr Rev.* 1998;56:S3–19.

24. Ferro-Luzzi A, Branca F. Mediterranean diet, Italian-style: prototype of a healthy diet. *Am J Clin Nutr.* 1995;61(suppl 6):1338–1345.

25. Arvola T, Holmberg-Marttila D. Benefits and risks of elimination diets. *Ann Med.* 1999;31:293–298.

26. Kestin M, Rouse IL, Correll RA, Nestel PJ. Cardiovascular disease risk factors in free-living men: comparison of two prudent diets, one based on lacto-ovo-vegetarianism and the other allowing lean meat. *Am J Clin Nutr.* 1989;50:280–287.

27. Kjeldsen-Kragh J, Haugen M, Borchgrevink CF, et al. Controlled trial of fasting and one-year vegetarian diet in rheumatoid arthritis. *Lancet.* 1991;338:899–902.

28. Potter JD, ed. *Food, Nutrition, and the Prevention of Cancer: A Global Perspective.* Washington, DC: American Institute for Cancer Research; 1997.

29. Berman BM, Larson DB, eds. *Alternative Medicine: Expanding Medical Horizons. A Report to the National Institutes of Health on Alternative Medical Systems and Practices in the United States.* Washington, DC: US Government Printing Office; 1995. NOH publication 94-066.

30. Block KI. Nutritional biotherapy. In: Jonas WB, Levin JS, eds. *Essentials of Complementary and Alternative Medicine.* Philadelphia, Pa: Lippincott Williams and Wilkins; 1999:490–521.

31. Vickers A, Zollman C. ABC of complementary medicine.

Jonas WB. Quantitative methods in research on complementary medicine: a methodological manifesto. *Med Care.* 1997;35:1079–1094.

Unconventional approaches to nutritional medicine. *BMJ.* 1999;319:1419–1422.

32. Food and Nutrition Board, Institute of Medicine. *Dietary Reference Intakes for Thiamin, Riboflavin, Vitamin B6, Folate, Vitamin B12, Pantothenic Acid, and Choline.* Washington, DC: National Academy Press; 1998.

33. American Dietetic Association. Vitamin and mineral supplementation—Position of ADA. *J Am Diet Assoc.* 1996;96:73–77.

34. Gaby AR. Orthomolecular medicine and megavitamin therapy. In: Jonas WB, Levin JS, eds. *Essentials of Complementary and Alternative Medicine.* Philadelphia, Pa: Lippincott Williams and Wilkins; 1999:459–471.

35. Werbach MR, Moss J. *Textbook of Nutritional Medicine.* Tarzana, Calif: Third Line Press; 1999.

36. Sarubin Fragakis A. *The Health Professional's Guide to Popular Dietary Supplements.* 2nd ed. Chicago, Ill: American Dietetic Association; 2003.

37. Douglas RM, Chalker EB, Treacy B. Vitamin C for preventing and treating the common cold. *Cochrane Database Syst Rev.* 2000;(2):CD000980. Review.

38. Wyatt KM, Dimmock PW, Jones PW, O'Brien PMS. Efficacy of vitamin B-6 in the treatment of premenstrual syndrome: systematic review. *BMJ.* 1999;318:1375–1381.

39. Mortensen SA. Perspectives on therapy of cardiovascular diseases with coenzyme Q10 (ubiquinone). *Clin Invest.* 1993;71(suppl):116–123.

40. Food and Nutrition Board, Institute of Medicine. *Dietary Reference Intakes for Calcium, Phosphorus, Magnesium, Vitamin D, and Fluoride.* Washington, DC: National Academy Press; 1997.

41. Anderson RA. Chromium in the prevention and control of diabetes. *Diabetes Metab.* 2000;26:22–27.

42. Marshall S. Zinc gluconate and the common cold. Review of randomized controlled trials. *Can Fam Physician.* 1998;44:1037–1042. Review.

43. Harris WS. n-3 fatty acids and lipoproteins: comparison of results from human and animal studies. *Lipids.* 1996;31:243–252.

44. Fortin PR, Lew RA, Liang MH, et al. Validation of a meta-analysis: the effects of fish oil in rheumatoid arthritis. *J Clin Epidemiol.* 1995;48:1379–1390.

45. Jonas WM, Levin JS. Introduction: Models of medicine and healing. In: Jonas WB, Levin JS, eds. *Essentials of Complementary and Alternative Medicine.* Philadelphia, Pa: Lippincott Williams and Wilkins; 1999:1–15.

46. Vincent C, Furnham S, Richardson P. *Complementary Medicine: A Research Perspective.* Chichester, England: John Wiley and Sons; 1997.

47. National Center for Complementary and Alternative Medicine. General information about CAM and the NCCAM. June 2000. Available at: http://nccam.nih.gov/nccam/an/general/index.html. Accessed June 11, 2001.

48. Lowe FC, Fagelman E. Cranberry juice and urinary tract infections: what is the evidence? *Urology.* 2001;57:407–413.

49. Margolin A, Avants K, Klieber HD. Investigating alternative medicine therapies in randomized controlled trials. *JAMA.* 1998;280:1626–1628.

50. Elwood M. *Critical Appraisal of Epidemiological Studies and Clinical Trials.* 2nd ed. Oxford, England: Oxford University Press; 1998.

51. Nahin RL, Straus SE. Research into complementary and alternative medicine: problems and potential. *BMJ.* 2001;322:161–164.

52. Gordis L. *Epidemiology.* Philadelphia, Pa: W.B. Saunders; 1996.

53. Bailey LB, Gregory JF III. Polymorphisms of methylenetetrahydrofolate reductase and other enzymes: metabolic significance, risks, and impact on folate requirement. *J Nutr.* 1999;129:919–922.

54. Ornish D, Scherwitz LW, Billings JH, et al. Intensive lifestyle changes for reversal of coronary heart disease. *JAMA.* 1998;280:2001–2007.

55. Beilin LJ, Burke V. Vegetarian diet components, protein and blood pressure: which nutrients are important? *Clin Exp Pharmacol Physiol.* 1995;22(3):195–198.

56. Appel LJ, Moore TJ, Obarzanek E, et al. A clinical trial of the effects of dietary patterns on blood pressure. DASH Collaborative Research Group. *New Engl J Med.* 1997;36:1117–1124.

57. Hrobjartsson A, Gotzsche PC. Is the placebo powerless? An analysis of clinical trials comparing placebo with no treatment. *N Engl J Med.* 2001;344:1594–1602.

58. Fielding JWL, Fagg SL, Jones BG, et al. An interim report of a prospective, randomized, controlled study of adjuvant chemotherapy in operable gastric cancer. *World J Surg.* 1983;7:390–399.

59. Masek K, Petrovicky P, Sevcik J, Zidek Z, Frankova D. Past, present, and future of psychoneuroimmunology. *Toxicol.* 2000;142:179–188.

60. Panush RS, Carter RL, Katz P, Kowsari B, Longley S, Finnie S. Diet therapy for rheumatoid arthritis. *Arthritis Rheum.* 1983;(4):462–471.

61. Ergil KV. China's traditional medicine. In: Micozzi MS, ed. *Fundamentals of Complementary and Alternative Medicine.* New York, NY: Churchill Livingstone; 1996:185–224.

62. Chapman EH. Homeopathy. In: Jonas WB, Levin JS, eds. *Essentials of Complementary and Alternative Medicine.* Philadelphia, Pa: Lippincott Williams and Wilkins; 1999:472–489.

63. Benor DJ. Spiritual healing. In: Jonas WB, Levin JS, eds. *Essentials of Complementary and Alternative Medicine.* Philadelphia, Pa: Lippincott Williams and Wilkins; 1999:369–382.

64. Federspil G, Vettor R. Can scientific medicine incorpo-

rate alternative medicine. *J Alt Comp Med.* 2000;6:241–244.

65. Vining EP. Clinical efficacy of the ketogenic diet. *Epilepsy Res.* 1999:37:181–190.

66. Ezzo J, Berman BM, Vickers MA, Linde K. Complementary medicine and the Cochrane Collaboration. *JAMA.* 1998;280:1628–1630.

67. Lee Y-K, Georgiou C, Raab C. The knowledge, attitudes, and practices of dietitians licensed in Oregon regarding functional foods, nutrient supplements, and herbs as complementary medicine. *J Am Diet Assoc.* 2000;100:543–548.

68. Mathai K. Integrative medicine and herbal therapy. In: Mahan LK, Escott-Stump S, eds. *Krause's Food, Nutrition and Diet Therapy.* Philadelphia, Pa: WB Saunders; 2000:415–430.

Further Reading

Messina M, Lampe JW, Birt DF, Appel LJ, Pivonka E, Berry B, Jacobs DR Jr. Reductionism and the narrowing nutrition perspective: time for reevaluation and emphasis on food synergy. *J Am Diet Assoc.* 2001;101:1416–1419.

Tonelli MR, Callahan TC. Why alternative medicine cannot be evidence-based. *Acad Med.* 2001;76:1213–1220.

23

Research in Foodservice Management

Jeannie Sneed, Ph.D., R.D., and Mary B. Gregoire, Ph.D., R.D., F.A.D.A.

Research is critical to the integrity and development of the field of foodservice management. There is a rich history of research related to foodservice management, dating back to the early years of the profession. Through research, the field has continued to change and develop. This chapter illustrates the historical development of research in the field, presents a matrix of foodservice management research areas, and discusses research techniques used in the field.

HISTORICAL DEVELOPMENT OF FOODSERVICE MANAGEMENT RESEARCH

The profession of dietetics formally began in 1917, and foodservice management always has been emphasized. Soon after the *Journal of the American Dietetic Association* was started in 1925, an article was published by Rush (1) on job analysis in lunchrooms and cafeterias. Thus, there is a long history of research in foodservice management.

In the 1930s, emphasis in foodservice management was on labor (2,3), cost control (4,5), and training (6). Research also was done on measuring effectiveness (7,8). The 1940s brought World War II, which had a dramatic impact on dietetics. The literature focused on the layout and design of kitchens, food cost control and rationing, and personnel management.

Much of the research in the 1950s focused on personnel management, with an emphasis on labor hours and costs (9,10) and work simplification (11). Related research also was done on layout efficiency in the kitchen (12). Much of the work on efficiency continued through the 1960s. Research in the area of work sampling and the use of computers in foodservice began in the 1960s (13). Computer simulations in cafeteria serving lines (14) were reported, as were computer applications for menu planning (15) and food cost accounting (16). It also was during this time that comparisons were initiated for food produced using different food production systems (17). Employee outcomes, such as job satisfaction, also were studied (18).

Research in the 1970s continued to focus on computer applications (10–21). It was during this decade that research related to Hazard Analysis and Critical Control Point (HACCP) and food safety (22,23) first appeared in the *Journal of the American Dietetic Association*. Research on food production systems continued (24). Behavioral science research, especially related to work values and job satisfaction, flourished (25–27). Research from the 1980s and 1990s will be used as examples of research techniques discussed in this chapter.

FOODSERVICE MANAGEMENT RESEARCH AREAS

There are many ways of organizing areas of foodservice management research. Olsen, Tse, and Bellas (28) developed a classification system for research and development in the hospitality industries. Other researchers have identified research needs related to specific areas of research, such as research related to school foodservice (29). Several years ago, we developed a foodservice management research area matrix (30) to provide a contemporary and comprehensive view of areas of research in the field. Table 23.1 is a revised version of this matrix that reflects current terminology and areas omitted in the earlier version. This matrix provides students, practitioners, and educators with a way to organize research and research needs in foodservice management.

RESEARCH TECHNIQUES IN FOODSERVICE MANAGEMENT

The research matrix in Table 23.1 illustrates the breadth of research areas in foodservice management. This breadth of research necessitates the use of multiple research techniques to answer research questions, develop a thorough understanding of research variables, and ultimately, improve practice in the field. This section of the chapter presents an overview of research techniques, along with examples of how each research technique has been used in foodservice management.

Research can be either qualitative or quantitative.

TABLE 23.1 Foodservice Management Research Area Matrix

Customer-Related Topics	Product and Process-Related Topics	Human Resources-Related Topics
Needs and preferences	Menu-related issues	Staffing
• Dietary Guidelines for Americans	• Nutrition	• Competencies
• ADA Guidelines	• Cost: food and labor	• Training and development
• Nutrition education	• Variety	• Compensation
	• Acceptability	• Retention
Behavior		
	Procurement	Performance
Marketing		• Productivity
• Product	Production	• Motivation
• Place	• Forecasting	• Satisfaction
• Price	• Production systems	• Organizational commitment
• Promotion	• Production scheduling	
	• Productivity	Safety and health regulations
Service	• Food preparation	• Americans With Disabilities Act
• Style	• Food safety/HACCP	• AIDS/HIV
• Institutional constraints	• Nutrition	
	• Equipment	Sociocultural factors
Environmental scanning	• Layout and design	• Multicultural diversity
• Political		• Organizational culture
• Economic	Cost	
• Technological		Leadership
• Sociological	Natural resources	
	• Waste management	
	• Water conservation	
	• Ventilation and air quality	
	• Energy conservation	
	Food Safety	
	• Microbiological	
	• Chemical	
	Environmental issues	

Qualitative research is used to build theory and generate hypotheses. Once a theory has been built and the hypotheses written, quantitative research methods are used to test the hypotheses. This testing may be an iterative process, in that results of quantitative research may lead the researcher to look at other aspects of qualitative research or to refine the proposed theory. Both qualitative and quantitative research techniques have been used extensively in foodservice management research, and specific examples will be given in the discussion of research methods. Perhaps the best way to understand the differences between these two types of data is to contrast them by their major characteristics:

- Qualitative research is inductive, whereas quantitative research is deductive. In other words, qualitative research examines facts about the real world in order to explain relationships among variables. Quantitative research provides an explanation of relationships among variables in an attempt to make predictions about the real world. Because of the inductive nature of qualitative research, it often precedes quantitative research. In some situations, there is a limited knowledge about the relationships among variables, and qualitative research may provide observations of the real world to help explain possible relationships.
- Qualitative research is theory building. Once a theory has been developed, quantitative research is used to test the theory. Results of the quantitative research will be used to refine the theory and may even provide evidence to the researcher that there is need to do additional qualitative research. Thus, the process is iterative.
- Qualitative research is used to generate hypotheses, whereas quantitative research is used to test hypotheses.
- Qualitative research focuses on process—how something happens or why a relationship exists. Quantitative research focuses on outcome or product—what is happening or what the relationships are among variables.
- Qualitative research is formative, whereas quantitative research is summative.
- Qualitative research does not yield discrete numerical data, whereas quantitative research does.
- The sample size for qualitative research is based on the number of observations required to obtain a full understanding of a characteristic, or the full range of variability. The sample size for quantitative research is related to the power required to test hypotheses.

Research can be further classified by six factors: type of data (qualitative or quantitative), research setting (laboratory or field), who records the data (observer, subject, or secondary sources), level of analysis (individual or group), number of observations (one-time or replicated observations), and research design (descriptive, preexperimental, quasi-experimental, and true experimental). Each of the factors should be considered when designing a research study. Also, as research develops in a field, multiple methods are required to gain a thorough understanding of the research problem and results.

Type of Data

Data collected can be either qualitative or quantitative. Both types of data can be useful for different purposes, and they often are used in complementary ways. Qualitative data are descriptive in nature and are collected in an effort to obtain a full range of explanation for a variable or a relationship between or among variables. Quantitative data are numerical and are collected from a large enough sample to be able to conduct statistical analyses for testing hypotheses.

Research Setting

Research may be conducted in a laboratory or in the field. There are advantages and disadvantages to conducting research in each of these settings. Laboratory research has the advantage that the researcher can control the research variables. A disadvantage is that the setting is not naturalistic, and in the real-world results might be very different. Field studies have the advantage of being naturalistic, but they have the disadvantage that the researcher cannot have as much control over the variables. Because of the inherent advantages and disadvantages of both research settings, it is important to conduct research on a topic both in the laboratory and in the field to fully understand the variables and their relationships.

Most of the examples of laboratory research focus on product development or equipment testing. One recent study (31), for example, examined the performance of various sweeteners in muffins, pound cakes, and cocoa cupcakes. A complete block experimental design was used, and products were compared using laboratory procedures to determine specific volume, surface area, tenderness, and percentage of water loss.

Many areas of research have been done in the field, including studies related to total waste composition (32) in a retirement community, food waste in a retirement community (33) and an elementary school (34), acceptance of foods (35,36) in a school and an employee cafeteria, and pricing strategy (37) in a high school. Field observational studies have been conducted to determine the time spent by schoolchildren eating lunch. In one such study, researchers timed meal service with stopwatches (38).

Who Records the Data

Data may be recorded by either an observer or the subject. Researchers may use existing databases and conduct secondary analyses of data. There are numerous examples in the foodservice management literature.

Lieux and Manning (39) observed workers in 8 senior centers at 5-minute intervals and recorded labor activities performed. Because they collected information on several operations, their results on minutes spent per meal performing various activities, such as service, processing, and cleaning, provided useful information for managers scheduling labor in similar operations. Research related to problems with salad bars (40) and tray error rates (41) also used observation techniques.

The subjects themselves may report data needed for a study. One example of self-reported data is a study conducted by Theis and Matthews (42) of time spent by dietitians performing functions. In this study, consultant dietitians were asked to estimate the time they spent performing selected functions. In a study conducted by Shanklin and coworkers (43), clinical dietitians documented actual time expenditures on specific client-related, administrative, professional, nonprofessional, and delay activities and transit time. Thus, data collected could be estimated or real time. Results of these studies could be used by current and prospective dietitians to estimate the amount of time required for various professional activities.

Sometimes data from secondary sources can be useful in answering research questions. Greathouse et al (44) obtained financial data (salaries, other direct costs, overhead, and total costs) from the Health Care Financing Administration to compare conventional, cook-chill, and cook-freeze foodservice systems. Cai (45) analyzed food expenditure patterns on trips and vacations, and Ham, and coworkers (46) studied expenditures on food away from home using Consumer Expenditure Survey data from the Bureau of Labor Statistics. Using yet another approach, Cheung and associates (47) obtained organization charts from college and university foodservice operations and used them to evaluate the organizational levels, position titles, and lines of reporting.

Level of Analysis

The level of analysis is based on the experimental unit, the smallest division of subjects that can be randomly assigned by the researcher and can respond independently. The experimental unit dictates the statistical analysis that can be used. Data can be analyzed at the individual or the group level, depending on the research question, the type of data, and how the data were collected. Some research has examined variables at the individual level, especially research related to job characteristics, job satisfaction, and organizational commitment. Much of the research in foodservice management has focused on the group level, particularly studies related to productivity and financial performance.

Number of Observations

Research may be done as a one-time observation or may be replicated. Most studies using survey research techniques represent one-time data collection. For example, O'Hara et al (48) asked geriatric patients to complete a survey to determine which of eight aspects of food and foodservice affected satisfaction. Wolf and Schiller (49) conducted a survey of dietetics and foodservice personnel to determine their readiness to contribute to team problem solving. In both examples, data were collected at one point in time.

Hackes et al (33) made observations to determine the amount of service food waste in a continuing-care retirement community. They observed service food waste for 7 days to get a good representation of the weight and volume.

Replications of observations will indicate the stability of data over time, whereas one-time observations provide "snapshots" of the variables studied. The use of one-time observations or multiple observations depends on the research questions and the variables studied.

Research Design

The research design can be descriptive, preexperimental, quasi-experimental, or true experimental. Simulations and mathematical modeling also are used fairly extensively in foodservice management research.

Descriptive Research

Delphi Technique. The Delphi technique and its modifications have been used for descriptive research in foodservice management. The Delphi technique is a group process using written responses rather than bringing individuals together. A group of individuals, often experts in their field, receive a series of questionnaires. The first questionnaire may be made up of a few very general questions. Based on the responses to the first questionnaire, a second questionnaire is developed. The process may include several iterations, depending on research objectives and data generated.

The Delphi technique has the advantages of being versatile, cost-effective, and time efficient for participants. When using the Delphi technique, it is important to have adequate time, high participant motivation, and participant skill in written communication (50).

Johnson and Chambers (51) used the Delphi technique with 11 expert panel members to identify activities and performance measures for benchmarking in foodservice operations. They used a two-round process. In round 1, panel members responded to open-ended questions about measures for benchmarking related to four areas: operations, finance, customer satisfaction, and human resources. These results were clustered and used as the basis for developing a list of performance measures used in round 2, in which the panel members were asked to indicate the importance of the measures for benchmarking.

Gregoire and Sneed (52) used a modified Delphi technique to develop an understanding of the barriers and needs of school foodservice practitioners attempting to implement the U.S. Dietary Guidelines for Americans. A select group of school foodservice practitioners attended a conference on procurement. As part of the conference, participants were divided into two discussion groups and asked to generate a list of barriers, research needs, and training needs. After the meeting, these lists were combined, and a written questionnaire was developed and mailed to participants to rate the importance of the items generated. This process developed consensus on the importance of barriers and needs and provided information to develop strategies to remove barriers. Using the true Delphi technique, the first step would have involved mailing an open-ended written questionnaire to participants. These researchers took advantage of having the foodservice practitioners together to conduct the first step.

Gregoire and Sneed (53) also used the Delphi technique to develop nutrition integrity standards. Participants were a group of 41 individuals, selected because of their knowledge and expertise in child nutrition programs. In round 1, panel members were asked to review, evaluate, add, and delete proposed nutrition integrity standards. Researchers compiled all responses and developed a revised list of standards. This list was mailed to panel members in round 2. For this round, panelists were asked to rate their level of agreement that each standard was important to include using a 5-point rating scale. An item was retained if at least 85 percent of the panel members agreed or strongly agreed that it should be included.

Focus Groups. Focus groups are used to collect qualitative information from a predetermined and limited number of individuals. Focus groups are carefully planned discussions designed to obtain perceptions and information from a small group of individuals (7 to 10 people) in a nonthreatening environment. Group members may influence one another's responses to open-ended questions posed by the leader of the focus group. The use of focus groups has several advantages. This method is socially oriented, offers flexibility, has high face validity, provides quick results, and is low in cost.

Focus groups, like other qualitative research methods, may be used to generate instruments to collect quantitative data. Focus groups have been used extensively for market research and more recently have been used in dietetics-related areas. There are some examples of the use of focus groups in foodservice management research. Parham and Benes (54) conducted focus groups of foodservice management educators to determine their preparation, factors that are either satisfying or frustrating about teaching, research involvement, and what would help them do their jobs better. The researchers combined focus groups, survey research, use of an advisory committee, and review of college catalogs to determine development needs of faculty in foodservice management.

Harp et al (55) used consumer and industry focus groups to develop a beef appetizer for casual dining restaurants. Three consumer groups were used: university students (aged 21 to 24), young professionals (aged 25 to 30), and midcareer professionals (aged 31 to 40). The industry group was made up of managers of casual dining restaurants. These researchers developed discussion guides for the consumer and industry groups. Consumer questions were posed to determine participants' habits and attitudes regarding beef consumption and their reactions to a beef appetizer. Industry participants' questions focused on quality of beef available to restaurants, appetizer consumption patterns, and appetizer preparation orientation.

Survey Research. Survey research is an important technique in descriptive research. Survey research can help the researcher understand a population, describe a population, or test hypotheses.

Many studies have been conducted using survey research to better understand and describe a population. For example, Sneed (56), Sneed and White (57), and Gregoire and Sneed (58) used survey methodology to determine continuing education needs of various groups of school foodservice employees.

There are many examples in the foodservice management research literature of the use of surveys to test hypotheses. Sneed (59), Duke and Sneed (60), and Sneed and Herman (61) tested hypotheses about relationships between job characteristics and job satisfaction and between organizational commitment and job satisfaction. Gilbert and Sneed (62) collected data about organizational commitment, job satisfaction, productivity, turnover, and absenteeism of employees in hospitals in the United States and Canada. Examples of research hypotheses tested included the following:

- There is no difference in job satisfaction of employees in foodservice operations with different types of organizational culture (bureaucratic, innovative, or supportive).
- There is no difference in organizational commitment of employees in foodservice operations with different types of organizational culture (bureaucratic, innovative, or supportive).
- Job satisfaction of foodservice employees is not related to gender, age, education level, or years of experience.

Multiple linear regression was used to test the research models.

Surveys used to test hypotheses are developed carefully to ensure the validity and reliability of the scales

used to measure the research variables. For survey scales, the Cronbach α (63) is used to determine the internal consistency (or reliability) of the measure. When available, developed scales with established validity and reliability are used. Many validated scales have been used in foodservice management research, including the Job Descriptive Index (64); Job Characteristics Inventory (65); and Organizational Culture Inventory (66).

Researchers often want to study variables with no established scale. In these cases, the researcher must establish the scale's validity and reliability. Dienhart and coworkers (67) developed a 50-item scale to determine the service orientation of restaurant employees. This scale was used in later research conducted by Groves and coworkers (68). In both instances, the reliability of the scales was determined using measures of internal consistency. Unklesbay et al (69) developed a scale to determine attitudes toward food safety. The Cronbach α and item-total statistics were used to determine the reliability of the scale. These analyses indicated that there were two subscales. Based on the items that were related to each other, the two scales were named "personal responsibility for food safety" and "external responsibility for food safety" (which included, for example, government, food processors, and restaurants).

Survey research data are collected through either an interview or a questionnaire. Usually, data are collected from a sample of members of a population. Occasionally, an entire population may be used for a survey. For example, Sneed and coworkers (70) did a study to develop financial management competencies for entry-level and advanced-level dietitians. The population of directors for Plan IV/V, AP4, and dietetics internship programs were included in the study. They used a random sample of practitioners, because the population for this group was very large.

In reviewing the literature in foodservice management, survey methods is the research technique that is used most often. Survey methods have been used to study a variety of foodservice areas, including computer use (71,72), customer satisfaction (48,73–75), equipment (76,77), food safety (69,78), management decision making (79,80), personnel issues (49,81), and purchasing (82).

Survey research has many advantages as a research technique. Written surveys are relatively inexpensive and can be distributed to large, geographically dispersed individuals by mail. Thus, nationally representative samples are easily accessed. Individuals can respond either anonymously or confidentially, which increases the likelihood that responses will be frank. The written survey format provides each individual with the same stimulus, so the variability in data collection is minimized.

There are several disadvantages of survey research as well. One concern is the response rate. Ideally, 100 percent of the surveys mailed would be returned to ensure that the results were representative of the sample. In reality, the response rate is less than 100 percent. The researcher needs to determine whether the respondents differed in some way from the people who did not respond. The smaller the response rate, the less generalizable the results. Another concern is reading levels of the study sample. Pilot testing is needed to ensure that the individuals in the sample getting the survey can read and understand the survey questions. The format of the survey form limits responses from individuals, so there are no explanations about a respondent's answers. Also, respondents may not answer all questions in a written survey, so the researcher must exclude surveys with missing data, thus reducing the response rate.

Preexperimental Designs

Preexperimental designs often are used in field studies. They do not have the experimental control of quasi-experimental or true experimental designs. Preexperimental designs, because they are done in the field, do have the advantage of a naturalistic setting.

There are several examples of the one-group pretest-post test design in the foodservice management literature. Getlinger et al (34) studied the impact of the timing of recess on food waste. Sixty-six students in grades 1 through 3 made up the study sample. A 5-week study was conducted, with data being collected in weeks 1 and 5. For week 1, students remained on their usual schedule of eating lunch for 15 minutes, followed by a 15-minute recess. In week 2, the schedule was reversed. A 3-week period was given for students to adjust to the new schedule. Plate waste data were collected for 4 days during weeks 1 and 5. The same menus were served during the 2 weeks of data collection. The researchers found that plate waste decreased when recess was given prior to meal time.

A waste composition study was conducted in one retirement community with two interventions (source reduction intervention and service delivery intervention) (32). Kim et al conducted a baseline waste stream analysis during the spring of 1994, and they performed follow-up analyses in the spring of 1995, following their first intervention, and in the fall of 1995, following the second intervention. They found that these interventions were ef-

fective in reducing the weight and volume of waste in the retirement community.

Perlmutter et al (36) examined the profitability and acceptability of fat- and sodium-modified hot entrees in one worksite cafeteria. Two interventions were done: entrees were reduced in fat and sodium, and marketing was done for the modified entrees. Sales data were collected for the 9-month study, and acceptability data were collected before and after entree modification. The researchers found that the interventions did not affect sales, and acceptability scores of some of the modified entrees decreased.

A variation of a preexperimental design was done by French et al (37). They selected two high schools for their study of a pricing strategy to promote fruit and vegetable consumption in high school cafeterias. These high schools were not equivalent; one was urban and one was suburban, and the two schools had very different socioeconomic, racial, and ethnic compositions. In both schools, researchers obtained baseline measures of the number of fruit pieces, carrot packets, and salad servings that were sold. They lowered the a la carte price of these items by approximately 50 percent and measured sales. A second baseline was obtained when prices were raised back to the original level. Sales for fruit and carrot packets increased dramatically when the price was lowered, but sales were not significantly different for the two baseline periods.

Preexperimental designs have both advantages and disadvantages. One advantage is that they are conducted in actual operations, so the setting is realistic or naturalistic. The questions studied are applied, needed to improve operations, and often difficult or impossible to study using more controlled research designs. A major disadvantage is that the researcher has little control over extraneous variables that might provide alternative explanations for the results. This design often is viewed as a case study. To be able to generalize findings, the study would need to be replicated in other operations or settings.

Quasi-Experimental Designs

Quasi-experimental research designs are conducted in field settings. The quasi-experimental design does not allow the researcher to randomly assign subjects to groups, because intact groups are used. It does allow the researcher to determine who gets measured and when the measurement takes place. A good example of a quasi-experimental research study is a study conducted by Costello and coworkers (83). These researchers randomly selected six stores of a quick-service restaurant chain and randomly assigned two stores as control (no treatment), two stores as stores where employees were trained in lectures, and two stores as stores where employees were computer trained. Food safety principles were taught in four of the stores, and the control and two treatment groups were compared. The researchers found that knowledge about food safety increased 29 percent for the lecture stores and 20 percent for the computer-trained stores.

Quasi-experimental designs have the advantage of occurring in a naturalistic setting. This research addresses actual operational research questions, and the results may only apply to that operation. The lack of control (because researchers lack the ability to randomly select participants and randomly assign them to treatment groups) means that there are other plausible explanations for the results of a study other than the treatment or intervention. As a result, theories cannot be proved, only explored. Quasi-experimental studies often have more external validity (generalizability) than internal validity.

True Experimental Designs

True experimental designs allow the researcher to manipulate the independent variable and determine the impact on the dependent variable. There are many examples of the use of true experimental designs in foodservice management. These research studies often have been conducted in a laboratory setting, but there are examples of studies in a field setting as well.

Energy consumption (84,85) and heat processing (86-88) have been studied using true experimental designs. Tutt et al (84) compared the energy consumption (dependent variable) of 110,000- and 100,000-BTU convection ovens in a university and a school, respectively. The independent variables were load (full loads of 16 pans versus partial loads of 8 pans) and preheating (no preheating versus preheating). Three trials for each treatment were conducted.

There also are many examples of true experimental design related to food product development and food quality. Goldmon and Brown (89) examined the effect of fat (15 and 20 percent) and the addition of soy fiber (0, 4, and 6 percent) on the quality of ground pork patties. The sensory attributes of the treatments were evaluated by a 10-member trained taste panel. The impacts of cooking methods and other treatments of food products, particularly meat, have been studied extensively using true experimental designs (90,91). Food safety issues also have

been studied using true experimental designs. For example, Ollinger-Snyder and Matthews (92) evaluated the coliform and aerobic plate counts of turkey slices reheated in a microwave oven.

True experimental designs have the advantage that all the variables are controlled, and the impact of the independent variable on the dependent variable can be determined. One major disadvantage is that many areas in which research is needed cannot be studied in a laboratory under tightly controlled conditions. Much of what we need to know occurs in operations where people work. Thus, the use of this design is not realistic for much of the needed research in foodservice management.

Simulations and Mathematical Modeling

Simulations. Computer simulations are used to help understand the behavior of systems and to evaluate strategies for the operation of a system. Simulations have many applications in foodservice management and provide a research model for predicting outcomes in a cost-effective manner. The use of computer simulation in foodservice dates back to the mid-1960s, when Knickrehm (93) used simulations to determine dining room seating capacity. Guley and Stinson (94) applied computer simulation techniques for production scheduling in a ready-foods system. Lambert and Kilgore (95) and Lambert and Lambert (96) used simulation techniques to examine seating policies on dining room productivity in the late 1980s. More recently, Nettles and Gregoire (97) used computer simulations to examine time required for tray-line flow in school foodservice.

Research on the use of computers to plan menus dates back to the early 1960s. Balintfy (98) and Eckstein (99) did much of the early work related to using computers for menu planning. More recently, artificial intelligence systems have been developed for computer-assisted menu planning (100).

Mathematical Modeling. Several mathematical modeling techniques, originally developed for use in business operations, have been applied successfully in foodservice management. These models use mathematical relationships to represent some aspect of reality. Using mathematical models allows the researcher to draw conclusions about the impact of various decisions by experimenting with the model instead of with actual operations. The advantages of mathematical models are that they are a less expensive, less time-consuming, and less risky way to examine the impact of a decision than implementing the decision in an actual operation and observing the impact.

Mathematical models have been used to assist with foodservice decision making related to forecasting (101), food expenditures (45,46), and customer seating (102). Miller and coworkers (103), for example, used simple mathematical models to forecast production quantity needs for a university residence hall. The models they developed provided more accurate forecasts than did the manual forecasting methods that had been used previously.

RESEARCH OUTLOOK

Many research techniques have been used to address foodservice management research questions. Much of the research conducted to date has used survey methodology to describe and compare foodservice operations. Future research should expand the use of qualitative techniques to better build theories and explore relationships. Experimental research methods in foodservice management have been limited to product development and equipment testing; expansion of the use of experimental methods in actual operational settings would be beneficial and move practice forward. Knowledge based in foodservice management grows best through the use of a variety of techniques to explore research hypotheses. Researchers are encouraged to expand their use of a variety of data collection and analysis techniques.

REFERENCES

1. Rush G. Job analysis of lunchroom and cafeteria management. *J Am Diet Assoc.* 1925;1:130–137.
2. Baker RT, Barlow M. Personnel study of dietary departments of hospitals. *J Am Diet Assoc.* 1931;6:356–359.
3. Augustine GM. Labor policies in college residence and dining halls. *J Am Diet Assoc.* 1939;15:254–272.
4. Gleiser FW, Severance GM. Budgeting the student's food dollar in a cooperative residence hall system. *J Am Diet Assoc.* 1938;14:692–696.
5. Leigh MJ. Management and food control in the college dormitory. *J Am Diet Assoc.* 1939;15:179–184.
6. Pendergast WS. Standards of postgraduate training in school lunchroom management for college graduates. *J Am Diet Assoc.* 1938;14:93–98.
7. MacDonald MF. Measuring effectiveness in the prepara-

tion and service of hospital food. *J Am Diet Assoc.* 1938;14:330–338.
8. Rogers MP. Operating lunchrooms with pupil satisfaction and financial success. *J Am Diet Assoc.* 1938;14:85–92.
9. Blaker GG, Harris KW. Labor hours and labor costs in a college cafeteria. *J Am Diet Assoc.* 1952;28:429–434.
10. Donaldson BD. Labor hours in the dietary department. *J Am Diet Assoc.* 1957;33:1239–1243.
11. McKinley MM, Augustine GM, Chadderdon H. Training employees in work simplification. *J Am Diet Assoc.* 1957;33:592–595.
12. Bloetjes MK, Gottlieb R. Determining layout efficiency in the kitchen. *J Am Diet Assoc.* 1958;34:829–835.
13. Wise BI, Donaldson B. Work sampling in the dietary department. *J Am Diet Assoc.* 1961;39:327–332.
14. Knickrehm ME, Hoffman TR, Donaldson B. Digital computer simulations of a cafeteria service line. *J Am Diet Assoc.* 1963;43:203–208.
15. Eckstein EF. Menu planning by computer: the random approach. *J Am Diet Assoc.* 1967;51:529–533.
16. Andrews JT, Moore AN, Tuthill BH. Electronic data processing in intra-departmental food cost accounting. *J Am Diet Assoc.* 1967;51:32.
17. Quam ME, Fitzsimmons C, Godfrey RL. Ready-prepared vs conventionally prepared foods. *J Am Diet Assoc.* 1967;50:196–200.
18. Tansiongkun V, Ostenso GL. Job satisfaction in hospital dietetics. *J Am Diet Assoc.* 1968;53:202–210.
19. Hoover LW, Moore AN. "Dietetic com-pak" an educational model simulating computer-assisted dietetics. *J Am Diet Assoc.* 1974;64:500–504.
20. Orser J, Mutschler M. A computer tallied menu system. *J Am Diet Assoc.* 1975;67:570–572.
21. Wilcox MM, Moore AN, Hoover LW. Automated purchasing: forecasts to determine stock levels and print orders. *J Am Diet Assoc.* 1978;73:400–405.
22. Bobeng BJ, David BD. HACCP models for quality control of entrée production in hospital foodservice systems: I. Development of Hazard Analysis Critical Control Point models. *J Am Diet Assoc.* 1978;73:524–529.
23. Bobeng BJ, David BD. HACCP models for quality control of entrée production in hospital foodservice systems: II. Quality assessment of beef loaves utilizing HACCP models. *J Am Diet Assoc.* 1978;73:530–535.
24. Zallen EM, Hitchcock MJ, Goertz G. Chilled food systems: effects of chilled holding on quality of beef loaves. *J Am Diet Assoc.* 1975;67:552–557.
25. Swartz RS, Vaden AG. Behavioral science research in hospital foodservice. I. Work values of foodservice employees in urban and rural hospitals. *J Am Diet Assoc.* 1978;73:120–126.
26. Swartz RS, Vaden AG. Behavioral science research in hospital foodservice. II. Job satisfaction and work values

of foodservice employees in large hospitals. *J Am Diet Assoc.* 1978;73:127–131.

27. Calbeck DC, Vaden AG, Vaden RD. Work-related values and satisfactions. *J Am Diet Assoc.* 1979;75:434–440.

28. Olsen MD, Tse E, Bellas C. A proposed classification system for research and development activities within the hospitality industries. *Hospitality Educ Res J.* 1984;9(2):55–62.

29. Matthews ME, Bedford MR, Hiemstra S. Report on school food service research needs—1985. *School Food Ser Res Rev.* 1986;10:35–39.

30. Sneed J. Research needs in foodservice management. In: Sneed J, Holdt C, eds. *Issues for the 1990s: Americans with Disabilities Act, Cultural Diversity, and Research. Proceedings of the 17th Biennial Conference of the Food-service Systems Management Education Council.* Hattiesburg, Miss: The University of Southern Mississippi; 1993:73–79.

31. Soliah L, Walter JM, Parks T. Laboratory performance of sweeteners: implications for recipe and menu development. *J Nutr Recipe Menu Dev.* 1998;3(1):53–66.

32. Kim T, Shanklin CW, Su AY, Hackes BL, Ferris D. Comparison of waste composition in a continuing-care retirement community. *J Am Diet Assoc.* 1997;97:396–400.

33. Hackes BL, Shanklin CW, Kim T, Su AY. Tray service generates more food waste in dining areas of a continuing-care retirement community. *J Am Diet Assoc.* 1997;97:879–882.

34. Getlinger MJ, Laughlin CVT, Bell E, Akre C, Arjmandi BH. Food waste is reduced when elementary-school children have recess before lunch. *J Am Diet Assoc.* 1996;96:906–908.

35. Borja ME, Bordi PL, Lambert CU. New lower-fat dessert recipes for the school lunch program are well accepted by children. *J Am Diet Assoc.* 1996;96:908–910.

36. Perlmutter CA, Canter DD, Gregoire MB. Profitability and acceptability of fat- and sodium-modified hot entrees in a worksite cafeteria. *J Am Diet Assoc.* 1997;97:391–395.

37. French SA, Story M, Jeffery RW, et al.. Pricing strategy to promote fruit and vegetable purchase in high school cafeterias. *J Am Diet Assoc.* 1997;97:1008–1010.

38. Bergman EA, Buergel NS, Joseph E, Sanchez A. Time spent by schoolchildren to eat lunch. *J Am Diet Assoc.* 2000;100: 696–698.

39. Lieux EM, Manning CK. Productivity in nutrition programs for the elderly that utilize an assembly-serve production system. *J Am Diet Assoc.* 1991;91:184–188.

40. Diaz-Knauf K, Favila E, Vargas D, Sommer R. Behavioral problems at a student managed salad bar. *J Coll University Foodserv.* 1993;1(3):55–62.

41. Dowling RA, Cotner CG. Monitor of tray error rates for quality control. *J Am Diet Assoc.* 1988;88:450–453.

42. Theis M, Matthews ME. Time spent in state-recommended functions by consulting dietitians in Wisconsin skilled nursing facilities. *J Am Diet Assoc.* 1991;91:52–56.

43. Shanklin CW, Hernandez HN, Gould RM, Gorman MA. Documentation of time expenditures of clinical dietitians: results of a statewide time study in Texas. *J Am Diet Assoc.* 1988;88:38–43.

44. Greathouse KR, Gregoire MB, Spears MC, Richards R, Nassar RF. Comparison of conventional, cook-chill, and cook-freeze foodservice systems. *J Am Diet Assoc.* 1989;89:1606–1611.

45. Cai LA. Analyzing household food expenditure patterns on trips and vacations: a tobit model. *J Hosp Tour Res.* 1998;22:338–358.

46. Ham S, Hiemstra SJ, Yang IS. Modeling U.S. household expenditure on food away from home (FAFH): Logit regression analysis. *J Hosp Tour Res.* 1998;22(1):15–24.

47. Cheung M, Gregoire MB, Downey RG. College and university foodservice organization charts. *NACUFS J.* 1990–91;15:5–11.

48. O'Hara PA, Harper DW, Kangas M, Dubeau J, Borsutzky C, Lemire N. Taste, temperature, and presentation predict satisfaction with foodservices in a Canadian continuing-care hospital. *J Am Diet Assoc.* 1997;97:401–405.

49. Wolf K, Schiller MR. Dietetics and foodservice personnel are ready for team problem solving. *J Am Diet Assoc.* 1997;97:997–1002.

50. Delbecq AL, Van de Ven AH, Gustafson DH. *Group Techniques for Program Planning.* Glenview, Ill: Scott Foresman and Company; 1975.

51. Johnson BC, Chambers MJ. Expert panel identifies activities and performance measures for foodservice benchmarking. *J Am Diet Assoc.* 2000;100:692–695.

52. Gregoire MB, Sneed J. Barriers and needs related to procurement and implementation of the Dietary Guidelines. *School Food Serv Res Rev.* 1993;17:46–49.

53. Gregoire MB, Sneed J. Standards for nutrition integrity. *School Food Serv Res Rev.* 1994;18:106–111.

54. Parham ES, Benes BA. Development needs of faculty in foodservice management. *J Am Diet Assoc.* 1997;97:262–265.

55. Harp SS, Hoover LC, Crockett KL, Wu CK. Development of a beef appetizer concept for casual dining restaurants: application of focus group interviews and consumer sensory evaluation. *J Hosp Tour Res.* 1998;21(3):43–60.

56. Sneed J. Continuing education needs of school food service supervisors. *School Food Serv Res Rev.* 1992;16:23–28.

57. Sneed J, White KT. Continuing education needs of school-level managers in Child Nutrition Programs. *School Food Serv Res Rev.* 1993;17:103–108.

58. Gregoire MB, Sneed J. Continuing education needs of

district school nutrition directors/supervisors. *School Food Serv Res Rev.* 1994;18:16–22.

59. Sneed J. Job characteristics and job satisfaction of school foodservice employees. *School Food Serv Res Rev.* 1988;12:65–68.

60. Duke KM, Sneed J. A research model for relating job characteristics to job satisfaction of university foodservice employees. *J Am Diet Assoc.* 1989;89:1087–1091.

61. Sneed J, Herman CM. Influence of job characteristics and organizational commitment on job satisfaction of hospital foodservice employees. *J Am Diet Assoc.* 1990;90:1072–1076.

62. Gilbert N, Sneed J. Organizational culture: does it affect employee and organizational outcomes? *J Can Diet Assoc.* 1992;53:155–158.

63. Cronbach L. Coefficient alpha and the internal structure of tests. Psychometrika. 1951;16:297–334.

64. Smith P, Kendall L, Hulin C. *The Measurement of Satisfaction in Work and Retirement.* Chicago, Ill: Rand McNally; 1969.

65. Sims HP, Szilagyi AD, Keller RT. The measurement of job characteristics. *Acad Manage J.* 1976;19:195–212.

66. Wallach EJ. Individuals and organizations: the cultural match. *Train Dev J.* 1983;37(2):29–36.

67. Dienhart JR, Gregoire MB, Downey R. Service orientation of restaurant employees. *Hosp Res J.* 1990;14(2):421–430.

68. Groves J, Gregoire MB, Downey R. Relationship between the service orientation of employees and operational indicators in a multiunit restaurant corporation. *Hosp Res J.* 1995;19(3):33–43.

69. Unklesbay N, Sneed J, Toma R. College students' attitudes, practices, and knowledge of food safety. *J Food Protect.* 1998;61:1175–1180.

70. Sneed J, Burwell EC, Anderson M. Development of financial management competencies for entry-level and advanced-level dietitians. *J Am Diet Assoc.* 1992;92:1223–1229.

71. Chien C, Hsu CHC, Huss JJ. Computer use in independent restaurants. *J Hosp Tour Res.*1998;22:158–173.

72. Yoon BJH, Huss JJ, Brown NE. Computer use and training preferences of school foodservice managers in Iowa. *J Child Nutr & Manag.* 1998;22:6–12.

73. Lau C, Gregoire MB. Quality ratings of a hospital foodservice department by inpatients and postdischarge patients. *J Am Diet Assoc.* 1998;98:1303–1307.

74. Meyer MK, Conklin MT. Variables affecting high school students' perceptions of school foodservice. *J Am Diet Assoc.* 1998;98:1424–1428, 1431.

75. Gregoire MB. Quality of patient meal service in hospitals: delivery of meals by dietary employees vs delivery by nursing employees. *J Am Diet Assoc.* 1994;94:1129–1134.

76. Meyer MK, Conklin M, Nettles MF, Carr D. School foodservice kitchens: Are they equipped to meet the challenges of the new millennium? Part one: equipment availability. *J Child Nutr Manage.* 1998;22:68–72.

77. Meyer MK, Conklin M, Nettles MF. School foodservice kitchens: Are they equipped to meet the challenges of the new millennium? Part two: age, condition, and frequency of equipment use. *J Child Nutr Manage.* 1998;22:73–78.

78. Giamalva JN, Redfern M, Bailey WC. Dietitians employed by health care facilities preferred a HACCP system over irradiation or chemical rinses for reducing risk of foodborne disease. *J Am Diet Assoc.* 1998;98:885–888.

79. Nettles MF, Gregoire MB, Canter DD. Analysis of the decision to select a conventional or cook-chill system for hospital foodservice. *J Am Diet Assoc.* 1997;97:626–631.

80. Myers EF, Gregoire MB, Spears MC. Quality delegation grid: A decision tool for evaluating delegation of management tasks in hospital departments. *J Am Diet Assoc.* 1994;94:420–424.

81. Barrios J, Boudreaux J. Foodservice managers' perceptions of issues related to the employment of individuals with disabilities. *J Child Nutr Manage.* 1998;22:3–5.

82. Wittenbach SA, Shanklin CW. Health care foodservice directors' perception of the importance of value-added services offered by foodservice distributors. *J Am Diet Assoc.* 1997;97:1152–1154.

83. Costello C, Gaddis T, Tamplin M, Morris W. Evaluating the effectiveness of two instructional techniques for teaching food safety principles to quick service employees. *J Foodserv Syst.* 1997;10:41–50.

84. Tutt M, McProud L, Belo P, Ferlin B, Neil C. Comparison of energy consumption of fully and partially loaded institutional forced-air convection ovens: preheated and nonpreheated. *School Food Serv Res Rev.* 1989;13:146–149.

85. Cremer ML, Pizzimenti KV. Effects of packaging, equipment, and storage time on energy used for reheating beef stew. *J Am Diet Assoc.* 1992;92:954–958.

86. Sandik K, Unklesbay N, Unklesbay K, Clarke A. Simulating convective heating with bentonite models. *J Foodserv Syst.* 1997;9:229–244.

87. Tsai S, Unklesbay N, Unklesbay K, Clarke AD. Effect of convective heating profiles on water absorption properties of restructured beef products. *J Foodserv Syst.* 1997;10:51–71.

88. Mahadeo M, Unklesbay N, Unklesbay K, Sandik K. Effects of alternate foodservice heat processing methods on thermophysical properties of restructured beef products. *J Foodserv Syst.* 1992;7:15–28.

89. Goldmon DC, Brown NE. Effects of fat level and addition of soy fiber on sensory and other properties of ground pork patties. *J Foodserv Syst.* 1992;7:1–14.

90. Berry BW. Effects of formulation and cooking method

on properties of low-fat beef patties. *J Foodserv Syst.* 1997;9:211–228.

91. Pringle TD, Williams SE, Johnson LP. Quality grade, portion size, needle tenderization and cookery method effects on cooking characteristics and palatability traits of portioned strip loin and top sirloin steaks. *J Foodserv Syst.* 1998;10:73–88.

92. Ollinger-Snyder PA, Matthews ME. Cook/chill foodservice system with a microwave oven: coliforms and aerobic counts from turkey rolls and slices. *J Food Protect.* 1988;51:84–86.

93. Knickrehm ME. Digital computer simulation in determining dining room seating capacity. *J Am Diet Assoc.* 1966;48:199–203.

94. Guley HM, Stinson JP. Computer simulation for production scheduling in a ready foods system. *J Am Diet Assoc.* 1980;76:482–487.

95. Lambert CU, Kilgore RA. An analysis of seating policies on dining room productivity. *Consultant.* 1989;22:40–42.

96. Lambert CU, Lambert JM. Setting reservation policies: a microcomputer-based simulation. *Hosp Educ Res J.* 1988;12:403–409.

97. Nettles MF, Gregoire MB. Use of computer simulation in school foodservice. *J Foodserv Syst.* 1996;9:143–156.

98. Balintfy JL. Menu planning by computer. *Commun ACM.* 1964;7:255–259.

99. Eckstein EF. Menu planning by computer: the random approach. *J Am Diet Assoc.* 1967;51:529–533.

100. Petot GJ, Marling C, Sterling L. An artificial intelligence system for computer-assisted menu planning. *J Am Diet Assoc.* 1998;98:1009–1014.

101. Messersmith AM, Moore AN, Hoover LW. A multi-echelon menu item forecasting system for hospitals. *J Am Diet Assoc.* 1978;72:509–515.

102. Luckhardt WE. A waiting line model: determining the number of seats needed in dining areas. *J Coll University Foodserv.* 1993;1(1):25–37.

103. Miller JL, McCahon CS, Bloss BK. Food production forecasting with simple time series models. *Hosp Res J.* 1991;14(3):9–21.

24

Research Techniques Used to Support Marketing Management Decisions

Sara C. Parks, Ph.D., R.D.

Today, more than ever before, dietetics professionals face marketing research problems that are at the very essence of the profession. Some typical examples follow:

- Lisa is a clinical dietitian in the outpatient services of Any General Hospital. One day Thomas, one of her patients with diabetes, comes to her office with a Clif Bar given to him by a friend. Thomas likes the bar because of its natural food composition and its energy-producing qualities. However, he does not know how to access information about the product or where to purchase it in his local community. Lisa is not familiar with the product but recognizes it as a nutraceutical. She wants to be helpful to Thomas by investigating the nutrient composition of the bar, who makes it, and how it is distributed in the local market area. Lisa does a quick search of on-line databases and then proceeds to counsel Thomas.

- To combat declining occupancy rates and increasing competition, hospital administrators hire a marketing research firm "to study population demographics, consumer lifestyles, and buyer behavior patterns" in their service delivery areas. They ask the head of the foodservice department to prepare a list of important consumer factors that she would like the marketing research firm to include in its study. What population characteristics in each of the three categories should she request? How

should she approach the task? What should she do with the information when it is provided?

- A dietitian has been offering a supermarket tour for the past several years. The tour was very popular at first, but recently consumer interest appears to be waning. The dietitian had expected the project to have a more enduring life cycle. How can she determine if supermarket tours still have market potential? What kind of information should she collect? How can she find out what customers really think about the tours, the pricing, and the competition? What information should go to potential customers to attract them?

- A dietetics consultant wants to begin to advertise professional services. How should she advertise—by using the Yellow Pages, the newspaper, the Internet, the radio, church bulletins, or perhaps her own Web page? What should the advertisements say? How can she measure the effectiveness of her advertising? How much does she know about present or potential customers? What do they read or listen to? How much are they willing to spend on nutrition services?

These are a few of the typical marketing research questions that dietetics professionals often address. Answers to these and similar questions are available to any manager or practitioner who understands market research techniques and how to access marketing information.

Even individuals with limited knowledge of current research methods can develop better solutions to questions similar to the ones just raised if they understand the critical role that marketing research plays in marketing decision making.

If it is true that the central focus of marketing (and, therefore, of any organization) is consumer satisfaction, then it is also true that every organization is constantly conducting market research. Managers within organizations face a constant stream of consumer-related questions that they must address. For example, a chef wonders whether a new menu item will be well received by cafeteria customers. A dietetics consultant who is successful at one location contemplates opening a second office on the other side of town. A hospital with a new wellness program for older patients must decide whether to continue to count on physician referrals or to look for new referral networks. A client wants to find a national company's sales channel for a particular product in a local market. These individuals ponder important marketing management decisions. The key to achieving appropriate answers to these questions is determining the needs and wants of target audiences and delivering consumer-responsive programs and services more effectively than competitors.

The purpose of this chapter is to help dietetics professionals improve their marketing decision-making ability through the effective use of primary and secondary research. To that end, a definition of *marketing research* will be presented, along with a discussion of the important role it plays in understanding consumer behavior. The chapter will discuss the steps in the marketing research process, secondary sources of marketing research data, the more prevalent primary research techniques used to support marketing management decisions, and how the research pieces fit together to help define consumer behavior and to show the relationship of market research to marketing decisions.

MARKETING RESEARCH DEFINED

There are many ways to approach the study of marketing research and to define the term. First, marketing research can be defined as a process to collect and analyze data and information about a specific market situation. Second, marketing research can be defined in terms of how it

is used. There are two widely accepted uses of marketing research: to build the theoretical framework for the discipline and to provide data to support marketing-related decisions. Finally, marketing research can be defined relative to the techniques used to collect primary and secondary data. Both qualitative and quantitative techniques will be discussed in this chapter.

The definitions presented by the American Marketing Association and by Kotler are the more widely accepted among the attempts to describe marketing research briefly and accurately. In 1987 the American Marketing Association approved the following definition:

> Marketing research is the function which links consumers, customers, and the public to the marketer through information—information used to identify and define marketing opportunities and problems; generate, refine, and evaluate marketing actions; monitor marketing performance and improve understanding of marketing as a process. Marketing research specifies the information required to address these issues; designs the method for collecting information; manages and implements the data collection process; analyzes the results; and communicates the findings and their implications (1).

This definition enlarges the role of marketing research to include marketing management decision support, as well as the development of theory. The definition has three important parts. First, it deals with all phases of marketing; second, it emphasizes the systematic gathering and processing of data; and third, it links consumers to environmental opportunities and challenges. Earlier definitions of marketing research were limited to the first two parts of this definition.

An additional definition of marketing research that has been widely accepted is one proposed by Kotler (2). He describes marketing research as "the systematic design, collection, analysis, and reporting of data and findings relevant to a specific marketing situation." The specific marketing situation usually involves a marketing decision, such as introducing a new product, changing a promotional appeal, or monitoring market conditions and competitive pressures. Another important dimension of the definition of marketing research was presented by Eugene Kelley, an early president of the American Marketing Association. Kelley describes marketing researchers as the "investigators, the eyes, and ears of our profession," and he predicts that marketing research will become the "strategic lifeline" for business decision makers (3).

MARKETING STRATEGY

Most marketing research evolves from a need to understand market potential and characteristics, and from the need to design the appropriate mix of price, product, place, positioning, and promotion to meet the needs and wants of consumers within a firm's target audience. Kress (4) identifies the most prevalent uses of marketing research to include measuring market potential, analyzing market share, and determining market characteristics. More specifically, market research on target audiences will forecast demand for existing and new products and services, provide information on general trends, and provide data needed to segment markets. Marketing research may be used for new-product or new-service testing, packaging evaluation, or comparison studies of competitive products or services.

Pricing research identifies price elasticities and cost analysis. It also tests alternative pricing strategies for various marketing segments. Research on place involves site analysis and distribution methods. Research on promotion involves testing of different advertising messages, establishing sales territories, and selecting and evaluating advertising effectiveness.

Marketing research related to corporate marketing functions and responsibilities is less important. Instead, the key outcomes of marketing research should be to help firms understand and satisfy consumers' needs, to provide input for marketing decisions, and to serve as key ingredients of marketing information systems.

To identify marketing opportunities, Burns and Bush (5) suggest obtaining answers to the following questions:

- What is the market?
- How do we segment the market?
- What are the needs and wants of the market?
- How do we measure the size of the market?
- Who are our competitors?
- What product (program or service) will best satisfy our market needs?
- What is the best price?
- What is the best and most cost-effective way to reach our market?

The American Dietetic Association's *The Competitive Edge: Advanced Marketing for Dietetics Professionals* provides specific applications and case studies to guide professionals in generating answers to each of these questions (6).

A FRAMEWORK FOR STUDYING CONSUMER BEHAVIOR

If marketers completely understood consumer behavior, poor decisions about marketing strategies would be rare. Unfortunately, product failures are commonplace, advertising campaigns are less than effective, and pricing strategies do not always reflect consumers' willingness to pay. Does this mean that marketers know little about buyer behavior? Although marketers probably will never have a complete grasp of consumer behavior, they do know a great deal about why people buy products or services. Research related to how knowledge of consumer behavior assists marketers in making better decisions regarding satisfying customer needs and wants is based in social and behavioral science literature—in particular, the literature of sociology, psychology, and anthropology.

Patti and Frazer (7) define *buyer behavior* as a "process that includes the actions, internal and external, involved in identifying needs, and in locating products and services." These authors go on to say that buying behavior consists of five steps: (1) recognizing that there is an unmet need, (2) searching for solutions, (3) evaluating alternative solutions, (4) making a purchase decision, and (5) evaluating the decision after the purchase. The length of time it takes a person to work through these five steps varies with need and with the overall market situation. A product or service such as health care may be more important if a health crisis exists than when a consumer might be seeking a health promotion program. However, each step might be influenced through the manipulation of one or more elements of the marketing strategy. For example, advertisers might attempt to shorten the search for appropriate solutions by letting consumers know how certain products or services will satisfy their needs. This strategy, of course, requires that advertisers know what factors most strongly affect purchase behavior.

Peter and Olsen (8) present a general framework that many researchers use to study consumer behavior. It consists of four major elements: cognition, behavior, environment, and relationship building. In this framework, cognition is referred to as "everything that goes on inside consumer minds, including rational, emotion, and subconscious processes" (8). Examples of cognitive behaviors studied by marketing researchers include memory, knowledge, beliefs, attitudes, and intentions.

The second element of the framework is behavior. A review of the literature reveals that little attention has been given to what consumers actually do. The focus of most consumer behavior research is on what consumers say they think and feel or what they report that they do; actual purchase behavior is rarely measured, in spite of its relevance to understanding consumers and developing appropriate marketing strategies. Because purchase behaviors are rarely the result of a one-step process, and because they are sometimes impulse decisions, designing and controlling a study aimed at measuring such behavior is difficult. This problem is one of the reasons why measuring purchase-related attitudes has become so important in the marketing research literature. When actual behavior is studied, it is generally done through personal observations of each of the steps in the buyer behavior process and of how various marketing strategies influence the process.

The study of environmental influences is the third element of the Peter and Olsen consumer behavior model. Broadly defined, the "social environment includes all human activities and interactions" of the consumer (8). The social environment is important because much of a consumer's knowledge about products, stores, prices, and advertising is influenced by the opinions of other people who are known as *key influentials*. This influence is why, for example, many consumers purchase the same products as parents or friends. Culture and reference groups—groups that serve as guides to shaping individual behavior—not only influence marketing strategies but also play an important role in creating a consumer's social and physical environments.

The Peter and Olsen model is unique in taking consumer behavior research beyond the one-way, cause-and-effect relationship between knowledge and behavior often discussed in the marketing research literature. Earlier models suggested that knowledge change would automatically lead to attitude change, which would then cause behavior change. Although these one-way causal approaches do have value, they often ignore the relationships among cognition, behavior, and environments.

The fourth element of the Peter and Olsen marketing framework is building relationships with consumers through carefully defined marketing strategies. According to the authors, marketing strategy provides the physical and social stimuli (products, promotional materials, price, and information) needed to attract consumer purchases. Marketing strategies are aimed at influencing future consumer cognitions and behaviors to purchase the products in question. Typically, marketing strategies are based on past cognitions and behaviors as defined or documented through marketing research, with the assumption that future cognitions and behaviors will be similar to those of the past. As a consumer's environment be-

comes increasingly saturated with promotional messages, the task of reaching a consumer with a single product, service, or message becomes considerably more complex and burdensome. The task becomes one of collecting appropriate research data to increase the probability that the best strategy will be selected.

CUSTOMER SATISFACTION AND SERVICE QUALITY

Recent emphasis on accountability in the health care industry has heightened the need for dietetics practitioners to look at measurement of customer satisfaction and service quality. Administrators, legislators, third-party payers, and the media continue to question the essential elements of quality health care. Similarly, providers of nutrition care are struggling to understand how consumers evaluate dietetics services and outcomes.

The consumer behavior and marketing literature has defined the relationships among service quality, consumer satisfaction, and behavioral intentions (5,9–11). The literature suggests, and has tested, the following relationships:

Expectations – Performance perceptions

$$= \begin{bmatrix} \text{Service} \\ \text{quality} \end{bmatrix} \rightarrow \begin{bmatrix} \text{Customer} \\ \text{satisfaction} \end{bmatrix} \rightarrow \begin{bmatrix} \text{Behavioral} \\ \text{intention} \end{bmatrix}$$

The service quality theory focuses on the process consumers use to measure overall service quality; that process is translated into the difference score between what was expected and what was actually received. The theory further states that there is a causal relationship between service quality and customer satisfaction. Positive customer satisfaction leads to positive intentions to repurchase a given service or program.

Despite the importance of measuring service quality in the health care industry, little is published on consumers' perspectives on what constitutes quality foodservice or nutrition care and how quality relates to customer satisfaction. This omission is significant, given the profound marketing problems and challenges of the profession today. The majority of research on quality factors of nutrition care consists of descriptive studies focusing on client characteristics; the context and characteristics of the nutrition intervention; and in some cases, the physical, social, or behavioral outcomes of the intervention. Few studies focus on quality factors from a consumer perspective, and none were found to address the relationship between quality, satisfaction, and intent to continue to use dietetics services. Given the competitive environment for dietetics services, this omission places nutrition professionals at a disadvantage.

One of the most popular models in the consumer behavior literature for measuring the relationships among the three variables (customer satisfaction, service quality, and behavioral intentions) is the SERVQUAL model (12). Parasuraman, Berry, and Zeithaml developed and tested a comprehensive instrument that measures service quality on five dimensions: tangibility, reliability, empathy, assurance, and responsiveness. The theory underlying this model suggests that consumers are either satisfied or dissatisfied with services, that satisfaction occurs as a result of meeting or exceeding consumers' expectations, and that dissatisfaction occurs when performance falls short of expectations.

The SERVQUAL instrument assesses an organization's performance along each of the five dimensions and provides a basis for comparing quality factors across organizations, programs, or services. Its developers also have provided guidelines for adapting the instrument to other programs or services (13). In the guidelines, the authors cautioned other researchers to use the SERVQUAL instrument in its entirety, with modifications to account for specific settings or contexts; items can be added to supplement SERVQUAL and can be categorized under the original five dimensions or treated separately.

The instrument has been subjected to rigorous validity and reliability testing by both the authors themselves and numerous researchers across various service industries. Babakus and Mangold (14) have tested the model with hospital services and found it to be a practical model for measuring patients' expectations and perceptions. Brown and Swartz (15) compared physicians' and patients' perceptions of quality medical services and found serious gaps.

Others have found limitations to the instrument. Cronin and Taylor found the definitions used in the model to be inadequate and suggested that service quality be measured as an attitude (16). Tess supported the results of Cronin and Taylor and further found the model to lack discriminate validity with respect to attribute importance (17). Although the model does have limitations, even the critics agree that it should continue to be tested and used as a basis for understanding the relationships among service quality, customer satisfaction, and behavioral intention. The model is suggested here as a means for dietetics practitioners and researchers to understand the relationship between consumer satisfaction with nutrition services and consumer intent to be a repeat customer. For a more complete review of the customer satisfaction literature, see Oh and Parks (18) and Oliver (9). Further, the reader is referred to a compilation of articles focusing on other variables influencing service quality in hospitality, tourism, and leisure (19); a critical review of the literature regarding the expectancy-disconfirmation paradigm (20); and an assessment of the role of brand value to customers (21).

CATEGORIES OF MARKETING RESEARCH

Most marketing research can be placed in one of three categories: basic research, applied research, and simple fact gathering (5). Basic research includes studies whose sole purpose is discovery of new knowledge or theory; applied research is used to support operational decision making; and simple fact gathering is collecting some predetermined data. The nature of marketing decision making determines the type of research to be done. For instance, if a dietetics professional planning a weight-management program wants to know how many competitors are in a given geographic area, the task is merely to collect data. Thus, simple fact gathering is the appropriate strategy. In contrast, if the same practitioner wants to measure the effectiveness of a promotional strategy in reaching a weight-management audience, applied research is probably the more appropriate research technique.

A more useful categorization is provided by Weiers (22), who uses the functional objective of the research investigation as the basis of categorizing four major research designs: exploratory, descriptive, causal, and predictive. Exploratory designs help one to become familiar with a problem situation, to identify important variables, and to establish which avenues of future research can be pursued within budgetary constraints. The literature survey, focus group analysis, and interviews of experts are all examples of exploratory techniques.

Descriptive designs are the most frequently used designs in marketing research. They describe or provide information about such issues as the characteristics of users of a given product and the use rates of various media sources by specific market profiles.

Causal and predictive studies are seen less often in marketing research; however, as the discipline of marketing research becomes more mature and more fully developed, it is expected that causal studies will become more important. The goal of causal studies is to determine cause-and-effect relationships between such variables as advertising and package design on sales.

Predictive studies are used to forecast sales based on the relationship of variables to sales. For example, the Ajzen-Fishbein model predicts consumer behavior by looking at the relationship of beliefs, attitudes, and subjective norms to a consumer's intention to make a purchase (23,24).

MARKET RESEARCH PROCESS: AN APPLICATION

Although each research problem imposes its own special requirements, the marketing research process can be viewed as a sequence of five steps, which are discussed here as they apply to a cafeteria manager (Table 24.1).

Step 1: Formulating the Research Problem and Question

The first step of the research process, formulating the marketing problem and research question, requires that the re-

searcher translate the decision problem into a research question (22). In our hypothetical example, a hospital cafeteria manager is faced with declining cafeteria sales. The manager must decide what to do to improve those sales records. If the cafeteria manager attributes the poor sales to inappropriate advertising, the research problem would include a hypothesis regarding the effectiveness of current advertising. In this example, the researcher might set up a comparative study and measure the customer responses to two different types of advertising strategies. The research question could be, Is a cafeteria Web page a more effective means of increasing cafeteria sales than flyers distributed to departments and units? Defining the problem situation and important variables often requires exploratory research. At a minimum, the research problem must be defined clearly enough to state the hypotheses and objectives or research questions for the subject.

Step 2: Determining Information Requirements and Sources

Determining information requirements and information sources, the second step in the research process, involves

TABLE 24.1 Application of the Market Research Process

Sequence of Steps	Application
1. Formulating the research problem and question	Research problem: • Cafeteria sales are declining; poor advertising is the potential cause. Research question: • Is a cafeteria Web page a more effective means of increasing cafeteria sales than flyers distributed to departments and units?
2. Determining information requirements and information sources	Information requirements: • Annual, monthly, weekly, and daily sales. • Source, frequency, and types of advertisements. • Customer reactions to advertisement strategies. Information sources: • Sales records. • Advertising copy and records. • Customers' responses.
3. Examining the decision implications of research findings	Decision implication: • Within the limited budget available for advertising, should change advertising type, source, or frequency.
4. Estimating time and cost requirements of the research	Time/cost proposal: • Collect customer reactions via comment cards and focus groups over a 2-week period. • Focus group incentives. • Cost: $500.
5. Determining the appropriate research design	Design: • Exploratory design. • Combination of qualitative and quantitative data.

listing the information needed to satisfy the research objectives. In our example, the cafeteria manager will have to collect annual, monthly, weekly, and daily sales records; review sales of individual menu items; and review what types of advertising were used over the same time period, how often they were used, what messages were highlighted, and their frequency. Finally, the cafeteria manager will have to obtain data regarding customer response to both the current and the proposed advertising strategies. Some information will not be available, making it necessary to make appropriate assumptions about the project. Additionally, caution must be exercised not to collect information that is interesting but not directly related to the project. In developing the list of information, the researcher becomes increasingly aware of the primary and secondary sources of data that are available.

Step 3: Determining Decision Implications of Findings

The third step in the process is examining the decision implications of potential findings. Whereas most market researchers agree that this step is the most difficult, it is nevertheless important to the final success of the project. Weiers (22) views this issue particularly strongly: "If the answer to a particular research question has no influence on the ultimate decision reached, then resources should not be expended on attempting to answer the question." Suppose that in our hypothetical case, there are limited funds for changing advertising type, source, or frequency. Under these circumstances, the collection of data regarding daily television advertisements is probably inappropriate. Similarly, if the hospital's foodservice director is unwilling to make changes, even in response to customer responses, a lengthy and costly research study probably is a waste of time and money.

Step 4: Estimating Time/Cost of the Research

Estimating time and cost requirements and preparing the research proposal make up the fourth step in the marketing research process. Both time and cost are critical to the decision context. Market research is extremely costly, as the number of study participants must be relatively large if the results are to be generalizable. Larger sample sizes are needed in research related to decision support, because those response rates are typically lower than for other types of research. It is not unusual for managers to use the results of studies that have 30 percent to 40 percent response rates. In basic research, this response would be cause for considerable concern. Nevertheless, the timing of data collection and the cost of continuing inappropriate marketing strategies often do not allow for the follow-up procedures usually conducted in other types of research. In our example, the cost of developing customer comment cards and collecting them over a 2-week period is minimal; the only cost is printing the cards and providing incentives (free lunches) for individuals participating in focus groups.

Step 5: Determining the Research Design

As stated earlier, there are four types of research design: exploratory, descriptive, causal, and predictive research. Exploratory research is often used to define the problem; it is intuitive and often used by managers who want to determine factors that influence their markets' purchase decisions. Descriptive research refers to designs that help describe marketing variables. These studies describe consumers' attitudes, intentions, and behaviors. Descriptive studies are common in marketing research and are the mainstay of marketing strategy, as they allow for drawing inferences. Causal research involves controlling various factors to determine which variable is causing a particular outcome. Causal designs generally involve experimental design. The cafeteria manager in our example has decided that the appropriate research design is exploratory, as it should collect both quantitative and qualitative data.

COMMON ERRORS IN MARKET RESEARCH

Burns and Bush (5) discuss common research errors that reduce the accuracy and usefulness of marketing research studies. Aaker et al (1) identify four categories of error: problem definition error, informational error, experimental error, and analysis error. The most time-consuming step in the research process is trying to define the "right" question to ask: If the problem is not well defined, the research results will not be useful. If the researcher studies consumers' reactions to the quality of hospital food, but it is actually the time when food is served that makes a difference to consumers, then the wrong question is being addressed. This is an example of a problem definition error.

There are two types of informational errors: sampling and nonsampling errors. Sampling errors arise in collecting data from an inappropriate sample; nonsampling errors occur when sample responses are distorted by a variety of conditions and yield does not reflect the actual population. Response and nonresponse biases are additional examples of nonsampling errors. Response bias occurs because of a subject's tendency to exaggerate an amount (for example, amount of income or amount of product used) or to underestimate use (for example, cigarette or alcohol consumption). Nonresponse bias occurs when the researcher does not attempt to document the differences (characteristics, actions, and attitudes) between segments of the sample respondents and nonrespondents.

Experimental errors are closely tied to validity, reliability, and objectivity (25). Validity refers to how well the research measures what it claims to measure; reliability identifies the stability of the results over time or different conditions; and objectivity addresses the researcher's ability to avoid preconceived notions as to the study outcome. These errors can be minimized by conducting the research under appropriate blinding conditions.

RESEARCH USING SECONDARY DATA SOURCES

To collect information about consumer lifestyles and competitors is not easy. Often, the researcher must rely on secondary sources, such as state and local government information, annual company or hospital financial reports, media reports, advertisements, and other formal and informal observations. The following example illustrates internal and external secondary data sources that might be readily available to a researcher.

EXAMPLE. Your facility has just initiated a new policy requiring marketing research proposals for all new food and nutrition projects under development. No one on staff is experienced with marketing research. Because you need information on the general characteristics of the proposed market area before completing a plan, you ask your facility's marketing department to provide data from internal records and your assistant to access on-line databases to collect external data available The alternative to doing the secondary data research yourself is to hire a marketing research consultant, but your budget does not provide for that luxury.

Internal Data

Internal secondary data that exist within an organization generally are collected for reasons other than the project at hand. In a hospital, for example, both the medical records and the admissions departments have excellent demographic data on the facility's current and past clients. Most hospitals also collect information on some health behaviors, disease status, and geographic location of its target audiences. This information is invaluable when segmenting markets for any new product, program, or service. The accounting department often collects revenue and expense data, usually according to the product or service lines offered by the facility. To the extent that the organization maintains a formal marketing department, the data are more likely to be in the format that is readily usable for the project at hand.

Other internal sources of secondary information include previous marketing studies, periodic reports on facility sales, customer correspondence and surveys, and reports from pertinent departments (for example, long-range plans and admissions data). Being able to access secondary data substantially reduces the cost and time needed to conduct the study.

External Data

One of the biggest problems in collecting secondary data is finding the key words needed to access the articles or periodicals to be used and determining which of the thousands of secondary data sources are relevant to marketing decisions. The sources listed in this chapter's Further Reading can make the task of external data collection easier.

Data should not be overcollected; in most cases, more data than needed will exist. Furthermore, bias may be present in secondary data, and it must be controlled if the data are used to support a research design. Sponsoring organizations, interviewees, researchers, and editors all bring a bias to data they present; thus, the user of secondary data has an obligation to identify in the study the bias that specific authors place on the data. Additionally, when selecting the data, care must be exercised to make sure the research methodology is sound. Questions such as the following must be considered: Is the sample size reliable for the level of accuracy desired? Is the statistical analysis consistent with the data set? Can the results be generalized? The answers to these questions and others will help avoid some of the pitfalls of using secondary data sources.

Steps in Collecting Secondary Data

Breen and Blankenship (26) provide tips for collecting general marketing information from secondary sources. The following are their tips, adapted to make them applicable to dietetics:

1. Start by consulting the most promising guides: *Reader's Guide to Periodical Literature, New York Times Index, Business Periodicals Index*, and *Index to Health Care Literature*. These indexes will provide access to current business literature.
2. Refer to the Standard Industrial Classification (SIC) manual to obtain SIC codes. These codes will allow you to access specific statistics regarding specific industries in both printed and on-line databases.
3. Use free government information sources (for example, the U.S. Department of Commerce, Bureau of the Census, U.S. Department of Aging, U.S. Department of Agriculture, and National Institutes of Health. The federal government prepares three census reports—on population, housing, and business. State, county, and local governments have similar statistics.
3. Learn about other government sources. *American Statistics Index, Statistical Abstract of the United States,* and *Survey of Current Business* are excellent sources of business and general economic statistics. All these sources are currently available on-line.
4. Check state and local (city or county) government sources. Start by going directly to the Web sites for state departments of commerce and development, as well as libraries. At the local level, try city or county planning offices and the economic development commission; they generally have data regarding present and future growth plans.
5. Use business and professional associations. The professional member database and other research studies available through the American Dietetic Association should be one of the first places to check.

The National Center for Nutrition and Dietetics and the National Agricultural Library also are excellent food and nutrition on-line sources.

6. Check on-line directories such as those of Dun and Bradstreet and Moody's, as well as *Thomas Register*. These sources will provide data on various organizations and businesses in a given market area.
7. Check other sources of commercial printed and on-line information. The *Sales Management Annual Survey of Buying Power* provides local information on population, income, and retail business (including eating and drinking establishments), as well as an index of market potential. *Restaurants and Institutions* is a magazine that publishes market surveys, generally in the July and October issues. Gallup Organization publishes studies about food, eating habits, and health trends on an annual basis.
8. Learn about existing databases and data banks that can provide useful demographic, buyer behavior, and psychographic data. More than 5,000 on-line data banks provide both general and specific information. To access them, check the *Directory of On-Line Information Resources* (CSG Press, Rockville, Maryland) and the *Database Catalog* (Dialog, Palo Alto, California).
9. Select the right specialist to work with. Information brokers provide such services on a fee basis. Many public and university libraries offer database searches for a minimal fee. At your local library you should at least be able to find out where to access the information.

Secondary Data Research in the Current Marketing Environment

There is little question that the marketing environment for dietetics professionals has changed dramatically over the past decade: the profession has shifted from a product orientation ("You must follow this diet prescription") to a customer-driven emphasis ("These are your options"). Changing consumer needs, more intense competition, and other factors have forced members of the profession to shift from identifying unique food and nutrition interventions and services and searching for potential users to focusing on target audiences, individual customer preferences, consumer demographics, and lifestyles prior to product development. Moreover, with greater competition for food and nutrition services, there is an increasing need to promote dietetics services and to motivate customers to purchase. More important is the dietetics profession's recognition of the need to improve market performance by "targeting" products and services to specific audiences. We can no longer define our audience as everyone.

These changes require vast amounts of data from a variety of sources: internal information about customers' purchase behavior and external segmentation data such as geo-demographic, psychographic, lifestyle, and financial data, as well as buyer behavior patterns. All these data are critical elements of the new marketing behaviors just described and serve as the basis for the following example.

EXAMPLE. Any General Hospital wants to develop a segmentation plan for a weight-management program recently developed by its dietetics staff. Its goal is to make the program a revenue-generating project. With limited advertising dollars, the hospital's marketing and nutrition departments have agreed that they should collect information about potential clients for the program. They are under time constraints, so they decide to rely primarily on secondary data sources.

The first step in searching out information abut potential markets is to decide on the project's research objectives. A typical research question might be, What percentage of women older than 25 years have purchased weight-management programs during the immediate past calendar year?

There are several ways to segment the weight-management market. A geographic sales analysis of other weight-management programs might be conducted. Demographic data (income, marital status, education, and so forth) could be studied. Product consumption (Weight Watchers, diet books, television programs, and so forth) could be evaluated. Additionally, hospital records could be explored to determine specific clients who are overweight or who have had weight-management programs prescribed during the period in question.

The following illustrates some of the most common segmentation characteristics in action. A study of geographic data shows that most women purchase weight management-programs close to their work or homes. Approximately 75 percent buy programs within a 3-mile radius of these two locations. Of prime importance is demographics. The external reports evaluated indicate that the majority of women interested in weight management, as opposed to weight loss, are college graduates, unmarried, and

employed in professional positions. Benefits sought by this market segment are time, convenience, and the ability to have reasonable weight-management options that can be adapted to busy lifestyles. Psychographic research shows that this market segment has a positive attitude toward a healthy lifestyle and a negative perception about returning to the local hospital to make the purchase. All data must be incorporated into the decision-making process when the segmentation strategies are developed.

The segmentation dimensions that have been mentioned represent some common data studied, but they are by no means all of the alternatives. The reader is cautioned against some common misconceptions that oversimplify the market research process. First, market segmentation is not a partitioning process. Rather, it involves gathering information about potential customers and then assembling this information around commonalities. Second, segmentation is not merely a marketing process; its real impact is what it brings to an organization's market plans and strategies. Finally, it is a myth to say that everyone is a part of a segment in a given market. It is likely that a small percentage of a population is unclassifiable based on specified segmentation criteria.

This section reviewed the common sources of internal and external secondary market research data available to food and nutrition decision makers and illustrated how a secondary data search might work. The benefits of secondary data sources—including timely and cost-effective data collection methods—probably override the negative aspects of this research type.

THE USE OF PRIMARY DATA

Most primary data used to support marketing decisions can be produced in one of two ways: by questioning people or by observing selected activities. A number of researchers also include experimental research designs. With surveys, "data are collected by asking questions of individuals thought to have the desired information" (8). A number of survey techniques generally are used to collect market research data: mail and telephone surveys, interviews, consumer panels, and focus groups. Observational research involves a researcher who "observes the objects or actions of interest—and [the observation process] can be performed by a human or mechanically" (8). In developing experiments, the researcher "controls or manipulates one or more independent variables and determines the effect of such manipulation(s) on the dependent, or outcome variable" (8).

There is general agreement among marketing researchers that the purpose or purposes of the research should determine the method used to collect primary data. Because it is often difficult to identify the appropriate research method, there are generally accepted criteria for making that determination: validity of findings, cost and timeliness, versatility, and accuracy (1). For example, if advertising expenditures and sales revenues are key variables in a given decision context, the method used to study these variables must provide sufficient data to test the relationship between advertising and sales. Researchers often rely on mail or telephone surveys to collect market research data because they usually meet the cost and timeliness criteria. Marketing research is costly, so cost and timeliness often take precedence over validity, versatility, and accuracy. Such a trade-off, especially with respect to validity issues, requires careful consideration of the data in using it to support costly decisions. Because marketing research projects generally seek information about more than a single variable, versatility becomes a third factor to consider in method choice. For that reason, the observation method is rarely used alone; it is often combined with the survey method. Finally, Kress (4) includes accuracy and representativeness in the criteria for selecting a research method. These factors assess the quality of the results and the extent to which results can be generalized from a small sample to a total population.

Methods Used to Collect Primary Data

There are numerous ways of collecting survey data. Five of these methods will be discussed here: mail surveys, telephone surveys, personal interviews, consumer panels, and focus groups.

Mail Surveys

The mail survey method is the most frequently used technique in collecting market research data, but it is also the most frequently misused. Various authors provide tips to increase the method's validity and reliability. Vichas (27) presents 10 criteria to consider for successful mail surveys:

1. Choose a sample that is homogeneous or has a common problem large enough to be representative.

2. Compose questions that reflect the objectives of the project.
3. Keep the questionnaire at a reasonable length (a maximum of 6 to 8 pages).
4. Code questions to ensure quick data entry.
5. Lay out the questionnaire with an interesting format.
6. Develop a professional, yet motivational, cover letter.
7. Test the questionnaire internally with coworkers and externally with a small number of sample respondents, and revise as needed.
8. Produce the questionnaire in a quality, upscale printed format.
9. Know how to increase participation rates.
10. Review examples of other mail questionnaires.

Other techniques used to increase the reliability and validity of mail surveys include expert reviewing for content validity, applying statistical methods to determine the instrument's reliability prior to use, and determining face validity by pretesting the instrument with sample respondents. The reader is referred to Vichas (27) and Salant and Dillman (28) for more specific details on each of the 10 steps just listed.

Telephone Surveys

Another way to collect qualitative and quantitative market research data is through telephone surveys. Like written surveys, this method is fraught with both sampling and nonsampling errors that are of concern to marketers. Sampling errors involve getting the right numbers and kinds of people to respond; nonsampling errors occur when the true intent of the variables under question is distorted by external factors or by the interviewer or interviewee. With the increased use of household telephone answering services and devices, reaching the appropriate sample can be difficult.

The following questions may help the researcher determine the existence of response errors: Is the true meaning of the question being reflected by the interviewer? Does the respondent know the right answer? Is the respondent willing to provide true answers? Is the wording of the question likely to elicit a biased response?

Computer-assisted telephone interviewing and mechanical computer surveys are two additional methods used successfully to obtain marketing data. Computer-assisted telephone interviewing involves programming a questionnaire into a computer; the interviewer reads the questions from the computer screen and records answers on the keyboard. Random-digit dialing helps overcome the problems caused by unlisted numbers or outdated directories. This method generates lists of possible numbers, either randomly or through some other systematic process, which means the survey will not exclude unlisted phone numbers, as a survey using numbers from a published telephone directory would.

Personal Interviews

Personal interviews are a third survey method for obtaining marketing information. Although written and telephone surveys are good ways to collect data, most marketing researchers say these methods should be supplemented by personal interviews. There are four basic types of interviews: structured and direct; unstructured and direct; structured and indirect; and unstructured and indirect (27). An unstructured interview appears to have no fixed pattern or order of questioning, but it does have a clear objective or purpose. Direct interviews are particularly valuable in helping researchers observe subtle feedback that otherwise would be unavailable.

Consumer Panels

Consumer panels are often used to test new products using the same persons in several tests. Marketing researchers assemble a group of study participants for a variety of projects. There are several problems with consumer panel designs: panel members do not always represent the buying population; seldom are all population segments represented on the panel; people who state their opinions for pay do not always give honest answers; and some panel members prevent others from expressing their true feelings (29).

Focus Groups

Focus groups continue to be one of the most used and abused marketing research techniques. This method is based upon the assumption that people feel more comfortable and provide more useful information in small groups. Focus groups have four primary purposes: to provide input on new products, new markets, and new packaging; to aid in identifying key variables used in more quantitative studies; to provide input into the development of new products and services; and to obtain research data quickly and inexpensively (29). To ensure some credibility of focus group results, the leaders must be well trained, the group composition should be homogeneous, and the procedures for running the group must be clearly defined. More specific details on setting up focus groups is given by Greenbaum (29).

ATTITUDE MEASUREMENT

This chapter has focused on research techniques used to collect data about the who, what, when, where, and how of making marketing decisions. Attitude research in marketing is particularly important. because it answers the question of why consumers buy a given product, what their preferences are, what factors motivate them toward repeat purchases, and why some consumers exhibit brand loyalty and others do not.

Attitudes are so important to the marketing process that millions of dollars per year are spent in advertising aimed at maintaining or changing consumer attitudes toward products and services of all types. Most attitude research is done either to measure consumer attitudes or, once those attitudes are known, to help devise strategies for shaping them. The California Raisin Advisory Board's "I Heard It Through the Grapevine" and Wendy's "Where's the Beef?" campaigns are often cited in the advertising literature as two promotional activities that had tremendous effects on attitude change. The raisin commercials took a product with a negative image and created a positive, upbeat feeling about it. Wendy's commercials, in contrast, were aimed at changing attitudes regarding competitive products.

Earlier in this chapter, attitudes were identified as cognitions, and they are often considered either strengths or weaknesses in marketing efforts. An *attitude* generally can be defined as "a person's point of view toward an object or an idea" (4). Kress goes on to say that determining attitudes in marketing is the process of identifying people's feelings about product attributes and how important those attributes are to them. Fishbein and Ajzen (23) are considered two of the leading researchers in the application of attitude theory to various marketing contexts.

Several types of scales are used to collect information on attitudes, including semantic differential scale, projective and expressive psychological techniques, and Likert Summated and Thurstone Differential scales (27). Of these techniques, Vichas and others identify the semantic differential scale as the most frequently used data collection method in marketing research (27).

Semantic Differential Scale

Vichas defines *semantic differential* as the "repetitious measurement of a concept compared against a series of descriptive polar-adjective scales" (27). It is a technique designed to look at how much customers like or dislike a company, product, sales force, or competitor. Vichas lists five steps to success in semantic differential measurement: defining study objectives, developing questions and responses, pretesting the questionnaire, administering the instrument, and analyzing the data (27).

Consumers' responses to advertisements are often measured with a semantic differential scale. In the Cogg-Walgren and Sleszynski (30) study of consumer reactions to physicians' Yellow Pages advertisements, a semantic differential scale was used to determine receptivity to a number of different advertisements. Consumers were asked to rate, on a scale, their perceptions of the advertisement and its specific attributes.

In step 1 of semantic differential measurement, the definition of objectives, the researcher asks the question relative to the purpose of the study. To arrive at the study purposes or purposes, Vichas (27) suggests that advertisements be reviewed, comparative advertisement studies be constructed, or consumer buying profiles be considered. Step 2 in the semantic differential methodology involves developing the questions and response scales. Table 24.2 provides an example of a question used on a modified semantic differential questionnaire on which the scale ranges in four steps from excellent to unsatisfactory. The

pairs of terms (for example, *high quality / low quality*) were identified in focus groups, employee panels, and foodservice publications. The questionnaire item was based on a study by Susskind et al in which the authors presented a model for the design and validation of measures used in describing customer behavior (31).

Table 24.3 provides a semantic differential scale used to define certain consumer characteristics relative to two weight-management programs. Four to seven levels of intensity are generally considered adequate for a semantic differential scale (4). To avoid end errors, scales should be expanded by one step on either side. There is considerable debate over whether the semantic differential scale should have even or odd numbers of responses; Vichas (27) contends that even numbers force respondents away from the middle or "safe" response categories.

The final steps in the semantic differential process are similar to the steps in almost any other research technique: pretesting to improve the questionnaire, administering the instrument, and analyzing data. The advantages of the semantic differential method are in the areas of cost, time, and improved validity and reliability. The im-

TABLE 24.2   A Four-Point Semantic Differential Question[a]

Question: What do you think of the foodservice in this hospital?

	Excellent	Satisfactory	Okay	Unsatisfactory	
High quality	4	3	2	1	Low quality
Large selection	4	3	2	1	Small selection
Friendly	4	3	2	1	Unfriendly
Low prices	4	3	2	1	High prices
Helpful employees	4	3	2	1	Unhelpful employees
Many specials	4	3	2	1	Few specials
Flexible	4	3	2	1	Inflexible

[a]Used as an example only; scale has not been validated.

TABLE 24.3   A Seven-Point Semantic Differential Question[a]

Question: What characteristics of a weight-management program are important to you?

Slow Weight Loss	1	2	3	4	5	6	7	Fast Weight Loss
Inexpensive	1	2	3	4	5	6	7	Expensive
Nonprofessional nutrition consultants	1	2	3	4	5	6	7	Professional nutrition consultants
Inconvenient	1	2	3	4	5	6	7	Convenient
Unfriendly	1	2	3	4	5	6	7	Friendly

[a]Used as an example only; scale has not been validated.

TABLE 24.4   A Likert Summated Scale Used to Measure the Effectiveness of Components of a Nutrition Consultation[a]

Question: How useful was the information provided?

	Very Useful	Somewhat Useful	Not Useful	Do Not Use
a. Consultation	1	2	3	4
b. Handout	1	2	3	4
c. Verbal instruction	1	2	3	4
d. Video	1	2	3	4

[a]Provided as an example only; scale has not been validated.

provement in validity and reliability is seen particularly when the adjectives are generated by consumer focus groups or panels.

Projective and Expressive Psychological Techniques

Vichas (27) identifies four projective and expressive psychological techniques currently used in marketing research: association, completion, expression, and construction. The purpose of each of these techniques is to induce study respondents to write, or to respond to verbally, their initial thoughts about a term, phrase, or comparison. Another variation of the projective technique is to ask subjects to respond to a series of terms, phrases, or comparisons just with words that come to mind, or to complete a sentence.

Are projective and expressive psychological techniques of value in developing marketing strategies? The answer is that these techniques, by themselves, are of very little value. When accompanied by other research techniques, psychological techniques may be useful in testing new products. These methods continue to provide excellent results when used in basic research and have made substantial contributions to the generation of knowledge. Additionally, these methods are generally valid only when prepared by trained psychologists, a fact that makes the method much more costly than other methods.

Likert Summated and Thurstone Differential Scales

In the Likert Summated Scale, respondents are given a series of statements and asked to rate each statement on the strength of their personal feelings toward it. The statements used in the survey usually are selected from a larger list generated through exploratory research with consumers. Table 24.4 provides an example of a questionnaire using a Likert Summated Scale for measuring the effectiveness of a nutrition consultant. A four-point scale is used as an example; however, the scale could have as many as seven descriptors. A particularly good feature of the Likert Summated Scale is the ability to separate respondents into three groups based on their total scores: favorable, somewhat neutral, and unfavorable. This separation allows for comparisons The Thurstone Differential Scale is a method in which respondents are asked to select from a list of 100 or more statements the 20 or 25 statements with which they most agree (27). Once again, the original list is generated by a panel of experts and confirmed by consumer focus groups. Respondents are asked to identify and rank the 20 or 25 statements that they most favor. The statements deal with the same subject; for example, they would deal with either the organization's products or its advertising, but not both. Most statisticians believe that this process only develops a set of ordinal data and thus cannot be used to predict other people's behaviors. Measures of central tendency can be applied to the data collected using this method.

REFERENCES

1. Aaker D, Kumar V, Day G. *Marketing Research*. New York, NY: John Wiley and Sons; 1995.
2. Kotler P. *Principles of Marketing*. 3rd ed. Englewood Cliffs, NJ: Prentice Hall; 1986.
3. Kelley E. Marketing researchers will become "strategic lifelines" of corporations. *Market News*. January 1983.
4. Kress G. *Marketing Research*. 3rd ed. Englewood Cliffs, NJ: Prentice Hall; 1988.
5. Burns A, Bush R. *Marketing Research*. 2nd ed. Upper Saddle River, NJ: Prentice-Hall; 1998.

6. Helm KK, ed. *The Competitive Edge: Advanced Marketing for Dietetics Professionals*. Chicago, Ill: The American Dietetic Association; 1995.

7. Patti C H, Frazer CF. *Advertising: A Decision-Making Approach*. Chicago, Ill: Dryden Press; 1988.

8. Peter J P, Olsen JC. *Consumer Behavior: Marketing Strategy Perspectives*. Homewood, Ill: Richard D. Irwin; 1987.

9. Oliver R. *Satisfaction: A Behavioral Perspective on the Consumer*. Boston, Mass: Irwin McGraw-Hill; 1997.

10. Crispell D. *The Insider's Guide to Demographic Know-How*. 3rd ed. Ithaca, NY: American Demographics Books; 1993.

11. Chakrapani C. *How to Measure Service Quality and Customer Satisfaction*. Chicago, Ill: American Marketing Association; 1998.

12. Parasuraman A, Berry L, Zeithaml V. SERVQUAL: A multiple item scale for measuring consumer perceptions of service quality. *J Retail.*1988;64(1):12–40.

13. Parasuraman A, Berry L, Zeithaml V. Re-assessment of expectations as a comparison standard in measuring service quality: implications for further research. *J Market.* 1994;58:111–124.

14. Babakus E, Mangold W. Adopting the SERVQUAL scale to hospital services: an empirical investigation. *Health Serv Res.* 1992;26(6):767–781.

15. Brown S, Swartz T. A gap analysis of professional service quality. *J Market.* 1989;53:92–98.

16. Cronin J, Taylor S. Measuring service quality: a re-examination and extension. *J Market.* 1992;56:55–68.

17. Tess R. Expectations as a comparison standard in measuring service quality: an assessment of reassessment. *J Market.* 1994;58:132–139.

18. Oh H, Parks S. Customer satisfaction and service quality: a critical review of the literature and research implications for the hospitality industry. *Hosp Res J.* 1997;20(3):35–64.

19. Kandampully J, ed. Managing service quality in hospitality, tourism, and leisure. *Managing Serv Quality.* 2000;10(6):339–419.

20. Yuksel A, Yuksel F. The expectancy-disconfirmation paradigm: a critique. *J Hosp Tour Res.* 2001;25(2):107–131.

21. Oh H. Effect of brand class, brand awareness, and price on customer value and behavioral intention. *J Hosp Tour Res.* 2000;24(2):136–152.

22. Weiers RM. *Marketing Research*. 2nd ed. Englewood Cliffs, NJ: Prentice Hall; 1988.

23. Fishbein M, Ajzen I. *Belief, Attitude, Intention, and Behavior: An Introduction to Theory and Research*. Reading, Mass: Addison-Wesley Publishers; 1975.

24. Ajzen I, Fishbein M. *Understanding Attitudes and Predicting Social Behavior*. Englewood Cliffs, NJ: Prentice Hall; 1980.

25. Churchill GA Jr. *Marketing Research: Methodological Foundation*. Chicago, Ill: Dryden Press; 1989.

26. Breen G, Blankenship AB. *Do-It-Yourself Marketing Research*. 3rd ed. New York, NY: McGraw-Hill; 1989.

27. Vichas RP. *Complete Handbook of Profitable Marketing Research Techniques*. Englewood Cliffs, NJ: Prentice Hall; 1982.

28. Salant P, Dillman DA. *Mail and Telephone Surveys: The Total Design Method*. New York, NY: John Wiley and Sons; 1995.

29. Greenbaum TL. *The Practical Handbook and Guide to Focus Group Research*. Lexington, Mass: Lexington Books Series, D.C. Health and Co; 1988.

30. Cogg-Walgren CJ, Sleszynski H. Responses to physician advertising in the Yellow Pages. In: Leigh J M, Martin CR, eds. *Current Issues and Research in Advertising*. Ann Arbor, Mich: University of Michigan Press; 1987.

31. Susskind A, Barchgrevnik C, Brymer R, Kacmar M. Customer service behavior and attitudes among hotel managers: a look at perceived support, functions, standards for service, and service process outcomes. *J Hosp Tour Res.* 2000;24(3):373–397.

Further Reading

Adapted from bibliography by Diane Zabel, Endowed Librarian for Business, Schreger Business Library, The Pennsylvania State University, University Park, Pennsylvania (unpublished). 2002. Used with permission.

Consumer Information: Sources on Demographics, Consumer Spending Patterns, Life Styles, and Social Trends

American Demographics [periodical]. Ithaca, NY: American Demographics; 1979. Provides descriptions of consumer market segments based on lifestyle, demographic, and psychographic factors.

American Forecaster Almanac. Ithaca, NY: American Demographics Books; 1994.

The American Marketplace: Demographics and Spending Patterns. 5th ed. Ithaca, NY: New Strategist Publications; 2001.

American Women: Who They Are and How They Live. 2nd ed. Ithaca, NY: New Strategist Publications; 2002.

Consumer Sourcebook. 15th ed. Detroit, Mich: Gale Group; 2002. This guide indexes over 18,000 agencies, associations, information centers, clearinghouses, and related sources in all fields.

The Gallup Poll Monthly. Princeton, NJ: The Gallup Poll; 1989– . Presents market research data on many consumer issues, including eating and dining behavior.

Generation X: The Young Adult Market. 2nd ed. Ithaca, NY: New Strategist Publications; 2001.

Americans 55 and Older: A Changing Market. 3rd ed. Ithaca, NY: New Strategist Publications; 2001.

Household Spending: Who Spends How Much on What. 6th ed. Ithaca, NY: New Strategist Publications; 2001.

Lifestyle Market Analyst. Wilmette, Ill: Standard Rate and Data Service; 1989– .

Mitchell S. *American Generations: Who They Are, How They Live, What They Think.* 4th ed. Ithaca, NY: New Strategist Publications; 2003.

Mitchell S. *American Attitudes: Who Thinks What About the Issues That Shape Our Lives.* 3rd ed. Ithaca, NY: New Strategist Publications; 2000.

Popcorn F. *Clicking: 16 Trends to Future Fit Your Live, Your Work, and Your Business.* New York, NY: HarperCollins; 1996.

Popcorn F. *EVEolution: The Eight Truths of Marketing to Women.* New York: Hyperion; 2000.

Russell C. *American Incomes: Demographics of Who Has Money.* 4th ed. Ithaca, NY: New Strategist Publications; 2001.

Russell C. *The Official Guide to Racial and Ethnic Diversity.* Biennial. Ithaca, NY: New Strategist Publications; 1996– .

The Sourcebook of Zip Code Demographics and Spending Patterns. Fairfax, Va: CACI; 1990– .

Statistical Abstract of the United States. Washington, DC: US Department of Commerce, Bureau of the Census; 1878– . Brings together statistics published by both governmental and private sources, including census data. The subject heading "Projections" is of particular interest.

U.S. Bureau of the Census. *1990 Census of Population and Housing.* Washington, DC: US Department of Commerce, Economics, and Statistics Administration, Bureau of the Census. For sale by the Superintendent of Documents, US Government Printing Office, 1993. (For 2000 Census data, see under Resources Available on the Internet, below.)

Valdes MI, Seoane MH. *Hispanic Market Handbook: The Definitive Source for Reaching This Lucrative Segment of American Consumers.* New York, NY: Gale Research; 1995.

Resources Available on the Internet (Some by Subscription Only)

American Demographics Web Site. Available at: http://www.demographics.com.

Census 2000 Gateway. Available at: http://www.census.gov. Provides summaries of the most frequently requested census data for states and counties. Users can also access tables and maps of 2000 Census data by geographical units, including the block level. Also includes detailed demographic profiles, special reports on demographic changes, tables showing rankings and comparisons, and selected data from previous censuses.

Factiva [database]. New York, NY: Dow Jones Inc. Provides over 3,000 publications, including The Wall Street Journal, Asian Wall Street Journal, Wall Street Journal Europe, Financial Times, New York Times, Washington Post, and Los Angeles Times. Also provides access to the most recent issues of Barron's, Forbes, Fortune, Far Eastern Economic Review, and Smart Money. Also gives current and historical stock quotes and company data. This database replaces Dow Jones Interactive.

LexisNexis Academic Universe [database]. Miamisburg, Ohio: LexisNexis. Provides full-text access to a wide range of news, business, legal, and reference sources. Covers many news sources for 20 years.

Polling the Nations [database]. Bethesda, Md: Silver Platter International.

Proquest Direct [database]. Ann Arbor, Mich: University Microfilms International. Indexes more than 5,000 periodicals and newspapers. Articles can be viewed in full-text, full-image format. Includes the ABI Inform database—a business-oriented database covering 1,400 trade, research, and popular journals in all fields of business.

U.S. Census Bureau Web Site. Available at: http://www. census.gov.

Marketing Research

American Business Climate and Economic Profiles. Detroit, Mich: Gale Research; 1994.

Markets of the U.S. for Business Planners: Historical and Current Profiles of 184 U.S. Urban Economies by Major Section and Industry, with Maps, Graphics, and Commentary. 2nd ed. Detroit, Mich: Omnigraphics; 1996.

Rand McNally Commercial Atlas and Marketing Guide. 133rd ed. Chicago, Ill: Rand McNally; 2002.

Sales and Marketing Management. Survey of Buying Power and Media Markets. New York, NY: Bill Brothers Publications; 2000– . Population, effective buying power, and retail sales estimates for state, county, and metropolitan areas. Includes special reports on most affluent markets and population shifts.

Site Selection. Norcross, Ga: Conway Data; 1994– .

The Sourcebook of Zip Code Demographics. Fairfax, Va: CACI; 1990– .

Standard Directory of Advertisers. Skokie, Ill: National Register Pub Company; 1964– .

Statistical Abstract of the United States. Washington, DC: US Department of Commerce, Bureau of the Census; 1878– . Recent editions available on-line at http://www.census.gov.

Resources Available on CD-ROM or the Internet (Some by Subscription Only)

Advertising Age [weekly]. Chicago, Ill: Crain Communications, Inc. Available at: http://www.adage.com.

Advertising World. Available at: http://advertising.utexas.edu.

American Demographics. Ithaca, NY. Available at: http://www.demographics.com.

Business Periodicals Index. New York, NY: H.W. Wilson Company. This index is useful for identifying major business journals from 1958 to present.

Choices II [CD-ROM]. Tampa, Fla: Simmons Market Research Bureau, Inc. Provides demographic and psychographic data on adult consumers of brand-name products and services. Data are based on a national survey conducted by a private research company.

KnowThis.com: Marketing Virtual Library. Available at: http://www.knowthis.com.

Mouse Tracks. Available at: http://nsns.com/MouseTracks.

PhoneDisc Powerfinder [database]. Bethesda, Md: Digital Directory Assistance, Inc. Includes more than 115 million U.S. business and residential listings. Searchable by name, mailing address, city, state, zip code, telephone number, distance, industry code, or Yellow Page heading. Can be used to identify potential customers.

The Right Site. Available at: http://www.easidemographics.com.

Sales and Marketing Management. Available at: http://www.salesandmarketing.com.

Tilburg University: Marketing and Marketing Research. Available at: http://www.tilburguniversity.nl/faculties/few/marketing/links/journal1.html.

Legislative Trends

Federal Regulatory Directory. Washington, DC: Congressional Quarterly; 1979– .

U.S. Government Manual. Washington, DC: Office of the Federal Register, National Archives and Records Services, General Services Administration; 1973– .

Industry Research

Directory of Corporate Affiliations. Skokie, Ill: National Register Publishing Company; 1973– .

Standard & Poor's Net Advantage [on-line database]. New York, NY: Standard & Poor's Corporation. Provides industry overiews and basic statistics for most industries.

Value Line Investment Survey. New York, NY: Value Line Publishing, Inc; 1995– .

Ward's Business Directory of U.S. Private and Public Companies. Detroit, Mich: Gale Research; 1989– .

Company Research

Almanac of Business and Industrial Financial Ratios. Englewood Cliffs, NJ: Prentice-Hall; 1970– .

American Big Business Directory. Omaha, Neb: Info USA; 2002.

Directory of Corporate Affiliations. Skokie, Ill: National Register Publishing Company; 1973– .

Industry Norms and Key Business Ratios, One Year. Murray Hill, NJ: Dun & Bradstreet Credit Services; 1989– .

RMA Annual Statement Studies. Philadelphia, Pa: Robert Morris Associates; 1977– .

Ward's Business Directory of U.S. Private and Public Companies. Detroit, Mich: Gale Research; 1989– .

Resources Available on the Internet (Some by Subscription Only)

Disclosure Global Access [database]. Enables users to access more than 5 million documents for company and industry research. Includes the Disclosure and Worldscope databases. Information includes company, financial, management data; SEC filings; annual reports; insider-trading filings.

EDGAR. Available at: http://www.sec.gov. A database of the U.S. Security and Exchange Commission filings for individual companies.

Factiva [database]. New York, NY: Dow Jones Inc. Provides over 3,000 publications, including The Wall Street Journal, Asian Wall Street Journal, Wall Street Journal Europe, Financial Times, New York Times, Washington Post, and Los Angeles Times. Also provides access to the most recent issues of Barron's, Forbes, Fortune, Far Eastern Economic Review, and Smart Money. Also gives current and historical stock quotes and company data. This database replaces Dow Jones Interactive.

FISonline [database]. Available at: http://www.fisonline.com. A subscription-based service offering information on 11,000 U.S. public companies and 17,000 non-U.S. public companies. Database is produced by Mergent, Inc, formerly known as Moody's.

Hoover's Online. Available at: http://www.hoovers.com. Web site includes information on company backgrounds, products and services, employment figures, finances, and stock quotes.

PC Quote. Available at: http://www.pcquote.com. Provides real-time securities quotations, recent related headlines, free delayed quotes, corporate profiles, and charts of stock performance.

Standard & Poor's Net Advantage [on-line database]. New York, NY: Standard & Poor's Corporation. Provides industry overiews and basic statistics for most industries.

Yahoo/Finance. Available at: http://quote.yahoo.com. Provides real-time securities quotations, recent related headlines, free delayed quotes, corporate profiles, and charts of stock performance.

Nutrition and Health Research

Resources Available on the Internet

The following Web sites provide information on nutrition, food safety, food service management, nutrition education, and consumer health. They also give links to national and international databases, professional associations, and related government organizations.

The Arbor Nutrition Guide. Available at: http://www. arborcom.com.

Arizona Health Sciences Library Nutrition and Health Page. Available at: http://www.ahsc.Arizona.edu/guides/ topics.

FDA Center for Food Safety and Applied Nutrition. Available at: http://www.cfsan.fda.gov/list.html.

Food and Nutrition Information Center (FNIC), United States Department of Agriculture. Available at: http://www. nal.usda.gov/fnic/.

IBIDS (International Bibliographic Information on Dietary Supplements Database). Available at: http://ods.od.nih. gov/databases/ibids.html.

IFIC (International Food Information Council). Available at: http://ific.org.

The Tufts University Nutrition Navigator. Available at: http://navigator/tufts.edu/about.html.

25

Dietetics Education Research

Mary B. Gregoire, Ph.D., R.D., F.A.D.A.

Dietetics education is defined by the Commission on Accreditation for Dietetics Education as "a dynamic and complex process that translates the theoretical and ideal into application and practice" (1[p3]). The formal education of dietitians began in the 1920s (2). At nearly the same time, research on dietetics education began as a way to find reliable answers to education questions, discover the best ways of educating future dietitians, and establish principles for dietetics education. The first issue of the *Journal of the American Dietetic Association*, published in 1925, contained a questionnaire from the education section of the American Dietetic Association (ADA) designed to solicit information on the courses given to student dietitians in hospitals (3).

This chapter categorizes research in dietetics education, discusses techniques used when conducting dietetics education research, and suggests future directions for dietetics education research. The chapter is not intended to be an exhaustive review of the research that has been conducted on dietetics education but rather will cite selected studies as examples within each section.

CATEGORIZATION OF DIETETICS EDUCATION RESEARCH

In Chapters 1 and 2 of this text, Monsen and Cheney categorize research as descriptive or analytic. Descriptive research describes what exists at a given point in time; analytic research involves testing hypotheses. Nearly all the research done in dietetics education would be categorized as descriptive, with only a small percentage of published research categorized as analytic.

Descriptive Research

Descriptive research studies include qualitative research, case reports, and survey research. The survey has been the predominant descriptive research design used in dietetics education research since its beginning in the 1920s. Surveys have been used to describe attitudes, beliefs, or practices related to dietetics education. These descriptive studies have focused on issues of concern to dietetics educators at particular points in time.

For example, Plan IV was adopted as the model for minimum competencies for dietetics education programs in 1974. Following its release, several survey projects were published addressing issues related to the determination of essential entry-level competencies (4–9). The introduction of the coordinated undergraduate program (CUP) prompted a series of descriptive studies to examine the quality of graduates from both the newer CUP and the traditional internship programs. Studies included evaluations of internship program (10,11) and CUP (12–16) graduates and comparisons of the graduates of both programs (17,18). More recent examples of descriptive studies include a focus on program content (19–23) and perceptions of cost-effectiveness (24).

Case studies also have been used to report results of descriptive studies related to dietetics education. These case studies (25–28) usually describe teaching techniques and innovative course content implemented at an individual dietetics education program.

Analytic Research

Very little of the dietetics education research could be categorized as analytic. The studies that have been structured as more experimental, with the goal of hypothesis testing, have focused primarily on the testing of methods for teaching information to students.

Only two analytic dietetics education research articles were published in the *Journal of the American Dietetic Association* between 1995 and 2000. Both (29,30) focused on evaluation of the effectiveness of computer-based simulations or instruction.

DATA COLLECTION TECHNIQUES

A variety of data collection techniques have been used in dietetics education research. Questionnaires have been the most common data collection technique used, but the use of tests, interviews, and observations also has been reported. This section gives examples of dietetics education research studies using each technique and discusses potential concerns.

Questionnaires

A questionnaire is a group of printed questions used to elicit information from respondents by self-report. The questions may be open ended, requiring respondents to answer in their own words; closed ended, requiring respondents to select one or more answers from among the answers provided; or a combination of the two. Questionnaires are the most common data collection technique reported in dietetics education research. Recent research studies have used questionnaires to collect data from students (19,31,32), preceptors (19,24,31), program directors (19–22), and practitioners (19,26) to address issues related to dietetics education.

Perkin discusses the design and use of questionnaires in Chapter 14 of this text. The accuracy of data collected using a questionnaire can be jeopardized when a question's meaning is misinterpreted. Guides for effective questionnaire development in Chapters 14 and 24 provide valuable information for individuals using this technique for data collection. Pretesting the questionnaire can help reduce the chances of misinterpretation of questions.

Tests

A test is any series of questions or exercises developed for assessing human performance. Standardized tests have consistent and uniform procedures for administration and for scoring and interpreting behavior and have been demonstrated to have strong validity and reliability (33). Moore (34) suggests that tests that are not standardized usually do not have an established procedure for administration and have not been constructed using procedures to minimize error.

Numerous standardized tests have been developed for measuring such things as personality, reading, intelligence, and achievement. The most common references that list standardized, commercially available measuring instruments are the *Mental Measurement* Yearbooks (35) and their companion volume, *Tests in Print* (36).

Standardized tests are not commonly used in dietetics education research. One recent example, however, was the work of McCabe et al (37). The authors used the Nelson-Denny Reading Test, a published reading skills test, in their research designed to assess and compare reading skills of dietetics interns with reading levels of internship references.

The use of researcher-developed tests is commonly reported in dietetics education research. Researchers who have developed their own tests have documented the steps taken to ensure the reliability and validity of the tests. A common use of researcher-developed tests is to measure knowledge or behavior before and after an educational program is initiated. Miller and Shanklin (38), for example, developed a test to measure behavioral objectives related to forecasting. The test was given before and after completion of a self-instructional module on foodservice forecasting, and data analysis focused on the change in test scores.

Dietetics education researchers collecting data using either standardized or nonstandardized tests must be concerned about the effect of retesting and test anxiety. The retesting effect is of primary concern in designs that use a pretest and a posttest as part of the methodology. The retesting effect is the improvement in test scores that occurs on subsequent tests because a previous test had been taken on the same material. The amount of this effect varies depending on the type of test, the sophistication of the test taker, and the amount of time between the two testings. Anderson et al (39) suggest that although reduction of the retesting effect may be difficult, having a control group that takes both the pretest and the posttest provides researchers with a way to statistically control for the effect of retesting.

Test anxiety is a concern because it may affect the meaning of test scores and thus influence inferences based on those scores. Dietetics education researchers can try to reduce the likelihood of test anxiety before data are collected, or they can try to assess the level of test anxiety and then take its influence into account in analysis and interpretation.

Interviews

Touliatos and Compton (40) define an *interview* as a verbal interaction in which an interviewer tries to obtain information from, and sometimes impressions about, an interviewee. Interviews vary in the amount of structure imposed and thus are categorized as structured or unstructured. Friebel and coworkers (41) used interviews of clients to obtain information on the effectiveness of students as nutrition counselors.

Dietetics educators using interviews must consider the possible increased cost involved using this technique and the bias the interviewer can create. Training and using skilled interviewers is expensive, and the time involved is often long. Interviewer training is critical, however, to help reduce bias. When several people serve as interviewers, interrater reliability must be assessed to reduce potential rater bias in the results.

Observation

As a data collection technique, observation allows researchers to document visual perceptions of behavior as it occurs rather than rely on self-reports of behavior in tests, questionnaires, and interviews. Research by Vickery and associates (42) is an example of the use of observation in dietetics education research. The authors videotaped students conducting diet counseling interviews. Trained observers documented 61 skills using a scale ranging from 0 (absent) to 3 (excellent).

Anderson et al (39) indicate that observation data can be collected using ratings, systematic observation, or sequential narratives. They define *ratings* as subjective assessments made on an established scale. They state that systematic observation instruments include two types of recording systems: sign and category. Sign systems list a large number of variables, and each variable that occurs during a given period of observation is marked. For example, a list of classroom behaviors might include the following: "student asks question," "teacher gives directions," and so forth. An observer using a sign system type of observation instrument would check each of the behaviors observed. Behaviors occurring more than once during the observation period are checked only once. Category systems generally include a more restricted number of variables. These variables are recorded continuously as often as they occur to produce an ongoing, moving record of behaviors. In the classroom example just cited, the observer would record continuous behavior, documenting each time the student asks a question, each time the teacher provides direction, and so on. Data collected using the category system of observation would include a sequence of events in the classroom and the frequency of occurrence of particular behaviors. Sequential narratives are a written description of all behaviors that occur during an observation session.

Dietetics education researchers who choose to use observation techniques for data collection must consider the Hawthorne and halo effects. The *Hawthorne effect* refers to changes in behavior that occur when subjects in an experiment or evaluation are aware of their special status. Students may work more eagerly or teachers teach more enthusiastically, perhaps because they feel they have been specially chosen. To help reduce the Hawthorne effect, researchers often need to minimize the newness of the program to students or find ways to make both the treatment and the control groups feel they are receiving something special. The halo effect occurs when raters allow their general impressions to influence their judgment when documenting observations. Thorough training of observers usually is needed to help reduce the impact of the halo effect.

FUTURE RESEARCH NEEDS

Dietetics education research has provided valuable information for dietetics educators. However, most of the research conducted to date has been descriptive. Some of the research has focused on results of an educational technique tried in a single program, which limits generalizing beyond that program.

Dietetics education researchers could benefit from the research and research strategies used in the field of education. Anderson (43) proposes four levels of educational research: descriptive, explanatory, generalization, and basic. Moving dietetics education research from its reliance on descriptive-level research toward the generalization and basic levels would improve its quality.

According to Anderson (43), descriptive research is used to describe either what has happened in the past or what is happening currently. Research methods such as case studies, needs assessment, program evaluation, and survey research are often used to describe past or current practice. Statistics often are used to quantify and simplify description by grouping observations.

The major questions addressed in explanatory research are, What is causing this to happen? and Why did it happen? Research methods used to address these questions often include case studies, comparative or correlational studies, observation, or time-series analysis. Explanation focuses on what is happening in a specific setting rather than on the implications for the world at large (43).

Determining whether the same thing will happen in different circumstances is the goal of generalization research. Experimental, quasi-experimental, meta-analysis, and predictive approaches are often used in this level of research (43). Very few dietetics education research studies reach the level of generalization research.

Basic or theoretical research attempts to determine whether there is an underlying principle to explain an observed phenomenon. Such research often involves experiments, meta-analysis, or time-series analysis (43).

Research in dietetics education is important to the growth and development of the profession of dietetics and is essential if the education of future dietitians is to be effective. The 1994 Future Search Conference (44) set forth the challenge for the dietetics profession, including dietetics education researchers, to create excellence. The 1998 ADA environmental scan (45,46) encouraged dietetics education researchers to look to the future and develop projects that would help provide the information needed to better guide dietetics education.

Nearly all the dietetics education research conducted to date has been very quantitative. Future research of a more qualitative nature might provide new insights into understanding the underlying intentions and feelings of students that affect the dietetics education process. Researchers in dietetics education must expand their research from the descriptive level to the generalization and basic levels. Continuing to explore the most effective ways to provide dietetics education and determining the underlying principles of how students best learn will be important. Interdisciplinary research projects conducted with education researchers could produce information on why students learn and factors that help motivate students in the learning process.

REFERENCES

1. The American Dietetic Association. *Accreditation/Approval Manual for Dietetics Education Programs*. 4th ed. Chicago, Ill: The American Dietetic Association; 1997.
2. Chambers MJ. Professional dietetic education in the US. *J Am Diet Assoc*. 1978;72:569–599.
3. Questionnaire for the education section. *J Am Diet Assoc*. 1925;1:31.
4. Loyd MS, Vaden AG. Practitioners identify competencies for entry-level generalist dietitians. *J Am Diet Assoc*. 1977;71:510–516.
5. Meeks DK, Zallen EM. Dietitians' perceptions of administrative competencies gained during professional education. In: Zallen EM, ed. *Structuring Education Experiences in Foodservice Systems Management: Proceedings of the Tenth Biennial Conference of the Foodservice Systems Management Education Council*. Norman, Okla: Oklahoma University; 1979.
6. Morales R, Spears MC, Vaden AG. Menu planning competencies in administrative dietetic practice: I. The methodology, II. Menu planning competencies. *J Am Diet Assoc*. 1979;74:642–650.
7. Parks SC, Kris-Etherton PM. Practitioners view dietetic roles for the 1980s. *J Am Diet Assoc*. 1982;80:574–577.
8. Holmes RW. Essential competencies for baccalaureate dietetic programs. *J Am Diet Assoc*. 1982;81:573–576.
9. Bedford MR. The affective domain: behaviors important in entry-level practice. *J Am Diet Assoc*. 1984;84:670–675.
10. Stanford JR, McKinley MM, Scruggs M. Graduates of hospital dietetic internships: I. Employment and administrative experiences in internships, II. Perceptions of administrative experiences in internships. *J Am Diet Assoc*. 1973;63:254–263.
11. Wenberg BG, Ingersoll RW, Donner CW. Evaluation of dietetic interns. *J Am Diet Assoc*. 1969;54:297–300.
12. Roach F, Hoyt D, Reed JG. Evaluation of a coordinated undergraduate program in dietetics. *J Am Diet Assoc*. 1976;68:154–158.
13. Johnson CA, Hurley RS. Design and use of an instrument to evaluate students' performance. *J Am Diet Assoc*. 1976;68:450–453.
14. Ingalsbe N, Spears MC. Development of an instrument to evaluate critical incident performance. *J Am Diet Assoc*. 1979;74:134–138.

15. Shanklin CW, Beach BL. Implementation and evaluation of a competency-based dietetic program. *J Am Diet Assoc.* 1980;77:450–454.

16. Fiedler KM, Beach BL, Hayman J. Dietetic performance evaluation: establishment of validity and reliability. *J Am Diet Assoc.* 1981;78:149–151.

17. Rinke WJ, David BD, Bjoraker WT. The entry-level generalist dietitian: I. Employers' general opinions of the adequacy of educational preparation in administration, II. Employers' perceptions of the adequacy of preparation for specific administrative competencies. *J Am Diet Assoc.* 1982;80:132–144.

18. Gregoire MB, Vaden AG, Hoyt DP. Comparative evaluation of graduates of internship and coordinated undergraduate programs. *J Am Diet Assoc.* 1986;86:1082–1889.

19. Marsico C, Borja M, Harrison L, Loftus M. Ratings of food courses and culinary training components in dietetics education. *J Am Diet Assoc.* 1998;98:692–693.

20. Gates G, Sandoval W. Teaching multiskilling in dietetics education. *J Am Diet Assoc.* 1998;98:278–284.

21. Hergenroeder A, Morrow S. Interdisciplinary adolescent health training in supervised dietetic practice programs across the southern United States. *J Am Diet Assoc.* 1999;99:1450–1452.

22. Scheule B. Food-safety educational goals for dietetic and hospitality students. *J Am Diet Assoc.* 2000;100:919–927.

23. Lorenz RA, Gregory RP, Davis DL, Schlundt DG, Wermager J. Diabetes training for dietitians: needs assessment, program description, and effects on knowledge and problem solving. *J Am Diet Assoc.* 2000;100:225–228.

24. Gilbride JA, Conklin MT. Benefits of training dietetics students in preprofessional practice programs: a comparison with dietetic internships. *J Am Diet Assoc.* 1996;96:758–763.

25. Brehn BJ, Rourke KM, Cassell C. Enhancing didactic education through participation in a clinical research project. *J Am Diet Assoc.* 1999;99:1090–1093.

26. Hampl JS, Herbold NH, Schneider MA, Sheeley AE. Using standardized patients to train and evaluate dietetics students. *J Am Diet Assoc.* 1999;99:1094–1097.

27. Litchfield RE, Oakland MH, Anderson JA. Improving dietetics education with interactive communication technology. *J Am Diet Assoc.* 2000;100:1191–1194.

28. Wolf KN, Dunlevy CL. Impact of preceptors on student attitudes toward supervised practice. *J Am Diet Assoc.* 1996;96:800–802.

29. Raidl MA, Wood OB, Lehman JD, Evers WD. Computer-assisted instruction improves clinical reasoning skills of dietetic interns. *J Am Diet Assoc.* 1995;95:868–873.

30. Turner RE, Evers WD, Wood OB, Lehman JD, Peck LW. Computer-based simulations enhance clinical experience of dietetic interns. *J Am Diet Assoc.* 2000;100:183–190.

31. Barrow EP, Jeong M, Parks SC. Computer experiences and attitudes of students and preceptors in distance education. *J Am Diet Assoc.* 1996;96:1280–1281.

32. Kobel KA. Influences on the selection of dietetics as a career. *J Am Diet Assoc.* 1997;97:254–257.

33. McMillan JH. *Educational Research.* 2nd ed. New York, NY: HarperCollins; 1996.

34. Moore GW. *Developing and Evaluating Educational Research.* Boston, Mass: Little Brown and Co; 1983.

35. Plake BS, Impara JC eds. *The Fifteenth Mental Measurements Yearbook.* Lincoln, Neb: University of Nebraska Press; 2003.

36. Murphy LL. *Tests in Print VI: An Index to Tests, Test Reviews, and the Literature on Specific Tests.* Lincoln, Neb: University of Nebraska Press; 2002.

37. McCabe BJ, Koury SD, Tysinger JW, Hynak-Hankinson MT, Foley S. Reading skills of dietetic interns and readability of dietetics literature. *J Am Diet Assoc.* 1995;95:874–878.

38. Miller JL, Shanklin CW. Status of menu item forecasting in dietetic education. *J Am Diet Assoc.* 1988;88:1246–1249.

39. Anderson SB, Ball S, Murphy RT. *Encyclopedia of Educational Evaluation.* San Francisco, Calif: Jossey-Bass Publishers; 1975.

40. Touliatos J, Compton NH. *Research Methods in Human Ecology/Home Economics.* Ames, Iowa: Iowa State University Press; 1988.

41. Friebel DM, Sucher K, Lu NC. University wellness program: the effectiveness of students as nutrition counselors. *J Am Diet Assoc.* 1988;88:596–598.

42. Vickery CE, Cotugna N, Hodges PA. Comparing counseling skills of dietetics students: a model for skill enhancement. *J Am Diet Assoc.* 1995;95:912–914.

43. Anderson G. *Fundamentals of Educational Research.* 2nd ed. Bristol, Pa: Falmer Press, Taylor & Francis; 1998.

44. Parks SC, Fitz PA, Maillet JO, Babjak P, Mitchell B. Challenging the future of dietetics education and credentialing—dialogue, discovery, and direction: a summary of the 1994 Future Search Conference. *J Am Diet Assoc.* 1995;95:598–606.

45. Maillet JO, Rops MS, Small J. Facing the future: ADA's 1998 environmental scan. *J Am Diet Assoc.* 1999;99:347–350.

46. Bezold C, Kang J. Looking to the future—the role of the ADA environmental scan. *J Am Diet Assoc.* 1999;99:989–993.

Part 8

—ɯɯ—

Useful Numbers in Research

All investigators find it a challenge to balance available resources and powerful research designs. For research to be beneficial, a sample size adequate to answer the research question and statistical analysis appropriate to evaluate the resulting data are critical. Chapters 26 and 27 address these two issues.

In determining sample size, a researcher must set the levels of two parameters: the desired statistical significance level (α) and the power to detect the magnitude of anticipated difference (β). A type I error, known also as an α or false-positive error, occurs when the researcher assumes that there is a difference or effect when none actually exists. A type I error is customarily set at 5 percent, or $P = .05$. In this example, the probability of correctly finding that there is no difference or effect is $1 - \alpha$ (that is, 95 percent, or $P = .95$).

A type II error, known also as a β or false-negative error occurs when one assumes that there is no difference or effect when there really is one. A type II error usually is set at 20 percent ($P = .20$). The power to find a real difference is $1 - \beta$ (that is, 80 percent, or $P = .80$). As sample size increases, the power to find a true effect increases. Increasing sample size also decreases the likelihood of a type II error.

Chapter 26 also discusses various formulas used to estimate sample size. The appropriate formula to select is based on the type of data to be analyzed (for example, continuous or proportion data) and the research design (for example, the sampling method). Economic constraints may require adjustment of the desired power and proposed significance level; however, these two terms cannot be modified drastically without jeopardizing the usefulness of the projected research. The text includes additional comments to aid the researcher in handling subject dropout or noncompliance, recalculating sample size during the study, or determining power after a study has been completed.

Once the data are collected, the researcher should look at them thoughtfully. Chapter 27 illustrates the process of devising various data plots during data analysis to enable effective visual inspection. If the data do not follow a normal distribution, the researcher should consider transforming the data (into logarithms, for example) or using nonparametric statistical methods. Although an investigator may graph and inspect the data in many different plots, none of the initial plots may be necessary when the research is reported or published.

After plotting the data, the researcher must develop summary statistics, estimate the magnitude of the data comparisons, and assess the differences by statistical analysis. Summary statistics, which include means, frequencies, ranges, and standard deviations (SDs), are useful in describing data sets. The SD must be differentiated clearly from the standard error (SE) of the mean. The SD indicates the distribution, spread, or variation around the mean; the SE indicates the precision of the measure. Because the SE is always a smaller number than the SD (the SE is derived by dividing the SD by the square root of the size of the sample), people may be tempted to report the SE, thinking that it connotes sharper control. The SD and SE are different statistics, however, and should be used knowledgeably.

Table 27.1 categorizes statistical methods appropriate for evaluating differences among groups. During the design phase, before data collection, the statistical tests by which the data will be analyzed are determined on the basis of four elements: the nature of the research question (comparative or relational), the scale of measurement of the data to be collected (discrete or continuous), the relationship between samples (dependent or independent), and the number of samples to be evaluated (one, two, or multiple). Multiple comparisons, or multiplicity, raises statistical problems in that the more

comparisons that are made, the more likely it is that false-positive results will be "detected." If the significance level were set at 5 percent, it would be expected that by chance alone, 1 out of 20 comparisons would appear to be significant (see Chapter 2). For example, if one compares the intake of 15 nutrients with 12 serum levels, one will find that by chance, approximately 9 of the 180 comparisons appear to be statistically significant. The mistaken appearance of statistical significance from multiple comparisons has been referred to as the "runaway P value."

A wise investigator uses statistics to evaluate whether the observed differences are significant, and then further evaluates whether the differences make a difference. As Thomas Carlyle said, "A judicious man looks at statistics, not to get knowledge, but to save himself from having ignorance foisted on him."

ERM, Editor

26

Estimating Sample Size

Carrie L. Cheney, Ph.D., R.D., and Carol J. Boushey, Ph.D., M.P.H., R.D.

THE LOGIC OF SAMPLE SIZE CALCULATIONS

Sample selection, discussed in Chapters 6 and 8, and sample size are two determinants of whether an investigation is worthwhile. An otherwise excellent study can fail to detect an important effect just because the sample size is too small. The results of such studies confuse the issue under investigation and can lead to misleading or patently wrong conclusions.

The process of estimating the required sample size involves several steps and can be technically complex; it is always wise to seek the help of a knowledgeable statistician. An understanding of the basic elements of estimating the sample size, which this chapter provides, will facilitate interaction with a statistician. This chapter highlights the issues underlying the logic of sample size calculations, outlines the general procedure that is common to all situations, describes the procedures specific to common research situations, and provides references for further information.

The use of statistics allows the investigator to estimate the unknown. By using statistics, the investigator can estimate characteristics of a population based on observations of a sample drawn from it. The size of the sample largely determines how accurate or precise the estimates from the sample are; the larger the sample, the more information about the population and the more precise the estimate. Uncertainty always exists. The investigator, however, can specify in advance the amount of un-

certainty that is acceptable for the study and perform appropriate sample size calculations.

Two hypotheses, the research hypothesis and the null hypothesis, provide the framework for the logic of sample size calculations. Before an investigation is undertaken, a research hypothesis that serves as the basis of the investigation is formulated. The null hypothesis—that there is no difference or effect—serves as a standard of comparison. Statistical analysis is conducted to determine whether the results of the study are consistent with the underlying null hypothesis. If the results do not demonstrate the presence of a difference or an effect, it is concluded that the data fail to refute the null hypothesis.

When drawing conclusions from statistical results, there are four possible outcomes—two correct and two incorrect (Table 26.1). First, one can correctly conclude that there is no difference or effect when there is none (probability = $1 - \alpha$; for convenience in sample size calculations, it is assumed that failure to reject the null hypothesis is the same as concluding that the null hypothesis is true; however, this assumption is not appropriate when interpreting results). Second, one can conclude that there is a difference or effect when there is none (probability = α, false-positive, type I error). Third, one can conclude that there is no difference or effect when there is one (probability = β, false-negative, type II error). Finally, one can conclude that there is a difference or effect, which is truly present (probability = $1 - \beta$, power). All four possible outcomes are expressed

TABLE 26.1   Possible Outcomes When Drawing Conclusions From Statistical Results

		Truth About Study Hypothesis	
		True (alternate, H_1)	**False** (null, H_0)
Statistical test results about hypothesis	**True** (reject H_0)	Correct ($1 - \beta$, power)	False positive (type I error, α error)
	False (do not reject H_0)	False negative (type II error, β error)	Correct ($1 - \alpha$)

statistically as probabilities of reaching the appropriate conclusions.

The type I error, or α error, is also known as the significance level of the study; its complement, $1 - \alpha$, is the correct conclusion if the null hypothesis is true. By convention, α is usually set at 5 percent, or $P = .05$. This means that the maximum acceptable risk of drawing a false-positive conclusion is 5 percent. Obviously, the smaller the α, the lower the risk of drawing a false-positive conclusion. The investigator specifies the α level during the planning of the study and compares the resulting P value with alpha at the end of the study. If the observed P value is less than α, the result is considered to be statistically significant.

The type II error, or β error, expresses the probability of missing a difference; its complement is power, or $1 - \beta$. If the null hypothesis is not true and a difference or effect exists, the β probability quantifies the risk of missing that difference, and power quantifies the chance of finding it. As β decreases, power increases. The investigator specifies β during the planning of the study, which then determines power. For example, if the risk of missing a difference were set at 20 percent ($P = .20$), the chance that the study would find a real difference would be 80 percent ($P = .80$).

The probability that if a true effect exists, a study will detect it (that is, power) largely depends on the sample size. Increasing the sample size increases the power. At the same time, increasing the sample size decreases the risk of a false-negative conclusion (that is, β or type II error), because the ability to detect a true difference is increased.

The power of a study also depends to some degree on the true magnitude of difference or effect under study. For any given power, a large difference can be detected with a smaller sample size more easily than can a small difference. Accordingly, for any given sample size, the

study will be more likely to detect a large difference than a small difference. The investigator determines in advance the magnitude of difference or effect that is important for the study to be able to detect, and this becomes the research hypothesis for the purposes of power and sample size calculations.

There is a general relationship among sample size, power, and the magnitude of the difference or effect sought. The required sample size is inversely related to the magnitude of the difference and the type I error rate, and it is positively related to the standard deviation and desired power. This relationship may be expressed as follows (1):

$$\text{Sample size } (n) > 2\left[\frac{(\alpha \text{ error} + \beta \text{ error} \times \text{SD})}{\text{Difference}}\right]^2$$

where the α and β errors are mathematically converted to the standardized normal deviates (Z values) for the probabilities, the SD equals the estimated standard deviation, and the difference is the absolute value of its magnitude. For example, a change in low-density lipoprotein cholesterol levels from 5.19 mmol/L to 4.87 mmol/L would be a difference of –0.32 mmol/L, or an absolute difference of 0.32 mmol/L.

If the sample size is not restricted, the investigator will want to determine the sample size required to ensure a high probability of detecting a meaningful difference or effect. If, in contrast, the sample size is limited (that is, predetermined), the investigator can use sample size calculations to determine the probability (power = $1 - \beta$) that the study will be able to detect a meaningful difference. In practice, the final determination of the size of the research project will be a judicious balance of power and economics.

GENERAL PROCEDURE FOR SAMPLE SIZE CALCULATIONS

Sample size estimates are based on a number of assumptions about the conditions of the study, Because it is not possible for an investigator to know in advance what the conditions of the study will be, the calculations provide only an estimate. The general procedure for calculating the required sample size involves seven steps, which are discussed in this section.

Step 1

Choose the main end point of interest and the method by which it is to be measured. A series of sample size calculations may be performed if there is more than a single important end point for the study. In such cases, the largest estimated sample size is generally used. Note that α may need to be adjusted for the increased number of simultaneous significance tests (see step 5 later in this section).

Step 2

Choose the statistical test that is appropriate for the data and the research question. It is best to consult with a statistician at this point (see Chapter 27).

Step 3

Specify the magnitude of the difference or effect that is meaningful to detect. The magnitude of the difference or effect selected should be practical—that is, an important difference in practice. Additionally, it should be sufficiently small that a negative study outcome (that is, no significant difference) would be assurance that if a true difference existed, it would be too small to be of practical importance.

Step 4

Estimate the expected variability—that is, the estimated SD. Preferably, this value comes from a pilot study conducted earlier. However, it can also come from published research results. Lacking either of these, a "best guess" must be made.

Step 5

Specify the maximum acceptable risk of a false-positive conclusion (α, or type I, error). Alterations in α concomi-tantly alter both power and β. As α is lowered, power decreases and β increases; as α is increased, power increases and β decreases. By convention, the α probability is set at .05, although the situation may warrant setting a lower or higher risk. The seriousness of a false-positive conclusion determines whether the maximum acceptable risk should be set lower. Only under rare circumstances is α set greater than .05, because to do so can compromise the ability of the results to be convincing. An increased α would be warranted, however, in circumstances in which there were serious consequences of a false-negative conclusion (β error) and it was desired to decrease β without increasing the sample size beyond what was feasible.

Another consideration in choosing α is whether the statistical test is to be one tailed or two tailed (see Chapter 27). A one-tailed α is more liberal than a two-tailed α, as it tests for a difference in only one direction. The more conservative approach of applying a two-tailed significance test enables the investigator to test for a difference in either direction from the null and is generally preferred.

When there is more than a single primary end point for the study, it is important to test each with the same level of rigor, that is, $\alpha = .05$ or lower. Some (but not all) statisticians believe that the appropriate way to ensure that the α level remains ≤ 0.05 (or desired level) for all significance tests is to account for more than one test. Accounting for more than a single primary outcome is usually achieved by dividing the desired α by the number of significance tests being conducted. For example, if we planned to test the difference between treated and control groups on three primary outcomes, and we chose $\alpha = .05$ as acceptable, we would compute the sample size based on $.05/3 = .017$ to preserve the type I error probability of .05.

Step 6

Specify the probability of successfully detecting the difference or effect, if it exists (power = $1 - \beta$). Alternatively, the probability of a false-negative conclusion can be specified (β, or type II, error). By convention, power is usually set at .80 to .90, and β is set at .20 to .10, respectively. Again, the seriousness of a false-negative conclusion guides the decision.

Step 7

Apply the appropriate calculations (see the following examples and calculations).

The estimated sample size may be larger than what is feasible under the actual circumstances and with available resources. If this is the case, the power of the study should be calculated according to the number of subjects feasible with available resources. The procedure for calculating the power of a study with a fixed sample size prior to undertaking it is similar to that just given. Steps 1 through 7 should be performed, substituting the fixed sample size for power in step 6 and solving for power instead of sample size in step 7.

Research design often requires a compromise of the ideal and the feasible; the goal of design is a practical and economic balance between power and sample size. However, in deciding to compromise power, the investigation must recognize that the ability of the study to accomplish its objective is also compromised. A study may not be worth doing if there is a low probability of detecting a meaningful effect.

SAMPLE SIZE DETERMINATION FOR SPECIFIC RESEARCH SITUATIONS

Continuous Data

All results from the following methods are based on the assumption that either the outcomes arise from a normal distribution or that the sample size is sufficiently large that the normal approximation is valid. These formulas can give improper results if the assumption of normality is not valid.

Paired Observations

A paired t test is usually used in an investigation in which a continuous response measure is observed before and after the subject receives a treatment or an investigation in which observations in two groups are linked by pairing. In this instance, the sample size formula accounts for the correlation between the measurements within the pairs (2,3).

An example might be a study to assess whether a particular intervention will decrease dietary cholesterol intake as measured by 3-day food records (step 1). For one sample, before and after study design, an experimental effect can be tested with a paired t test (step 2). Using the data of Cohen and associates (4), it can be determined that a change of −75 mg would be meaningful and practical (step 3). Furthermore, the SD of the difference (SD_{diff})

can be estimated (step 4) as 158.9 mg, according to the study of Van Horn and coworkers (5), which used 3-day food records.

α is specified in advance with a two-tailed test (step 5) as .05. The decision is made to set power, or $1 - \beta$, at .80, making $\beta = .20$ (step 6). The appropriate calculations (step 7) can now be applied. The calculation of the sample size needed to conduct a test with a significance level of α and a power of $1 - \beta$, follows:

$$n = [(Z_{1-\beta} + Z_{1-\alpha}) \times SD_{diff}/Mean_1 - Mean_2)]^2$$

$$[26.1]$$

The quantities $Z_{1-\alpha}$ and $Z_{1-\beta}$ are values from the standard normal distribution that correspond to the desired probabilities of type I (α) and type II (β) errors. Table 26.2 gives selected values of $Z_{1-\alpha}$ and $Z_{1-\beta}$ corresponding to commonly used values of α and β. Using the values previously given, $SD_{diff} = 158.9$ mg, and $Mean_1 - Mean_2 = 75$ mg. Therefore, using formula 26.1, the sample size for a two-sided test can be estimated as follows:

$$n = [(Z_{1-\beta} + Z_{1-\alpha}) \times SD_{diff}/Mean_1 - Mean_2)]^2$$
$$= [(0.84 + 1.96) \times 158.9/75]^2$$
$$= [444.92/75]^2$$
$$= 35.2, \text{ or } 36 \text{ subjects}$$

If the investigators also planned to measure the difference in other nutrients (for example, saturated fat intake), these calculations would be repeated for each nutrient of interest, using $\alpha = 0.05/k$, where k = number of nutrients of interest. The final sample size would corre-

TABLE 26.2 Unit Normal Deviates Z_α and Z_β for Selected Values of α and β

α or β	Two-sided Test[a]	
	$Z_{1-\alpha/2}$	$Z_{1-\beta}$
0.01	2.58	2.33
0.025	2.24	1.96
0.05	1.96	1.64
0.10	1.64	1.28
0.20	1.28	0.84
0.30	1.04	0.52

[a]If using a one-sided test, the $Z_{1-\alpha}$ values would be the same as in the $Z_{1-\beta}$ column.

spond to the calculation with the highest n. Finally, when they recruited subjects, the investigators would enroll extra participants to allow for attrition during the intervention without compromising the study's power (see the later discussion of dropout rates and noncompliance).

Tables are available by which sample size and power can be estimated for a variety of differences and levels of α and β errors (2,6). An increasingly wide variety of choices of computer programs for performing sample size calculations are also available. (Examples are nQuery Advisor by Statistical Solutions, Saugus, Massachusetts, and the program offered by Dupont and Plummer [7].)

The examples in this section use continuous variables; for discrete variables, the formulas would be slightly different (8) and are discussed later. Chapter 27 again clarifies the issue of continuous versus discrete variables.

Independent Groups

Study designs addressing nutrition questions usually involve a comparison of two samples. Investigations often are planned to observe the response measures on subjects who receive either of two treatments, typically an experimental treatment and a control treatment. The response variable (for example, high-density lipoprotein cholesterol) is measured on a continuous scale. A specified magnitude of difference is set at a level thought to be important with a particular power. The comparison is usually made by t test for independent samples.

An example might involve members of the dietetics department of a health maintenance organization (HMO) who are concerned that the agency's current screening criteria for anemia using the hemoglobin value may need to be revised. The article by Nordenberg and colleagues (9) suggests that hemoglobin cutoff values should be adjusted upward for smokers. The HMO collects detailed smoking information on each new enrollee and determines hemoglobin value as well, so an investigation is planned to determine whether women smokers and nonsmokers between the ages of 18 and 44 years have significantly different hemoglobin values. One of the study components involves comparing the mean hemoglobin values of a random sample of smokers with a random sample of nonsmokers.

In this case, the main end point of interest is hemoglobin, a continuous variable (step 1). To compare the means of the two randomly selected groups, an independent t test can be used (step 2). The results reported by

Nordenberg and colleagues (9) indicate that the mean hemoglobin value among female smokers is 137 g/L and is 133 g/L among female nonsmokers. The calculated difference of interest is 4 g/L (step 3). A standard error of 0.4 g/L for smokers and 0.5 g/L for nonsmokers was reported (9). By converting these values (step 4) to their corresponding SDs (standard error = SD/square root of n), setting α at the conventional .05 (step 5) and power at 90 percent (step 6), and applying the appropriate formula, the sample size for the two groups can be determined. The formula for a two-sided test (assuming unequal variances) is as follows (8).

$$n = (SD_1^2 + SD_2^2)(Z_{1-\beta} + Z_{1-\alpha/2})^2/(Mean_2 - Mean_1)^2 \quad [26.2]$$

The values for $Z_{1-\beta}$ and $Z_{1-\alpha/2}$ can be found in Table 26.2. The SDs for smokers and nonsmokers are 12.37 and 17.37, respectively. The difference of interest, $Mean_2 - Mean_1$, is 4 g/L. According to formula 26.2, the sample size is as follows:

$$n = (17.37^2 + 12.37^2)(1.28 + 1.96)^2/(-4)^2$$

$$= (454.7338)(10.4976)/16$$

$$= 298 \text{ in each group (596 total)}$$

However, the funding is limited to 175 subjects in each group (350 total). Lack of sufficient funds is common. As a consequence of various constraints, a sample size analysis often begins with a fixed value for n. In this case, the resulting power $(1 - \beta)$ can be determined by rearranging formula 26.2 and solving for $Z_{1-\beta}$:

$$Z_{1-\beta} = \sqrt{\frac{(Mean_2 - Mean_1)^2 \times n}{(SD_1^2 + SD_2^2)}} - Z_{1-\alpha/2} \quad [26.3]$$

Using all the values determined previously, but substituting 175 for n, the study power is calculated as follows:

$$Z_{1-\beta} = \sqrt{\frac{(4)^2 \times 175}{(17.37^2 + 12.37^2)}} - 1.96$$

$$= \sqrt{6.157} - 1.96$$

$$= 2.48 - 1.96$$

$$= 0.52$$

Table 26.2 indicates that $Z_{1-\beta} = 0.52$ corresponds to $\beta = .30$, so $1 - \beta = 0.70$, or 70 percent power. The investigators conclude that the 175-subject sample size will provide adequate power, and they continue with plans for the study.

Because the actual formula for calculating sample size based on the t test can be solved using computational iterative methods, tables have been constructed for use (2,6). These tables provide sample sizes necessary to detect a range of differences with varying degrees of power. Additional tables indicate the power provided by various sample sizes and magnitudes of differences, and the text that accompanies them describes their use in detail (2). As has been mentioned, various statistical software manufacturers offer computer software for determining sample size and power analyses. Investigators should review products carefully and consult with a statistician before using unfamiliar statistical software.

Three or More Independent Groups

Studies that compare a continuous response measure in more than two groups usually use an analysis of variance model for data analysis rather than several t tests. Based on analysis of variance, Day and Graham (10) provide a nomogram to estimate the required sample size when comparing three or more treatment groups.

More Complex Designs

Nutrition studies commonly employ designs, such as prospective cohort or retrospective case-control designs, that evaluate the association of a risk factor with some outcome of interest. The measure of association estimated from these studies is the relative risk or odds ratio. Procedures appropriate for the prospective cohort study are given by Phillips and Pocock (11), and procedures appropriate for the case-control study, by Lubin and co-workers (12).

In some nutrition studies, especially certain clinical trials, the time when an end point occurs is important. It is especially important if it is believed that an intervention may result in a shorter duration of illness or that the desired outcome may occur sooner. Such studies are called *time-to-event investigations*. Usually the analysis uses survival analysis methods instead of more simple statistical approaches. Sample size procedures for such studies using a specialized computer program are described by Shih (13).

Reliability Studies

Reliability studies—for example, studies of the reliability of methods of assessing dietary intake—are also common in nutrition and dietetics. In these studies, reliability is often estimated by the coefficient of intraclass correlation from an analysis of variance. Sample size requirements for reliability studies are discussed by Donner and Eliasziw (14) and by Walter et al (15). Both references provide either power contours or tables to guide in the planning. Donner (16) provides sample size formulas and tables for the design of studies that compare two or more coefficients of interobserver agreement. For inferences regarding agreement for dichotomous variables, the κ statistic is used; Donner and Eliasziw (17) present a discussion of sample size procedures for studies using the κ statistic.

Proportions

Independent Groups

In an investigation in which a dichotomous or categorical response measure is observed in two independent groups, the frequencies of response are compared between groups, usually by the chi-square test in a two-way contingency table. As with the procedure for the t test, the investigator must guess about an unknown quantity—in this case, one of the proportions. The investigator then is asked, as usual, to specify the smallest difference from this amount that is important to detect, as well as the α and β errors that are acceptable. With these quantities, the investigator can estimate the required sample size. A major distinction between power calculations for the t test and comparing two proportions is that for discrete outcomes, the variance (or standard deviation) is a function of the proportions being compared. In other words, with discrete outcomes, the variance is a function of the mean.

For the example of anemia (hemoglobin < 120 g/L) among smokers and nonsmokers, a two-way contingency table based on the data reported by Nordenberg and colleagues (9) can be constructed (Table 26.3). The proportions can be quantified; for example, $46/956 = 4.8$ percent prevalence of anemia among smokers. The prevalence of anemia among nonsmokers is 8.4 percent; therefore, the difference of interest could be 3.6 or any value specified as meaningful in the population.

Although formulas are available to calculate sample size (3,18,19), a simpler and perhaps more informative

TABLE 26.3   Two-way Contingency Table
Anemia Among Women Smokers and Nonsmokers

		Anemia (hgb[a] < 120 g/L)		
		+	–	
Smoker	+	46	910	956
	–	101	1106	1207
		147	2016	2163

[a]hgb = hemoglobin value.

Data are from Nordenberg et al (9).

method is to use graphs (20,21) or tables (22,23). Tables and graphs have the advantage of providing, at a glance, the required sample sizes for several combinations of proportions and differences. Several computer programs, such as the one by Dupont and Plummer (7), also perform the required calculations. A public domain program available through the Centers for Disease Control and Prevention, Epi Info, is available on-line; investigators can download the software at no charge (see http://www.cdc.gov/publications.htm). A function within Epi Info includes calculations designed for studies in which the results are proportions. Additional formulas and tables are compiled and carefully reviewed by Sahai and Khurshid (24).

EXAMPLE.   A trial has been planned to use available tables to assess the efficacy of vitamin C in preventing the common cold. The subjects, employees in a large machinery plant, have agreed to be assigned randomly to receive a vitamin C supplement or a placebo daily for the duration of the winter season. A previous survey has shown that the usual incidence of colds during winter is 50 percent. The investigators think that a reduction in the incidence by half (that is, to 25 percent) would result in a meaningful economic benefit to the company and the employees. The investigators adhere to convention and set α at .05. Because a number of trials have shown negative results (with questionable statistical power), the investigators also want to be reasonably certain to avoid a false-negative conclusion and to have sufficient power for the results to be conclusive; thus, they set b at .10, giving 90 percent power. Using the tables provided by Fleiss (22), they find that a sample size of 85 per group, or a total of 170, is needed for a two-tailed test of the difference in proportions in this study.

After discussions with the company administration, the investigators are told that funds are available to support a study of only 120 subjects, or 60 per group. Referring to the tables by Fleiss (22), they find that 60 subjects per group will provide power of 75 percent at an α of .05. The investigators decide that this level of power is acceptable and proceed with plans for the study.

Paired Observations

An investigation that employs a matched design, pairing observation from a case with observation from a control (that is, a matched case-control study), is analyzed in a manner that accounts for pairing, such as McNemar's test for paired studies (25). Procedures for sample size determination are provided by several authors (22,25,26) and reviewed by Lachenbruch (27).

More Complex Designs

The analysis and sample size determination are more complicated when the investigation involves more than two groups and more than one response measure. The analysis generally uses some form of the chi-square test in a multiway contingency table. Lachin (28) provides the statistical rationale and methods for determining the required sample size for such studies for the statistically inclined investigator; investigators who are less mathematically inclined should consult a statistician.

Related classes of studies common in nutritional epidemiology are studies of more than two risk factors that are dichotomous measures, such as cohort or case-control studies of the association of several risk factors with a chronic disease. Clinical trials can also evaluate more than two treatments simultaneously. Studies of this type generally employ discrete multivariate analysis methods (for example, multivariate contingency tables and unconditional logistic models). A general method for sample size determination in this class of study is described by Greenland (29). A modified method is applied to prospective studies by Phillips and Pocock (11) and to cohort and case-control studies by Lemeshow and associates (30). Again, investigators who are unfamiliar with these techniques should consult a statistician.

Performance Characteristics of Laboratory Tests

It is frequently useful in dietetics to employ tests to classify persons or to screen them for certain characteristics or risks. The use of anthropometry to assess nutrition status and screen for patients at risk of malnutrition at hospital admission is one example. Tests are often compared with one another to determine their performance characteristics and relative usefulness in classifying persons, especially when one test is more expensive or labor intensive. The important performance characteristics are the positive and negative predictive values (described in Chapter 8), two proportions that determine the practical usefulness of tests (31,32). Power and sample size requirements of studies of this nature are presented by Arkin and Wachtel (32).

Additional Considerations

Loss of Subjects From Dropouts and Noncompliance

It is rare that investigators can manage a study in which all participants are able to complete the study with total compliance to the study protocol. Knowing this, it is wise to anticipate some rate of noncompliance when determining sample size. Investigators can look to past experience with similar studies—their own or the studies of others—to estimate dropout rate and noncompliance *(R)*. Sample size can be adjusted by the simple method of Lachin (3), $N_d = N/(1 - R)^2$, where N_d is the sample size needed to account for dropouts, and N is the sample size calculated without accounting for dropouts.

Repeated Measures or Longitudinal Designs

When the outcome is measured at a single point in time, the equations given previously can be relied upon to give useful estimates of sample size. They are not useful, though, when the outcome is measured more than once (repeated measures) or for longitudinal study designs. Repeated measures designs are efficient in determining treatment effect in many applications (33); that is, they can require smaller sample sizes than comparable studies that do not employ repeated observations. Because repeated observations on the same individual are usually positively correlated, sample size estimates and data analysis must account for this correlation. Procedures related to sample size estimation are provided for both continuous (34) and discrete or binary outcome variables (34,35).

Recalculating the Sample Size During the Study

Sometimes investigators have no pilot data or published studies upon which to base a variance of the outcome or response. Researchers then simply guess about the variance for sample size calculations, and thus the experiment is based on a guess. The result may be an underpowered study. In an effort to correct for this situation, statisticians developed sequential study designs—that is, designs in which data are analyzed when preset numbers of responses have occurred. Underlying this class of designs is the practical effect that after gathering an initial sample, the investigators recalculate the final sample size based on the current observed variance in the response (36). Investigators interested in this type of design should consult a statistician. Background on this design and considerations for sample size estimates are presented by Betensky and Tierney (36).

Determining Power Retrospectively

The ability of a study to detect a difference that truly exists is power, as has been described. Determining the power of the study after a study is completed is crucial for interpreting the findings when the results are negative (for example, concluding that the intervention had no effect or that there was no association between variables). As readers, we want to know the likelihood that this finding was the result of a type II error. An author's claim that there was no difference in response between groups or that groups were equivalent in some characteristic may be based on a study that was underpowered to detect a meaningful difference. Readers (and investigators) can apply the previously described procedures to either (1) compute the sample size that would have been required to show a difference and compare this number with the study sample size or (2) calculate the power of the study with the reported sample size (37). With either procedure, the reader can then determine whether the negative findings reflect the lack of a meaningful difference or simply insufficient study power.

Clinical and Statistical Significance

It is necessary to emphasize that sample size and power calculations incorporate the concepts of both clinical and statistical significance. Of these two concepts, clinical significance is more important. The finding that the effect of two treatments is statistically significantly different is of little value if the size of the difference is of no practical importance. When planning a study, clinical or practical significance should be the driving force (38,39).

There are several methods to determine the degree of difference or strength of association needed to obtain clinical significance. Commonly, investigators use information from published reports or references, or data from pilot studies recently conducted. Lacking either of these, investigators can look to their own experience or that of colleagues as a basis for a meaningful outcome. Lindgren et al (39) describe a procedure for choosing a size of treatment effect that is based on the underlying distribution of the measurement of interest in the target population. This procedure has the benefit of minimizing any subjectivity in selecting clinical significance and is useful in generating a range of values to use for the size of the effect.

REFERENCES

1. Armitage P. *Statistical Methods in Medical Research.* London, England: Blackwell Scientific Publications; 1971:186.

2. Dixon WJ, Massey FJ Jr. *Introduction to Statistical Analysis.* 3rd ed. New York, NY: McGraw-Hill; 1969:269.

3. Lachin JM. Introduction to sample size determination and power analysis for clinical trials. *Control Clin Trials.* 1981;2:93–113.

4. Cohen NL, Laus MJ, Stutzman NC, Swicker RC. Dietary change in participants of the Better Eating for Better Health course. *J Am Diet Assoc.* 1991;91:345–346.

5. Van Horn L, Moag-Stahlberg A, Liu K, et al. Effects of serum lipids of adding instant oats to usual American diets. *Am J Public Health.* 1991;81:183–188.

6. Pearson ES, Hartley HO. *Biometrika Tables for Statisticians.* 3rd ed. Cambridge, England: Cambridge University Press; 1970.

7. Dupont WD, Plummer WD Jr. Power and sample size calculations: a review and computer program. *Control Clin Trials.* 1990;11:116–128.

8. Rosner B. *Fundamentals of Biostatistics.* 2nd ed. Boston, Mass: Duxbury Press; 1986:264, 322.

9. Nordenberg D, Yip R, Binkin NJ. The effect of cigarette smoking on hemoglobin levels and anemia screening. *JAMA* 1990;264:1556–1559.

10. Day SJ, Graham DF. Sample size and power for comparing two or more treatment groups in clinical trials. *BMJ.* 1989;299:663–665.

11. Phillips AN, Pocock SJ. Sample size requirements for prospective studies, with examples for coronary heart disease. *J Clin Epidemiol.* 1989;42:639–648.

12. Lubin JH, Gail MH, Ershow AG. Sample size and power for case-control studies when exposures are continuous. *Stat Med.* 1988;7:363–376.

13. Shih JH. Sample size calculation for complex clinical trials with survival endpoints. *Control Clin Trials.* 1995;16:395–407.

14. Donner A, Eliasziw M. Sample size requirements for reliability studies. *Stat Med.* 1987;6:441–448.

15. Walter SD, Eliasziw M, Donner A. Sample size and optimal designs for reliability studies. *Stat Med.* 1998;17:101–110.

16. Donner A. Sample size requirements for the comparison of two or more coefficients of inter-observer agreement. *Stat Med.* 1998;17:1157–1168.

17. Donner A, Eliasziw M. A goodness of fit approach to inference procedures for the kappa statistic: confidence interval construction, significance-testing and sample size estimation. *Stat Med.* 1992;11:1511–1519.

18. Casagrande T, Pike MC. An improved approximate formula for calculation sample sizes for comparing two binomial distributions. *Biometrics.* 1978;34:483–486.

19. Fleiss JL, Tytun A, Ury HK. A simple approximation for calculating sample sizes for comparing independent proportions. *Biometrics.* 1980;36:343.

20. Feigl P. A graphical aid for determining sample size when comparing two independent proportions. *Biometrics.* 1978;34:111–122.

21. Aleong J, Bartlett DE. Improved graphs for calculating sample sizes when comparing two independent binomial distributions. *Biometrics.* 1979;35:875.

22. Fleiss JL. *Statistical Methods for Rates and Proportions.* 2nd ed. New York, NY: John Wiley and Sons; 2000.

23. Cohen J. *Statistical Power Analysis for the Behavioral Sciences.* 2nd ed. New York, NY: Academic Press; 1977.

24. Sahai H, Khurshid A. Formulae and tables for the determination of sample sizes and power in clinical trials for testing differences in proportions for the two-sample design: a review. *Stat Med.* 1996;15:1–21.

25. Schlesselman JJ. *Case-control Studies: Design, Conduct, Analysis.* New York, NY: Oxford University Press; 1982:160, 207.

26. Fleiss JL, Levin B. Sample size determination in studies with matched pairs. *J Clin Epidemiol.* 1988;41:727–730.

27. Lachenbruch PA. On the sample size for studies based upon McNemar's test. *Stat Med.* 1992;11:1521–1525.

28. Lachin JM. Sample size determinations for r × c comparative trials. *Biometrics.* 1977;33:315.

29. Greenland S. Power, sample size and smallest detectable effect determination for multivariate studies. *Stat Med.* 1985;4:117–127.

30. Lemeshow S, Hosmer DW Jr, Kiar J. Sample size requirements for studies estimating odds ratios or relative risks. *Stat Med.* 1988;7:759–764.

31. Weiss NS. *Clinical Epidemiology. The Study of the Outcome of Illness.* 2nd ed. New York, NY: Oxford University Press; 1996.

32. Arkin CE, Wachtel MS. How many patients are necessary to assess test performance? *JAMA.* 1990;263:275–278.

33. Jensen DR. Efficiency and robustness in the use of repeated measurements. *Biometrics.* 1982;38:813–825.

34. Rochon J. Application of GEE procedures for sample size calculations in repeated measures experiments. *Stat Med.* 1998;17:1643–1658.

35. Lipsitz SR, Fitzmaurice GM. Sample size for repeated measures studies with binary responses. *Stat Med.* 1994;13:1233–1239.

36. Betensky RA, Tierney C. An examination of methods for sample size recalculation during an experiment. *Stat Med.* 1997;16:2587–2598.

37. Streiner DL. Sample size and power in psychiatric research. *Can J Psychiatry.* 1990;35:616–620.

38. Baumgardner KR. A review of key research design and statistical analysis issues. *Oral Surg Oral Med Oral Pathol Oral Radiol Endod.* 1997;84:550–556.

39. Lindgren BR, Wielinski CL, Finkelstein SM, Warwick WJ. Contrasting clinical and statistical significance within the research setting. *Pediatr Pulmonol.* 1993;16:336–340.

Further Reading

Arkin CE. The t-test and clinical relevance. Is your *Beta* error showing? *Am J Clin Pathol.* 1981;76:416–420.

Detsky AS, Sackett DL. When was a "negative" clinical trial big enough? How many patients you needed depends on what you found. *Arch Intern Med.* 1985;145:709–712.

Diamond GA, Forrester JS. Clinical trials and statistical verdicts: probable grounds for appeal. *Ann Intern Med.* 1983;98:385–394.

Ellenberg SS. Biostatistics in clinical trials: part 2. Determining sample sizes for clinical trials. *Oncology.* 1989;3:39–46.

Hall JC. A method for the rapid assessment of sample size in dietary studies. *Am J Clin Nutr.* 1983;37:473–477.

Lwanga SK, Lemeshow S. *Sample Size Determination in Health Studies.* Geneva, Switzerland: World Health Organization; 1991.

Marshall JA, Scarbro S, Shetterly SM, Jones RH. Improving power with repeated measures: diet and serum lipids. *Am J Clin Nutr.* 1998;67:934–939.

Pagano M. Interpretation of clinical studies in relation to malnutrition. *Nutr.* 1995;11(suppl 2):210–212.

Young MJ, Bresnitz EA, Strom BL. Sample size nomograms for interpreting negative clinical studies. *Ann Intern Med.* 1983;99:248–251.

27

Statistical Applications

Carrie L. Cheney, Ph.D., R.D.

Selecting the statistical method to apply to research data can be a challenge for the nonstatistician. Guidance from a statistician during the planning of the research project and as necessary throughout the research effort is useful. To facilitate communication with a statistician, the investigator should be familiar with the fundamentals of statistics and their applications. This chapter reviews the fundamentals of statistical analysis, outlines the general procedure involved, provides suggestions for analysis of several common research situations, and illustrates the procedure with a detailed example of applying statistical methods to a typical study design. Readers are encouraged to take advantage of the References, especially for the technical aspects of statistical calculations, which are not presented here.

FUNDAMENTALS OF STATISTICAL ANALYSIS

Four elements of the study design help guide the selection of statistical method: the research question, the scale of measurement in which the data are collected, the relationship among samples, and the number of samples to be evaluated. Additional considerations relate to characteristics of the statistical test and include the test's assumptions about the normal distribution (frequently referred to as the *Gaussian distribution*) and whether the test should be applied as a one-sided or two-sided test of significance.

The Research Question

Most, if not all, research questions in dietetics can be categorized into one of two main categories of questions: comparative or relational. In operational terms, the research is concerned with drawing comparisons or examining relationships. The distinction is largely a result of the sampling method and study design chosen. The statistical methods for these two types of research questions are not the same, because the purposes of the analyses differ. The comparative question asks the statistical analysis to determine whether differences exist; the relational question asks the statistical analysis to determine whether associations exist. Statistical analysis methods for comparative questions detect differences in means or medians, for example, and may use tests such as the Student *t* test or the Wilcoxon rank sum test. Methods for relational questions assess correlations or associations, for example, and may use tests such as Pearson correlation or the chi-square test.

Comparative Research Question

One example of a comparative research question is, Does vitamin C supplementation elevate serum oxalate levels in patients with renal disease? In a hypothetical study designed to answer such a question, patients could be randomized to receive either the standard vitamin preparation that includes vitamin C (the preparation currently in use in the clinic) or a similar vitamin preparation that excludes vitamin C. The analysis evaluates the difference, particularly the amount of increase, in serum oxalate levels between patients who receive vitamin C supplementation and patients who do not receive vitamin C supplementation.

Relational Research Question

A relational research question might be, Is vitamin C supplementation associated with an increased risk of hyperoxalemia among patients with renal disease? In a study designed to answer this type of question, all patients in a given clinic could be examined to determine serum oxalate levels and interviewed about use of vitamin C supplements. The analysis evaluates whether vitamin C supplement use is associated with the presence of hyperoxalemia.

Scale of Measurement (Type of Data Collected)

The measurements collected in research are referred to as *variables*. Variables can be classified in a number of ways to help determine the method of data analysis to use. Variables that are not inherently numerical—that is, for which only a few possible values exist, as would be the case for gender—have a distribution that is *discrete*. If the distribution is *continuous,* the variables have numerical meaning, as would be the case for blood pressure. The statistical methods used for discrete variables differ from the methods used for continuous variables.

Discrete Variables

Although the symbol used to represent discrete information may be a number, these data are categorical—that is, they represent or name categories. A discrete datum may be further classified by whether it is nonordered, termed *nominal,* or ordered, termed *ordinal*. Nominal data correspond to a limited number of categories that have no ordered meaning. Nominal variables that fit into two categories, such as "present" and "absent," are termed *binary*. Ordinal data are ordered by categories, but the space between the categories is undefined. Treatment groups may be considered ordinal if the different treatments differ by dosage of a particular supplement. For example, binary measurements might include gender (female, male) and disease status (present, absent). Race (several categories, no order) is a nominal measure. Clinical stage of cancer (1 through 4) is an ordinal measure.

Continuous Variables

Continuous variables have a numerical value (a numerical "category"), and the space between the values is defined and can be measured. Continuous data fit into a theoretically unlimited number of categories with equal spaces between the categories. Common examples of continuous data are height, weight, and energy intake.

The Relationship Among Samples

Independent Samples

The assumption underlying many statistical tests is that the measurements among samples are independent. Samples are independent when the data points in one sample are unrelated to the data points in the second sample. For example, an investigator may be interested in the relationship between smoking and hemoglobin levels in women between the ages of 18 and 44 years. If the investigator identifies a group of smokers and a group of nonsmokers from a prepaid health plan and measures their hemoglobin levels, the two samples would be completely independent, because the data were obtained from unrelated groups of women.

Dependent Samples

Measurements in samples that are related are dependent; that is, they are inherently correlated. A number of situations in research produce related measurements and thus do not meet the assumption of independence.

Pairing and Matching. Pairing or matching in the study design can relate samples. An example of a common study design that uses pairing is the crossover trial, a study that uses subjects as their own controls. In a crossover trial, an initial observation is compared with a second observation measured on the same subject after the completion of some intervention by the investigator.

Related observations are also obtained when the subjects are matched. In the usual matched study, each subject in one group is matched with a subject in another group by one or more factors, such as age and gender. Specially designed statistical tests that account for the pairing and its resulting dependence among measurements must be used. Examples of such tests are the paired test and the sign test, which are described by standard statistics textbooks.

Serial Measurements. Besides matching and pairing, another situation giving rise to dependent measurements is the practice of obtaining repeated or serial measurements on individual subjects. It is common to repeat measurements of a variable at several points in time and to evaluate the change from baseline or how the measurement varies over time. In the study of more than one group, the variation over time must also be compared between groups.

The dependence inherent in serial measurements is not widely appreciated in the nutrition literature. Such studies are frequently analyzed by applying *t* tests at each time period. Because the measurements are related, this procedure is not appropriate. This approach also may present the problem of multiplicity (see the following section on the number of samples). A simple approach to the analysis described by Matthews and associates (1) is a two-stage method that summarizes the observations of the individual responses over time and then analyzes the summary measure by standard techniques. Another method would be to use repeated measures analysis of variance to determine whether groups differ in their responses over time. Investigators who are not familiar with this procedure should consult a statistician.

Replicate Measurements.   Replicate measurements, or several measurements taken without regard to time, are also related observations. Analysis of variance can be used for replicate measurements of a continuous variable, provided the number of observations is the same for each subject. If this is not the case, the analysis is more complex, and statistical advice should be obtained (2). The distribution-free Friedman test is useful to analyze several related discrete observations or continuous data that are not normally distributed (see the later discussion of the assumption of normality).

Number of Samples

Statistical tests are designed to compare one sample, two samples, or more than two samples. Tests are so designed because as the number of groups increases, the number of possible pair-wise comparisons increases. For 2 groups, only 1 comparison is possible; for 3 groups, 3 comparisons are possible; for 4 groups, 6 comparisons are possible, and for 5 groups, 10 comparisons may be made. The chances of finding a spurious significant result increases as the number of tests applied to a single set of data increases, giving rise to the statistical problem of *multiple comparisons,* or *multiplicity.*

More Than Two Groups

In the multiplicity situation, the level of statistical significance, or α level, increases dramatically with the number of groups compared. Instead of the chances of a false-positive result at the conventional 5 percent level ($\alpha = 0.05$), the chance of a false-positive "significant" result is greater—almost 15 percent in the case of 3 groups (3 comparisons) and up to 40 percent in the case of 5 groups (10 comparisons) (3). Clearly, the possibility is great that conclusions will be incorrect.

For this reason, the common procedure of using the *t* test to examine each pair in such studies is not appropriate, because the *t* test does not account for multiplicity present in the study design. Multiple comparisons techniques are described by Godfrey (3) and detailed in standard statistics texts. In general, when more than two samples are being compared, the appropriate statistical procedure is to first determine whether an overall difference is present using a test designed to do so, such as analysis of variance. After finding that a statistically significant difference does exist, the appropriate multiple comparison technique should be applied to determine which individual pairs of samples differ. Examples of multiple comparisons methods are the Bonferroni, Scheffe, Tukey, Newman-Keuls, and Duncan tests.

Unrestrained Significance Testing

Multiplicity is also present in a situation in which group comparisons are done on a large number of variables, as is common in nutrition research. In fact, inappropriate methods for multiple comparisons, particularly the unrestrained repeated use of *t* tests, are frequently seen in nutrition literature and are no doubt responsible for a number of the claims of statistically significant results (4). If many variables are compared—for example, all the dozens of nutrients assessed by a nutrient analysis program of dietary intake—the problem of multiplicity will be present. The multiplicity problem exists because there is a 1-in-20 chance of finding a significant difference at a .05 significance level, even if no true difference exists. Furthermore, the chances of spurious significant findings (false-positive results) increase as the number of tests increases.

To avoid this problem, the conventional α level should be applied only to tests that address the research questions. Results of significance tests applied to the hypotheses that serve as the basis of the study should carry the greatest weight (2). If other tests are performed, they should be regarded as exploratory, and a more conservative α level should be used. Adjusting the criterion of statistical significance downward will reduce the chances of spurious false-positive results. This downward adjustment can be made using a technique such as the Bonferroni, in which the α level is made more conservative by dividing it by the number of comparisons (5,6). For example, if 20 comparisons were made, the significance level would be .05/20 = .0025 instead of the conventional .05.

Other Considerations

Assumption of Normality

The validity of many statistical tests depends on the assumptions that the data are from a normal distribution and that the variability within groups is similar. Tests that depend on these assumptions are termed *parametric* and are, to some degree, sensitive to violations of those assumptions. Violating the assumptions does not necessarily rule out the use of parametric statistical methods, but the nonstatistician usually does not know the consequences of doing so. In general, parametric statistical procedures applied to data that form a skewed distribution can yield misleading results (7). When parametric assumptions are clearly not met, it is better to be cautious and choose a method that accounts for the violations. There are two common options for doing so: transformations and nonparametric methods.

Transformations. One option in accounting for violations in parametric assumptions is to transform the data to induce normality in the distribution, and then apply the statistical test to the transformed data (8). A data set that has extreme observations may be transformed to an approximately normal distribution by scale transformation, such as a logarithmic conversion (for example, natural or log base 10). Plotting the transformed data using a histogram to determine whether the transformation is appropriate, that is, whether it results in an approximately normal distribution. The drawback of this option is that interpretation of the results may not be straightforward.

Nonparametric Methods. The second option in accounting for violations in parametric assumptions is to use a nonparametric or distribution-free statistical method. Nonparametric statistical tests do not depend on the normal distribution and thus are valid with skewed data or with data that are collected in categorical form. These tests are easy to apply, and most require minimal calculation. The major disadvantage is that nonparametric tests

are usually somewhat less powerful than their parametric counterparts, especially if the assumptions for the parametric tests are met and the parametric method can be applied. Nonparametric tests generally are less sensitive in finding effects and produce wider confidence intervals. However, nonparametric statistical methods are useful and should be considered when the sample size is small, when the distribution is skewed, or when categorical data are used. Siegel and Castellan (9) provide details on the use of nonparametric methods.

One-Sided and Two-Sided Significance Tests

Departures from the mean (or other parameter of interest) can occur in two possible directions: either above or below it, or in the observed direction and its opposite. A one-sided significance test evaluates departures in only one direction, whereas a two-sided significance test evaluates departures in both directions.

In the majority of situations, the two-sided test should be used. A one-sided test is justified only when the difference is expected to be in a specified direction (stated in advance), and a difference in the opposite direction is either not possible or of no interest. Because one-sided tests are less stringent, the validity of their results should be questioned if the results are marginally significant and the conclusions would change if a two-sided test were applied (10).

GENERAL PROCEDURE FOR STATISTICAL ANALYSIS

Whether the research question is comparative or relational, the investigator first describes the data and then makes inferences about the population from which the sample was drawn. This procedure is performed statistically by use of descriptive statistics, followed by the application of inferential statistical tests. The procedure involves three steps: summarize, estimate, and assess statistical significance.

First, the observations are summarized using a summary statistic or set of statistics (for example, the mean, frequency, or range of the observations in the sample or samples). Summary statistics show the distribution of experiences or characteristics and provide information about the characteristics of the underlying population from which the sample was drawn.

Second, the investigator uses the observations to estimate the magnitude of the difference in the comparison or the strength of the relationship (for example, how large the difference is or how strong the association is). The estimate provides information about the clinical or practical importance of the difference or association. A small difference may be of no consequence, whereas a large difference may make a major impact.

Third, the answer is assessed by determining its statistical significance—in other words, how likely it is that the observed difference or association would be obtained if no difference or association existed. The assessment provides information about the probability that the answer is due to chance alone rather than a true condition.

Step 1: Creating Statistical Summaries

Plotting the Data

Regardless of the type of data collected, plotting the data first and then summarizing it numerically is the best approach to summarizing observations. For comparative questions, construct a frequency distribution of the data, and examine its shape. For relational questions, construct a scatter plot of the two variables of interest (see the hypothetical clinical example later in the chapter).

Summarizing the Plot

The shape of the distribution or plot may clarify the correct summary statistic to use. The idea of summarizing is to convey concisely and accurately the characteristics of the shape of the distribution curve or scatter plot.

Summarizing Discrete Observations. For discrete variables, nominal or ordinal data, summarize the frequency distribution by simply providing a single number: the frequency. The frequency describes the distribution of the group completely. Often the frequency is presented as a proportion of the total observations. If the sample size is sufficient (at least 100), a percentage can be presented, along with the numerator and denominator from which the percentage was derived. Differences among groups can be expressed simply as the difference between the group frequencies or group proportions.

Summarizing Continuous Observations. Statistical summaries of continuous variables are more complex than statistical summaries of discrete variables. The frequency distribution or histogram forms a shape, usually approximating a curve. It is clear from examining the shape of the distribution that a single number does not describe any curve adequately. In this case, it is better to describe the distribution of observations by using at least

two numbers—one describing the curve's height (central location, for example, mean or median) and another describing its width (variation, for example, standard deviation or range).

Determining the Standard Deviation. The shape of the distribution determines the appropriate summary statistic. If the distribution is generally normal, with a shape approximating a normal bell-shaped curve, summarize it by using the mean and standard deviation (SD). A normal distribution has the convenient property that 95 percent of the sample observations lie within the mean ±2 SD. If the distribution is asymmetrical or skewed, as is common in nutrition research, the mean and SD are less accurate summary statistics. For skewed distributions, more than two summary statistics may be necessary. The median and the range are helpful additional summaries, as are the values of the 5th and 95th percentiles.

Step 2: Estimating in Statistics

Statistical procedures are concerned with estimates and uncertainties. Because it is rarely feasible for an entire population to be measured, it is generally agreed that characteristics about populations cannot be determined directly but must be estimated from samples drawn from the population. The summary statistics—such as mean, median, correlation coefficient, and relative risk—are single-value or point estimates derived from samples.

Because a point estimate varies to some extent even among samples drawn from the same population, it is useful to quantify the "precision" of the estimate in some manner. Precision is measured statistically by calculating the standard error and the confidence interval.

Determining the Standard Error

If a number of random samples of sufficient size (usually $n > 30$) were taken from a population, the sample means would determine a normal distribution. The height or center of the distribution of sample means—the mean of the means—would be near the true population mean. The width of the distribution—the SD of the means—expresses the variation among the sample means. As with any normal distribution, 95 percent of all the sample means are within 2 SDs of the population mean.

The standard deviation of the means is estimated from the sample by the standard error of the mean (SEM) or the standard error (SE). The SE is calculated by dividing the sample SD by the square root of the sample size. Consequently, the SE is inversely related to the sample size, a convenient property of a measure of precision. As the sample size increases, the SE decreases; that is, as the amount of information about the population increases, the variation in the estimate of the mean, although not the mean itself, decreases.

The SD is used to describe the variation among individual subjects in a sample, whereas the SE is used to describe the uncertainty in a sample estimate about a population parameter, such as a mean (11). They are not used interchangeably. When describing a sample distribution, the SD is a more useful statistic than the SE. However, when comparing differences among samples, the SE is helpful. The SE allows probability statements about the population mean (or other estimated parameter) to be made—that is, Given the sample data, how likely is it that the population parameter is the value estimated by the sample? This question is best answered using the SE to calculate a range of probable values, the confidence interval.

Determining the Confidence Interval

The confidence interval (CI) is the estimated range within which it is likely (for example, with 95 percent probability) that the point estimate (for example, the true mean, difference, or correlation coefficient) exists. Because the CI is calculated using the SE derived from the study sample, it is dependent in part both on the variation in the factor of interest and on the sample size. The CI is also dependent on the degree of confidence assigned to the results, conventionally placed at the 95 percent level (α = .05). Mathematically, the CI is generally expressed as shown in Formula 27.1:

CI = Point estimate ± "Confidence (1 — α) level" × SE

[27.1]

The CI shows the range from the smallest to the largest values of that parameter that is consistent with the sample data. It is presented alone with the point estimate. A wide CI indicates that the sample's point estimate (for example, mean or correlation coefficient) lacks precision, and the true value could actually be any one of a large range of values. A narrow CI indicates that the sample's point estimate is relatively precise, and the true value is likely to be one of a few possible values. The width of the CI is inversely related to the sample size, indicating that as the amount of information about the population increases, the precision in the estimate increases.

The CI provides additional information about magnitude that is useful for interpreting results. For example, it answers the questions, By how much did the diet alter the hemoglobin levels? and What was the increase in risk associated with cholesterol intake? Instead of offering a single value (the point estimate) by which to interpret the magnitude of a difference or association, the CI offers a range of values that are plausible, given the data in hand. This information is especially helpful when evaluating the practical importance of results. The use of the CI is illustrated in the hypothetical clinical example. Gardner and Altman (11) provide an excellent review of the importance of the CI in reporting and interpreting study results and show methods for calculating the CI for a number of situations. Guyatt and colleagues point out the importance of the CI in interpreting the results of clinical studies (12).

Step 3: Assessing Statistical Significance

Statistical procedures are concerned with uncertainties, so an investigator makes assumptions—hypotheses—about the underlying populations prior to initiating the study. The investigator then tests the hypotheses using the research observations. Formally, the hypotheses are known as the *statistical hypothesis* and the *working hypothesis.*

The research question generates the statistical hypothesis. This hypothesis defines the distributions in the populations under study. An example would be the hypothesis that a parenteral amino acid solution rich in branched-chain amino acids enhances nitrogen retention, as compared with a standard parenteral solution.

The null hypothesis is the working hypothesis. The null hypothesis states that there is no difference or no relationship among the factors under investigation, or there is no difference in the distributions in the study populations. In an investigation of a parenteral amino acid solution rich in branched-chain amino acids and its effect on nitrogen retention, the null hypothesis (H_0) would be that the branched-chain solution has the same effect on nitrogen retention as a standard amino acid solution. The study or alternative hypothesis (H_1) would be that the branched-chain solution enhances nitrogen retention as compared with a standard amino acid solution.

Testing Hypotheses

Because the two hypotheses assume different characteristics about the underlying population distributions, the hypothesis-testing procedure employs statistical tests to compare the expected distribution, defined by the null hypothesis, with the observed distribution, estimated by the study results. The statistical test assesses statistical significance (that is, the probability, or *P,* value) that the results are consistent with the null hypothesis. The statistical significance test asks the question, How likely is it that the values for the distribution characteristics given by the sample will be observed if the null hypothesis is true?

Results yielding a *P* value that is less than α indicate that the study data provide evidence to reject the null hypothesis and to support an alternative hypothesis. Results yielding a *P* value that is greater than α indicate that the study was unable to detect evidence that is contrary to the null hypothesis.

Interpreting Statistical Probability Values

Caution and common sense must guide the use and interpretation of statistical probability values. Although statistical significance is important to assess, it is not the primary result of a data analysis. Statistical hypothesis testing is used to determine whether results are consistent or not consistent with the null hypothesis and, as noted by Rothman and others, artificially classifies results into a dichotomous outcome of significant or not significant (12–14). This answer is not adequate as a guide for decisions in many practical situations (12). It completely ignores the size of any effect that was observed and whether the study was able (had sufficient power) to detect statistically significant results. A finding of statistically nonsignificant results does not mean the findings are necessarily insignificant. Likewise, a finding of statistically significant results does not mean the findings are necessarily meaningful.

Significance values must be interpreted in relation to other aspects of the study, including design characteristics, sample size, missing values, biases in sampling and measurement, and compliance to study requirements and treatment, if given. In addition, the size of the differences or effects must be considered when interpreting results. The CI provides the information about size, and the CI, along with *P* values and point estimates, should be presented to allow a meaningful conclusion to be made.

ANSWERING THE RESEARCH QUESTION

This section describes in general terms how the three-step process just described would be applied to several of the most common research situations. Because readers are most familiar with studies of differences, these applications are briefly outlined in a format that will serve as a ready reference for future use. Methods used for evaluating associations are provided in a more detailed, narrative form. The reader is urged to use these descriptions and suggested applications as a foundation for further study of the topic; to refer to the References to determine whether a suggested statistical method is appropriate for the application at hand; and when possible, to consult with a statistician. An example illustrating both comparative and relational applications follows in a hypothetical clinical example.

Comparisons and Differences

When comparing differences between samples or groups, select the statistical method based on the type of variable considered (for example, binary, ordinal, or continuous). Suggested statistical methods for evaluating differences for these types of variables are outlined in Table 27.1.

Relationships and Associations

Relationships are summarized by a variety of procedures. If the data are discrete, frequency plots that are classified by categories can be used. Such plots are summarized simply by constructing contingency tables (2×2 tables or $R \times C$ tables [tables with more than 2 rows and columns]) of the cross-category frequencies. See Table 27.3, presented later in this chapter, for an example of a 2×2 table. The association between variables in a 2×2 table (that is, the hypothesis that the rows are independent from the columns) can be assessed statistically by the chi-square statistic described in standard statistics texts.

As previously noted, the statistical assessment of the association is not adequate by itself. It conveys no information about the degree of association or its practical importance, and because the *P* value is dependent in part on the sample size, an association of little strength may be statistically significant if the sample is large enough. For this reason, it is also important to estimate a measure of the strength of the association.

Discrete Data

The strength of the association among binary variables can be measured by various methods, depending on the type of study design. For behavioral and educational studies, the φ coefficient is popular despite its deficiencies. Calculated from a 2×2 table, the φ coefficient is interpretable as a correlation coefficient ranging from −1 to +1, with values near 0 indicating little or no association between the two variables. However, Fleiss (15) cautions that the φ coefficient has serious deficiencies and should

TABLE 27.1   Suggested Statistical Methods for Evaluating Differences Between Samples or Groups[a]

Sampling Situation	Variable Type	Hypothesize	Summarize	Estimate	Assess	References
Two independent samples	Binary	Proportions are equal	Frequency table (2 × 2 table)	Difference in proportions with its CI	x^2	11,15,16
	Ordinal	Medians are equal	Median, interquartile range	Difference in medians with its CI	Mann-Whitney Test, Wilcoxon rank sum test	16–18
	Continuous	Means are equal	Mean SD	Difference in means with its CI	Independent t test	11,16
Several independent samples	Binary	All proportions are equal	Group frequencies (contingency table)	Difference in proportions; pairwise CI from multiple comparisons	Global x^2 followed by multiple comparisons analysis	15
	Binary, but groups are ordered	Proportions are equal	Group frequencies (contingency table)	Difference in proportions	Bartholomew's test	15
	Ordinal	All medians are equal	Medians, interquartile range	Difference in medians	Kruskal-Wallis (Jonckheere), nonparametric test	18
	Continuous	All means are equal	Group means, SDs	Difference in means; pairwise CI after multiple comparison analysis	One-way analysis of variance followed by multiple comparisons methods	3,16
Crossover, measures taken at two times in a single group	Nominal or ordinal	Means of time periods do not differ	Medians, interquartile range	CI for median change	Wilcoxon sign rank test	16,18
	Continuous	Medians of time periods do not differ	'Means, SD	Difference in means with its CI	Paired t test	16
Two independent groups, change in measures taken at two times (e.g., before and after treatment)	Binary	Proportion improved is equal	Group frequencies (2 × 2 table)	Difference in proportions with its CI	Normal approximation to binomial or x^2 test; matched study—McNemar's test	11,15
	Continuous	Change in measures is equal	Mean, SD of changes	Difference in mean change with its CI	t test of mean changes, or analysis of covariance (see hypothetical clinical example)	19–21
Two independent groups, serial measures, difference in the response over time	Continuous	Response over time is equal	Plot response over time to determine how it changes over time (peaked or growth curves) then select appropriate summary	If appropriate, difference with its CI	t test of mean difference (from summary), or repeated measures analysis of variance, or multivariate analysis of variance	1,22

[a]CI indicates confidence interval; SD, standard deviation.

be avoided in areas of research requiring a comparison of findings among investigations.

Fortunately, better measures of association exist. Two of the most useful measures are the relative risk and the odds ratio. The relative risk is used when the investigation is a cohort or prospective design, and the odds ratio is appropriate for investigations that are of case-control or cross-sectional design. Both measures describe the degree of association between an antecedent factor and an outcome event, such as morbidity (23,24), so both are important in observational analytic studies that evaluate potentially causal relationships. Methods for calculating and interpreting the relative risk and the odds ratio are discussed in Chapter 6 Readers are also referred to Fleiss (15) for details on deriving the CIs for both measures and for assessing statistical significance.

Continuous Data

The relationships among continuous variables are commonly explored by scatter plot and summarized with linear regression or correlation coefficients. Although they are related, regression and correlation analysis are used for different purposes and thus are interpreted differently. Linear regression expresses the relationship between two variables by a mathematical model describing a straight line. The correlation coefficient measures the degree of linear association between the two variables. Regression analysis is used most commonly to quantify the association between two variables and to make predictions based on the linear relationship. The correlation coefficient is used to measure the strength of the linear association and provides little other descriptive information. Guyatt et al provide helpful illustrations of the use of regression and correlation in the medical literature (25).

The first step in regression or correlation analysis is to plot the data. In regression analysis, a scatter plot is constructed with the dependent (predicted) variable on the vertical axis (y-axis) and the independent (predictor) variable on the horizontal axis (x-axis). The plot will help determine whether a straight-line model is appropriate for the data. In both regression and correlation analysis, any outlying observations can seriously affect the analysis, and a scatter plot assists in detecting those observations. If the scatter plot appears to be nonlinear, methods other than linear regression should be used. (Consult with a statistician.)

Regression Analysis. In regression analysis, after plotting the data, the regression equation to summarize the

plot is calculated. This method is particularly useful when an investigator wishes to predict the value of one variable from that of another. The regression equation summarizes the straight-line relationship between two variables by the equation $y = a + bx$. The equation is expressed conceptually as follows:

$$\left[\begin{array}{l}\text{Predicted}\\\text{variable}\end{array}\right] = \text{Intercept} + (\text{Slope} \times \text{Predictor variable})$$

The equation provides coefficients for the intercept (a), slope (b), and the correlation. The intercept is the estimated value of y when $x = 0$. The slope describes the average value of y at each value of x and is thus dependent on the units in which x and y are measured. Therefore, the slope can be used to predict the change in y that is associated with each unit change in x. Both the intercept and slope have error terms (variances) that are used to calculate additional significance tests and CIs for the coefficients.

The correlation coefficient has a special interpretation in regression analysis. When squared (R^2), it expresses the proportion or percentage of the variation in y that is explained by the linear regression with x. This interpretation is different from that of the correlation coefficient (r), which will be covered later.

In addition to the coefficients, the degree to which the data points cluster around the regression line is also important to quantify. The difference between the actual observed value of y and the value predicted by the regression equation is known as the *residual* (Figure 27.1); thus, the quantity of interest is the *residual variance*. The residual variance measures the amount by which the actual values of y differ from the predicted values. A good regression equation minimizes the residual variance.

It is important to verify, at least roughly, that the regression equation accurately summarizes the data (26). Briefly, the procedure involves examining the residuals by plotting them on the x-axis with the predicted values on the y-axis and determining whether a pattern exists. A relatively accurate regression equation exhibits no distinctive pattern, whereas a less accurate equation shows a systematic trend, such as a V-shaped spread. The regression equation requires further refinement if a trend is detected. Details on residual analysis are provided by Kleinbaum et al (27) and Godfrey (26); the procedure usually is done by computer analysis. The important summary statistics of regression analysis are the regression equation, the coefficients and variances of the slope and intercept, the variance of the residuals, and the

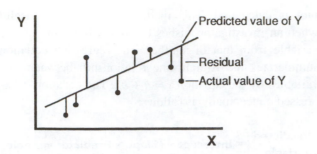

FIGURE 27.1 The difference between the observed values of Y and the fitted regression line (predicted values of Y).

proportion of the variation in the dependent variable explained by the regression equation (R^2).

Correlation. The product moment, or linear correlation coefficient *(r),* is a measure of the strength of the linear association between two variables. It is dependent on the slope and the sample size and does not depend on the units of measurement of the original observations. The correlation coefficient ranges from –1 to +1. When the correlation coefficient is 0, the slope of the regression line is also 0. A value of either –1 or +1 indicates that the data approximate a straight line and that the slope of the line is not 0. A positive coefficient indicates a positive relationship: that y increases as x increases. A negative coefficient indicates the opposite: a negative or inverse relationship in which x increases as y decreases.

The correlation coefficient can be useful in indicating whether y is related to x, but it provides no other quantitative information to describe the linear relationship. It does not describe the amount of change in y that occurs for each unit change in x, as did the previously described coefficients in the regression equation. Furthermore, because of its dependence on the slope and variance, the correlation coefficient can be influenced by both the steepness of the line and the degree to which the data points cluster about the regression line. Because it does not distinguish between these two components, it is difficult to interpret the correlation coefficient correctly when it is presented alone (28). A large value can be misleading. For example, it is possible for a correlation coefficient to be large simply because the axes are scaled in such a way that the slope is steep. For this reason, it is better to interpret the correlation coefficient when it is paired with a plot of the data or with the regression equation, including the slope and variances. The purpose of the analysis determines which statistical analysis method

to include. If the purpose of the analysis is predicting y, regression analysis is used; if the purpose is determining whether a linear relationship is present, correlation analysis is used.

Correlation analysis assumes that the observations are independent. Observations of x and y are taken on each subject, but each subject contributes only one x-y pair. A common error in correlation analysis is to compute correlation coefficients on data that are related. A frequently seen example of this error is the correlation analysis of serial measurements. For example, if serum magnesium and magnesium intake are measured on each subject at several points in time, it is not valid to pool all the data to calculate the correlation coefficient for the relationship between magnesium intake and serum magnesium, because measurements taken on the same person are related.

Correlation for Discrete Variables. A scatter plot also can be used for ordinal, or ordered, categorical data. Unlike continuous data, however, ordinal data should not be analyzed by the product moment correlation normally used. Data of these types are better summarized with a distribution-free correlation procedure, such as the Spearman or Kendall correlation coefficients.

A HYPOTHETICAL CLINICAL EXAMPLE

The application of the statistical methods described in this chapter can be demonstrated using a study undertaken to determine whether the use of a glucose polymer could enhance magnesium absorption as determined by serum magnesium levels. (Charuhas and coworkers [29] reported such a study, and their results are modified here for the purposes of illustration.) The subjects were 40 patients with hypomagnesemia who required daily magnesium supplementation until their serum magnesium levels were normal. The patients were randomized into two groups ($n_1 = 20$, $n_2 = 20$) to receive their magnesium supplementation with either a solution containing a glucose polymer or a placebo solution that was identical in appearance and taste. Measuring the patients' serum magnesium levels after 7 days of treatment and comparing the increase in serum magnesium of the patients receiving the glucose polymer with that of the patients receiving the placebo determined the effectiveness of the glucose polymer. The hypothetical raw data are presented in Table 27.2.

TABLE 27.2 Example of Study Data on Serum Magnesium Levels

Subject	Baseline (mmol/L)	Final (mmol/L)	Change[a] (mmol/L)	% Change
Placebo group				
1	0.51	0.56	0.05	10.6
2	0.55	0.58	0.03	4.5
3	0.59	0.62	0.03	4.9
4	0.54	0.60	0.06	11.5
5	0.59	0.64	0.05	8.3
6	0.55	0.61	0.06	11.2
7	0.55	0.59	0.04	8.3
8	0.56	0.59	0.03	5.9
9	0.50	0.58	0.08	14.8
10	0.57	0.60	0.03	5.8
11	0.59	0.64	0.05	8.3
12	0.50	0.59	0.09	17.2
13	0.52	0.57	0.05	10.2
14	0.58	0.62	0.04	7.8
15	0.55	0.61	0.06	10.4
16	0.54	0.58	0.04	8.4
17	0.53	0.60	0.07	12.4
18	0.56	0.61	0.05	9.6
19	0.58	0.62	0.04	6.4
20	0.60	0.69	0.09	14.4
mean =	0.55	0.60	0.05	9.5
SD =	0.031	0.029	0.017	3.40
Glucose polymer group				
1	0.59	0.62	0.03	4.2
2	0.52	0.58	0.06	11.1
3	0.51	0.59	0.08	15.2
4	0.58	0.67	0.09	15.7
5	0.60	0.65	0.05	8.2
6	0.52	0.61	0.09	17.5
7	0.51	0.62	0.11	22.0
8	0.54	0.64	0.10	19.2
9	0.58	0.66	0.08	13.4
10	0.56	0.65	0.09	15.3
11	0.52	0.64	0.12	22.0
12	0.56	0.67	0.11	19.1
13	0.58	0.68	0.10	17.0
14	0.58	0.69	0.11	19.3
15	0.51	0.63	0.12	22.4
16	0.55	0.64	0.09	17.3
17	0.59	0.69	0.10	17.6
18	0.53	0.62	0.09	17.8
19	0.57	0.64	0.07	12.9
20	0.57	0.67	0.10	17.4
mean =	0.55	0.64	0.09	16.2
SD =	0.031	0.030	0.023	4.57

[a]Change = final value − baseline value

Comparison of Proportions

A number of approaches to the analysis of this study are possible. The calculations, figures, and tables that follow are useful in assessing the data, but for the most part would not be submitted for publication. A simple method would be to describe the proportion of patients in the two groups whose serum magnesium levels improved to at least 0.65 mmol/L (Table 27.3).

The simple difference in the proportions is calculated in this instance as follows:

$$\text{Difference} = \frac{9}{20} - \frac{1}{20}$$

$$= \frac{8}{20}, \text{ or } 0.40, \text{ or } 40\%$$

Confidence intervals for differences between two proportions can be constructed similarly to those for continuous variables (see Formula 27.1) using as the SE:

$$SE_{diff} = \sqrt{(P_1Q_1)/n_1 + (P_2Q_2)/n_2} \qquad [27.2]$$

where P_1 = proportion improved in group 1, $Q_1 = 1 - P_1$, P_2 = proportion improved in group 2, and $Q_2 = 1 - P_2$.

This procedure is useful for samples of sufficient size—say, 50 per group—and with proportions within the range 0.1 to 0.9 (10). Smaller sample sizes require more accurate, but complex, procedures that may necessitate consultation with a statistician. Readers are referred to Gardner and Altman (11) and Fleiss (15) for details and examples of the usual procedure. Because the example data do not meet the size requirement, a CI is not constructed for this point estimate (that is, difference in proportions).

To assess statistical significance, the usual approach when the sample size is large would be to apply the z test (normal approximation to the binomial distribution) or

TABLE 27.3 Number of Patients Showing Improvement by Treatment Group

Treatment	N improved (no./n)	Total (n)
Glucose polymer	9 (0.45)	20
Placebo	1 (0.05)	20
Overall	10 (0.25)	40

the chi-square test, described in standard statistics texts. However, if an expected frequency is small (for example, approximately 5), the chi-square test may not be accurate (7).

To compute the expected frequencies for the glucose polymer response trial, refer to Table 27.4, which gives the observed values for these data. The row totals are 20 and 20; the column totals are 10 and 30; and the grand total is 40. Thus,

E_{11} = Expected number of units in the (1,1) cell

= 20(10)/40 = 5

E_{12} = Expected number of units in the (1,2) cell

= 20(30)/40 = 15

E_{21} = Expected number of units in the (2,1) cell

= 20(10)/40 = 5

E_{22} = Expected number of units in the (2,2) cell

= 20(30)/40 = 15

Because the expected frequency of two cells is small (no greater than 5), a more accurate significance test is given by use of the Fisher exact test. Although the assumptions of this test—that all marginal frequencies are fixed—is rarely met in nutrition research, the test is commonly used for studies in which two of the marginal frequencies are fixed, as in this study ($n_1 = n_2 = 20$). Details of the Fisher exact test for 2×2 tables are given by Matthews and Farewell (30) and others (7,15), and computer programs are available to complete this test. When applied to this table as a two-tailed test, the P value is .008.

The statistically significant result indicates that it is unlikely that a difference of this magnitude (40 percent) would be observed if there were no true difference in the underlying populations. The magnitude, 40 percent, implies that of every 100 patients given a placebo (in whom

an improvement of 5 percent is expected), an additional 40 percent would be expected to achieve serum magnesium levels of at least 0.65 mmol/L within 1 week had they been given the glucose polymer instead. This degree of improvement was considered important by the clinic staff, which concluded that glucose polymer is superior to the standard therapy (placebo) as an adjunct to magnesium supplementation in the treatment of patients with hypomagnesemia.

Analysis of Continuous Variables

Another approach to the analysis would be to evaluate the response as a continuous variable. First, summarize the baseline magnesium levels by graphing them using a histogram, and examine the shape of the curve (Figure 27.2). The histogram helps assess whether the two groups are similar in the distribution of baseline measurements. Figure 27.2 shows that the distributions of the two groups are also similar, indicating that randomization was successful in making the two groups comparable in this baseline measure. The distributions appear to be approximately bell shaped, indicating that parametric statistical methods are appropriate for these data. If the distributions were not bell shaped, the use of nonparametric methods would be preferable.

A simple analysis of the difference in group means of the final serum magnesium measurement by an independent t test may be misleading (for example, 0.60 versus 0.64 in Table 27.2), because the final measurement may be related to the initial measurement. For example, the final value for patients with low baseline levels may be lower than the final value for patients with higher baseline levels. It is best to plot (scatter plot) the final measure with the baseline measure to determine whether they are related (19). As is evident in the scatter plot of these data (Figure 27.3), this is the case.

The final measurement of serum magnesium is linearly related to the baseline measurement. The correlation coefficients (r) are also indicative of the relationship; $r = .70$ ($P = .0006$) and $r = .83$ ($P = .0001$) for the glucose polymer and placebo groups, respectively. Because the purpose was to determine whether a linear relationship existed, the correlation coefficient was adequate when presented along with the scatter plot.

When the two measurements are related, some adjustment for the baseline measurement is necessary. A common approach is to compute the change value—the difference between the final and first measurements—and

TABLE 27.4 Data for Patients Receiving Magnesium Supplementation With and Without Glucose Polymer

Treatment	Response Improved (serum magnesium level ≥0.65 mmol/L)		
	+	−	Total
Glucose polymer	9	11	20
Placebo	1	19	20
Total	10	30	40

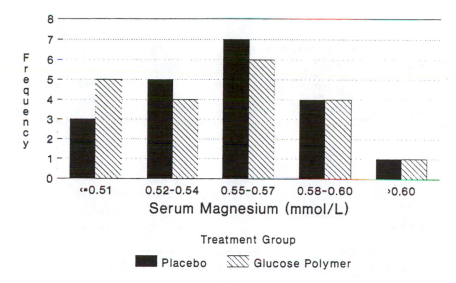

FIGURE 27.2   Histogram of baseline magnesium measurements (n = 20 subjects per group).

then apply statistical methods to this value. The difference computed for each subject is shown in Table 27.5, and a histogram for these values is presented in Figure 27.4

In some situations, investigators may be tempted to use percentage change instead of the value of the change between the two measurements. The choice between change and percentage change is not arbitrary. Kaiser (19) provides guidance on choosing between the two values. Briefly, plot change and percentage change versus the baseline for each treatment group, and then choose the one that shows little dependence on the baseline value (19). Scatter plots for the study data are shown in Figures 27.5 and 27.6.

The scatter plots and r values shown in Figures 27.5 and 27.6 indicate that the value of change is less dependent on the initial values than percentage change, so it is this value that should be compared between groups. Compute the CI for the difference in the mean change, and assess its statistical significance by the usual *t* test. Results are shown in Table 27.6.

From the standard tables of the *t* distribution, the value of the Student *t* at α = 0.05 and 38 degrees of freedom (*df*) is 2.021. The 95 percent CI of the difference between the means can be calculated using Formula 27.1:

$$95\% \text{ CI} = \text{Difference} \pm t \times \text{SE difference}$$
$$= 0.04 \pm 2.021 \times 0.0065$$
$$= 0.027, 0.053 \text{ or } (0.03, 0.05)$$

The pooled variance is used, because the sample variances are similar. (As a general rule, variances may be considered to be similar if the ratio of the sample variances is less than 2.) (7) The statistical significance test for the hypothesis that the mean change is the same for both groups is given by the standard two-tailed Student *t* test, which results in

$$t = 5.652 \quad \text{and} \quad P < .0001$$

These results provide evidence to reject the null hypothesis and to conclude that the mean change in serum magnesium levels differs between the groups. The size of the difference is estimated from the study to be 0.04 mmol/L, although the data are consistent with a difference of as little as 0.03 mmol/L and a difference as large as 0.05 mmol/L. It is a matter of judgment by the investigators and the readers whether this is a clinically meaningful difference.

Analysis of Covariance

Although the *t* test of the difference between initial and follow-up measurements among groups is the most common approach to analyzing data from a study of this type, another method of analysis should be considered here as well. Analysis of covariance is generally a more efficient statistical significance test than the *t* test when the response measurement is related to the initial measurement, as is the case with these data (19–21). Briefly, analysis of covariance involves computing the linear regression of

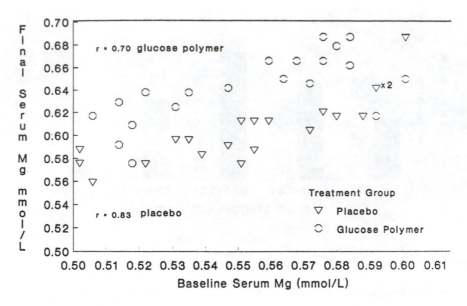

FIGURE 27.3   Scatter plot of the final measurement with the baseline measurement.

TABLE 27.5   Analysis of Covariance Results for Example Data

Source	df^a	Sum of Squares	Mean Square[b]	F Value[c]
Regression $(X)^d$	1	0.019762	0.019762	27.38
Residual	38	0.027418	0.000722	
Regression $(X, Z)^e$	2	0.0333357	0.016679	44.60
Residual	37	0.013823	0.000374	
Regression $(X, Z, XZ)^f$	3	0.033443	0.011148	29.18
Residual	36	0.013737	0.000382	

[a]df = degrees of freedom
[b]mean square = (sum of squares/df)
[c]F value = (regression mean square/residual mean square)
[d]where X = initial serum magnesium value (mmol/L)
[e]where Z = 0 if placebo group, if glucose polymer group
[f]where XZ = interaction term X × Z (ie, 0 for placebo, initial serum magnesium for glucose polymer group)

the final measurement data (dependent variable) versus the initial measurement data (independent variable) and testing the difference between groups by comparing the distance between the regression lines (20). The procedure, described for medical investigators by Egger and associates (20), produces a parallel-lines analysis of covariance model by first testing whether the slopes of the regression lines for the two groups are equal and then, if

the slopes are not significantly different, testing whether the intercepts of the two lines differ (Figure 27.7). This procedure warrants consideration and at times may be preferred to the more common analysis previously described. Readers are referred to Egger and associates (20) for details regarding its use and misuse, although readers who are unfamiliar with analysis of covariance also should consult a statistician.

Analysis of covariance is applied to these data to illustrate this powerful technique. Kleinbaum et al (27) present the topic with an emphasis on application rather than theory, and their text is particularly helpful for the nonstatistician investigator.

The results of analysis of covariance for the example study data are shown in Table 27.7. Three questions are relevant to the analysis, and three regression models are constructed from these data to provide the components for answering the questions. The regression coefficients (β_1, β_2, and β_3) are associated with the independent variables: baseline serum magnesium *(x)*, treatment group indicator *(z)*, and an interaction variable *(xz)* that is a product of the other two variables. This relationship can be shown by the following equation:

$$y = \beta_0 + \beta_1 x + \beta_2 z + \beta_3 xz + \textbf{Error term}$$

The first question is this: Is the relationship between the initial value and the final value the same for both groups? This question is answered by determining if

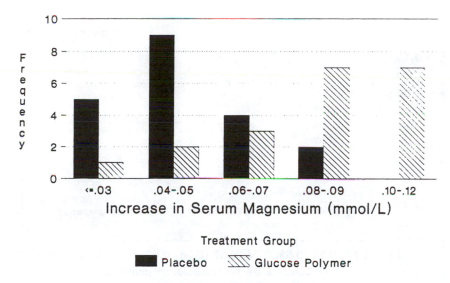

FIGURE 27.4 Histogram of change in serum magnesium from baseline to final value (n = 20 subjects per group).

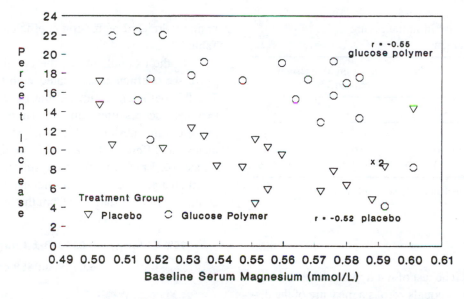

FIGURE 27.5 Scatter plot of percentage change in serum magnesium and baseline measurement.

the lines are parallel or nearly parallel, because if they were not, another method of analysis would be necessary (seek statistical advice). A test of the hypothesis that the regression coefficient β_3 is equal to zero assesses whether the regression lines are parallel. The testing procedure is detailed by Kleinbaum et al (27). The results, as shown in Table 27.7a ($F = 0.22$; 2,36 *df*, $P > .10$), indicate that there is no evidence to show that the two lines are not parallel. Figure 27.7 also shows that the lines appear parallel.

The second question is, Are both the slopes and intercepts the same in the groups? It is important at this step to determine whether the two lines are actually the same line. The test of the hypothesis that both regression coefficients β_2 and β_3 equal zero assesses whether the lines are coincident. The results in Table 27.7b ($F = 17.91$; 1,36 *df*; $P < .001$) provide strong evidence that the two lines are not coincident.

The third question is, Is there a difference in the mean scores? The first and second questions indicate that the lines are parallel but not coincident, so the logical next step is to determine whether the distance between the lines is great enough to provide evidence of a differ-

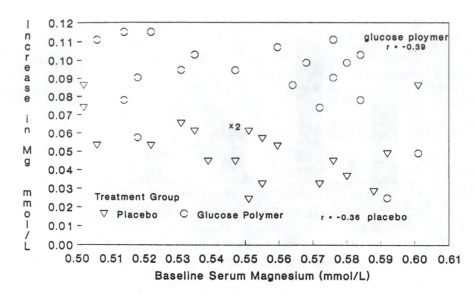

FIGURE 27.6   Scatter plot of the change and baseline measurements.

TABLE 27.6   Increase in Initial Serum Magnesium Measurement

Group	Increase in Serum Magnesium (mmol/L)		
	Mean	SD	SE
Placebo	0.05	0.017	0.004
Glucose polymer	0.09	0.023	0.005
Difference	0.04	0.0206[b]	0.0065[b]

[a]SD indicates standard deviation; SE, standard error.
[b]Pooled SD or SE.

ence between them. The test of the hypothesis that the regression coefficient β_2 equals zero is a measure of the distance and determines whether there is a difference in means between the groups. The results in Table 27.7c ($F = 36.35$; 1,37 *df; P < .001*) indicate that the means of the placebo and glucose polymer groups are significantly different. These results confirm the results of the *t* test and reject the null hypothesis at the level of less than 1 percent.

As with all methods of analysis, assessing statistical significance is only one part of data analysis in the analysis of covariance; estimating the size of the difference is also important. Analysis of covariance is a linear regression procedure, so it produces coefficients that express the linear relationship of the variables of interest. The parameters resulting from analysis of covariance (omitting

xz and its related regression coefficient, β_3) are shown in Table 27.8.

In the example study, the coefficient of interest is β_2, or the coefficient associated with the group variable. The β_2 coefficient estimates the difference between the two mean scores after removing (in part) the influence of the initial magnesium value. Analysis of covariance estimates the difference to be 0.037 mmol/L, close to the estimate (0.04 mmol/L) from the simple analysis using the mean change values. The confidence interval can also be computed in the usual way from the SE of the coefficient:

$$\text{95\% CI for } \beta_2 = 0.036873 \pm 1.96(0.06112)$$
$$= 0.0249, 0.0488 \text{ or } (0.03, 0.05)$$

These results are nearly identical to those derived by the previous method and would be interpreted in the same way. The benefit of using analysis of covariance, however, is that it can be a more efficient analysis than the *t* test (as indicated by the narrower CI) when the initial and final measurements are linearly related and the sample size is sufficient (approximately greater than 20) (20,21).

It is useful to consider the conclusions possible if the significance test resulted in a statistically nonsignificant *P* value. As pointed out by Rothman (13) in 1978, and more recently by Guyatt and colleagues (12), the CI becomes key to the interpretation in such a case. The CI shows the readers the range of values that are plausible, given the data in hand. If the CI were to range from −0.02

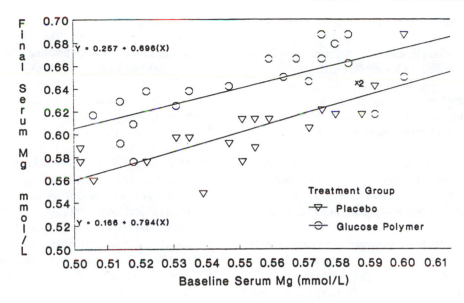

FIGURE 27.7   Plot of serum magnesium values for completing analysis of covariance.

TABLE 27.7   ANOVA Tables for Analysis of Covariance Models (Using Results from Table 27.5)

Source		df^a	Sum of Squares	Mean Square	F Value
A. With the Interaction Variable					
Regression	(X, Z)	2	0.033357	0.016679	43.66
	(XZ / X, Z)	1	0.000086	0.000086	0.22
Residual		36	0.013737	0.000382	
Total		39	0.047180		
B. For Coincident Lines					
Regression	(X, Z)	1	0.019762	0.019762	51.73
	(XZ / X, Z)	2	0.013681	0.006841	17.91
Residual		36	0.013737	0.000382	
Total		39	0.047180		
C. For Difference of Means Between Groups					
Regression	(X, Z)	1	0.019762	0.019762	52.84
	(XZ / X, Z)	1	0.013595	0.013595	36.35
Residual		37	0.013823	0.000374	
Total		39	0.047180		

$^a df$ indicates degrees of freedom.

TABLE 27.8   Parameters from the Analysis of Covariance

Variable	Coefficient	Estimate	SE Estimate^a
Intercept	β_0	0.193257	0.056963
Initial magnesium level	β_1	0.744974	0.102725
Group	β_2	0.036873	0.006112

^{a}SE indicates standard error.

tation of the data is possible when the CI is reported along with the *P* value. Readers then have the information to consider whether the position of the interval warrants a conclusion other than "not significant." In reporting the results, it is sufficient to present a simple table of descriptive statistics and a statement of the analysis of covariance statistics (*F* value, *df,* and *P* value).

to +0.10, the interval would include 0, which corresponds to a nonsignificant *P* value. However, most of the values extend into the range of increased mean values. The CI shows that although the data are consistent with no real difference, the data are also consistent with an increase in serum magnesium levels that generally suggests a favorable result of the treatment. A more meaningful interpre-

REFERENCES

1. Matthews INS, Altman DG, Campbell MJ, Royston P. Analysis of serial measurements in medical research. *BMJ.* 1990;300:230.
2. Altman DG, Gore SM, Gardner MI, Pocock SI. Statistical guidelines for contributors to medical journals. *BMJ.* 1983;286:1489.

3. Godfrey K. Comparing the means of several groups. *N Eng J Med.* 1985;313:1450.

4. Ried M, Hall IC. Multiple statistical comparisons in nutritional research. *Am J Clin Nutr.* 1984;40:183.

5. Tukey W. Some thoughts on clinical trials, especially problems of multiplicity. *Sci.* 1977;198:679.

6. Guyatt G, Jaeschke R, Heddle N, Cook D, Shannon H, Walter S. Basic statistics for clinicians: 1. Hypothesis testing. *Can Med Assoc J.* 1995;152:27.

7. Armitage P, Berry G. Statistical Methods in Medical Research. 3rd ed. London, England: Blackwell Scientific Publications; 1994.

8. Gore SM. Assessing methods—transforming the data. *BMJ.* 1981;283:548.

9. Siegel S, Castellan NJ Jr. *Nonparametric Statistics for the Behavioral Sciences.* New York, NY: McGraw-Hill College Division; 1988.

10. McKinney WP, Young MI, Hartz A, Bi-Fong Lee M. The inexact use of Fisher's exact test in six major medical journals. *JAMA.* 1989;261:3430.

11. Gardner MI, Altman DG. Confidence intervals rather than P values: estimation rather than hypothesis testing. *BMJ.* 1986;292:746.

12. Guyatt G, Jaeschke R, Heddle N, Cook D, Shannon H, Walter S. Basic statistics for clinicians: 2. Interpreting study results: confidence intervals. *Can Med Assoc J.* 1995;152:169.

13. Rothman KJ. A show of confidence. *N Engl J Med.* 1978;299:1362.

14. Poole C, Lanes S, Rothman KI. Analyzing data from ordered categories. *N Engl J Med.* 1984;311:1382-1383.

15. Fleiss JL. *Statistical Methods For Rates and Proportions.* 3rd ed. New York, NY: John Wiley and Sons; 2003.

16. Rimm AA, Hartz AJ, Kalbfleisch JH et al. *Basic Biostatistics in Medicine and Epidemiology.* New York, NY: Appleton-Century-Crofts; 1980.

17. Moses LE, Emerson ID, Hosselini H. Analyzing data from ordered categories. *N Engl J Med.* 1984;311:442.

18. Forrest M, Anderson B. Ordinal scale and statistics in medical research. *BMJ.* 1986;292:537.

19. Kaiser L. Adjusting for baseline: change or percentage change? *Stat Med.* 1989;8:1183.

20. Egger MI, Coleman ML, Ward IR, Reading IL, Williams HI. Uses and abuses of analysis of covariance in clinical trials. *Control Clin Trials.* 1985;6:12.

21. Samuels ML. Use of analysis of covariance in clinical trials: a clarification. *Control Clin Trials.* 1986;7:325.

22. Morrison DE. *Multivariate Statistical Methods.* 2nd ed. New York, NY: McGraw-Hill; 1976.

23. Cornfield I. A method of estimating comparative rates from clinical data. Applications to cancer of the lung, breast, and cervix. *J Natl Cancer Inst.* 1951;11:1269.

24. Jaeschke R, Guyatt G, Shannon H, Walter S, Cook D, Heddle N. Basic statistics for clinicians: 3. Assessing the effects of treatment: measures of association. *Can Med Assoc J.* 1995;152:351.

25. Guyatt G, Walter S, Shannon H, Cook D, Jaeschke R, Heddle N. Basic statistics for clinicians: 4. Correlation and regression. *Can Med Assoc J.* 1995;152:497.

26. Godfrey K. Simple linear regression in medical research. *N Engl J Med.* 1985;313:1629.

27. Kleinbaum DG, Kupper LL, Muller KE, Nizam A. *Applied Regression Analysis and Other Multivariable Methods.* 3rd ed. Boston, Mass: Brooks/Cole Publishing; 1997.

28. O'Brien PC, Shampo MA, Anderson CF. Statistics in nutrition. Part 4: regression. *Nutr Intl.* 1986:2:331.

29. Charuhas PM, Cheney CL, Aker SN, Stern JM, Barale KM. Effect of glucose polymer on serum magnesium in adult allogeneic marrow transplant recipients. *FASEB.* 1989;3:A1071.

30. Matthews DE, Farewell VT. *Using and Understanding Medical Statistics.* 2nd ed. New York, NY: Karger; 1988.

Part 9

—ꝳ—

Presentation of Research Data

The exuberance of completing one's research fuels the next step in the research process: communicating the findings effectively and ethically. Chapters 28 through 30 guide researchers in preparing presentations, devising effective tables and graphs, and addressing issues related to research journals and peer review. Part 9 also addresses the perspectives of reviewers (the researcher's peers and guardians of scientific literature) and readers (the ultimate recipients and users of the research findings).

Original research can be presented in may ways: as technical reports (interim, summary, and evaluation reports), abstracts (to introduce a report, summarize projects, and submit a report for presentation consideration), posters at technical and scientific meetings, oral presentations, videotape and film presentations, and manuscripts prepared for publication in professional and research journals. The specific format should fit the purpose, the type of presentation, and, of course, the audience. All presentations are enhanced by thoughtful, clear organization.

Oral presentations, discussed in Chapter 28, are frequently orchestrated with supportive slides, overhead transparencies, or multimedia computer projections (e.g., Powerpoint). These visual materials are designed to aid, not distract, the listener. They should be readable from anywhere in the room; thus, they should be simple and composed of large letters and large num-

bers. Although slides should be intelligible by themselves, they lose effectiveness if they contain long titles, elaborate footnotes, or multiple data columns, all of which would be acceptable in tables for written presentation but not for projection with oral reports. Slides must be visually strong; two or more may be needed to support the oral presentation of material that would be summarized in a single written table. In general, effective slides should encompass no more than 42 to 50 characters and spaces horizontally and no more than 7 to 12 lines vertically, including lines used in double-spacing. The "rule of seven" is another useful, and more stringent, guide to consider: there should be no more than 7 words per line and no more than 7 lines on a slide. The individual giving an oral presentation is cautioned to prepare for every possible occurrence. For example, if a computer is used for a slide presentation, the presenter should be familiar with the software and be able to project only slides for the audience, not the originating desktop—a particularly distracting way to begin a presentation.

Visibility is equally important in poster presentations. The material must be arranged so that the entire audience can read it easily. It is customary to lead the eye from top to bottom, moving from the left to the right panels. Within this construct, the most important material should be placed at or above eye level, where it is easiest to read. Although all the information is of interest to the people attending poster sessions, the abstract, key data, and conclusions and recommendations are particularly favored.

Chapter 29 discusses how researchers can illustrate their research effectively. The decision of whether to create a table or a graph depends on what is to be presented and the intended audience. The investigator's purpose is to inform, so he or she should consider several formats and revise for clarity. Information should be presented in a logical order, such as from highest to lowest or from most recent to least recent. The presentation should avoid acronyms uncommon to the audience. Consistency of scale should be maintained within the various tables in the text. All tables and graphs should be intelligible by themselves: The number of samples should be indicated, and the key characteristics of the subjects should be stated. Additionally, the units of measure should be indicated clearly.

Bar graphs should be reserved for exhibiting frequency data (for example, the number or proportion of discrete scales), whereas point graphs are superior for displaying parameters of continuous variables, such as means, medians, standard deviations, standard errors, or percentiles. A clever strategy in designing graphs is to maximize the ratio of data to ink. Another good strategy is to present two-dimensional data on an x-axis and a y-axis, and three-dimensional data on an x-axis, a y-axis, and a z-axis; in other words, when using only the x-axis and the y-axis, the data should be two-dimensional, not three-dimensional.

Chapter 30 examines research publications from the point of view of the writer, the reviewer, and the reader. The writer's goal is to communicate logically, clearly, accurately, and ethically. In designing the research and in presenting the findings, the researcher is advised to consult a statistician. Issues related to responsible authorship are delineated clearly (see also Chapter 4). The reviewer plays a prominent role in maintaining the quality of scientific literature. Peer review is a serious business and a professional responsibility. Peer reviewers must respect the work of their colleagues and maintain its confidentiality. Thoughtful, conscientious review gives clear, constructive direction to authors. The third critical corner of the presentation triangle is the readers. Guidance is provided to aid them in developing skills to evaluate the scientific literature critically. Understanding basic statistics (Chapter 27) speeds the interpretation of scientific articles. Suggestions are made to enhance efficiency in reading the vast scientific literature: look at the title and the list of authors; determine the article's intent; and read the abstract, methods, results, discussion, and recommendations. The skilled reader avoids overgeneralizing the findings by assessing the research design, sample selection, and data collected. A study's findings may be generalized to a population other than the specific study sample only if the study controls well the many variables of the research. The triangular support—researcher, reviewer, and reader—form a strong base for research.

ERM, Editor

28

Techniques and Approaches for Presenting Research Data

Ronni Chernoff, Ph.D., R.D., F.A.D.A.

Conceiving, designing, conducting, and analyzing research studies and data provide answers to previously unanswered questions and give a sense of accomplishment to investigators and their colleagues. In previous chapters, the skills needed to plan, implement, and evaluate research have been discussed. The link between the work completed and the audience with whom it needs to be shared is the essence of research data presentation. There are as many methods and forums for presenting research information as there are audiences to whom to present it (1). The method chosen to share the results of a research project should be matched carefully to the intended audience, and the same research results may be presented in many different ways to suit the interests of different audiences. The many and varied techniques and approaches that can be used to present the findings from research projects will be discussed in this chapter.

TECHNICAL REPORTS

Dietitians are called upon, with increasing frequency, to present clinical or outcomes research or technical information within their organizations, to funding agencies, and in professional forums. The current focus on justifying expenditures, new programs, resource use, personnel, and research projects requires both oral and written presentations of data, including data on cost benefits and recovery, production figures, anticipated income, and expected outcomes. Buying a new piece of equipment, requesting additional staff, proposing a new program, requesting funds to support a pilot research project, or remodeling space all require a technical paper that provides the rationale for the request, justification of the expenditure, potential cost recovery or efficiencies, anticipated benefits or outcomes, evaluation plan, and proposed time line. The more complete the technical report, the easier it will be for the recipient to understand what you are going to do or have done, why, and what the outcomes or results are.

Technical papers also may be reports to grant or contract agencies (federal or state agencies, foundations, professional organizations, pharmaceutical or nutrition companies, academic institutions, or others) on the progress or outcomes of grants and contracts. Written proposals or contracts to do work usually are accompanied by requirements for periodic progress reports. Information on the progress, completion, and evaluation of the project is often a requirement of the commitment to perform the work.

Writing clear, concise, and thorough technical reports, whether the audience is within an organization or external to it, is a challenge (2,3). The process may not allow for great creativity, but it does provide excellent opportunities to hone writing skills and to learn how to present data clearly, concisely, and in a straightforward manner. Technical reports should be written in direct, precise terms for their audience. They should set out the purpose and objectives of the project, what was done, why it was done, how it was done, what was accomplished, and what outcomes were measured (3). In evaluation reports, the implications of the outcomes are discussed thoroughly; the reports explain how the results are related to the purpose of the project and how they can be applied to future projects or activities.

Interim Reports

Written reports generally have a clearly defined structure; reports usually follow the outline of the original grant or proposal, and many granting agencies provide forms or guidelines to follow. Interim reports chart progress to date and are written at specified points in the course of the research or project; these reports may be part of midcourse, or formative, evaluations. An interim report starts with a summary or abstract that describes the study under way. It should recap the rationale for the project, what the target outcomes are for subject accrual, what interventions are being used, what data are being collected, or what progress has been made toward accomplishing feasibility studies or marketing goals. If impediments to achieving goals or difficulties with planned interventions have been encountered, an interim report is a reasonable place to explain the problems and discuss alternative plans to achieving the project's goals.

Graphs and figures that chart advancement toward achieving goals may be an effective way to present progress visually (see Chapter 29). This technique may depict how the study or project has progressed and may determine midcourse corrections. Time lines for projects often are laid out in the proposal. Charting the achievement of activities compared with the time line is an effective visual presentation of accomplishments.

Interim reports should be well structured, concise, clear, and focused. Their purpose is to restate the objectives of the research study or project, review the methods used to collect and analyze data, describe the progress made toward the stated objectives, and discuss the problems encountered and the solutions attempted. The conclusion of an interim report should summarize what has been stated and project future accomplishments and achievement of the study objectives.

Summary Reports

Summary reports follow the same format as interim reports; however, they can be used to present completed projects or studies. They should recap the study or project objectives, review the data collection methods, describe the data analysis methodology, and report the results. A discussion section can be used to recount problems, difficulties, or unplanned occurrences and to report the solutions that corrected or resolved them. Summary reports are required at the completion of a contract or grant and often are needed when a project is concluded. If a researcher prepares interim reports conscientiously, summary reports will be fairly easy to write.

Evaluation Reports

Evaluation reports have an added dimension in comparison with summary reports: they must include a section of analytic discussion to interpret the results. Interim evaluations are referred to as *formative evaluations*, and final evaluations are called *summative evaluations*. This analytic section transcends presentation of data, discussing implications and evaluating results. The impact of the outcomes should be analyzed, and the application of the results interpreted within the context of the objectives of the study. Evaluation reports are challenging to write because they go beyond the presentation of facts, requiring analysis and evaluation.

ABSTRACTS

Abstracts often serve as the introduction to, or an executive summary of, technical reports and manuscripts. They provide the first impression that an editor, a review board, a meeting participant, or a journal reader will have of the research reported. They may also stand alone as concise publications of work conducted or of oral presentations that cannot be published verbatim. Abstracts are succinct summaries of research that are submitted for consideration for the presentation of short papers or posters at scientific meetings (4). They may serve as an advertisement for the presentation or for the published article that they precede. In addition, they can be used as brief summaries of the content of formal papers in tables of contents or as succinct descriptions in computerized or printed literature summations (5).

Abstracts have all the basic components and organizational structure of longer manuscripts reduced to include only essential information. Abstracts usually are limited by space (Figure 28.1) or by the number of words

ABSTRACT FORM

All abstract information must be typed in this original form, remain within the border, and be *postmarked on or before April 4, 2003*. Please complete all areas of the form, referring to the abstract example and the *Formatting and Typing of the Abstract* section on the previous page for detailed information. Complete this form neatly as, if accepted, will appear in the September Supplement to the *Journal of the American Dietetic Association* exactly as submitted.

Limit title to 25 words

Use first & middle initials separated with a period and no spaces. Delete from blinded copies only.

Text limited to 250 words.

TITLE

AUTHOR(S)

LEARNING OUTCOME

TEXT

Please select the abstract details below, referring to the accompanying pages for definitions and topic categories. (This information must also appear on the blind copies.) If nothing is selected, abstracts will be reviewed as a project/program report for a poster presentation.

ABSTRACT TOPIC
Primary #_____
Secondary #_____

TYPE (must select one)
☐ Research
☐ Project/Program Report

PRESENTATION TYPE
☐ Original Contribution
☐ Poster
☐ I would be willing to change my presentation type to a poster should the reviewers request it.

DO NOT FOLD OR STAPLE ORIGINAL FORM

FIGURE 28.1 Sample abstract application form.

allowed, so every word must contribute to the clarity of the message. In reading an abstract, the reader should understand what was done, how it was done, and what the results or outcomes were (5).

Organization of Abstracts

Abstracts, like longer manuscripts, should contain a brief introduction that states the purpose of the work, a description of the methodology used, a report of the results found, and a succinct statement of conclusion. Occasionally, a brief table may be included, but most authors prefer to use the space to present written information; tables often consume a lot of space. There is no need for references to be included in an abstract. Abbreviations can be used if they are defined or common. If the abstract is being prepared for a journal or scientific meeting, guidelines for authors usually specify the abbreviations that are acceptable (5,6).

Writing abstracts is not easy (7,8). It often takes many drafts before an abstract is the correct length for the space or fits the allocated number of words. The first draft of an abstract should focus on including the information needed to present a complete report. Once the first draft is completed, extraneous words can be edited, sentences restructured, and abbreviations devised for recurrent terms. Usually abbreviations that are most useful describe the study groups or treatment methods; for example, *long-term tube-fed patient group* may be abbreviated as *LTF.* Common abbreviations include *mg, dL, kg, mmol, cm, yr,* and other frequently used units of measure.

It is wise to allow time for colleagues to read the abstract and suggest changes, and for the author to gain some perspective on it. Writing an abstract is an intellectual challenge similar to completing a crossword puzzle. The right words will fit into the space allocated. Writing abstracts takes some skill, but when the skills are mastered the author has the satisfaction of having chosen the best words according to the designated space or word limits.

Submitting Abstracts

Abstracts are published as a summary of work accomplished and can be cited as a publication. Submissions should be clean, clear, and camera ready, because they frequently are printed just as they are submitted (directly from the abstract form). The blue-line border found on some abstract submission forms to define space allocation or margins for the abstract does not copy or photograph.

POSTERS

Many professional organizations have both short oral presentations and poster sessions. The presentation of posters is different from short oral presentations (4,9). Posters are more visual than abstracts and allow for more interaction between the author or presenter and the audience (10). Posters that address the same or similar themes are presented during a specified period.

Posters sessions provide a professional forum for presenting to colleagues a research project, clinical case, technique or skill demonstration, new approach to practice, or investigation of a professional issue. They offer a unique setting for interaction with colleagues who have similar interests. Posters are flexible, can be used in many settings, are easily updated, and are relatively inexpensive to produce (9,10). Poster presentations should tell the whole story of the research being described, and the author should be available to answer questions and elaborate on theory, method, rationale, results, and conclusions for the interested observer.

When an abstract is accepted for a poster session, the organizing institution provides guidelines for preparation. Posters may be mounted on boards usually 4-ft high by 6-ft wide or on tabletop displays divided into panels; the boards or panels are usually made from soft materials so the poster pieces can be mounted using pushpins or thumbtacks. Posters should be constructed from lightweight cardboard, poster board, or other materials that are easily transported, because the author will have to carry them from home to the meeting site. It is wise to transport posters in carry-on luggage to ensure that they arrive at the meeting with the author.

A poster should follow the outline of the abstract by presenting the purpose of the research; the subjects, materials, and methods used; the results, with data; and the conclusions. Because posters are visual presentations of work performed, they should be illustrated with graphs, tables, figures, photographs, and illustrations. They should be visually interesting; a poster that consists of only text will not be very interesting to the viewer. The layout should direct the viewer's eye through the information, starting at the introduction and ending with the conclusions. A title board, often put together in segments, should run across the top of the poster. It should include the paper's title, authors, and their affiliations. The title

1. Remember that your illustrations and information will be viewed from a distance of 3 feet or more; all lettering should be at least 1/2-inch high, if possible.
2. Illustrations, charts, graphs, and photos used may be similar to those you would use in making slides, although the lettering should be large and easy to read. The format should be kept as simple as possible.
3. Do not mount artwork or lettering on heavy board that may be difficult to keep pinned to the tackboard. Please do not write or paint on the tackboards.
4. Be sure that all items, including your title sign, will fit in an area 4-feet high by 6-feet wide.
5. A sample poster layout is shown below.

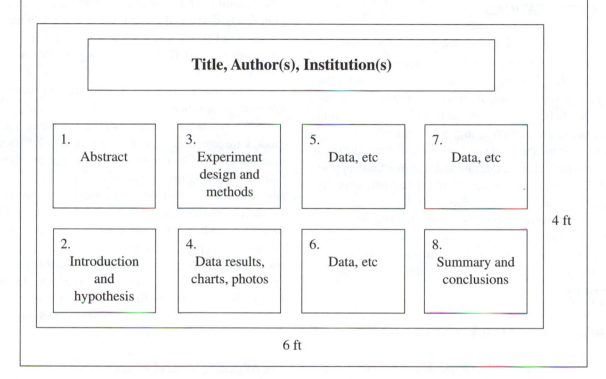

FIGURE 28.2 Tips for preparing posters.

should be large enough to be seen from 40 ft away, and each panel should be clearly legible from 2 ft away. Figure 28.2 shows the arrangement of elements in a poster and gives tips for preparing posters.

Posters are visual, so they should consider graphic principles in presenting their messages. Posters should be free of clutter; readable, with a print size that can be easily seen from a distance (title lettering, 2 in to 3 in; subtitles, 11/2 in to 2 in; narratives, 1 in); colorful; interesting; and balanced. There should be space between the panels or sections of the poster so the flow of the presentation is easy to follow. A succinct, descriptive title will attract people to the poster by piquing their interest. Color helps draw attention to the poster and can highlight points or concepts. Primary color combination usually work best;

black on white or white on red, green, or blue usually provide the best contrast. Colored lines on graphs make the comparison of data instantly understood (9). Pictures, diagrams, graphs, or charts add visual interest and may save space for supporting narrative. Balance can be achieved through careful layout and planning (10).

Before a poster session, the elements should be laid out on the floor or a conference table in a space that approximates the size of the display area board and marked for sequence and spacing. When the spacing looks good, the pieces should be numbered or coded on the back. A picture or drawing of the layout will assure proper placement when the poster is being set up. Having colleagues review the material and ask questions is a reasonable rehearsal.

Prepare for every potential occurrence. Bring all the material you think you may need, even if the meeting organizers have told you what materials will be available. Include pushpins; thumbtacks; tape; pens; pencils; staplers; glue; copies of the abstract and other handout materials; wrapping paper or cloth to cover a discolored mounting board; and business cards to give to people who may be interested in obtaining more information, collaborating on future projects, or obtaining advice (10,11).

ORAL PRESENTATIONS

Among the earliest steps in preparing an oral presentation is to be absolutely clear about the message that will be transmitted (12). It is also very important to consider the forum in which the presentation will be given and the anticipated audience for the message (12,13). Presenting data at a scientific gathering minimizes the effort needed to define the character and needs of the audience, the time frame allocated, and the audiovisual and handout support needed. By being at the meeting and participating in the organization's activities, attendees have a common interest. Most organizations exist as special-interest groups to disseminate content- or profession-specific information, so the audience for a poster or short paper session will have been defined by the forum in which the data are to be presented.

Organization of Oral Presentations

An oral presentation of abstracted data provides an opportunity to elaborate on the details and the rationale for the research, the methods used, the results obtained, and the applications possible. A brief review of the literature to provide the background for the research being presented helps engage the listeners in the presentation. If they understand the purpose of the study, they will listen more carefully to the information being offered. They will want to know about subject selection criteria, data collection methods, data analysis methods, results of the study, what conclusions can be drawn from the information presented to them, and what future research is planned. Too much data overwhelms listeners; therefore, significant results should be the focus of an oral presentation. The data in their entirety can be presented in a published manuscript. If the oral presentation is based on a submitted abstract, the abstract should serve as an outline for the organization of the presentation.

Planning and Preparation of Oral Presentations

Because of the time required to plan a scientific meeting, where most research data are presented, authors will have advance notice that they need to prepare a talk. Notification of acceptance for a scientific paper or poster session is usually sent at least 3 months before the meeting dates. An expanded outline of the presentation should be constructed from the material that has already been prepared (12–14). An analysis of appropriate visuals or illustrations should be made; research data will be clearer if it is graphically displayed. An author can decide what should be described verbally and what will benefit from a visual presentation. Relationships among variables will be clearer if they are graphically displayed, as will the impact of an intervention on an important variable. Major points in an oral presentation can be presented on slides.

When the presenter has a firm idea of the background information and research data to be presented, note cards can be prepared for the major points and slides, or poster illustrations can be made. Oral presentations can be written and rehearsed, but the presenter should be familiar enough with the study and its findings that the speech is conversational and not read. A certain spontaneity in presentation is more engaging for the audience and demonstrates confidence on the part of the speaker (12–14). It is wise for the presenter to rehearse the presentation several times prior to the actual event to coordinate visual support with verbal descriptions (15).

Developing Visual Materials

Both short paper (abstract) and poster presentations are visual events, and strong visual support must be developed. For oral presentations, the visual support should highlight important points, present complex data, and elucidate relationships among variables. Various techniques can be used for the effective visual presentation of information.

Overhead Projectors and Transparencies

Transparencies displayed by an overhead projector can be used in the same way slides are used to highlight important points of an oral presentation. Transparencies are easy and fast to prepare and easy to transport. Overhead projectors are readily available in most meeting places (15). Using a computer graphics program or a clean copy of an image to be displayed, the visual aid can be copied onto an acetate sheet.

Sequential transparencies can be overlaid to demonstrate progressive or multiple relationships (15). Figures, graphs, tables, and other illustrative material should be centered on the transparency, with wide margins to avoid distortion during projection. Print should be large enough to be read easily from the back of the room when projected. The print used should be clear and have high contrast with the background, which is frequently white. There should not be too many words or too much data on a transparency, or it will be difficult to read. Legends on graphs, tables, and figures should be easy to read. The guidelines provided for the development of graphics in Chapter 29 apply to transparencies a well.

It may be difficult to use an overhead projector with transparencies for short paper presentations, because transparencies have to be placed and replaced manually. Short paper presentations are often held in large auditoriums where the presenter is at a podium, and there may be some distance between the podium and the overhead projector. Presenting data with overhead projectors may be more appropriate in a small room, with a more interactive lecture or workshop.

Transparencies have a unique advantage: a skilled speaker can write on them with wax pencil to emphasize points made while speaking or to demonstrate complex relationships. The wax pencil marks are easily removed with a mild solvent, allowing the transparencies to be used again.

Slides

Slides frequently are used as visual support for short paper research presentations, and they offer the most effective visual support for an oral presentation of research data (15). Slides can visually demonstrate the relationships among variables and make complex data more comprehensible by displaying them graphically. Slides can be used to make specific points and effectively show data. However, slides that contain rows and columns of data that are illegible to everyone, including the speaker, are obviously not effective. If it is necessary to use complex slides, a handout of the table or chart should be prepared so the audience can follow the speaker's points.

Effective slides are an adjunct to the verbal presentation of research data. The title of the presentation, the study design, a succinct description of subject selection and exclusion criteria, a description of the research methods, an explanation of the statistical analyses used, the data results, and the conclusions drawn can be put on slides. Lists can be highlighted with bullets and key phrases. Slides do not have to be written in complete sentences. Trigger words, which may serve as headings for persons who are taking notes, can be effective.

Most academic institutions have instructional media departments that provide support for making scientific presentation graphics. Many investigators use computer graphics packages to construct figures, graphs, and tables (16). Laser printers yield the sharpest images. Paper images must be photographed, and the best copy will produce the best slides. Virtually all experienced presenters use computer-generated slides that can be printed from many presentation packages. More sophisticated computer users make their presentations directly from their laptop computers.

Slides also can be made using less technically sophisticated methods. These methods are no longer commonly used but may be handy in the face of technological failure. The message can be typed in a space that approximates the dimensions of a standard slide. A typewriter that uses a film ribbon and a simple typeface will produce the most legible slides; the darker and sharper the typed version, the clearer the slide. A piece of carbon paper can be placed face-up behind the page so that the carbon image comes out on the back of the typed page, making the contrast between type and paper greater. Graphs, figures, and illustrations can be drawn with India ink on plain, nonerasable paper, preferably by a graphic artist.

Presentations can be delivered using multimedia devices if the speaker is computer literate (16–18). Sophisticated multimedia presentations require advance development and storage of the presentation on a computer, along with a multimedia software package that enables the use of different media and the integration of sound, still images such as slides, video images, or animation. Always bring your own computer if you are planning on using this method for presentation, and prepare for a backup if the equipment malfunctions. Inform the meeting organizers that you will need a projection device that has a computer connection and a large screen for proper viewing (18). Experienced presenters with computer skills can make adjustments and alterations immediately before or during their presentations, but this option is risky and not recommended.

Check your slides carefully before you leave for the meeting. Although almost all meeting sites provide slide carousels, bring your own carousel if your slides are unusual in size or mounting. Slides can be stored in slide holders; keep the slide holders in a closed envelope to prevent loss. Most meeting facilities have remote-control slide advancement capabilities so that the verbal description does not have to be interrupted by asking an audiovisual support person for the next slide. Guidelines for slide production are listed in Figure 28.3.

Giving an oral presentation of research data using slides as visual support requires practice. A presenter should allow sufficient time in slide preparation for the rehearsal of the synchronization between slides or other

- A horizontal format, using a ratio of 2 units of height for 3 units of width (eg, 6 cm × 9 cm), makes the best slides.
- Capital letters in a bold, simple typeface are easiest to read.
- Make sure type is large enough to be easily read from the back of the presentation room.
- Illustrations, graphs, and figures should be drawn in black ink on a white background.
- Use a simple design: do not put too much information on one slide.
- Do not exceed 50 spaces (including letters, spaces, and punctuation) per horizontal line.
- Do not exceed 7–10 lines of lettering or numbers per slide.
- Use maximum contrast between lettering and background: black on white, black on light yellow, white on blue.
- Limit each slide to one idea, even if it takes several slides to make your point.
- Allow an adequate margin on all sides.
- Legends on graphs, tables, and figures should be clear and legible.
- Color can be used to highlight points or accent different data sets.
- Complicated data can be supported with handouts.
- Proofread all material to avoid misspellings, which are distracting.
- Place a red dot or number in the lower left-hand corner of the slide when you hold it so that you can read it.
- Important features on an x-ray or photomicrograph should be pointed out with arrows or other symbols.
- Illustrations and photographs should be easily recognizable.

FIGURE 28.3   Guidelines for preparing slides.

graphics and oral presentation. Before any presentation it is wise to preview the slides or other media to ensure that they are right side up, in the proper sequence, and are not backward. Larger meetings provide a slide preview room for presenters.

Videotapes and Films

Videotapes and films can be effective adjuncts to oral presentations. Multimedia presentations are becoming more common and can be effective if used properly and appropriately (18). They are expensive methods of audiovisual support, however, unless you plan on using them multiple times. Certainly for a brief abstract presentation, videotapes and films can effectively demonstrate procedures or depict events that require motion. A few brief minutes of film can save thousands of words of explanation. For example, a real-time presentation (filmed using an X-ray device) of subclavian catheter placement will more effectively illustrate the procedure than any number of verbal explanations or a sequence of slides. Similarly, the impact of vitamin deficiency on altered gaits in chickens or an exercise regimen in stroke rehabilitation will be remembered better if actually seen by the learner.

The use of videotape or film can enhance a poster presentation by attracting attention and running continuously. However, the decision to use film should be made only after considering its cost versus its usefulness in making a point, describing an intervention, or demonstrating results. Films and videotapes are expensive to produce and require special equipment to present. The relative contribution that a film will make to a presentation should be very high to justify the extra cost and effort involved in using this technology to present the data. A film should be used because it is necessary to show activity or movement that cannot be conveyed through slides or still photographs. Videotapes imbedded in slide presentations avoid the need to pause to change or refocus equipment. Sophisticated speakers who are computer literate can present very polished, professional presentations (18). It is important to let the meeting organizers know you will need a videocassette recorder or projection equipment as early as possible so arrangements can be made to have the equipment available.

Handout Materials

Printed handout material is a useful, inexpensive adjunct to a short oral presentation or poster presentation and is frequently requested by meeting organizers. The short paper or poster abstract is published in a program book or supplement to the organization's official publication, so it is not necessary to duplicate it as handout material. An expanded summary, however, can be written and provided as handout material at a poster session. Other effective handouts include a bibliography or reference list on the topic, reproductions of complex slides, complex diagrams such as metabolic pathways, examples of questionnaires or survey instruments, tables of product comparisons, an outline of the presentation, a list of definitions of abbreviations or unfamiliar terminology, sources of equipment, ordering forms for pamphlets or other resource materials, and other information that would be too time-consuming or complex to describe verbally.

Printed material should be legible, neat, and attractive; have adequate margins and appropriate headings; and be set in an easy-to-read typeface. Colored paper can be used to distinguish among different handouts or to make one page of a handout more noticeable. The rules about maximum contrast between type and background colors for slides and transparencies apply to printed handout materials as well. Black print on a light background is the most commonly used combination. Grammatical conventions and correct spelling should be checked carefully, and drawings or illustrations should be simple, clear, and well labeled.

Handouts are effective in reminding the observer of a particular poster after the meeting or scientific session is over. They may also be saved for future reference for prospective new research studies.

Oration Techniques

Many people feel anxiety when speaking in front of a large crowd of people. One way to reduce the anxiety and give a cohesive, coherent presentation is to rehearse it so that it becomes familiar and comfortable (13). It may help to write out the discussion of your research so you can accurately estimate its length when read. However, one of the most important rules of oral presentation is never to read a speech. Writing it down, though, helps to organize it, ensure that all the major points are included, determine what visual support is needed, and make notes from which to actually talk. Key points can be typed in boldface type or set off with bullets.

Speaking well in public requires a great deal of practice and development of self-confidence. Experience and rehearsal make this process easier. Practicing a speech in front of a mirror, before a friend, before col-

leagues, or into a tape recorder can help make the presenter more comfortable. Researchers who present their own research should be the most confident. The relevant literature has been reviewed, the work has been conducted, the data have been analyzed, the results have been assessed, the implications have been discussed, and the abstract has been written and accepted for presentation. No one knows the work better than the researcher; it just takes some practice to present the research well to an audience.

Techniques for securing the interest of the audience include displaying a high level of enthusiasm for the topic, introducing conversational vocal inflections, pacing the presentation so that it is not too fast or too slow, using effective visual support, and appearing relaxed. Speaking in a monotone and appearing nervous distracts the audience from the message. Some eye contact with the audience should be attempted rather than looking only at notes or talking to a spot on the wall; it may be reassuring to the speaker to spot an audience member who is listening raptly or nodding in agreement.

It is important to stay within the time limits established for the presentation. Many organizations provide timers on the podium with a green light that turns yellow when there are 3 minutes to 5 minutes left, and red when there is no time left. If appropriate, the speaker should build in time for a question or two. If there is no time for questions with the presentation, the presenter should remain available after the session so that members of the audience can ask their questions.

Giving any type of oral presentation can be uncomfortable for some people. However, with practice, preparation, planning, and good visual support, giving a talk to an audience of interested colleagues can be educational and fun for everyone.

PUBLISHING A RESEARCH ARTICLE

The researcher who has had an opportunity to present data in a brief published form, such as an abstract, and to present it orally as a short paper may be ready to write an article for publication consideration by a peer-reviewed journal. This step is the most difficult in the continuum of presenting research data. Writing for publication is time-consuming, is repetitive, and demands commitment to producing a quality product (19). Nevertheless, writing for publication can be the most satisfying experience in the research process.

Selecting the Journal

Selecting the journal that might publish the article should be one of the first steps in getting ready to write (19). Journals have specific readerships defined by profession or subject interest; if an abstract or poster has been presented at a professional meeting, the official publication of the professional organization might be the first choice. Other journals that address the same topic areas might also be considered for manuscript submission.

Selecting the journal to which a not-yet-written article will be submitted may seem premature, but there are advantages to making this decision before writing anything. Many journals, such as the *Journal of the American Dietetic Association,* have several different types of articles with different formats, including research reports, short papers, case studies, continuing education articles, literature reviews, and others. The format used to present information determines how the article should be developed. Every journal has its own set of guidelines for its authors, and they may vary depending on the type of article being submitted.

Reading the journal's most current guidelines for authors is important and may save considerable time in manuscript preparation. Margins, page numbering, heading and subheading rules, acceptable abbreviations, line spacing, punctuation guidelines, bibliographic style, number of copies needed for submission, rules for figures and tables, and manuscript length are indicated in the guidelines. It is much easier to start with proper directions than it is to reformat a manuscript after it has been written and revised (20).

Planning an Article

The first step in planning an article is to decide on the set of data to be published. Often research studies generate more data than can or should be presented in one article. If the research data have been reported in abstract form, the focus may already have been identified. The article to be written will address one main theme, which will make it easier to develop thoroughly. If data are sufficient, additional articles may be considered; having one manuscript completed provides a basic structure and some important information in already written form.

The next step after selecting the data that will be used is to outline the article in broad terms. As previously mentioned, the guidelines for authors for the selected journal may provide a broad structural outline for the article. If this information is not specifically given in the guidelines, reviewing a few issues of the selected journal can reveal how published articles are organized. Most journals have a preferred format that includes the following sections: Introduction, Methods, Results, and Discussion.

The Introduction should include a presentation of the problem, a concise review of pertinent literature, the investigators' hypothesis, and the motivation for conducting the research being reported. It also should tell the reader the purpose of the study, explain why it was conducted, and describe its scientific context.

The Methods section tells the reader how the study was done. It should describe the subject groups and their selection or exclusionary criteria, the research design, the methods or instruments used to collect data, and the data analysis methods used.

The Results part of the article includes the outcomes of the study, without interpretation; it also may include the final numbers of completed subjects, reasons for subject dropout or loss, a description of the variables, and the data collected. The results should be described objectively, with an explanation of the statistical analyses. Results may be supported by tables, charts, or figures that demonstrate data and their relationships.

The Discussion is where the author interprets the data (19,20). Results are compared and contrasted with similar research done by others or with previous work performed by the author. The implications and applications of the reported research can be explored in this part of the article. Conclusions can be drawn and future research suggested.

An outline, following the selected journal's format, is the most logical way to approach the planning of the article. The outline can be filled in with phrases and notes on what should be covered under each major heading. As ideas are formulated and noted, the first draft can begin. A well-developed outline makes it easier to write a thorough, organized, comprehensive article.

During this phase of development, the author might develop a working title for the article, which should help focus on the main theme. The title should be informative, brief, and to the point; some journals restrict the number of characters allowed. Such a limitation is noted in the guidelines for authors.

Writing the Article

The first draft gets everything down on paper and is probably the most difficult of all the stages of writing. Notes of references to be used, ideas for tables and figures, possible placement of tables and figures, and headings and sub-headings can be penciled in when the first draft is completed. The manuscript then should be put away for a few days. An author needs some distance from the first draft to develop a clear perspective on the article, reflect on what has been written, and allow new ideas to percolate.

After a few days, the author can read the first draft with a fresh, objective view. It is a good idea to reread the journal's guidelines for authors to review the appropriate sections, length, and bibliographic style. The writing style should be examined and the article evaluated for appropriate paragraph breaks, one-sentence paragraphs, misplaced modifiers, dangling participles, and other grammatical problems. The logical sequence of paragraphs, development of themes, relevance of cited literature, and inclusion of pertinent data can be assessed.

A second draft offers an opportunity to evaluate whether each of the article's sections provides adequate information to explain to the reader why the research was undertaken, how it was conducted, what was accomplished, and what implications and applications can be derived from the outcomes reported. Tables and figures should be drafted at this stage, with consideration given to the contribution each will make to the final product. Data described in the text of the article do not need to be repeated in tables, and some information described in the text may be better presented in a table format. References should be inserted into the text and the bibliography written using the journal's preferred style. The spelling should be checked using a word processing program and the draft then carefully read to correct properly spelled but incorrect words (for example, *their* versus *there*).

After the second draft has been completed to the author's satisfaction, it is time to have the article read by coauthors and colleagues. The article is being written for others to read, and having it read first by friendly eyes should be minimally stressful. Criticism should be assumed to be constructive, serving to improve the clarity and quality of the article. Coauthors want their names on work that reflects excellence, so they will offer suggestions that will make the article better. It is important to remember that writing is an iterative process and that published journal articles often go through multiple revisions and rewriting. Nothing that appears in print is a first or even second draft of a manuscript. An article should be regarded as a work in progress.

Future drafts of the manuscript, integrating suggestions from coauthors and colleagues, should refine and polish the article. A final manuscript should tell a clear, concise, cohesive, and complete story; it should have a beginning, a middle, and an end. Each section should flow into the next, explaining the why, what, where, how, and who of the research being reported. The final manuscript should be well written; avoid jargon; and demonstrate consistency in language, grammar, and verb tense.

Experienced authors know that writing research reports or articles for publication does not get easier with time (19,20). The advantage of experience comes in knowing what to expect when starting the process of writing and in gaining the ability to accept constructive criticism with equanimity.

Submitting the Article

Preparing an article for submission means giving some attention to the details of publishing. Reference style should be checked, along with the completeness of each citation. Pages should be numbered, and page numbers should be in the designated position (for example, the lower left corner or the upper left corner). Figure legends often are required to be on a separate page; figures should be drawn in India ink on white paper or produced by a laser or other high-resolution printer. All symbols used in tables and figures should have easily spotted explanations in footnotes.

Many journals provide a checklist for the author to ascertain that everything required for submission is included with the manuscript. All the required paperwork should be reviewed for completeness. If a figure that appeared elsewhere is to be used, written permission to reprint it from the copyright holder must accompany the article. Journal articles usually contain original figures; using already published figures is more common in books.

Each journal requires an original and several copies of the manuscript. In peer-reviewed journals, two or more reviewers read and critique each article, and each needs a copy.

A letter of transmission to the editor of the journal should accompany the package consisting of an original manuscript; the correct number of copies; glossy prints of figures; permissions to reprint; and other documents, such as copyright release forms, as required by the journal. Letters of transmission initiate a dialogue between author and editor.

Peer Review

Having an article read by two or more content or practice experts can be very valuable. These experts read the manuscript for scientific accuracy, clarity, completeness, and contribution of new knowledge. Their criticism and comments are designed to make the article clearer and more complete. They ask questions and make suggestions that are designed to help the author see what is missing or unclear. Depending on the journal, articles may be reviewed anonymously. Reviewers are rarely made known to the authors, but some journals allow the reviewers to know who the authors are. After the review process, revisions often have to be made and the article resubmitted before it is accepted for publication. This process may take several months.

Between Acceptance and Publication

There usually is a lag of several months between the final acceptance of an article and publication. During this period, the manuscript is copyedited for style, grammar, and conventions specific to the journal. A copy of the edited manuscript is returned to the author with the typeset version of the article. It is important that these galley proofs be read carefully for typographical errors. Publishers often require that galleys be returned quickly—sometimes within 48 hours—so that publishing deadlines can be met. Depending on the publication, two sets of galleys may be sent so that the author can keep one. Typeset tables also need to be compared carefully against the original manuscript to ensure that numbers have not been transposed, columns and rows have been maintained, and headings properly aligned.

During this time, permission to reprint figures can be secured if that step has not yet been accomplished. Additional figures or graphic materials may need to be produced in camera-ready form. The final details of publication are addressed to ensure a polished product. Many journals provide a copy of the issue for the author prior to its mailing date.

Authorship

Issues of authorship are among the most difficult to resolve in publishing (21). However authorship is determined, it should be decided before an article has even been written. This topic is discussed in Chapter 4.

There is a great deal to be gained by participating in research and by presenting the research data in public forums, whether verbally or in print. Research in nutrition and dietetics can contribute to the discovery of new knowledge that can make positive changes in health. The difficult process of presenting research data to interested colleagues can be well worth the effort, resulting in personal satisfaction, career advancement, and professional pride.

REFERENCES

1. Teel CS. Completing the research process: presentations and publications. *J Neurosci Nurs.* 1990;22:125–127.
2. Hayes P. "De-Jargonizing" research communication. *Clin Nurs Res.* 1992;1(3):219–220.
3. Rogers B. Readability in research. *AAOHN J.* 1995;43(4):220–221.
4. Coulston A, Gottschlich M. Writing brief communications. In: Chernoff R, ed. *Communicating as Professionals.* 3rd ed. Chicago, Ill: The American Dietetic Association. In press.
5. Brazier H. Writing a research abstract: structure, style, and content. *Nurs Stand.* 1997;11(48):34–36.
6. Eason JM, LaPier TK. Research corner. The "how to" of writing and submitting an abstract. *Cardiopulm Phys Ther J.* 2000;11(3):105–108.
7. Cole FL, Koziol-McLain J. Writing a research abstract. *J Emerg Nurs.* 1997;23(5):487–490.
8. Haddock N. How to write an abstract. *Managing Clin Nurs.* 1998;2(4):127–128.
9. Cantrell J, Bracher L. How to design and present a poster. *Adv Clin Nurs.* 1999;3(2):91–92.
10. Maltby HJ, Serrell M. The art of poster presentation. *Collegian.* 1998;5(2):36–37.
11. Bergren MD. Professional presentations with posters. *J Sch Nurs.* 1995;11(2):6–7.
12. Garon JE. Presentation skills for the reluctant speaker. *Clin Lab Manage Rev.* 1999;13(6):372–385.
13. Chernoff R. Presentation to professional audiences. In: Chernoff R, ed. *Communicating as Professionals.* 3rd ed. Chicago, Ill: The American Dietetic Association. In press.
14. Koop PM. Reflections on research. How to develop informative, interesting, and organized conference presentations. *Can Oncol Nurs J.* 2000;10(4):154–156.
15. Walker M. A survival guide to paper presentation. *Br J Occup Ther.* 1997;60(1):26–28.
16. Marks LS, Penson DF, Maller JJ, et al. Computer-generated graphical presentations: use of multimedia to enhance communication. *Urology.* 1997;49(1):2–9.
17. Savel TG. Computers. Make your presentations more powerful. *Fam Pract Manage.* 1999;6(1):58–59.
18. Bergeron BP. Digital doc. What you'll need to give all-electronic presentations: slide shows are giving way to video clips and sound. *Postgrad Med.* 1999;106(2):21–22, 27–28.

19. Kris-Etherton PM. Peer-reviewed journal articles. In: Chernoff R, ed. *Communicating as Professionals*. 3rd ed. Chicago, Ill: The American Dietetic Association. In press.

20. Lawrence DJ, Mootz RD. Research agenda conference 3: editor's presentation: streamlining manuscript submission to scientific journals. *J Neuromusc Syst*. 1998;6(4):161–167.

21. Stern EB. The issue is. Authorship criteria: opening a dialogue. *Am J Occup Ther*. 2000;54(2):214–217.

29

Illustrating the Results of Research

Carol West Suitor, D.Sc., R.D., and Carrie L. Cheney, Ph.D., R.D.

The effective presentation of research results poses a challenge to even the most experienced investigator. This chapter addresses the use of illustrations—tables, graphs, distribution maps, photographs, algorithms, and flowcharts—to enhance communication of research results. It emphasizes the most widely used types of illustrations—tables and graphs—as they are used in published works. The usefulness of illustrations in enhancing text (especially for textbooks and their readers) has been the subject of considerable study (1–4); however, an extensive search of the literature reveals that relatively little research has been directed toward the types of illustrations used in reporting research results.

PURPOSES OF ILLUSTRATIONS

Illustrations are used to make information more understandable; depict relationships; add needed emphasis; or allow the presentation of important, exact data in a clear and compact form. Types of illustrations and their functions are presented in Table 29.1.

In a set of guidelines for statistical reporting in medical journals, Bailar and Mosteller (5) state, "Restrict tables and figures to those needed to explain the argument of the paper and to assess its support. Use graphs as an alternative to tables with many entries; do not duplicate data in graphs and tables." These noted statisticians argue for economy in presentation as a method of increasing the chances that an article will be read. Regardless of the type of illustration used, it should contain enough information to be understandable without referring to the text.

Illustrations for published works, posters, slides, or transparencies should be prepared differently. Although all types of illustrations are suitable for inclusion in research articles if they fulfill one of the purposes just outlined, many are unsuitable for display in a poster or on a screen unless they are greatly simplified. Guidelines for preparing materials for posters (6–8) and slides (9–11) focus on simplicity and clarity.

MESSAGES TO BE CONVEYED BY ILLUSTRATIONS

In deciding on illustrations for research articles, investigators should focus on the messages they wish to convey concerning the data, both in general and illustration by illustration. Different kinds of illustrations send different messages and serve different functions, as will be discussed. Thus, it is inappropriate to use different methods for illustrating similar data sets just to introduce variety in an article.

ILLUSTRATIONS AS A SET

The number of illustrations included in a research article should be kept to a minimum so that the reader can easily

TABLE 29.1 Functions of Different Types of Illustrations

Type	Function
Table	Representation of exact data in compact form
Graph	Display trends or relationships in quickly interpretable form
Distribution map	Display of the location of data
Photograph	Accurate representation of the appearance of the subject (e.g., a clinically observable disorder, microorganisms, newly developed equipment)
Algorithm, flow chart	Display of the steps in a procedure that lead to one or more outcomes
Other diagrams	Simplified representation of the subject

comprehend the article's overall message and the data that support it. More extensive illustration may be appropriate for monographs, technical reports, and some types of scientific books (13).

Consistency adds clarity. Scientific journals therefore specify a style for tables and require its use. However, many do not have rigid specifications for graphs and other figures. Because these journals reproduce the figures submitted with the manuscript, authors are advised to give special attention to consistency, accuracy, and scale when preparing a set of figures. A consistent use of symbols is recommended, along with similar proportions and style. For example, a series of graphs comparing food use by Mexican Americans and Puerto Ricans should represent these ethnic groups using consistent symbols in line graphs or types of fill in bar graphs. More suggestions for achieving consistency among graphs are given later in the chapter.

When deciding the order in which comparison groups are to be presented, as in tables or bar graphs, consistency is often undesirable. Instead, the order of presentation ordinarily should be determined by the message to be conveyed, as illustrated in Figure 29.1 (12). The preferred order appears in Figures 29.1c and 29.1e, because this order makes it easy to compare the relative rankings of the different groups. (The category "Other" remains at the end because it includes many different groups with low individual rankings.)

GUIDELINES FOR PREPARING USEFUL TABLES

Many style manuals, such as the *Chicago Manual of Style* (14), give extensive guidelines for preparing tables. How-

ever, these manuals tend to deal only superficially with substantive issues in handling data. Day (15) provides a number of examples of poorly designed and well-executed tables. Colton (16) and Ehrenberg (17), both statisticians, and Clark (18), a noted editor, present complementary suggestions for making the data in tables more understandable. Many of these suggestions are listed in Figure 29.2 (16–19).

Essential Categories of Information

Clark specifies the categories of information that should be included in a table to provide a complete picture of the data (18). She recommends organizing information before actually preparing a table by producing a descriptor set using the categories in the far left-hand column of Table 29.2, which includes examples of Clark's approach using a hypothetical data set. Missing from the list is identification of the sample size, which is necessary for interpretation of the generalizability of the data.

Stages of Table Reading

According to Clark (18), there are three stages of table reading: scanning, reading and primary comparisons, and second-level comparisons. In the scanning stage, the reader looks across the column heads and down the stub. Additional scanning practices appear to depend on the experience of the reader. Clark asserts that, in the reading stage, readers read across the rows of data; and they assume that the column heads are the categories being presented for comparison, even if that was not the intent of the author. If this assertion about readers is true, it directly conflicts with Ehrenberg's advice to present the numbers to be compared in columns rather than in rows (17). No scientific basis was found for choosing one approach over the other. Table 29.3 (20) shows the effects of applying some of these recommendations, including the effect of transposing the rows and columns. The data in these tables are easy to transpose, because the same units are used throughout.

One of the major advantages of placing the data to be compared in columns is that it often facilitates labeling. It is preferable to use consistent units of measure for all items in a column. In the dietetics literature, however, listing nutrients down the stub may keep a table from becoming excessively wide and favors comparisons across the rows.

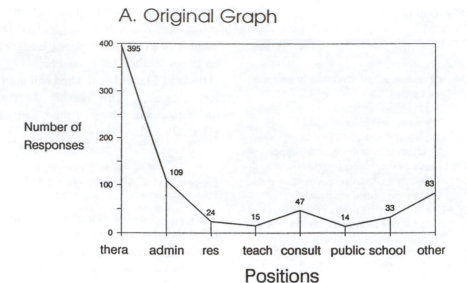

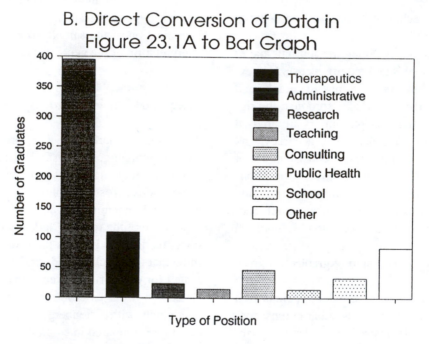

FIGURE 29.1 Examples of undesirable and improved methods of depicting the same data. Example A is not a recommended method for several reasons: it appears to be a frequency polygon, but it is not; it uses abbreviations that are not standard and may not be clear to all readers; there is no logical order to the arrangement of the data; and the actual frequencies are given on the graph. Example B is an improved version of the same graph. However, it would be even better if the order were changed so that the positions (type of employment) appeared in descending order of frequency, if the shading reflected the relative frequency, and if the vertical axis displayed the percentage of graduates in each type of position, rather than absolute numbers. Example A reprinted from Fiedler KM, Raguso A, Morgan G, Renker L. A retrospective study of graduates of a coordinated internship/master's degree program. *J Am Diet Assoc.* 1990;90:591–596. Reprinted with permission from Elsevier Science.

C. Improved Bar Graph

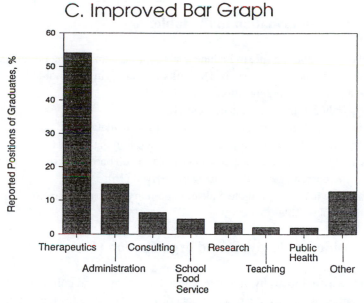

D. Revised Bar Graph (Preliminary)

Type of Position

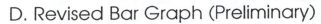

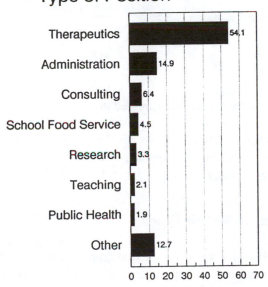

Reported Positions
of Graduates, %

E. Revised Bar Graph (Preferred)

Type of Position

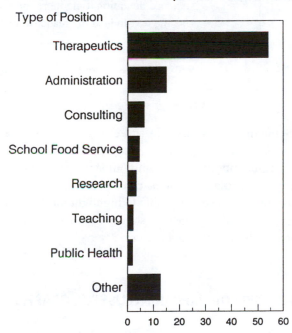

Reported Positions of Graduates, %

FIGURE 29.1 (continued) Example C depicts some of these changes and uses an alternative approach for labeling. The names of the positions have been changed slightly to be more consistent in style and more informative. Example D shows how a vertical bar graph can aid in labeling. This graph was made with default settings. Example E shows the same graph customized by deleting vertical grid marks and data labels, which cluttered the graph and were therefore considered undesirable (13).

Provide complete information in the table:

- Label clearly, making sure to include a label for the stub list (the far left-hand column of the table) and the column heads. Difficulty in identifying a suitable label is likely to indicate a problem in organization of the data (18).
- Clearly indicate units of measurement (16).
- Indicate totals, where applicable, to summarize the data in the table and to help reconcile the data with that in other tables and material in the text (16).
- Show in which direction the percentages add to 100 percent in order to inform the reader how the percentages in the table were derived (16).
- Use tables when they promote a clearer summary of results than would prose.
- Avoid complex tables.

Carefully consider table layout and organization (17):

- Provide a visual focus by giving averages for the rows and columns. (Often this procedure is not possible for the types of data displayed in dietetics journals.)
- Arrange the columns and rows in a logical order; facilitate comparisons when relevant.
- Round appropriately to reflect the precision of the data collection instrument (i.e., round the mean to no more than one decimal place beyond the data it summarizes and the standard deviation to no more than two decimal places (19).
- Use the text to lead the reader to important patterns and exceptions.

FIGURE 29.2 Tips for creating clear tables.

Sometimes it is possible and effective to set up a table to convey a strong visual message. For example, because incompatibility of vitamin/mineral preparations with enteral feeding mixtures can be of real concern, symbols might be used in a table to highlight this kind of problem. A visual approach is shown with a more standard approach in Table 29.4 (21).

GUIDELINES FOR PREPARING USEFUL GRAPHS

Many of the shortcomings of graphs published in the nutrition and dietetics literature appear to result from individuals who use computer graphics programs routinely rather than taking the time to customize a graph for a particular application and carefully inspecting the result. One common mistake is to present data three-dimensionally, implying a z axis, when the data are plotted only along the x and y axes. Suggestions for avoiding unintentional misrepresentation of data or other common problems that may be associated with the routine use of graphics software are incorporated in this section. Figure captions include additional tips.

When adding text to graphs, use initial capital letters only, rather than all uppercase letters. Words written in lowercase letters are easier to read (13,22,23).

Choice of Graph Type

Standard graph types include line graphs, scatter graphs, histograms, frequency polygons, bar graphs, stacker bar graphs, and pie charts. Texts such as *Illustrating Science: Standards for Publication* (13) are good sources of information on the appropriate use of each type of graph. Investigators should not choose the type of graph to use simply based on the choices offered by their graphics software package.

Graphs serve two general purposes: to examine data and to communicate data to others. Stem and leaf diagrams and scatter plots are types of graphs that are useful for finding out if a few data points are strongly influencing measures of effect. Such graphs are very useful

TABLE 29.2 Categories of Information Necessary for a Complete Representation of Data in Tables

Category	Definitions	Examples (Comments)
Current source of the table	Author, publication date	From Smith et al 1990 (necessary only for data taken from sources apart from an original research effort; especially necessary in review articles)
Source of the data	Data collector and period of data collection	Statewide Preschool Nutrition Survey, 1981–1982
Observer	Respondents: Who reported the values?	Food intakes by preschoolers as reported by their mothers and day care providers
Matter	Entities involved in the event covered in the table	Preschoolers aged 3–5 yr; milk consumption
Function	Nature of the event covered and factors that may influence it	Milk intake; race; income
Space	Location of the event	Large state; USA
Time	Period when the event occurred	1981–1982 (in studies examining past events—or exposures, as in case-control studies—this time may be much earlier than the time given by the period of data collection)
Aspect	What was measured and to what topic does this point?	Mean intake in grams in a single 24-hr period; points to weight of all forms of fluid milk
Domain	Range of values	$0, \ldots, 790$ g
Sample size	Number of subjects (total and in subgroups)	$n = 100$; males = 60, females = 40

Data are from Clark (18).

for data interpretation, but they are seldom used in communicating the results of studies. Box plots depict important aspects of the distribution of data (24). (See Figure 29.3 for a generic example of a box plot, and see articles by Hebert and Waternaux [25] and by Worthington-Roberts and associates [26] for examples of the use of this type of graph in reporting the results of nutrition research.)

Important Characteristics of Graphs

According to Tufte (23), "graphical excellence is the well-designed presentation of interesting data—a matter of substance, of *statistics,* and of *design.*" He demonstrates ways to achieve clear, precise, and efficient communication of complex ideas and emphasizes displaying truthful messages with the data. He objects to graphs that have a small ratio of data to ink—as is the case with many bar graphs, for example. (See Figure 29.4 [27] for a superior alternative to such bar graphs.) Tufte compiled a useful list of suggestions for enhancing the visual display of statistical information:

- Choose proper format and design.
- Use words, numbers, and drawing together (for example, little messages that help explain the data).

- Produce a balanced, well-proportioned graph with a relevant scale.
- Display complex detail (the data) in a simple manner (avoiding abbreviations and elaborate codes).
- Tell a story with the data, if appropriate.
- Draw the graph in a professional manner.
- Avoid decorations and moire effects (as from hatched lines).

Colton (16), in turn, emphasizes three important characteristics of graphs:

- Graphs should aid the reader's comprehension of the material. They are unlikely to help if they include a large number of variables, even with ingenious graph design.
- The axes of graphs should be clearly labeled and include the units of measure. A glance should suffice for alerting the reader to what is being illustrated and in what units. Cryptic labeling of the vertical axis of graphs (for example, only the word *Percentage*) is common; more complete labeling (for example, *Percentage of Iron Absorbed*) helps convey the message.
- Graphs should be scaled to represent the data and their importance accurately.

TABLE 29.3   Series of Tables Containing the Same Data in Different Formats

a. Reproduction of a table as it appeared in a journal article

Comparison of Responses from Experimental ($n = 22$) and Control ($n = 19$) Groups to the Nutrition Knowledge Test (NKT) Prior to and Following the Nutrition Education Module[a]

Group	% Correct Mean ± SD Scores on NKT Pretest	% Correct Mean ± SD Scores on NKT Posttest	% Correct Adjusted Mean[b,c] Scores on NKT
Experimental ($n = 22$)	54.0 ± 14.4	65.3 ± 14.6	64.4[x]
Control ($n = 19$)	51.2 ± 11.4	53.3 ± 12.8	54.2[y]

[a]SD indicates standard deviation.
[b]Values within a column with superscripts x and y are significantly different at the $P \leq .01$ level.
[c]Percentage of correct posttest scores in this column are adjusted based on percentage of correct pretest scores.

b. The same data displayed with simplified caption and column heads, deletion of redundancies, and the qualifier of "missionaries." The organization facilitates comparison of pretest and posttest scores in reading across rows.

Comparison of Percentage Correct of Pretest, Posttest, and Adjusted Scores on the Nutrition Knowledge Test by Experimental and Control Groups of Missionaries

Group	Pretest Score	Posttest Score	Adjusted Mean Score[d]
	-----------------Mean ± SD-----------------		
Experimental ($n = 22$)	54.0 ± 14.4	65.3 ± 14.6	64.4[x]
Control ($n = 19$)	51.2 ± 11.4	53.3 ± 12.8	54.2[y]

[d]Adjustments are based on percentage of correct pretest scores. Values within a column with superscripts x and y are significantly different at the $P \leq .01$ level.

c. The data arranged to favor comparison of controls with module participants when reading across the rows; this version also adds clarifying information about the experimental group.

Comparison of Control and Experimental[e] Group Scores Achieved by Missionaries on the Nutritional Knowledge Test

Type of Test Score	Mean Test Score by Group Controls ($n = 19$)	Module Participants ($n = 22$)
Pretest	51.2 ± 11.4[f]	54.0 ± 14.4
Posttest	53.3 ± 12.8	65.3 ± 14.6
Adjusted mean score[g]	54.2	64.4[h]

[e]Experimental group members were required to attend a nutrition education module.
[f]Mean ± standard deviation
[g]Posttest scores in this row are adjusted based on percent correct pretest scores.
[h]$P < 0.01$

All three tables adapted from Hart PC, Alford BB, Gorman MA. Evaluation of a nutrition education module as a component of the career orientation of foreign missionaries. *J Nutr Educ.* 1990;22:81–88. Used with permission from *J Nutr Educ,* Society for Nutrition Education.

TABLE 29.4 Alternate Approaches to Presenting the Same Information in Tabular Form

a. Slightly modified excerpt from a table by Burns PE, McCall L, Wirsching R (21).

Physical Compatibility of Vitamin/Mineral Preparations With Products X, Y, and Z

	Degree of Compatibility[a]		
Medication	Product X	Product Y	Product Z
Vitamin/mineral preparations			
Feosol®	4	4	C
Gevrabon liquid	4	4	C
KCl elixir	C	C	C
Fleets phosphosoda	1	4	C
Neucalglucon syrup	3	4	C
Theragran liquid	C	C	C
Zinc sulfate capsules	4	4	C

[a]C indicates compatible. Incompatibility is measured on a scale of 1 to 4, with 4 being the most incompatible or hardest to unclog.

b. Example of a More Visual Presentation of the Same Data.

Physical Compatibility of Vitamin/Mineral Preparations With Products X, Y, and Z

	Degree of Compatibility[b]		
Medication	Product X	Product Y	Product Z
Vitamin/mineral preparations			
Feosol®	• • • •	• • • •	C
Gevrabon liquid	• • • •	• • • •	C
KCl elixir	C	C	C
Fleets phosphosoda	•	• • • •	C
Neucalglucon syrup	• • •	• • • •	C
Theragran liquid	C	C	C
Zinc sulfate capsules	• • • •	• • • •	C

[b]C indicates compatible. Incompatibility is measured on a scale of 1 to 4, with 4 dots (• • • •) being the most incompatible or hardest to unclog.

Both tables adapted from Burns PE, McCall L, Wirsching R. Physical compatibility of enteral formulas with various common medications. *J Am Diet Assoc.* 1988;88:1094–1096. Adapted with permission from Elsevier Science.

Improper or misleading scaling often occurs unintentionally, especially when using graphics programs. Such programs include default settings—computer-selected settings for the range, the scales of the x-axis and y-axis, the typeface, and so forth—that are intended to

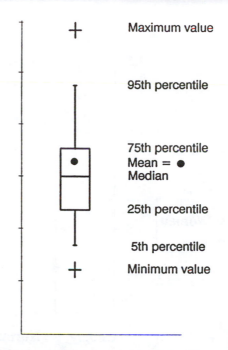

FIGURE 29.3 Example of a single box plot. The elements define the mean, median 50th percentile), first and third quartiles (25th and 75th percentiles, respectively), and minimum and maximum values. Note that this plot depicts data that are skewed toward high values; the mean exceeds the median; there is considerable spread between the median and the 95th percentile; and there is at least one serious outlier. Several box plots may be presented on the same graph to allow comparison of the effects of three different treatments and to provide information about the distribution of data. Adapted with permission from Worthington-Roberts BS, Breskin MW, Monsen ER. Iron status of premenopausal women in a university community and its relationship to habitual dietary sources of protein. *Am J Clin Nutr.* 1988;47:275–279. Reproduced with permission by the *American Journal of Clinical Nutrition.* © Am J Clin Nutr. American Society for Clinical Nutrition.

make it easy to produce standard graphs that look good (at least to the casual observer). Default settings for the range of the vertical axis are based on the range of the data being displayed. Therefore, they minimize unused space—a desirable practice. However, the net result is that they often use an inappropriately high scale that makes minor changes appear major, as illustrated by Figure 29.5. The researcher should make sure that it is easy to tell if a scale does not start at zero and if the scales represent arithmetic or mathematical (for example, logarithmic) change; the investigator also should make sure that scales correspond exactly if graphs are to be compared (see the discussion later in the chapter). Chapter 3

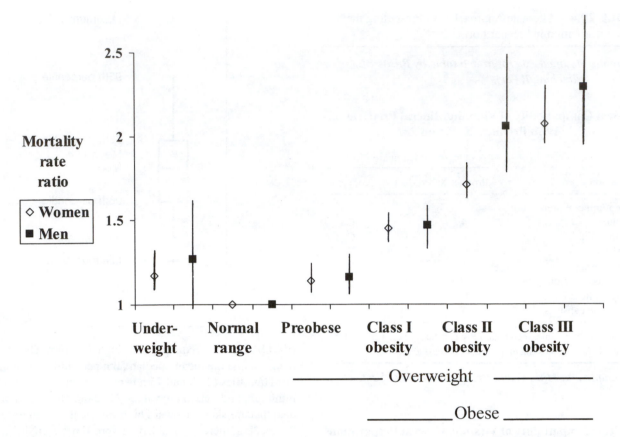

FIGURE 29.4   Rate ratios for death from all causes in white men ($n = 57{,}073$) and women ($n = 240{,}158$) by World Health Organization body mass index categories (underweight = 18.4 or less; normal range = 18.5 to 24.9; preobese = 25.0 to 29.9; class I obese = 30.0 to 34.9; class II obese = 35.0 to 39.9; class III obese = 40+). Values were adjusted for age, education, and physical activity. All values were significantly different from normal range at $P < .001$.

This graph illustrates the display of comparisons of means along with standard error (SE) among different categories of a factor. This graph is superior to bar graphs in displaying parameters of continuous variables, such as means, medians, and the accompanying standard error, standard deviation, or percentiles. Note that the parameters of interest are clearly shown, as is the range of values within the error bars, and that the graph does not distort the size of the differences between categories; it provides a maximum ratio of data to ink, as recommended by Tufte (23). A bar graph, in contrast, uses a small ratio of data to ink; the bars do not represent data points or any specific parameter from the data, and the relative size of the bars is not proportional to the difference among the categories compared. A bar graph is useful for frequency data (i.e., number or proportion of a discrete scale variable). A point graph, as shown, more clearly shows the parameters of interest (here, the rate ratios along with SE) (27). Reprinted with permission from Stevens J et al. Evaluation of WHO and NHANES II standards for overweight using mortality rates. *J Am Diet Assoc.* 2000;100:825–827.

presents information about scale transformations. In all cases, the researcher must inspect all graphs visually for completeness, clarity, and accuracy before using them.

Achieving Consistency in Graphs

To achieve visual consistency, it is advisable to use the same computer software to prepare all the graphs for a given report. If two or more programs must be used, spe-

cial steps may be required to achieve consistency in the use of symbols, fill, and lettering. Even if the same software is used to prepare all the graphs in a set, there must be consistency of scale for graphs that are likely to be compared. For example, the linear distance in millimeters between tick marks on graph A should be identical to that on graph B. To achieve this consistency, the preparer of the graphs must avoid the use of default settings for the vertical axis and be sure to specify the same range for all graphs to be compared (for example, "0 percent to 100

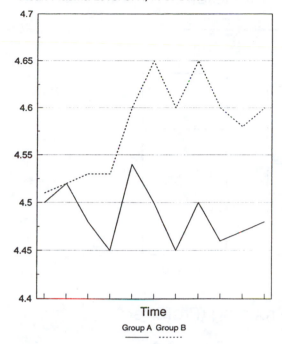

Mean Plasma Level of X, in SI Units

Time

Group A Group B

FIGURE 29.5 Inappropriate graph that overemphasizes the importance of this data. This graph was produced using default settings in a graphics program. The scaling of the Y axis is inappropriate; there is no break in the Y axis to show that the scale does not start at zero, and the lettering is too small to be reduced for publication.

percent" or "2.0 mmol to 6.0 mmol"). Some graphics software allows the user to change the size of the graph. If this feature is used, identical changes in size should be made in all graphs that are to be compared. Furthermore, the authors must specify that identical reductions be made in preparing the art for printing.

Illustrating Science: Standards for Publication (13) contains an outstanding set of guidelines for the preparation of graphs, including very detailed methods for improving visual clarity. The book advises individuals preparing graphs to choose symbols for data points that reproduce clearly and can be easily discerned. The recommended symbols are ● ▲ and ■. The actual choice of symbols depends on what they represent and where they will appear in the graph. When only two symbols are required, black (filled) and white (open) circles are preferred; these symbols might be used to represent black and white subjects, respectively. Similarly, white (open) symbols could be used to represent two groups before interventions and black symbols to represent them after the interventions (in this case, circles and triangles would be

preferred). Although all these symbols are acceptable, it is preferable if circles do not appear next to squares, because these two shapes are difficult to distinguish, especially after reduction. If only one symbol is needed, black circles are recommended, because they are most like data points and are prominent.

Graphical Perception

Graphical perception involves the way graphical information is visually decoded (28). Because a graph is successful only if it is accurately and efficiently decoded, researchers should keep abreast of new developments in this field of study. According to Cleveland and McGill (28), the elementary tasks in graphical perception can be ranked from most to least accurate, as shown in Table 29.5.

These investigators provide experimental evidence that specific graph types are interpreted more accurately than are certain other types. In particular, they recommend dot or bar charts in place of pie charts, and dot or bar charts with grouping in place of stacked bars (Figure 29.6). Component (stacked) bar graphs merit special attention because they are widely used to depict the components of a whole and are easy to create with graphics software. A major problem with these graphs is that they require estimation of length along nonaligned scales. Thus, Figure 29.6b is clearly easier to interpret than Figure 29.6a.

Cleveland and McGill further recommend the direct display of the differences between two curves in place of

TABLE 29.5 Elementary Tasks in Graphical Perception in Decreasing Order of Accuracy

Elementary Estimation Task	Examples
1. Position along a common scale	Height or length of a bar that is part of a bar graph
2. Position along non-aligned scales	Heights of segments in identical closed rectangles
3. Length, direction, angle	Comparison of line lengths without any point of reference; relative sizes of segments in a pie chart
4. Area	Difference in size of two charts
5. Volume, curvature	Difference in volume of two or more spheres
6. Shading, color saturation	Differences in shading on distribution maps

Data are from Cleveland WS, McGill R (28).

A. Stacked Bar Graph (Not Preferred)

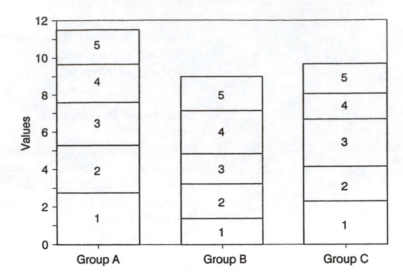

B. Dot Chart With Grouping (Preferred)

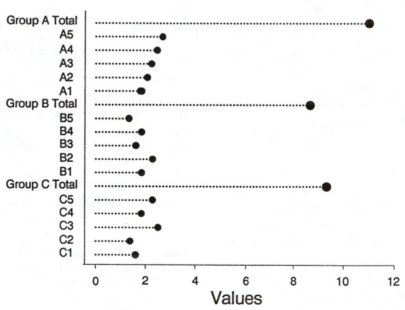

FIGURE 29.6   Stacked bar graph (A) compared with dot chart with grouping (B). Using Part B it is easier to estimate the relative frequencies of the items within groups. The program used to produce the stacked bar graph used different kinds of hatching to denote the different groups; the hatching was deleted to avoid a cluttered graph with moire (shimmering or wave-like) effects. Adapted with permission from Cleveland WS, McGill R. Graphical perception: theory, experimentation, and application to the development of graphical methods. *J Am Stat Assoc.* 1984;79:531–554.

the curves themselves (Part d in Figure 29.7). As can be seen in Figure 29.7, the messages conveyed by curve-difference graphs are greatly different from those conveyed by graphs that depict the two curves separately. If the object is to show that one treatment consistently produces

better results than another, it is more appropriate to use a graph like the one in Figure 29.7a or 29.7b. In contrast, if the difference between values at various time points is important, curve-difference graphs (Figure 29.7c or 29.7d) or a table of differences would be superior.

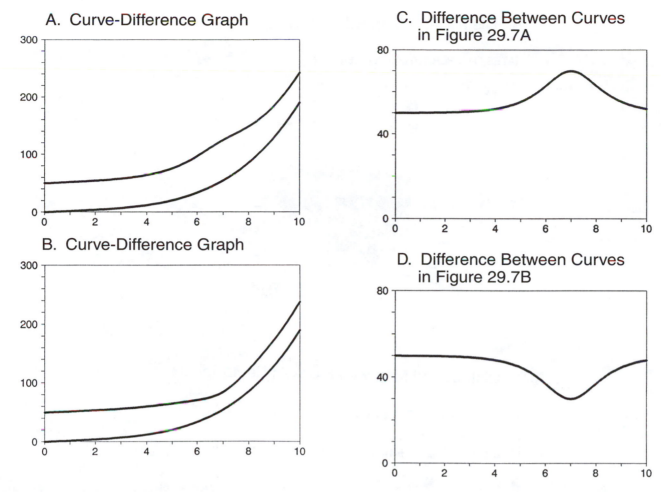

FIGURE 29.7   Curve difference graphs. A and B depict data for each treatment over time, whereas C and D depict the absolute difference between the treatments over time. Note the difference in message; the author should determine whether the difference between the curves warrants emphasis. Some readers who compare the two types of graphs suspect an error because of the great difficulty of visually perceiving absolute differences between two adjacent curves. Adapted from Cleveland WS, McGill R. Graphical perception: theory, experimentation, and application to the development of graphical methods. *J Am Stat Assoc.* 1984;79:531–554.

Other common pitfalls can be ave of the flowchart in Figure 29.9 had been to provide a complete description of the methods, the diagram would have included a much longer series of steps.

The same symbol should not be used to represent two different variables. For example, if N is used in the legend to denote the number of an activity node, a different symbol, such as T, should be used to denote the time required for the activity. In Figure 29.9, which represents hypothetical data, different codes (for example, C1 and C2) were used to denh are acceptable. Horizontal bar graphs (Figure 29.1e) make it possible to use complete labels rather than abbreviations or other, sometimes awkward strategies.

Increased computer capabilities have resulted in rapid developments in the graphic display of results from multidimensional modeling. Although such displays are favorably described (29), there is little information about how well these complex graphs convey messages to readers who are not specialists in the area.

OTHER FORMS OF ILLUSTRATIONS

Distribution Maps

Distribution maps focus on the location of data and can be useful in depicting differences in rates, ratios, total amounts, or percentages by area. For example, a map of

A. Distribution Map with Shading

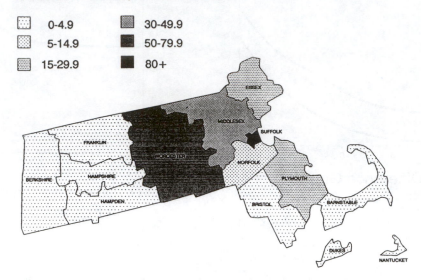

B. Distribution Map with Blocked Rectangles

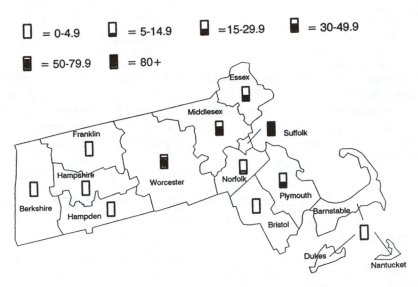

FIGURE 29.8 Distribution maps. A depicts the conventional approach of using different intensities of shading to denote different rates of X in various counties. The computer program automatically uses all upper-case letters for the county names, and all upper-case letters were used for the legend title for consistency. B depicts the framed (blocked) rectangle approach. In this approach, the area of the county has little or no effect on interpretation of the extent of the problem. Note the improved readability when only the initial letters are capitalized.

the United States in which states are grouped by census regions can be used to depict differences in breastfeeding rates in different parts of the country. A state map can be used to identify counties with an unusually high or low prevalence of obesity, and a city map can be used to identify census tracts where members of an ethnic minority reside in large numbers. Shades from light to dark are often used to depict numerical values from low to high, as in Figure 29.8a. This practice has some serious drawbacks: regardless of the numerical value, large areas tend to appear more important, and there is a tendency to overestimate differences in the shades of gray and thus in the numerical values (13). If such maps are used, seven intervals for the data should be the maximum number.

Cleveland and McGill (28) suggest the use of framed rectangle (blocked rectangle) charts as replacements for distribution maps in which shading denotes quantitative information. Figure 29.8b is a framed rectangle chart that depicts the same data used in Figure 29.8a. Both figures were prepared with Freelance Plus computer

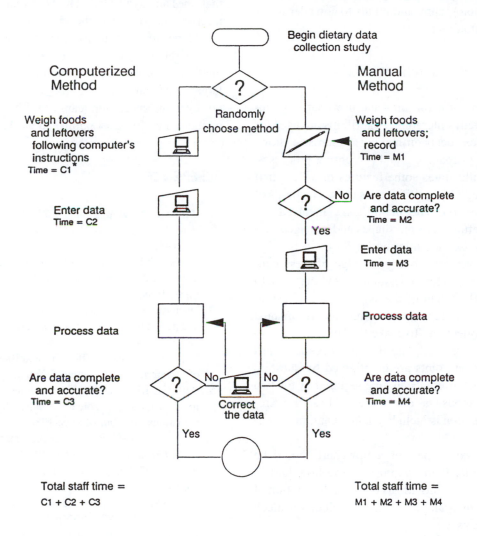

FIGURE 29.9 Example of a flow chart. Adapted from Fong AKH, Dretsch MJ. Nutrition evaluation scale system reduces time and labor in recording quantitative dietary intake. *J Am Diet Assoc.* 1990;90:664–670. Adapted with permission from Elsevier Science.

software (Lotus Development Corporation, Cambridge, MA 02142).

Photographs

Photographs bring the element of reality to the reader. A photograph showing clinical signs of a rarely seen nutrient deficiency reinforces the author's statement that a specific treatment can lead to serious nutrition problems. *Illustrating Science: Standards for Publication* (13) and *A Guide to Medical Photography* (30) contain detailed information on photography and points to consider in the reproduction of photographs.

Algorithms and Flowcharts

Increasing numbers of algorithms and flowcharts are appearing in the dietetics literature. Algorithms are used for clarifying complex decision-making processes; flowcharts are used for organizing and presenting processes. Figure 29.9 (31) illustrates some features of a flowchart designed to highlight basic differences of two methods of dietary data collection. The major tasks involved are placed within carefully selected shapes and arranged logically. The shapes used are informative for those familiar with standard conventions, but knowledge of these conventions is not required for understanding the diagram. In Figure 29.9, the alignment of the steps makes it easy to identify where extra steps are required by the manual method of data collection. To make the diagram easy to read, active verbs are used, and the sentences are short and simple. Decision points are highlighted by question marks. Because the difference in time required by the two data collection methods was one of the reasons for the research, this information is included in the diagram in concise form.

Drawings used as part of a flowchart should be readily recognizable. If the purpose of the flowchart in Figure 29.9 had been to provide a complete description of the methods, the diagram would have included a much longer series of steps.

The same symbol should not be used to represent two different variables. For example, if N is used in the legend to denote the number of an activity node, a different symbol, such as T, should be used to denote the time required for the activity. In Figure 29.9, which represents hypothetical data, different codes (for example, C1 and C2) were used to denote times at various steps so that the reader would realize that each time might be different.

Other Diagrams

Marcus (32) describes principles of visual organization and the limits of perception that can be useful to know in developing clear displays of complex relationships. Among his recommendations are the use of sans serif typefaces; simplified imagery; open spaces; and consistency of design, including reliance on a grid of implied lines. Marcus recommends that similar things be arranged in similar ways and that they be positioned to make the visual hierarchy clear. He further recommends that lines and symbols in charts have a relationship to the information to which the chart refers. For example, it would be appropriate to represent relatively imprecise data by relatively thin, rather than thick, lines. Visual emphasis can be achieved through the use of heavier lines, larger type, and gray levels. These recommendations, however, are more applicable to illustrations for posters or slides than for most published works.

REFERENCES

1. Willows DM, Houghton HA. *The Psychology of Illustration: Basic Research.* Vol 1. New York, NY: Springer-Verlag; 1987.
2. Goldsmith E. *Research Into Illustration: An Approach and a Review.* Cambridge, England: Cambridge University Press; 1984.
3. Duchastel PC. Research on illustrations in text: issues and perspectives. *Educ Commun Technol J.* 1980;28:283–287.
4. Levie WH, Lentz R. Effects of text illustrations: a review of research. *Educ Commun Technol J.* 1982;30:195–232.
5. Bailar JC III, Mosteller F. Guidelines for statistical reporting in articles for medical journals: amplifications and explanations. *Ann Intern Med.* 1988;108:266–273.
6. Jackson K, Sheldon L. Poster presentation: how to tell a story. *Paediatr Nurs.* 1988;10(9):36–37.
7. Warmuth JF. Perspectives on research. *J Nurs Staff Dev.* 1988;4:192–193.
8. Ryan NM. Developing and presenting a research poster. *Appl Nurs Res.* 1989;2:52–55.
9. Kroenke K. The 10-minute talk. *Am J Med.* 1987;83:329–330.
10. Garson A Jr, Gutgesell HP, Pinsky WW, McNamara DG. The 10-minute talk: organizations, slides, writing, and delivery. *Am Heart J.* 1986;111:193–203.
11. Johnson V. Picture-perfect presentations. *Training Dev J.* May 1989;45–47.
12. Fiedler KM, Raguso A, Morgan G, Renker L. A retrospective study of graduates of a coordinated internship/

master's degree program. *J Am Diet Assoc.* 1990;90:591–596.

13. Scientific Illustration Committee of the Council of Biology Editors. *Illustrating Science: Standards for Publication* Bethesda, Md: Council of Biology Editors; 1988.

14. *The Chicago Manual of Style.* 14th ed. Chicago, Ill: University of Chicago Press; 1993.

15. Day RA. *How to Write and Publish a Scientific Paper.* 5th ed. Philadelphia, Pa: ISI Press; 1998.

16. Colton T. *Statistics in Medicine.* Boston, Mass: Little Brown and Co; 1974.

17. Ehrenberg AC. The problem of numeracy. *Am Statistician.* 1981;35:67–71.

18. Clark N. Tables and graphs as a form of exposition. *Scholarly Publishing.* 1987;19:24–42.

19. Lang TA, Secis M. How to Report Statistics in Medicine: Annotated Guidelines for Authors, Editors, and Reviewers. Philadelphia, Pa: American College of Physicians; 1997:48.

20. Hart PC, Alford BB, Gorman MA. Evaluation of a nutrition education module as a component of the career orientation of foreign missionaries. *J Nutr Educ.* 1990;22:81–88.

21. Burns PE, McCall L, Wirsching R. Physical compatibility of enteral formulas with various common medications. *J Am Diet Assoc.* 1988;88:1094–1096.

22. Hartley J. Planning the typographical structure of instructional text. *Educ Psychol.* 1986;21d:315–332.

23. Tufte ER. *The Visual Display of Quantitative Information.* Cheshire, Conn: Graphics Press; 1998.

24. Williamson DF, Parker RA, Kendrick JS. The box plot: a simple visual method to interpret data. *Ann Intern Med.* 1989;110:916–921.

25. Hebert JR, Waternaux C. Graphical displays of growth data. *Am J Clin Nutr.* 1983;38:145–147.

26. Worthington-Roberts BS, Breskin MW, Monsen ER. Iron status of premenopausal women in a university community and its relationship to habitual dietary sources of protein. *Am J Clin Nutr.* 1988;47:275–279.

27. Stevens J, Cai J, Juhaeri, Thun MJ, Wood JL. Evaluation of WHO and NHANES II standards for overweight using mortality rates. *J Am Diet Assoc.* 2000;100:825–827.

28. Cleveland WS, McGill R. Graphical perception: theory, experimentation, and application to the development of graphical methods. *J Am Stat Assoc.* 1984;79:531–554.

29. Graedel TE, McGill R. Graphical presentation of results from scientific computer models. *Science.* 1982;215:1191–1198.

30. Hansell P, ed. *A Guide to Medical Photography.* Baltimore, Md: University Park Press; 1979.

31. Fong AKH, Dretsch MJ. Nutrition evaluation scale system reduces time and labor in recording quantitative dietary intake. *J Am Diet Assoc.* 1990;90:664–670.

32. Marcus A. Computer-assisted chart making from the graphic designer's perspective. *Comput Graphics.* 1980;14:247–253.

The authors wish to thank Marian M.F. Millstone for her assistance with the preparation of this chapter.

30

Research Publications: The Perspectives of the Writer, the Reviewer, and the Reader

Judith A. Ernst, D.M.Sc., R.D.

The writer, the reviewer, and the reader have different perspectives. The writer might say, "I'm an expert in my area of research. I have something of value to contribute to the scientific community that advances knowledge, and I want it published as soon as possible." The reviewer would say, "I assist the writer, the reader, and the editor. I volunteer my time to help ensure the quality and clarity of research in the literature in as timely a fashion as possible." The reader has still another point of view: "I read in part to learn. I am not as familiar with some areas of research and have limited time to read. Therefore, I expect articles to represent quality research and to be communicated in simple, logical terms that I can understand and apply."

The dietitian has the opportunity to assume the roles of writer, reviewer, and reader of research publications. Meaningful research that is original, well organized, meticulously conducted, and effectively communicated characterizes the ideal within the perspectives of all three roles. Guidelines have been developed that assist the writer, the reviewer, and the reader in the implementation, interpretation, and communication of meritorious research. Today's computers, World Wide Web-based literature archives, and on-line publishing provide writers with enhanced access, reduced costs, flexible publication formats, and faster publication of articles. These developments, however, have raised some issues related to intellectual property, the peer-review process, and the dissemination of research findings to populations without access to current technology (for example, most of the developing world) (1–4).

THE WRITER'S PERSPECTIVE

The writer is responsible for scrupulous behavior in the design and completion of research studies, intellectual honesty, and responsible coauthorship (5). The writer, as scientist, has an idea that emerges from an area of interest, from professional experience, or from the literature. He or she develops this idea into a research protocol and fosters it through the stages of implementation, data collection, and data interpretation. The author has an ethical obligation to society to design research that furthers the advancement of the science. Intellectual honesty, a responsibility of medical authors, is essential for the continued professional and public trust of scientific research (5). Scientific dishonesty was defined in 1830 (6) as "trimming," "cooking," or "forging" data, and that definition still applies to published literature today. The following three suggestions can lead to rational inquiry and intellectual honesty: (1) write only what you mean, and mean what you write; (2) provide all the evidence (including negative findings) honestly obtained, and reason logically from the evidence; and (3) be aware of, and discuss, all substantive counterclaims (based on evidence) to your claim (based on evidence) (5).

Consultation with a statistician during the design phase and when results are analyzed is essential to prevent the collection of potentially worthless data that do not fit into an appropriate design for statistical analysis (7,8) (see also Chapter 3). It may be necessary to establish a network within one's institution and work with identified people who have statistical expertise. It is important to identify a statistician who meets the research needs—that is, a statistician who understands biomedical research if the research involves clinical subjects or who understands statistics related to epidemiology if the research involves that type of study. Chapters 1, 2, and 3 review methods for design, data analysis, and presentation of research methods in nutrition and dietetics, as well as providing a review and update for the researcher with a background in basic statistics.

The 1997 (printed) and 2001 (on-line, updated) editions of the *Uniform Requirements for Manuscripts Submitted to Biomedical Journals* (9,10) should be familiar to authors. This text, created by the International Committee of Medical Journal Editors (ICMJE), describes the format in which editors agree to receive articles and includes guidelines for presenting statistical aspects of scientific research in ways that are clear and helpful to readers (Figure 30.1).

The writer, as communicator, needs to be logical, clear, and accurate in describing the methods and relating the results and conclusions of the research. He or she should read the literature and learn which journals would be likely to publish a text on a particular topic, have a particular readership, and publish quality research. Tailoring the format of the manuscript to suit the chosen journal and following that journal's guidelines for authors can expedite the reviewing process (9–17).

Submitting a manuscript for peer review can be an invaluable educational experience for the author. Authors are entitled to expect a consistent response from the editor and prompt and courteous treatment of their articles. They should feel free to question why a paper has been turned down. Frequently, authors complain that the months of time spent in reviewing and fine-tuning a paper delays the transmission of knowledge. The time spent refining a manuscript, however, is well spent and relatively minor when compared with the time spent completing the research and writing (18). A review can be facilitated by the author's inclusion of page and line numbers throughout the manuscript.

An author can best interpret and respond to reviewers' and editors' comments by putting emotions aside.

Adherence to the following suggestions can facilitate communication between the author and editor about a particular manuscript, as well as future manuscripts (19):

- Consider and respond to all comments and suggestions made by both the editor and the reviewers.
- Do not resubmit a manuscript to the same journal if it is refused for publication; instead, consider the reviewers' and editor's comments and submit to another journal.
- Avoid priority comments, as almost no study is "the first"; this claim most likely indicates a failure to review the literature.
- Do not call the editor directly, unless invited to do so.
- Do not approach the editor personally at the annual meeting or elsewhere to discuss a particular manuscript.
- Use restraint in the last paragraph of the manuscript; do not to make naive policy recommendations or generic calls for more research.

Irresponsible authorship and wasteful publication in scientific publishing is considered offensive and perhaps far more damaging than fraud or plagiarism (20). Irresponsible authorship is identified as the inclusion, as authors, of persons who made little or no contribution to the work reported or the omission of persons who made major contributions. The responsible writer, as collaborator, acknowledges the complexity of modern medical research, which may require a variety of skills and techniques available only from the joint efforts of several people. Principles that can be used for justification for multiple authorship are included in the *Uniform Requirements for Manuscripts Submitted to Biomedical Journals* (9) (Figure 30.2).

Abuse with regard to authorship has been attributed in part to the system of academic promotion and reward (21,22). Many peer-reviewed journals provide clear guidelines for authorship. A summary of policies of several medical journals regarding author criteria and responsibilities indicates that issues related to the ordering of authors and alternative forms of recognition are not addressed by the current guidelines of the ICMJE (23). A new system has been proposed that would require that all participants be named as contributors with the intent "to eliminate the artificial distinction between authors and acknowledge and enhance the integrity of publication" (24). Compared to the ICMJE's suggested guidelines for

- Describe statistical methods in enough detail to enable a knowledgeable reader with access to the original data to verify the reported results.
- When possible, quantify findings and present them with appropriate indicators of measurement error or uncertainty (such as confidence intervals).
- Avoid sole reliance on statistical hypothesis testing, such as the use of P values, which fails to convey important quantitative information.
- Discuss the eligibility of experimental subjects.
- Give details about randomization.
- Describe the methods for, and success of, any blinding of observation.
- Report treatment complications.
- Give numbers of observations.
- Report losses to observation (e.g., dropouts from a clinical trial).
- When possible, for study design and statistical methods use as references standard works (textbooks or review papers with pages specified) rather than papers in which designs or methods were originally reported.
- Specify any general-use computer programs used.
- Put general descriptions of statistical methods in the "Methods" section. When data are summarized in the "Results" section, specify the statistical methods used to analyze them.
- Restrict tables and figures to those needed to explain the argument of the paper and to assess its support. Use graphs as an alternative to tables with many entries. and do not duplicate data in graphs and tables.
- Avoid nontechnical uses of technical terms in statistics, such as *random* (which implies a randomizing device), *normal, significant, correlations*, and *sample*.
- Define statistical terms, abbreviations, and most symbols.

FIGURE 30.1   Guidelines for statistical reporting in articles for medical journals. Data are from reference 7.

author acknowledgement in manuscript submission (9,10), the new system proposes using more complex, detailed, and accurate descriptions of contributors that better define the efforts of the individuals involved in the work and publication (24). The new system substitutes the word *contributor* for *author*. It also designates the role of *guarantor* to contributors who are responsible for the integrity of the entire work. Furthermore, the new system helps the reader by identifying for each contributor the following job descriptions with regard to the work and publication:

- Design of the review, the literature search, the data extraction, the data analysis, the production of the first draft, the revision of subsequent drafts, and the coordination of communication among all investigators.
- Literature search, retrieval of articles, creation of data extraction forms, data extraction, data analysis, comments on first draft, creation of first draft of tables, and comments on subsequent drafts.
- Generation of the idea for a review on this topic,

design of the review, and financial support comments on drafts.

Also within the new system, contributors are listed in order of percentage of contribution to the entire project, and a scale to determine the order of contributors in a work that involves multiple investigators and contributors has been described (25). Agreements about contributor order at the beginning of collaboration may change by the time the work is ready for publication, based on the actual contributions of collaborators rather than intended activities (26).

Authors should avoid wasteful publication, which includes reporting the results of a single study in two or more papers (or as Huth puts it, "salami science") and republishing the same material in successive papers that differ only in format and how the content is discussed. Wasteful publication also includes blending data from one study with additional data that are insufficient to stand on their own to create another paper, or "meat extending" (20).

The author is required to sign a copyright form stat-

- All persons designated as authors should qualify for authorship. Each author should have participated sufficiently in the work to take public responsibility for the content.
- Authorship credit should be based only on substantial contributions to (1) conception and design, or analysis and interpretation of the data; and to (2) drafting the article or revising it critically for important intellectual content; and (3) final approval of the version to be published. Conditions 1, 2, and 3 must all be met. Participation solely in the acquisition of funding or the collection of data does not justify authorship. General supervision of the research group is not sufficient for authorship. Any part of an article critical to its main conclusions must be the responsibility of at least one author.
- Editors may ask authors to describe what each contributed; this information may be published.
- Increasingly, multimember trials are attributed to a corporate author. All members of the group, who are named as authors, either in the authorship position below the title or in a footnote, should fully meet the above criteria for authorship. Group members who do not meet these criteria should be listed, with their permission, in the Acknowledgements or in an appendix.
- The order of authorship should be a joint decision of the coauthors. Because the order is assigned in different ways, its meaning cannot be inferred accurately unless it is stated by the authors. Authors may wish to explain the order of authorship in a footnote. In deciding on the order, authors should be aware that many journals limit the number of authors listed in the Table of Contents and that the U.S. National Library of Medicine (NLM) lists in MEDLINE only the first 24 plus the last author when there are more than 25 authors.

FIGURE 30.2   *Uniform Requirements for Manuscripts Submitted to Biomedical Journals* from the International Committee of Medical Journal Editors (9).

ing that the article being submitted is exclusive and has not been published elsewhere. This procedure is designed to prevent the problem of repetitive publication (20).

The MEDLINE database has made literature review for authors easier and far less time-consuming. MEDLINE, however, indexes only the top 4,000 journals and includes only articles from 1966 onward; therefore, the author is responsible for finding and referencing the primary source of the information upon which the submitted work is based (27). For authors without access to a medical library, a list of medical/health sciences libraries on the World Wide Web is available. Pub Med is a freely accessible Web resource for searching the biomedical literature (28,29). Assistance can also be obtained through the National Network of Libraries of Medicine (30).

Direct on-line publication (originally named E-biomed and now known as Pub Med) was proposed in May 1999 by the director of the National Institutes of Health to "accelerate the dissemination of information, enrich the reading experience, deepen discussions among scientists, reduce frustrations with traditional mechanisms for publication, and save substantial sums of public and private money" (31). Since January 2000 the site has accepted papers in every area of biomedicine, and it provides free access to the full text of these papers to all readers

(32). In July 1999 *The Lancet* electronic research archive (ERA) in international health was launched. Also available to authors is the e-print server, an alternative route to formal publication in *The Lancet*. An author can request that a paper appear as an e-print, which is formally peer reviewed. Formal comments from the readership are directed back to the author, as well as the editor. The accepted paper—after revision, if necessary—will be available in both print and electronic format; if rejected, the paper will be removed from the site, and the author will be free to submit it elsewhere (1,33). Guidelines to authors for the citing of electronic references and for readying their own data figures for digital publication in both print and on-line journals are found in several sources (34–38).

The advancement of technology during the past decade has created controversy around the issue of copyright control between authors and publishers involved in scholarly communication. Academic authors historically have viewed their work as having "barter value" only—value in achieving tenure, obtaining time and money for research, and building and maintaining a reputation (4). Four arenas where academic authors are beginning to seek copyright control over scholarly communication have been identified. The first area is electronic prepublication, which allows anyone to see preprinted work and work that has not yet been peer reviewed. The second area is emerging knowledge environments in which the literature of an entire discipline or subdiscipline is brought together digitally for convenience. Authors in these environments are interested in securing the greatest possible flexibility in publishing. The third area in which authors seek more copyright control is personal or laboratory Web sites, where they can post original writings for teaching purposes. The final area is distance education, which requires printed material and streaming video (transmission to a personal computer via the Internet of audio or video content that is seen and/or heard as the content is received) in lieu of the traditional verbal classroom lecture. Advancements in technology and the changing marketplace for education will likely increase the need for authors to negotiate copyright agreements that will allow the widest possible dissemination of their work and ensure that authors, rather than the publishers, have control over, and barrier-free access to, the accumulating body of scholarship on which future teaching and research will build (4).

There is a wealth of resources that address the issue of copyright. Many are electronically available to writers interested in learning about authors' intellectual property rights (4,39–43).

THE REVIEWER'S PERSPECTIVE

Peer review plays a critical role in determining the nature and level of clinical practice. Approximately three-quarters of the major scientific journals use some sort of peer review (18). A historical perspective of peer review and guidelines for the reviewer presented by Lock (18), editor of the *British Medical Journal,* is of interest to authors and critical readers, as well as reviewers. In his guidelines for the reviewer, Lock emphasizes that the unpublished manuscript is a privileged document and should be protected from any form of exploitation. Reviewers are expected not to cite a manuscript or refer to the work it describes before it has been published, as well as to refrain from using the information it contains for the advancement of their own research. The reviewer, as confidant, must not plagiarize or use in any form the work that is being reviewed during the lengthy editorial process (44). Therefore, the reviewer, as impartial referee, may be faced with important ethical questions, because the author and reviewer often are competitors.

The peer review is a positive, usually constructive critical process that allows the author to enhance the publication. In comments to the author, the reviewer should present criticism dispassionately and avoid abrasive remarks (18). The reviewer assesses organization, originality, scientific reliability, clinical importance, clarity, correct and current referencing, and suitability for publication. Figure 30.3 presents the Guidelines for Manuscript Review used by reviewers for the *Journal of the American Dietetic Association* when they critique Perspectives in Practice articles, review articles, and Research and Professional Briefs, and when they review manuscripts presenting original research.

At the end of the process, the reviewer makes a recommendation to accept the paper for publication, accept it for publication after modification, or reject it for publication in a particular journal. The reviewer may recommend that the manuscript be submitted to another journal and may cite a particular journal (44). Specific statements about the acceptability of a paper are directed to the editor in a confidential cover letter or on a form provided for that purpose. The editor gratefully receives a reviewer's recommendations. However, editorial decisions are usually based on evaluations derived from several sources, and a reviewer therefore should not expect the editor to honor every recommendation (45).

The peer review not only influences the content of medical literature but also directly affects medical education in the classroom and at the bedside. The process influences the use or rejection of various medical innovations (45). Peer review also benefits the readership by reducing the number of gross errors that appear in the literature, enforces some set of standards for practice, exerts a mechanism for quality control, and stimulates efforts to produce better work and better writing. Potential risks of peer review include delay in transmission of helpful information, as well as the exclusion of new ideas or approaches that conflict with orthodoxy, which can retard progress (45).

Even though the current referee system may fail from time to time, it represents today's single greatest protection of scientific integrity and excellence (44). If the reviewer accepts the role of teacher by giving constructive criticism and remains open to feedback from the investigator, as in the case of a rebuttal, both investigator and reviewer are provided an educational experience. This effective communication within the editorial review process makes a good paper better and an excellent paper superb (44). Nearly 50 percent of rejected manuscripts that had the benefit of additional peer review eventually have been accepted for publication (45).

The current peer review process has been chal-

The following questions may guide you when critiquing Perspectives in Practice and review articles. Your comments will be most useful to the author if they are constructive and informative.

1. Does the *article,* in your opinion, make a valuable contribution to the field of dietetics?
2. Is that contribution clearly conveyed in the article?
3. Is the *title* clear and informative?
4. Is the *abstract* intelligible by itself? Does it summarize the purpose, content, and conclusions of the article?
5. Does the *introduction* state the intention of the article?
6. Is the *text* developed in logical order?
7. Is each *table/figure* intelligible by itself, concise, and necessary to the article? Are the legends understandable? Is the information in the text and tables/figures non-repetitious?
8. Are the *implications/applications/recommendations* logical, well considered, and pertinent, yet far-sighted?
9. Are the *references* appropriate, current, and sufficient in number and scope?
10. Considering each of the *above sections,* is each presented concisely? Is the information relevant and non-repetitious?

The following questions may guide you in critiquing Research and Professional Briefs. Criteria for a Research and Professional Brief are 1500 words or less (approximately three and one-half to four pages, double-spaced), plus one to two short tables/figures, and pertinent references from the scientific literature. Your comments will be most useful to the author if they are constructive and informative.

1. Does the *Research and Professional Brief* in your opinion, make a valuable contribution to the field of dietetics?
2. Is the *title* clear and informative?
3. Is the *abstract* intelligible by itself? Does it summarize the purpose, content, and conclusions of the brief?
4. Does the introduction state the intention of the article?
5. Is the text developed in logical order?
6. If the Research and Professional Brief is research oriented, please consider the following two points:
    a. Are the *materials and methods* straightforward, well-conceived, and scientifically accurate? Is the research design appropriate to test the hypothesis? Is the sample selection appropriate? Is the sample size sufficient? Are suitable statistical tests applied?
    b. Are the *results* clear and appropriately analyzed? Do the *results* follow the same order presented under *methods?*
7. Is each *table/figure* intelligible by itself, concise, and necessary? Are the legends understandable? Is the information in the text and *tables/figures* non-repetitious?
8. Are the *implications/applications/recommendations* logical, well-considered, and pertinent, yet far-sighted?
9. Are the *references* appropriate, current, and sufficient in number and scope?
10. Considering each of the *above sections,* is each presented concisely? Is the information relevant and non-repetitious?

The following questions may guide you when reviewing manuscripts presenting original research. Your comments will be most useful to the author if they are constructive and informative.

1. Is the *article* of importance to the field of dietetics? Is that import clearly conveyed in the article?
2. Is the *title* clear and informative? Does it convey the major findings of the research?
3. Is the *abstract* intelligible by itself' Does it summarize the purpose, methods, sample, results, and conclusions of the article?
4. Does the *introduction* state the intention of the article?
5. Are the *materials and methods* straightforward, well-conceived, and scientifically accurate? Is the research design appropriate to test the hypothesis? Is the sample selection appropriate? Is the sample size sufficient? Are suitable statistical tests applied?
6. Are the *results* clear and appropriately analyzed? Do the *results* follow the same order presented under *methods?*
7. Is each *table/figure* intelligible by itself, concise, and necessary to the article? Are the legends understandable? Is the information in the text and *tables/figures* non-repetitious?
8. Is the *discussion* relevant to the findings? Are the results interpreted appropriately and compared with other published data of a similar nature?
9. Are the *implications/applications/recommendations* logical, well-considered, pertinent yet far-sighted?
10. Are the *references* appropriate, current, and sufficient in number and scope?
11. Considering each of the *above sections,* is each presented concisely? Is the information relevant and nonrepetitious?

FIGURE 30.3 Guidelines for Manuscript Review for the *Journal of the American Dietetic Association.* Reprinted with permission from Elaine R. Monsen, author.

lenged by some as an area "ripe for systematic research and review" (46). In a recent study, reviewer performance was evaluated using a preconceived manuscript into which purposeful errors were placed; the study showed that reviewers failed to identify two-thirds of the major errors (47). An International Congress on Peer Review in Biomedical Publications, sponsored by the American Medical Association, emphasized responsibility as it applies to authors and editors and the improvement of quality control over the entire peer review process, the intent being to improve the process (48).

Electronic publication does allow a path for the peer review process to continue. However, concern has been expressed that immediate unreviewed publication, even if only temporary while the peer review process is ongoing, "is risky and might well fill the clinical data bases with misleading and inadequately evaluated information." Furthermore, "the few weeks saved between acceptance and print would not justify the confusion and misunderstanding that would attend the immediate electronic posting and subsequent publicizing of clinical studies" (49).

THE READER'S PERSPECTIVE

People read reports of research in the literature to keep abreast of current findings in their profession and areas of specialty. In 1981 more than 20,000 different biomedical journals were published, and it was projected that the biomedical literature would double every 10 years to 15 years and increase 10-fold every 35 years to 50 years. The clinician, who has limited time available for reading, was estimated to need to read 200 articles and 70 editorials per month to keep up with the 10 leading journals in internal medicine (50). A more current estimate of more than 100,000 bioscience journals in the world that cover a broad range of bioscience subjects shows that it is no longer possible to keep up to date (49).

The reader, as student and critic, looks for scholarly articles that contribute to the scientific knowledge base, are clearly communicated, can be applied, and promote individual professional development. University-gained knowledge is significantly outdated after a few years; professionals must review and update their knowledge regularly through journal publications.

Students generally receive little exposure to any organized method for reading articles in the literature. Critical evaluation of journal articles, however, can be taught to medical students by presenting methodological criteria

for determining the validity and usefulness of published data. The critical evaluation of medical literature can be incorporated into a course in biostatistics and clinical epidemiology in the second year of medical school (51). A 1990 survey of dietitians identified scientific journals as one of the most valuable resources for keeping current with the professional literature (52). Several of the respondents emphasized the need for a basic understanding of statistics to interpret adequately the information presented in scientific journals. Educators in dietetics are currently incorporating critical thinking into the dietetic internship experiences at the undergraduate level. Likewise, dietetics students are encouraged to incorporate a course in statistics in their undergraduate studies. The reader who is trained to be more critical and skeptical of the printed word recognizes the limitations of individual papers, as well as the limitations of the scientific method as applied to a given discipline (45).

Strategies mentioned for keeping current with the literature included a journal club at work, allowing professional colleagues and students to share research articles. Another strategy was to read only articles specific to one's interest or area of expertise.

The following steps serve as a guide to readers for the critical selection of articles from the printed literature.

- Look at the title, and determine whether the article is of interest or use to you. If not, go on to the next article.
- Review the list of authors and/or the institution where the research was completed. If the authors are well-known authorities in the subject area and have a good track record of careful and thoughtful work, read on.
- Determine the intent of the article as a Perspectives in Practice piece, a review article, an original research article, or a research or professional brief. If it tweaks your interest and meets your needs, read on.
- For a Perspectives in Practice piece, review article, or original research article, read the abstract. Then decide whether the brief descriptions of the purpose, methods, and sample seem reasonable and the results and conclusions seem valid and useful. If further reading would be of value to you, read on.
- For a Perspectives in Practice or review article, read the text and check it for clarity. Check also the references for appropriateness and sufficiency in number and scope.
- For a research article, read the materials and methods section, and critically review it for scientific ac-

curacy, research design, sample selection, and suitability of applied statistical tests.

- For a research article, read the results and discussion sections, and critically review them for clarity and appropriateness in interpretation. Check the references for appropriate incorporation into the discussion.
- For all types of articles, read the sections on conclusions, implications, and recommendations, and critically review them for relevant application into practice.

At present, most biomedical journals have a Web site from which readers can obtain limited parts of the printed journal's content shortly before, or on the date of, publication. Full-text versions, however, generally require a subscription. PubMed and ERA do not require a subscription (2). Some on-line journals allow readers to review the archives of all papers published by the journal on a particular topic and inform the journal of select topics about which they want to be kept routinely updated. Readers are then alerted by the on-line journal when articles are published that match their interests; a significant time-saving service. In its first 16 months on-line, this feature attracted 20,000 subscribers to the *British Medical Journal*. Delamothe suggests that on-line Letters to the Editor and the on-line publication of full articles with abridged versions in the paper journal should be pursued as a dual publishing strategy. Authors will automatically receive editorial responses to their work by e-mail (3). The future of on-line articles will also include the publication of abridged forms as hyPer papers (electronic texts with "clickable" [hyperlinked] phrases that take the reader to areas of interest within the paper) (3). This approach is likely to be instituted for all original papers in the *British Medical Journal*.

The Internet may soon make information readily available worldwide. For the foreseeable future, however, clinicians in developing areas of the world will continue to rely on printed media. Professional development infrastructures in developing countries should expand to include the delivery of Internet resources to support medical education and clinical practice decisions (53).

FUTURE OPPORTUNITIES

Dietitians have the opportunity to be viewed as the expert resources for nutrition knowledge and the primary communicators of that knowledge to their scientific and ad-

ministrative colleagues, as well as the lay public. The tools needed to fulfill these challenging roles lie in the development of a critical readership, a responsible authorship, and an invested group of peer reviewers. Critical readers will become critical reviewers of noteworthy information. Responsible authors will continue to be stimulated to research worthwhile ideas and effectively communicate the findings. Peer reviewers, through their efforts and expertise, guarantee high-quality, valid published knowledge. Journals are, and will continue to be, the most current source of nutrition knowledge; therefore, personal commitment to develop and maintain skills in all aspects of the periodical arena is necessary for dietitians to become the readers, writers, and reviewers that they are called on to be.

REFERENCES

1. McConnell J, Horton R. Lancet electronic research archive in international health and eprint server. *Lancet.* 1999;354:2.
2. Anonymous. Biomedical research publishing: radical changes ahead. *Bull World Health Organ.* 1999;77(7):610.
3. Delamothe T, Smith R. The joy of being electronic. The BMJ's website is mushrooming [editorial]. *BMJ.* 1999;319:465.
4. Bennett S. Author's rights. *J Electronic Publishing* [serial online]. 1999;5(2). Available at: http://www.press.umich.edu/jep/05-02/bennett.html. Accessed January 21, 2003.
5. Schiedermayer DL, Siegler M. Believing what you read. Responsibilities of medical authors and editors. *Arch Intern Med.* 1936;146:2043.
6. Babbage C. *Reflections on the Decline of Science in England and on Some of Its Causes.* London, England: Gregg International; 1969.
7. Bailar JC, Mosteller E. Guidelines for statistical reporting in articles for medical journals. *Ann Intern Med.* 1988;108:266.
8. Gardner MJ, Machin D, Cambefl MJ. Use of checklists in assessing the statistical content of medical studies. *BMJ.* 1986;292:810–812.
9. International Committee of Medical Journal Editors. Uniform requirement for manuscripts submitted to biomedical journals (a.k.a. "Vancouver Style"). *Ann Intern Med.* 1997;126:36.
10. International Committee of Medical Journal Editors. Uniform requirements for manuscripts submitted to biomedical journals (updated October 2001). Available at: http://www.icmje.org. Accessed February 24, 2003.
11. Monsen ER. The Journal adopts SI units for clinical laboratory values. *J Am Diet Assoc.* 1987;87:356.

12. Now read this: the SI units are here [editorial]. *JAMA*. I 986;255:2329.

13. Chernoff R, ed. *Communicating as Professionals*. 2nd ed. Chicago, Ill: The American Dietetic Association; 1994.

14. Day RA. *How to Write and Publish a Scientific Paper*. 4th ed. Phoenix, Ariz: Oryx Press; 1994.

15. Huth EJ. *How to Write and Publish Papers in the Medical Sciences*. 2nd ed. Baltimore, Md: Williams and Wilkins; 1990.

16. Huth EJ. *Scientific Style and Format: The CBE Manual for Authors, Editors, and Publishers*. 6th ed. New York, NY: Cambridge University Press; 1994.

17. Journal of the American Dietetic Association Guidelines for authors. *J Am Diet Assoc*. 2002;102:26. Available at: http://www.eatright.org/journal.

18. Lock S. *A Difficult Balance: Editorial Peer Review in Medicine*. Philadelphia, Pa: SI Press; 1985.

19. Samet JM. Dear author—advice from a retiring editor. *Am J Epidemiol*. 1999;150:433.

20. Huth El. Irresponsible authorship and wasteful publication. *Ann Intern Med*. 1986:104:257.

21. Marusic A, Marusic M. Authorship criteria and academic reward. *Lancet*. 1999;353:1713.

22. Horton R. A fair reward. *Lancet*. 1998;352:892.

23. Gaeta TJ. Authorship: "law" and order. *Acad Emerg Med*. 1999;6:297.

24. Rennie D, Yank V, Emanuel L. When authorship fails: a proposal to make contributors accountable. *JAMA*. 1997;278(7):579.

25. Ahmed SM, Maurana CA, Engle JA, Uddin DE, Glaus KD. A method for assigning authorship in multiauthored publications. *Tam Med*. 1997;29:42.

26. Baughman AL. Invited commentary: what can we infer from author order in epidemiology? *Am J Epidemiol*. 1999;150(6):663.

27. Baum GL. MEDLINE-induced blindness. *Chest*. 1999;115(5):1224.

28. Medical/Health Sciences Libraries on the Web. Available at: http://www.lib.uiowa.edu/hardin-www/hslibs.html. Accessed January 21, 2003.

29. PubMed. Available at: http://www.ncbi.nlm.nih.gov/PubMed/. Accessed January 21, 2003.

30. National Network of Libraries of Medicine. Available at: http://www.nnlm.nlm.nih.gov. Accessed January 21, 2003.

31. E-BIOMED: A Proposal for Electronic Publications in the Biomedical Sciences. Available at: http://www.nih.gov/welcome/director/pubmedcentral/ebiomedarch.htm. Accessed January 21, 2003.

32. Marshall E. NIH's online publishing venture ready for launch. *Science*. 1999;285:1466.

33. ERA International Health Guidelines for Authors and Readers. Available at: http://www.thelancet.com/era/guidelines. Accessed January 21, 2003.

34. American Psychological Association. Electronic references. Available at: http://www.apastyle.org/elecref.html. Accessed January 21, 2003.

35. Emory University Health Sciences Center Library. A field guide to sources on, about, and on the internet: citation formats. Available at: http://www.emory.edu/WHSCL/citation.formats.html. Accessed January 21, 2003.

36. Purdue University Online Writing Lab. On-line resources for documenting electronic sources. Available at: http://owl.english.purdue.edu/handouts/research/r_docelectric.html. Accessed January 21, 2003

37. Electronic Reference Shelf. Available at: http://www.np.edu.sg/library/ref.htm. Accessed January 21, 2003.

38. Schenk MP, Manning RJ, Paalman MH. Going digital: Image preparation for biomedical publishing. *Anat Rec*. 1999;257:128.

39. Bailey CW Jr. 5.1 Legal issues: intellectual property rights. In: *Scholarly Electronic Publishing Bibliography*. Houston, Tex: University of Houston Libraries; 1996–2001. Available at: http://info.lib.uh.edu/sepb/1copyr.htm. Accessed January 21, 2003.

40. Rozenberg P. Developing a Standard for Legal Citation of Electronic Information. Available at: http://www.murdoch.edu.au/elaw/issues/v4n4/rozen44.html. Accessed January 21, 2003.

41. EFF "Intellectual Property Online: Patent, Trademark, Copyright" Archive. Available at: http://wwww.eff.org/pub/Intellectual_property/#files. Accessed January 21, 2003.

42. The Center for Advanced Research and Study on Intellectual Property (CASRIP) of the University of Washington School of Law. Available at: http://www.law.washington.edu/casrip/. Accessed January 21, 2003.

43. US Copyright Office, The Library of Congress. Available at: http://lcweb.loc.gov/copyright. Accessed January 21, 2003.

44. Soffer A. Proponent view. *Chest*. 1987;91:255.

45. Robin ED, Burke CM. Peer review in medical journals. *Chest*. 1987;91:252.

46. Jones R. Publish or perish. The debate from a global perspective [news]. *Aust Fam Physician*. 1999;28(5):425.

47. Baxt WG, Waeckerle JF, Berlin JA, Callaham ML. Who reviews the reviewers? Feasibility of using a fictitious manuscript to evaluate peer reviewer performance. *Ann Emerg Med*. 1998;32(3):310.

48. Rennie D. Guarding the guardians: a conference on editorial peer review. *JAMA*. 1986;256:2391.

49. Relman AS. The NIH "E-Biomed" proposal—a potential threat to the evaluation and orderly dissemination of new clinical studies. *N Engl J Med*. 1999;340(23):1828–1829.

50. Sackett DL, Haynes RB, Tugwell P. *Clinical Epidemiology: A Basic Science for Clinical Medicine*. Boston, Mass: Little Brown and Co; 1985.

51. Radack KL, Valanis B. Teaching critical appraisal and application of medical literature to clinical problem-solving. *J Med Educ.* 1986;61:329.

52. Wellman NS. The well-read dietitian [President's Page]. *J Am Diet Assoc.* 1990;90:996.

53. Haddad H, MacLeod S. Access to medical and health information in the developing world: an essential tool for change in medical education. *Can Med Assoc J.* 1999;160:63.

Coda

—ᴍ—

Applications of Research to Practice

Research advances practice and allows effective decision making. In turn, questions arising from practice provide a practical focus for research. Quality of care may be improved and treatment modalities evaluated. Research may be extended and augmented through collaborative projects. The many techniques and guidelines presented in this book can lead individuals toward successful research that will pleasurably enhance their profession and practice.

Research opportunities exist in every facet of professional life. The following list can serve as a springboard to research projects that propel science forward and fascinate active investigators:

- Translate good science to good client care, and evaluate the devised protocol.
- Devise dietary intake methods for enhanced precision and validation through biochemical measurement (biological markers).
- Design and evaluate treatment modalities and dietary interventions appropriate to clinical practice (for example, in treating infants and children with HIV infection and cancer, elderly people in ambulatory care settings, and adolescents with eating disorders; or in determining the effects of dietary supplementation).
- Examine relevant gene-diet interactions in disease etiology and treatment.
- Conduct food composition research to supply data currently missing from existing databases (for example, data on trace minerals, engineered foods, therapeutically designed foods, culturally specific foods, individual fiber categories, phytochemicals, and food contaminants).
- Examine the roles and effects of specific food components and nutrients in delaying the onset of cardiovascular disease, in lowering the risk of cancer, or in maintaining gut function through nutrition support.
- Evaluate the safety and suitability of medical foods.
- Assess the bioavailability of nutrients, and estimate the impact on specific populations.
- Estimate the prevalence and interrelationships of health and nutrition characteristics through integration of population surveys and record-based surveillance.
- Conduct sensory evaluation research to encompass intake, nutrition status, attitudes, and psychosocial information; assess the development, maintenance, and modification of sensory preferences.
- Examine gustatory, olfactory, texture, and other complex real food stimuli in controlled laboratory settings, as well as in realistic eating situations.
- In foodservice research, apply marketing techniques, devise effective staff training and retention techniques, incorporate robots, and address solid waste management.

- Examine service quality, evaluate decision support systems, and enhance computer applications, including the use of artificial intelligence techniques.
- Document cost-effectiveness and perform cost-benefit analyses of nutrition and dietetics services, including the extent to which illness is prevented, the severity of illness is decreased, the duration of illness is curtailed, and the patient's rehabilitation is facilitated and quality of life is improved.
- Substantiate cost savings from nutrition and dietetics intervention (for example, make recommendations for using less costly products that have similar value in the healing process, improving lifestyle through patient education, establishing the number of visits appropriate for each diagnostic group, and evaluating the cost-effectiveness of alternative foodservice production systems).
- Improve methods to manage confounding variables in attributing improved health status to nutrition care.

- Conduct marketing research to enhance one's competitive position, evaluate audience readiness for new products and services, and evaluate available avenues for the promotion of services and products.
- In dietetics education research, devise cost-effective curricula, identify factors that enhance the educational process, determine what motivates an individual's career choice, and devise and evaluate continuing education opportunities.
- Using meta-analysis research, address proposed hypotheses, observe the magnitude of an intervention, and determine the factors that influence an intervention.

A productive research environment encourages everyone to investigate, compare, document, validate, evaluate, refine, analyze, and design—that is, to study.

ERM, Editor

31

Bridging Research to Practice

Judith A. Gilbride, Ph.D., R.D., F.A.D.A., and Margaret D. Simko, Ph.D., R.D., F.A.D.A.

To integrate research into practice, resources must be skillfully mobilized and managed. The profession of dietetics needs a much broader practical research base. This chapter—and indeed, this book—has been designed to provide background and technical information that will further this effort. It is the authors' hope that practitioners will be motivated and inspired to approach research questions in practice with renewed vigor and self-confidence and thus contribute to a progressive and productive future.

The discovery of new knowledge is the foundation and framework of the dietetics profession (1–3). Research helps dietitians develop professionally and allows them to integrate findings into their work. Nutrition professionals who work with the public must keep up to date on nutrition science and be able to interpret scientific research accurately and thoroughly and correct misinformation (4). In all practice settings, the generation of scientific data keeps practitioners accurate and gives credibility to what they say (3,5).

Research helps practitioners solve problems they face every day. It is useful in monitoring ongoing activities in all areas of dietetics and provides feedback that serves as the basis for changing procedures to improve the general health of clients. Well-designed studies can also provide data to improve food and nutrition services, ensure quality management, determine effectiveness of medical nutrition therapy, and lower health care costs. Monsen stated that "stronger links must be built between research and practice to strengthen our profession be-cause research is driven by practice, and practice is supported by research" (6).

Although "most problems in practice can be addressed through research," job demands, limited resources, and time constraints may hamper investigators' efforts to solve practice problems (7). Practitioners are often so busy concentrating on meeting their routine responsibilities that they have little time to begin a research project or become involved in an ongoing study. Sometimes practitioners, in their eagerness to solve clinical problems, attempt to incorporate findings that have not been studied and tested adequately (5). Collaborating with dietitians in academic settings and finding research mentors have been identified as helpful ways clinical dietitians can increase their participation in research (7).

INTEGRATION OF RESEARCH INTO DIETETICS

Dietetics research, based on an understanding of food composition, nutrition, metabolism, and management principles, is used to demonstrate the application of knowledge in the field to help people choose a healthy diet and lifestyle. The American Dietetic Association (ADA) set a goal in 1993 to increase member involvement in dietetics research in four practice arenas: disease prevention and health promotion, acute and long-term care, foodservice, and consumer education (8). Research topics and priorities were established by the ADA

Research Agenda and by a National Academy of Science report (9). New practice initiatives and publications have recognized the importance of supporting the research efforts of dietetics professionals (10–13). In addition, the ADA has been developing practice guidelines that can apply to both research and practice definition (7).

All dietitians are encouraged to incorporate research into their professional responsibilities. Indeed, one of the six tenets of professional practice in dietetics is the application of research. The ADA Quality Management and Research Team has identified several activities in which practitioners can become involved in research:

- Review of original and current research related to one's specific area of practice.
- Documentation of service outcomes compared with goals and expectations.
- Development of research protocols for students.
- Publication of research findings and provision of services.
- Participation in data collection.
- Reporting of results to colleagues on the team (14).

The revised ADA Standards of Education supports the development of research skills by dietetics students, including a basic knowledge of research methods, needs assessment, and outcomes research, as well as an in-depth knowledge of the scientific method and quality improvement methods (15). Educators have increased the research content in dietetics curriculums and have initiated novel approaches to applied research skills (16–18). The criteria for evaluating dietetics education programs rely on the ability of graduates to interpret current research and basic statistics.

According to Parks et al, "we need new knowledge, scholarship, and research to stay ahead of the trends shaping our customers' actions and the science upon which the profession has been built" (19[p1159]). They consider scholarship a way of life for today's professionals, thus encouraging the creation of new knowledge and building the foundation for future dietetics practice. Besides conducting original research, we are challenged to use the scientific method in everyday practice, keep up to date on the scientific literature, formulate problems for quality improvement, devise protocols to test interventions, evaluate and validate findings, and give presentations on the latest research (19).

In the spring of 2001, the ADA House of Delegates adopted a motion to strengthen members' abilities to understand and interpret research and to increase research opportunities in all practice settings. The group endorsed practice-based research to measure outcomes that may affect reimbursement and future legislation. Delegates supported broader dissemination and implementation of research findings to add value for clients of dietetics professionals and to enhance overall quality of care.

Practice-based studies can document dietetics and assess the effectiveness of nutrition procedures and treatment (20–25). Once effectiveness is determined, it is possible to evaluate the costs of intervention procedures and measure them against the efficacy of outcomes. Outcome evaluation will keep dietetics competitive as a profession (26–28). The need for more nutrition science has also been addressed by the National Institutes of Health through increased support of randomized controlled nutrition trials, often with required input from dietetics practitioners. In this era of shrinking financial resources in health care, the evaluation of the provision of dietetics care and intervention can demonstrate the value of nutrition services as they compete for limited funds (29).

APPLICATION OF RESEARCH TO PRACTICE

Research encompasses facts that are not ends in themselves but merely components of a unified effort "to control and dictate the acquisition of data" and "extract meaningfulness from them" (30). After all, "unless there is a discovery of the meaningfulness of the data, there is no research" (30[p9]). Research studies do not always have immediate, practical application but rather build on what was learned in previous studies. The application of sound research principles can confirm impressions or observations about patient care. Research is a systematic process of deductive-inductive reasoning to provide answers to questions and to develop theories (31). Such answers may be abstract and general in qualitative studies; they may be concrete and specific in clinical trials. In both descriptive and analytic research, the investigator uncovers facts and then formulates a generalization based on the exploration, description, and explanation of those facts (31).

Linking Research and Practice

The application of research techniques to practice focuses on everyday operations and problem solving (32,33). Data collection and its interpretation can provide insight and direction for doing collaborative projects with other

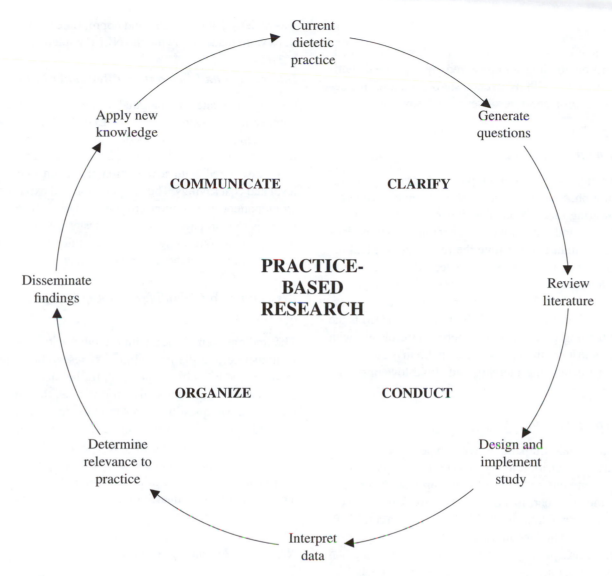

FIGURE 31.1 Cycle of Research in Dietetic Practice. Model adapted from Leedy PD (30); Rinke WJ, Berry MW (32); Eck LH et al (33).

colleagues and health care professionals (34). Figure 31.1 demonstrates the interactive relationship between practice and research. The cycle begins with questions generated by practice; a workable research question is clarified through an extensive literature search, and the research methods are refined. The design and implementation of the research project seeks to answer unresolved problems in practice. Conducting the project produces new facts that necessitate careful analysis. However, integrating that new information into practice requires determining its practical relevance to current procedures. The final steps are disseminating findings to colleagues and other practitioners and applying the new knowledge to improve

practice. Thus, the cycle is completed and starts again as other practice questions are raised and solutions to new, perplexing problems are sought.

Illustration of the Cycle of Research in Practice

A nutrition intervention study can illustrate the cycle of research. The following discussion illustrates these interactions through the study entitled, "Medical Nutrition Therapy Lowers Serum Cholesterol and Saves Medication Costs in Men with Hypercholesterolemia" (35).

The Problem

The problem in the study is stated as follows: Does medical nutrition therapy administered by registered dietitians for patients with hypercholesterolemia lead to a decrease in serum cholesterol level and save medication costs?

Clarifying the Question

The investigators developed a protocol in the dietary intervention phase of a clinical trial using an experimental lipid-lowering medication. The dietary protocol required at least two (and a maximum of four) intervention visits with the dietitian to determine the following: (1) Did the medical nutrition therapy sessions lead to a reduction in serum cholesterol level and low-density lipoprotein cholesterol (LDL-C)? (2) How many medical nutrition therapy sessions improved the clinical outcome? and (3) Is the cost of treating patients with hypercholesterolemia with medical nutrition therapy from a dietitian significantly less than treating the patients with lipid-lowering drug therapy?

Conducting the Study

Ninety-five male outpatients with hypercholesterolemia took part in a nutrition intervention program prior to beginning treatment with a lipid-lowering medication. The participants took part in a 6-week to 8-week program using the National Cholesterol Education Program (NCEP) Step I diet. Patients' records were reviewed retrospectively to determine plasma lipid levels at the beginning and end of the program, as well as the number and length of sessions with a dietitian. Participants returned at weeks 6, 7, and 8 for blood lipid evaluations to qualify for the lipid-lowering drug therapy using NCEP criteria. Initial and final evaluations for total cholesterol, LDL-C, high-density lipoprotein cholesterol (HDL-C), triglycerides, and weight were recorded. Height, number of dietitian visits, and estimated dietitian intervention time (in minutes) were also noted. Costs for the intervention and medication costs were also calculated and compared. Later, a sensitivity analysis was done to calculate cost-effectiveness ratios for medical nutrition therapy that varied for differing dietitian consultation charges.

Intervention

The medical nutrition therapy protocol was administered by the dietitian in at least two 60-minute and two 30-minute sessions in some instances. A 4-day food record

was reviewed at each visit, and appropriate recommendations were made following the NCEP guidelines.

Interpreting and Determining Relevance to Practice

Findings indicated a marginal difference between the number of visits and change in LDL-C. By estimating cost savings by avoiding medications, it was concluded that three or four sessions with a dietitian over 7 weeks were associated with a reduction in serum cholesterol level and cost savings. The continuation and expansion of an outpatient intervention program is indicated by these findings to help patients lower cholesterol levels. A case for sufficient counseling sessions by a dietitian could be supported by data generated by this study.

Dissemination of Findings and Application to Practice

The findings were shared with the intervention team and administrators in the lipid clinic. As research results are incorporated into clinical practice, further questions arise that warrant additional study. In this case, the investigators raised two questions: (1) Are individuals who do not respond to medical nutrition therapy in need of more intense intervention, or are they resistant to diet? and (2) What are the optimal number and frequency of intervention visits by dietitians to maintain normal lipid levels? Thus, new research questions are devised, and the practice-research-practice cycle continues.

Related or Follow-up Studies

A cost-effectiveness analysis was piloted with a subset of patients in a lipid intervention study comparing diet alone with diet and medication for treating patients with hypercholesterolemia (36). The researchers made several recommendations for a cost-effectiveness analysis in a clinical setting, including a well-controlled pilot study and detailed documentation for use in a prospective economic analysis. Monitors to measure compliance with both diet and drug regimens were also encouraged. Follow-up studies (37,38) were conducted to examine the long-term outcomes for these patient populations.

Porter and Matel recommend that practice management decisions be made only with sufficient evidence (39). Using an evidence-based approach, the current "best evidence" should be weighed in a conscientious, judicious, and explicit manner. The recommendations rely on assessing the integrity, accuracy, and relevance of studies in the literature; balancing the risks and benefits for the patient or client; and judging whether the evidence is substantial enough to support decision making. Evidence-based decisions are made by considering the available resources; patient or client needs and preferences; current best evidence in the scientific literature and practice arena; and the practitioner's knowledge, skills, and experience. The authors encourage a critical appraisal and thoughtful application of the best evidence available to dietetics practice and suggest ways to examine the strength of evidence—for example, What is the weight of evidence that developing a medical nutrition therapy protocol for hypertensive older adults will have positive outcomes? What are the outcomes measures and the limits of the data and conclusions in similar studies?

Evidence-based medicine and evidence-based practice are particularly important to today's dietitians and require both clinical judgment and valid research to guide decisions on patient care. Evidence-based medicine encourages the production of valid summaries of the best available evidence on clinical topics (40) that are systematically evaluated according to uniform scientific criteria. (See Chapter 12 for further definitions and guidelines.)

READING RESEARCH LITERATURE

As dietitians read research studies in the literature, they should look for ways to integrate findings into practice and carefully weigh the scientific evidence (41). When reading and examining reports, questions should come to mind—for example, Are there practical applications for these investigative findings? What is the impact of this study on patients or the setting? Can I apply this information to my setting?

Knowledge of research methods is required to understand articles in the scientific literature (42). Critical analysis is useful when reading investigative reports to determine whether the purpose and need of the study are supported, the methods are appropriate, the conclusions indicate accurate interpretation of the data, and the references are well chosen and up to date. Some published research studies may contain limitations or gaps in knowledge. Practitioners should evaluate the quality of each report and determine whether the study has weaknesses that limit its application to a particular health care setting. After a literature search from a myriad of information sources, a clear clinical question should be devised that includes the patient or problem; the intervention (cause, prognostic factors, and treatment); the compari-

son intervention, if appropriate; and the outcomes to be measured (40).

EXAMPLE. A comparison study was designed to test a quantitative food frequency method of obtaining dietary intakes by telephone and to contrast the telephone method with face-to-face interviews. Establishing a method for assessing diets by telephone would save time and money and allow better access to geographically dispersed populations. Three hundred and twenty participants completed the randomly assigned sequence of 2 interviews within 4 months to 6 months. The participants were able to use photographs for estimating amounts in both interviews. The paired t test was used to compare mean daily intakes of the two methods and revealed somewhat higher means of energy and nutrient content on the first interview, irrespective of the method.

Based on these findings, the estimation of dietary intakes from telephone interviews can be completed satisfactorily using a 115-item survey and trained interviewers. The telephone method for assessing usual intake is conducive to increasing sample size in geographically dispersed areas. Regardless of the method used, the first interview generally produced more information than the second. Further exploration of interview methods and timing could provide the practitioner with greater confidence in estimating dietary intakes through telephone interviews (43).

EXAMPLE. A descriptive survey was conducted to identify the variables associated with high satisfaction of food and foodservice in a continuing-care hospital. Data were collected from 65 patients using an 8-item questionnaire measuring various dimensions of satisfaction. Findings indicated "satisfaction with presentation of the meal" as the best overall predictor of satisfaction. The taste of food and appropriate coldness of cold foods indicated satisfaction more than 80 percent of the time. As part of a quality assurance system, dietitians and foodservice managers should focus on taste and temperature characteristics of meals and how food is presented, rather than patient-specific variables, to maximize patient satisfaction with hospital food (44).

Based on these findings, food satisfaction surveys provide baseline data for future study. Well-constructed surveys can be used to improve foodservice and help optimize the quality of life for people in continuing-care settings. Two recent surveys have been conducted to examine foodservice practices perceived by foodservice directors—one on benchmarking (45) and another on current and future practices in hospital foodservice (46).

SOME USES OF RESEARCH IN THE PRACTICE SETTING

Research to Assess and Analyze a Setting

To develop a framework for investigating nutrition intervention, grounded research// theory—an inductive approach to understanding a phenomenon built on actual data—can be employed to collect data about the patient population, the institution, and the community. This information is vital in planning and testing the most efficient and effective delivery of nutrition services. Questions such as the following can be asked: What is the population serviced by this institution or agency (numbers, age, gender, economic status)? What are the nutrition needs of this population (diagnosis, health status, mobility)? What resources are available to help deliver nutrition services (infrastructure, time, funds, personnel, other health care professionals)?

An instrument can be developed to collect pertinent information, or a model may be found in the literature and adapted to a specific setting. This kind of investigation can precede a research design and assists in formulating appropriate, practical research questions—for example, How are resources organized to meet the needs of the population? Starting with a needs assessment can be very useful, because the problem selected for study depends on the needs in the practice setting, as well as funding sources, constraints of time and personnel, and answers to the question, Will method X or method Y be more effective in solving problems relating to this population?

In the past 2 decades we have experienced an increase in randomized clinical trials that include nutrition. Research sponsored by the National Institutes of Health and pharmaceutical companies has given new responsibilities to dietitians as study managers and coordinators (47), as investigators in clinical research centers (48), and as employees in independent research organizations (49). For dietitians who are entering these positions or embark-

ing on research in clinical settings, Castro and Walsh emphasize in-depth analysis of published research data to determine clinical relevance before changing treatment protocols (11). Data should be carefully scrutinized to determine the validity of the study, the controls, and the relevance to clinical and patient outcomes.

Outcomes research has been touted by the medical and dietetics professions in recent years to have a positive effect on delivering patient care, economic factors, and controlling clinical and functional outcomes in intervention trials. Outcomes research is the rigorous determination of what works and what does not work (21). Its purpose is to help patients, providers, payers, and administrators determine appropriate choices regarding medical treatment options and health care policy. Enthusiastically adopted by the dietetics community, the application of outcomes research has stimulated a new way to show effectiveness of medical nutrition therapy. Positive benefits have been presented at ADA meetings and published in the *Journal of the American Dietetic Association*.

Research to Measure Practice

Documentation and measurement of practice standards can provide evidence of the effectiveness of nutrition care being delivered. Practice guidelines are intended to help dietitians make decisions on how various nutrition-related conditions are most effectively prevented and treated (50). If effectiveness is not demonstrated, the findings can provide a framework for further study that can change practice and produce more positive outcomes.

EXAMPLE. A study was conducted to examine the effectiveness of a food safety curriculum with 227 children in 14 rural low-income counties in southern Illinois. Children aged 8 years to 12 years were recruited to participate in a 1-week Youth Cooking School to learn healthy eating behaviors and safe food handling. A pretest measured baseline data and food behaviors. A posttest and 3-month follow-up test assessed knowledge gained and self-reported behavior changes. After the nutrition education, which combined a lecture and daily hands-on activities, more children reported following safe food practices, employing food preparation skills, and selecting foods according to the Food Guide Pyramid. The children continued to report changes after 3 months (12).

EXAMPLE. Enrichment status and nutrient analysis of 368 gluten-free cereal products were assessed to determine whether these foods contain amounts of thiamin, riboflavin, and niacin similar to the amounts in the enriched wheat products that they replace in a diet. Only 35 of the gluten-free products were enriched. Nutrient analysis revealed that a gluten-free diet designed for individuals with celiac disease may be deficient in one or more of the nutrients generally present in enriched grains and cereals. Dietitians are encouraged to carefully evaluate the dietary intake of these vitamins in persons following a gluten-free diet (51).

EXAMPLE. Intense dietary counseling was employed to lower LDL-C in 59 men with coronary artery bypass grafts in the recruitment phase of a 5-year clinical trial. During the first visit, 24-hour dietary recalls were obtained and analyzed for total energy; total, saturated, monounsaturated, and polyunsaturated fat; and dietary cholesterol. Participants were instructed on the Step I diet, and additional counseling was provided monthly during the second and third visits. Another dietary recall and a biochemical analysis were done on the third visit. The diet intakes were improved to adhere more closely with the NCEP Step II diet, and participants decreased their total cholesterol and LDL-C levels after intervention (52).

Research to Change Practice

Research is useful to monitor activities or procedures, solve problems, and change practice by finding a better way to deliver nutrition services.

EXAMPLE. A patient survey was administered to assess the appropriateness of postoperative diets for 31 short-stay surgery patients. Variable postoperative symptoms, food tolerances, and food preferences suggested the inappropriateness of regular meals for the first meal after surgery. The study found that a first meal consisting of a variety of simple solid and fluid foods, which can be tailored to a patient's needs before consumption, reduces food waste and increases meal acceptance with fewer requests for alternative foods. A new postoperative diet protocol was developed and is in continued use. This study, which involved a change in practice by the dietary department, demonstrated a positive patient outcome, as well as a cost savings (53).

EXAMPLE. An outcomes study assessed the acceptance and effectiveness of Nutrition Practice Guidelines for insulin-dependent diabetes mellitus when used by dietitians in a variety of practice settings. Participating dietitians from across the United States were randomly assigned to provide care to a total of 54 patients, either by traditional methods or the new practice guidelines over 3 months. Dietitians using practice guidelines spent 63 percent more time with patients and were more likely to assess and review results with them than dietitians providing traditional care. Glycosylated hemoglobin levels improved in 88 percent of patients utilizing the new guidelines, compared with 53 percent of patients getting traditional care. Dietitians were positive in adopting the new guidelines because of improved dietary adherence and self-management by patients (54).

EXAMPLE. A descriptive study was conducted to evaluate the quality of nutrition care provided to patients with traumatic injuries at risk for multiple organ dysfunction syndrome. The medical files of 8 critically ill patients were reviewed for the first 15 days of hospitalization. Despite dietitians recommending feedings consistent with estimated energy needs, patients were fed, on average, 4 of the first 15 days. The majority of the time, patients were either underfed or not fed at all; overfeeding occurred on only a few days. It was concluded that overfeeding and underfeeding may be detrimental to the patients' conditions and that overall nutrition care had identifiable weaknesses. Further exploration is needed to identify ways to improve efficiency of care and measure patient outcomes, staff practices, and costs (55).

Research to Document Cost Outcomes

Dietetics professionals are producing more and more research studies and projects that exemplify the documentation of patient and cost outcomes with nutrition therapy intervention.

EXAMPLE. A cost-effectiveness analysis was conducted for 66 patients undergoing bowel resections who were fitted with a jejunal feeding tube during surgery. The treated patients were tube fed within 12 hours after surgery, whereas 129 control patients received usual care. Successful treatment was defined as a patient discharged from the hospital without a complicating infection. Patients with tube placements received immediate nutrition assessments and monitoring by a dietitian as part of the early feeding protocol, whereas patients in the control group received a dietitian's visit only upon request by a physician.

Results showed a 7.5 percent reduction in nosocomial bacteremia in the treatment group compared with the control group. In addition, a reduction in variable costs of $1,531 per successful treatment patient and $4,450 total cost savings per treatment group success were demonstrated. In this study, changes in critical pathways for patients undergoing bowel resection, through the implementation of early postoperative enteral feeding, have decreased initial patient days without feeding and have shortened hospitals stays, thus reducing costs (56).

EXAMPLE. An investigation was done to determine whether, within a low-income population serviced by the Special Supplemental Nutrition Program for Women, Infants, and Children (WIC), breast-feeding was associated with a reduction in Medicaid expenses during the first 6 months of life. The study participants included 470 formula-fed infants and 406 exclusively breast-fed infants who were tracked prospectively for 6 months to determine WIC costs and Medicaid expenditures. Using economic analyses, the comparison showed that breast-feeding of infants saved an average of $478 in WIC costs and Medicaid expenditures or $161 after considering the manufacturer's rebate. The researchers concluded that the promotion of breast-feeding in WIC programs was cost-effective (57).

USING RESEARCH REPORTS TO HELP SOLVE PROBLEMS

The earlier discussion of the practice-based research model drew on the study of Sikund et al (35) to illustrate the implications of the model. An examination of the other steps in developing a research project helps to clarify further the process of incorporating research into practice.

Planning the Project

When confronting a practice problem, some steps may facilitate planning the project and moving it along. Among them are appointing a committee or work group; defining the problem and subproblems; making assignments to committee members; setting a time frame; and organizing ongoing meetings to discuss progress, refocus if necessary, and keep the project progressing toward completion.

EXAMPLE. Collaborative teamwork is illustrated in the development of a research project by dietitians at the Cleveland Clinic. They had made a commitment to outcomes research by putting it in the departmental strategic plan. A team of 11 inpatient dietitians worked jointly to examine the effect of their training on patients and their families and to identify potential areas for improvement (58).

The problem was to examine the outcomes of patients who received home enteral feeding training. The first step was to establish a committee of dietitians to determine the research design, methods of data collection, and responsibilities. The committee met and defined their research objective—to "examine the outcomes of patients who received home enteral nutrition training by dietitians." The first phase included a literature search by committee members to learn what had been reported and to refine the project design.

To obtain consistent and accurate data, it was important to train all the dietitians on how to collect and document patient outcomes. The follow-up telephone survey had to be drafted so that the same information was collected on all patients and their caregivers. The project was completed in 1 year, with meetings held at intervals during that time. When the project was completed, the researchers disseminated the results to their colleagues at a meeting and to nurses, physicians, and other health providers in their institution using an agreed-upon outcomes report format.

Defining the Problem

Research begins with a problem or question: what a practitioner wants to know about his or her practice that would be useful. The question should be clearly defined at the outset, and it should have an answer that is measurable. After putting the question in writing, the practitioner should work on refining and clarifying it. With further thought, the question usually expands and evolves into a broader statement; however, an effort should be made to tighten and focus the problem and allow measurement of very specific variables. Coulston (48[p30]) summarizes three prototypical formats for research questions in clinical dietetics practice: (1) What is the nutrition status of patients with, or at risk of developing, specific diseases? (2) What are the nutrient requirements of patients with specific diseases, and how do they differ from the requirements of the healthy population? and (3) What is the efficacy of nutrition intervention in the prevention of disease, as adjunctive therapy, and as primary treatment for specific diseases?

The Literature Search

Literature related to the selected problem provides the foundation for the planned study. A review of the literature provides ideas for methodology and shows how other researchers have handled a similar question. It can disclose sources of information that may not be known. A literature review can assist in evaluating the proposed project and comparing it with other studies. For dietitians embarking on new ventures, electronic databases and search engines have greatly expanded access to current investigations and researchers worldwide. A literature search can provide information on descriptions of participants, sample selections, inclusion and exclusion criteria for participants, outcomes or end points used, validated instruments or researcher-designed tools, reported results and significance, and gaps and limitations of previous studies (21).

In reviewing the literature, it may be useful to pose some questions to clarify the problem and develop the study—for example, Can this information help solve the problem? A literature review sometimes provides the information that answers the question without further study in an evidence-based practice summary—an efficient use of existing research.

Another useful question in a literature review is whether there is a model that can be used to study the problem. Some studies may provide such a model and eliminate steps in the research process. Can the information in the literature be modified or adapted for the case in question? Other models, findings, methodology, or instruments appropriate for the study under consideration may be discovered through a literature review and discussion with peers, especially peers with research experience. Rebovich and her colleagues devised a model for partnering educators, researchers, and practitioners to design studies that could benefit the local community and advance research initiatives at the local university (18).

Implementing the Plan

After developing the question and conducting the literature search, a design for the study is selected. Preparation of a proposal or research protocol is necessary to delineate clearly the procedures and processes for data collection. A pilot study is useful to test for any problems in the methodology and provide an opportunity to make adaptations prior to undertaking the larger investigation.

Analysis of Results

The procedures for analysis of data should be planned at the beginning of the study, not after the data are collected. In conducting research in the practice setting, resources for collection, analysis, and interpretation of data may be limited. The process may need to be simplified to complete the project with the resources available in the health care setting. Assistance can often be obtained from a statistician or academician interested in practice-based research. Babbie warns researchers to be careful of certain pitfalls in interpreting data, including inaccurate observations, poor reasoning, overgeneralization, and selective observations (59).

BARRIERS TO QUALITY RESEARCH

Getting started with research in the practice setting is the first giant step. Reading the research literature and one's own curiosity help generate ideas. Identifying possible questions to address is a good starting point. Assessment of the needs of the population and the resources available to implement investigations are crucial to productive planning. Creativity and imagination are useful tools to assist with conducting research and managing the barriers that may impede the implementation of practice-related research projects. These barriers involve time, staffing, money, permissions, and knowledge.

Time Constraints

Time must be found to conduct practice-related research. Unfortunately, sufficient time for research generally must be carved out of an already full schedule. An evaluation of existing responsibilities to determine if some can be simplified, delegated, or eliminated may open up some blocks of time. Reading articles on time management may help.

An attempt should be made to conduct the study within the working day. Structuring professional reading time into the work day is positive time management. It not only helps keep the practitioner informed about professional development but also helps generate research ideas. However, a willingness to devote some personal time in the early stages of a research investigation is usually necessary.

Staffing Constraints

Staff members may not be available or interested in assisting the principal investigator when she or he is planning a research project. Enlisting other staff members to collaborate in at least some part of the project is crucial, however. It may be easier to motivate staff members if the investigation has the potential to make their jobs easier or more efficient. Other health care personnel within an institution may be interested in the project, and volunteers or students sometimes may be eager to participate.

Money Constraints

A practitioner must recognize that funds generally are not allocated for his or her first efforts at research, so a simple design is in order. Selecting data that are readily available is desirable; the researcher should ask, for example, What laboratory values are already collected that could be used for end points? Are data analysis systems in place in the institution? Working through a pilot study may be an excellent method of learning how to utilize an existing data analysis program. The project should be planned to keep within the resources available. If data analysis must be done with a hand calculator, for example, the study design should reflect this limitation.

Need for Permission and Cooperation

Implementing any research necessitates permission from supervisors or superiors. The reorganization of duties or staffing must be authorized. Cooperation and permission are needed to make use of facilities such as computer time. Permission from physicians and patients is necessary for human subject research. The practitioner must go through the appropriate channels to organize the project, or the barriers could lead to frustration. Explaining the potential patient benefits of the study or potential higher productivity will encourage cooperation.

Knowledge Constraints

Learning how to conduct research is essential for success. Taking courses is a good way to learn. However, reading the current research literature (60–62) and talking with researchers is also very helpful. Many people are afraid to initiate investigations, but involvement usually builds confidence. Published and tested protocols and validated practice guidelines are very useful for developing a research project. Naglak and colleagues (36) and Assell and colleagues (63) shared their experiences in developing and conducting cost-effectiveness analyses in the hope that by knowing some of the problems in advance, practitioners would avoid some of the pitfalls and be encouraged to develop successful economic analyses.

SUGGESTIONS FOR FUTURE RESEARCH

A vast array of topics (5,8) could be studied by the practitioner to improve practice and open up new vistas for the profession. The following research topics might be used to expand the dietetics database:

- Documentation of clinical practice and assessment of the effectiveness of medical nutrition therapy in selected nutrition-related diseases.
- Investigation of the team approach to determine what aspect of care provided by the dietitian contributed to improved patient or client outcomes.
- Comparison of different prevention and treatment models of nutrition intervention and the outcomes for clients over time.
- Evaluation of the achievement of quality improve-

ment methods of foodservice systems in various settings.

- Evidence-based practice analyses that examine the strength of evidence for continuing or changing usual practices or services.
- Expansion and extension of some of the studies presented in this chapter.

REFERENCES

1. Sims LS, Simko MD. Applying research methods in nutrition and dietetics: embodiment of the profession's backbone. *J Am Diet Assoc.* 1988;88:1045–1046.
2. Fitz P, Winkler MF. Education, research, and practice: bridging the gap. *J Am Diet Assoc.* 1989;89:116–117.
3. Smitherman AL, Wyse BW. The backbone of our profession [President's Page]. *J Am Diet Assoc.* 1987;87:1394–1396.
4. Broihier K. Communicating nutrition research to the public: the dietitian's role. *Top Clin Nutr.* 2000;15:1–9.
5. Dwyer JT. *Scientific Underpinnings for the Profession: Dietitians in Research. Challenging the Future of Dietetic Education and Credentialing Proceedings.* Chicago, Ill: American Dietetic Association; 1993.
6. Monsen ER. New practices and research in dietetics. The 1988 Journal. *J Am Diet Assoc.* 1988;88:15.
7. Slawson DL, Clemens LH, Bol L. Research and the clinical dietitian: perceptions of the research process and preferred routes to obtaining research skills. *J Am Diet Assoc.* 2000;100:1144–1148.
8. *The Research Agenda for Dietetics Conference Proceedings.* Chicago, Ill: American Dietetic Association; 1993.
9. Hunt JR, Mullis RM, Woteki CE. The Council on Research: investment in dietetics research. *J Am Diet Assoc.* 1994;94:1104.
10. Ireton-Jones CS, Gottschlich MM, Bell SJ. *Practice-Oriented Nutrition Research: An Outcomes Measurement Approach.* Gaithersburg, Md: Aspen Publishers; 1998.
11. Castro J, Walsh J. Evaluating published clinical research trials. *Support Line.* 1997;XIX:7–10.
12. Winter MJ, Stanton L, Boushey CJ. The effectiveness of a food preparation and nutrition education program for children. *Top Clin Nutr.* 1999;14(2):48–59.
13. Ireton-Jones CS, Garritson B, Kitchens L. Nutrition intervention in cancer patients: does the registered dietitian make a difference? *Top Clin Nutr.* 1995;10(4): 42–48.
14. Quality Management and Research Team. *Implementing the Standards of Professional Practice: A Trainer's Guide.* Chicago, Ill: American Dietetic Association; 1998:18.
15. *Accreditation/Approval Manual for Dietetics Education Programs.* 4th ed. Chicago, Ill: American Dietetic Association; 2000.
16. Hynak-Hankinson MT, Martin S, Wirth J. Research competencies in the dietetics curricula. *J Am Diet Assoc.* 1997;97(suppl 2):102–106.
17. Guyer LK, Roht RR, Probart CK, Bobroff LB. Broadening the scope of dietetic practice through research. *Top Clin Nutr.* 1993;8(3):26–32.
18. Rebovich EJ, Wodarski LA, Hurley RS, et al. A university-community model for the integration of nutrition research, practice, and education. *J Am Diet Assoc.* 1994;94:179–182.
19. Parks SC, Schiller MR, Bryk J. Investment in our future—the role of science and scholarship in developing knowledge for dietetic practice [President's Page]. *J Am Diet Assoc.* 1994;94:1159–1161.
20. Biesemeier CW. Demonstrating the effectiveness of medical nutrition therapy. *Top Clin Nutr.* 1999;14(2):13–24.
21. Schiller MR, Moore C. Practical approaches to outcomes evaluation. *Top Clin Nutr.* 1999;14(2):1–12.
22. Lorenz RA, Gregory RP, Davis DL, et al. Diabetes training for dietitians: needs assessment, program description, and effects on knowledge and problem solving. *J Am Diet Assoc.* 2000;100:225–228.
23. Brody RA, Touger-Decker E, VonHagen S, Maillet JO. Role of registered dietitians in dysphagia screening. *J Am Diet Assoc.* 2000;100:1029–1037.
24. Barr SI, McCarron DA, Heaney RB, et al. Effects of increased consumption of fluid milk on energy and nutrient intake, body weight, and cardiovascular risk factors in healthy older adults. *J Am Diet Assoc.* 2000;100:810–817.
25. Schwartz DB, Gudzin D. Preadmission nutrition screening: expanding hospital-based nutrition services by implementing earlier nutrition intervention. *J Am Diet Assoc.* 2000;100:81–87.
26. August DA. Outcomes research, nutrition support, and nutrition care practice. *Top Clin Nutr.* 1995;10(4):1–16.
27. Kaye GL. *Outcomes Management: Linking Research to Practice.* Columbus, Ohio: Ross Products Division, Abbott Laboratories; 1996.
28. Braunschweig C, Gomez S. Impact of declines in nutritional status on outcomes in adult patients hospitalized for more than 7 days. *J Am Diet Assoc.* 2000;100:1361–1324.
29. Gallagher-Allred C, Voss AC, Gussler JD. *Nutrition Intervention and Patient Outcomes: A Self-Study Manual.* Chicago, Ill: The American Dietetic Association and Ross Products Division of Abbott Laboratories; 1995.
30. Leedy PD. *Practical Research: Planning and Design.* 6th ed. Upper Saddle River, NJ: Merrill; 1997.
31. Best JW, Kahn JV. *Research in Education.* 8th ed. Boston, Mass: Allyn and Bacon; 1998.
32. Rinke WJ, Berry MW. Integrating research into clinical

practice: a model and call for action. *J Am Diet Assoc.* 1987;87:159–161.

33. Eck LH, Slawson DL, Williams R, et al. A model for making outcomes research standard practice in clinical dietetics. *J Am Diet Assoc.* 1998;98:451–457.

34. Wylie-Rosett J, Wheeler M, Krueger K, Halford B. Opportunities for research-oriented dietitians. *J Am Diet Assoc.* 1990;90:1531–1534.

35. Sikund G, Kashyap ML, Yang I. Medical nutrition therapy lowers serum cholesterol and saves medication costs in men with hypercholesterolemia. *J Am Diet Assoc.* 1998;98:889–894.

36. Naglak M, Mitchell DC, Kris-Etherton P, et al. What to consider when conducting a cost-effectiveness analysis in a clinical setting. *J Am Diet Assoc.* 1998;98:1149–1154.

37. Sikund G, Kashyap ML, Wong ND, Hsu JL. Dietitian intervention improves lipid values and saves medication costs in men with combined hyperlipidemia and a history of niacin noncompliance. *J Am Diet Assoc.* 2000;100:218–224.

38. Naglak MC, Mitchell DC, Shannon BM, et al. Nutrient adequacy of diets of adults with hypercholesterolemia after a cholesterol-lowering intervention: long-term assessment. *J Am Diet Assoc.* 2000;100:1385–1388.

39. Porter C, Matel JLS. Are we making decisions based on evidence? *J Am Diet Assoc.* 1998;98:404–407.

40. Kolasa KM. Evidence-based medicine: what is it and how does a dietitian use it? *Top Clin Nutr.* 2000;15:19–30.

41. Mattes R. To read or not to read original research articles: it should not be a question. *J Am Diet Assoc.* 2000;100:171–174.

42. Glore S. Show me the science. *J Am Diet Assoc.* 2001;101:186.

43. Lyu L, Hankin JH, Liu LQ, et al. Telephone vs face-to-face interviews for quantitative food frequency assessment. *J Am Diet Assoc.* 1998;98:44–48.

44. O'Hara PA, Harper DW, Kangas M, et al. Taste, temperature, and presentation predict satisfaction with foodservices in a Canadian continuing-care hospital. *J Am Diet Assoc.* 1997;97:401–405.

45. Johnson BC, Chambers MJ. Foodservice benchmarking: practices, attitudes, and beliefs of foodservice directors. *J Am Diet Assoc.* 2000;100:175–182.

46. Silverman MR, Gregoire MB, Lafferty LJ, Dowling RA. Current and future practices in hospital foodservice. *J Am Diet Assoc.* 2000;100:76–80.

47. Schmidt L. A new career for dietitians: study coordinators. *J Am Diet Assoc.* 1993;93:749–751.

48. Coulston AM. Make a career of clinical nutrition research. *Top Clin Nutr* 1995;10(3):29–33.

49. Peterson DA, Albers JE, Mertz JR, McCoy RA. Broadening career opportunities in dietetics: employment in independent research. *J Am Diet Assoc.* 1999;99:799–801.

50. Franz MJ, Splett P, Monk A, et al. Cost-effectiveness of medical nutrition therapy provided by dietitians in the management of non-insulin dependent diabetes mellitus. *J Am Diet Assoc.* 1995;95:1018–1024.

51. Thompson T. Thiamin, riboflavin, and niacin contents of the gluten-free diet: is there cause for concern? *J Am Diet Assoc.* 1999;99:858–862.

52. Shenberger DM, Helgren RJ, Peters JR, et al. *J Am Diet Assoc.* 1992;92:441–445.

53. Travis KA, Barr SI. Rethinking postoperative diets for short-stay orthopedic surgery patients. *J Am Diet Assoc.* 1997;97:971–974.

54. Kulkari K, Castle G, Gregory R, et al. Nutrition practice guidelines for type I Diabetes mellitus positively affect dietitian practices and patient outcomes. *J Am Diet Assoc.* 1998;98:62–70.

55. Klein CJ, Wiles CE III. Evaluation of nutrition care provided to patients with traumatic injuries at risk for multiple organ dysfunction. *J Am Diet Assoc.* 1997;97:1422–1424.

56. Hedberg AM, Lairson DR, Aday LA, et al. Economic implications of an early postoperative enteral feeding protocol. *J Am Diet Assoc.* 1999;99:802–807.

57. Montgomery DL, Splett PL. Economic benefit of breast-feeding infants enrolled in WIC. *J Am Diet Assoc.* 1997;97:379–385.

58. Carr-Davis E, Polisena C, Austhof S, et al. The effectiveness of instruction of home enteral nutrition [abstract]. *J Am Diet Assoc.* 1997;97(suppl):A30.

59. Babbie E. *The Practice of Social Research.* 8th ed. Belmont, Calif: Wadsworth Publishing Company; 1998.

60. Delahanty LM, Sonnenberg LM, Hayden D, Nathan DM. Clinical and cost outcomes of medical nutrition therapy for hypercholesterolemia: a controlled trial. *J Am Diet Assoc.* 2001;101:1012–1018.

61. Wylie-Rosett J, Swencionis C, Ginsberg M, et al. Computerized weight loss intervention optimizes staff time: the clinical and cost results of a controlled clinical trial conducted in a managed care setting. *J Am Diet Assoc.* 2001;101:1155–1164.

62. Kwon J, Gilmore SA, Oakland MJ, Shelley MC. Clinical dietetics changes due to cost-reduction activities in healthcare systems. *J Am Diet Assoc.* 2001;101:1347–1353.

63. Assell C, Skipper A, Gregoire MB, Lafferty LJ. Cost-effectiveness strategies for enteral product distribution in health care facilities. *Top Clin Nutr.* 2000;16(1):43–49.

Index